Geriatric Neuropsychology

STUDIES ON NEUROPSYCHOLOGY, NEUROLOGY AND COGNITION

Series Editor:

Linas Bieliauskas, Ph.D.
University of Michigan, Ann Arbor, MI, USA

Other titles in this series:

Geriatric Neuropsychology
Practice Essentials

Edited by
Shane S. Bush & Thomas A. Martin

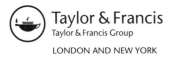

Taylor & Francis
Taylor & Francis Group

LONDON AND NEW YORK

Published in 2005
by Taylor & Francis
270 Madison Avenue
New York, NY 10016
www.taylorandfrancis.com

Published in Great Britain
by Taylor & Francis
27 Church Road
Hove, East Sussex BN3 2FA
www.taylorandfrancis.co.uk

Typeset in Times by Macmillan India, Bangalore, India
Printed and bound in the USA by Sheridan Books, Inc., Ann Arbor, MI, on acid-free paper
Cover design by Jim Wilkie

British Library Cataloguing in Publication Data
A catalogue record for this book is available from the British Library

Library of Congress Cataloging-in-Publication Data
  Geriatric neuropsychiatry : practice essentials / Shane S. Bush & Thomas A. Martin, editors.
    p. cm.
  Includes bibliographical references and index.
  ISBN 1-84169-443-6 (hardback : alk. paper)
  1. Geriatric neuropsychology. I. Bush, Shane S., 1965– . II. Martin, Thomas A., 1965–
  RC451.4.A5G468 2005
  618.97′68–dc22
                                                                      2005012733
ISBN 1-84169-443-6

This book is dedicated to:

Dana, Sarah, and Megan

S.B.

My parents, whose support knows no bounds.
My brother, Brad, whose spirit is with me always.
And Rhoda, Lauren, Dalton, and Kyle who have brought
  unimaginable joy to my life.

T.M.

Contents

Section I

Introduction   **1**

Introduction   **3**

SHANE S. BUSH AND THOMAS A. MARTIN

Section II

Assessment   **9**

1   The clinical interview   **11**

JACOBUS DONDERS

9   **Cerebrovascular disorders: Neurocognitive and
     neurobehavioral features**   **219**

STEPHEN N. MACCIOCCHI, AMY L. ALDERSON, AND SARA L. SCHARA

10   **Neuropsychology of Parkinson's disease and its dementias**   **243**

ALEXANDER I. TRÖSTER AND STEVEN PAUL WOODS

List of plates and figures

echo time, 90° flip angle, 5 mm thick, 0 spacing) (courtesy of
H. Michael Gach, University of Pittsburgh)

7.10 Regional CBF in the posterior ingulate cortex among AD patients
with a better response to cholinesterase inhibition

7.11 FDG scans of brain metabolism in AD and DLB. The left-hand
image shows an AD patient with decreased glucose metabolic
activity in the right parietal cortex, and preservation of occipital
metabolism. The right-hand image shows the metabolism of a DLB
patient with more severe (and bilateral) metabolic reductions, most
prominent in the parietal and the occipital cortices (courtesy of
N. Bohnen, University of Pittsburgh)

7.12 Example of visualization of beta-amyloid using the Pittsburgh
Compound-B, and brain metabolism as shown by FDG
(courtesy of W. Klunk, University of Pittsburgh)

7.13 Coregistered PET and MR images of a healthy 74-year-old man,
showing the distribution of 5-HT1A receptors, including midbrain
region of the raphe and hippocampus (top row, middle image).
Lack of binding in the cerebellum, where there are negligible
5-HT1A receptors, is also demonstrated (top row, left image)
(courtesy of C. C. Meltzer, University of Pittsburgh)

Figures

List of tables

About the editors

Shane S. Bush, PhD, ABPN, ABPP, is in independent practice in Smithtown NY. He is board certified in Neuropsychology by the American Board of Professional Neuropsychology and in Rehabilitation Psychology by the American Board of Professional Psychology. He is president of the Neuropsychology Division of the New York State Psychological Association. He serves on the editorial boards of *The Clinical Neuropsychologist* (coediting the Ethical and Professional Issues section), the *Journal of Forensic Neuropsychology*, and *Applied Neuropsychology*. He is coeditor of the book *Ethical Issues in Clinical Neuropsychology*, editor of *A Casebook of Ethical Challenges in Neuropsychology*, and coauthor of *Health Care Ethics for Psychologists: A Casebook*. He has presented at national psychology, neuropsychology, and rehabilitation psychology conferences. He is a veteran of both the US Marine Corps and Navy.

Thomas A. Martin, PsyD, ABPP, is Chief of Psychology Services at Missouri Rehabilitation Center and a Clinical Assistant Professor in the Department of Health Psychology at University of Missouri–Columbia. He earned his doctoral degree from the Adler School of Professional Psychology and completed a postdoctoral fellowship in Clinical Neuropsychology and Rehabilitation Psychology at the University of Missouri–Columbia. He is board certified in rehabilitation psychology by the American Board of Professional Psychology. He currently serves on the Board of Directors of the Brain Injury Association of Missouri, is a member of the Social and Ethical Responsibility Committee of APA's Division of Rehabilitation Psychology, and is a member of the Education Committee of the National Academy of Neuropsychology. He has published in the areas of clinical neuropsychology and rehabilitation psychology, and is currently conducting research in the area of traumatic brain injury and treatment outcomes.

List of contributors

Howard Aizenstein, M.D., Ph.D., University of Pittsburgh School of Medicine, Pittsburgh, PA

Amy Alderson, Ph.D., Shepard Center, Atlanta, GA

Teresa Ashman, Ph.D., Mount Sinai School of Medicine, New York, NY

Bradley N. Axelrod, Ph.D., John D. Dingell DVAMC, Detroit, MI

James T. Becker, Ph.D., ABPP, University of Pittsburgh School of Medicine, Pittsburgh, PA

Sabrina Breed, Ph.D., Mount Sinai School of Medicine, New York, NY

Nicole R. Burkett, B.A., Southern Illinois University School of Medicine, Springfield, IL

Shane S. Bush, Ph.D., ABPN, ABPP, Independent Practice, Smithtown, NY

Meryl A. Butters, Ph.D., University of Pittsburgh School of Medicine, Pittsburgh, PA

Desiree A. Byrd, Ph.D., Columbia University, New York, NY

Bruce Caplan, Ph.D., ABPP, Lankenau Hospital, Wynnewood, PA

John DeLuca, Ph.D., ABPP, Kessler Medical Rehabilitation Research and Education Corporation, West Orange, NJ

Jacobus Donders, Ph.D., ABPP, Mary Free Bed Hospital, Grand Rapids, MI

Maureen Gibney, Psy.D., Independent Practice, Philadelphia, PA

Efrain A. Gonzalez, Psy.D., MS ClinPharm, ABPP, University of Miami School of Medicine, Miami, FL

Manfred F. Greiffenstein, Ph.D., ABPP, Psychological Systems, Inc., Royal Oak, MI

Mary Hibbard, Ph.D., ABPP, Mount Sinai School of Medicine, New York, NY

Felicia Hill-Briggs, Ph.D., ABPP, Johns Hopkins University School of Medicine, Baltimore, MD

Anjeli B. Inscore, Psy.D., Johns Hopkins University School of Medicine, Baltimore, MD

Jennifer Jacobson Kirk, Psy.D., Johns Hopkins University, Baltimore, MD

Doug Johnson-Greene, Ph.D., ABPP, Johns Hopkins University School of Medicine, Baltimore, MD

Brick Johnstone, Ph.D., ABPP, University of Missouri-Columbia, Columbia, MO

Jeffrey S. Kreutzer, Ph.D., ABPP, Virginia Commonwealth University Medical Center, Richmond, VA

Jean Lengenfelder, Ph.D., Kessler Medical Rehabilitation Research and Education Corporation, West Orange, NJ

Lee A. Livingston, Psy.D., Virginia Commonwealth University Medical Center, Richmond, VA

Stephen N. Macciocchi, Ph.D., ABPP, Shepherd Center, Atlanta, GA

Jennifer J. Manly, Ph.D., Columbia University, New York, NY

Thomas A. Martin, Psy.D., ABPP, Missouri Rehabilitation Center, Mt. Vernon, MO

Paul J. Moberg, Ph.D., ABPP, University of Pennsylvania Medical Center, Philadelphia, PA

Margaret M. Mustelier, Independent Practice, Miami, FL

Jose A. Rey, Pharm.D., BCPP, Nova Southeastern University, Fort Lauderdale, FL

Sara Schara, Ph.D., Shepherd Center, Atlanta, GA

Philip Schatz, Ph.D., Saint Joseph's University, Philadelphia, PA

Judith A. Shechter, Ph.D., Independent Practice, Wynnewood, PA

Laura A. Taylor, Ph.D., Virginia Commonwealth University Medical Center, Richmond, VA

Alexander I. Tröster, Ph.D., University of North Carolina School of Medicine, Chapel Hill, NC

Stephen T. Wegener, Ph.D., ABPP, Johns Hopkins University, Baltimore, MD

Deborah D. West, B.A., Virginia Commonwealth University Medical Center, Richmond, VA

Julie Williams, Psy.D., Mount Sinai School of Medicine, New York, NY

John L. Woodard, Ph.D., Rosalind Franklin University of Medicine and Science, North Chicago, IL

Steven Paul Woods, Psy.D., UC San Diego, San Diego, CA

Ronald F. Zec, Ph.D., ABPP, Southern Illinois University School of Medicine, Springfield, IL

From the series editor

While there are a number of available texts which discuss issues in geriatric neuropsychology, there is a paucity of information to address the practical impact of newly acquired knowledge in the field. In keeping with the translational emphasis of our series, *Geriatric Neuropsychology: Practice Essentials*, edited by Shane Bush and Thomas Martin, admirably fills this gap. As has been pointed out by many clinicians and researchers, there are issues of assessment and treatment which differ significantly between younger and older adults. It is clearly a mistake to assume that the nature of test performance, the impact of the context of assessment, medication-related effects, and neurophysiological and psychological response to injury and disease are the same in the elderly as they are in younger populations.

Geriatric Neuropsychology: Practice Essentials employs the contributions of well-known clinicians and researchers in examining age-related considerations in the construction of test batteries and conduction of interviews, necessary test accommodations, the relationship between test results and neuroimaging findings, common disease conditions, and specific practical issues related to sleep disorders, pain, psychiatric impairment, and substance abuse. Addressing of common referral questions such as decision-making capacity and consideration of pertinent ethical issues also provides solid clinical advice to clinical practitioners and students.

Bush and Martin have put together a valuable resource to the practicing clinician as well as the student preparing for specialized service in geriatric neuropsychology and it is a worthy and welcome addition to our series.

Linas A. Bieliauskas
Ann Arbor
September, 2005

Preface

Purpose of the book

Neuropsychologists working with older adults and their support systems must remain abreast of advances in multiple, interrelated health care and scientific fields. Depending on the specific context in which services are provided, geriatric neuropsychologists must maintain working knowledge of relevant areas of psychology, medicine, pharmacology, genetics, geriatrics, and other disciplines. Acquiring and integrating such information can be a time- and energy-intensive process.

The goal of this book was to draw together recent research and information from neuropsychology and related disciplines that is essential for clinical practice with older adults and those involved in their lives. While the content of this book is intended to be as specific to older adults as possible, some of the information provided is relevant to adults of all ages.

Format of the book

The book is comprised of four sections: Introduction, Assessment, Neurological Disorders, and Clinical Considerations.

- *Section I.* The Introduction provides an overview of neuropsychological practice issues relevant to older adults, including work settings, referral questions, diagnostic and treatment issues, and consumer education and prevention.
- *Section II.* The Assessment section presents current considerations in the selection and use of neuropsychological methods, technology and test accommodation issues, cultural considerations, and neuroimaging applications relevant to older adults.
- *Section III.* The section on Neurological Disorders is comprised of four chapters: Alzheimer's disease and other dementias, cerebrovascular disorders, Parkinson's disease, and traumatic brain injury. These topics were chosen due to the frequency with which they are encountered in clinical practice.

- *Section IV*. This section, on Clinical Considerations, presents wide-ranging issues relevant to the practice of geriatric neuropsychology, including comorbid medical and psychiatric conditions, psychophar-macology, family treatment issues, decision-making capacity, and ethical issues. Adequate understanding of these issues is necessary for the provision of competent and meaningful neuropsychological services to older adults and those involved in their lives.

Conclusion

A thorough, comprehensive text on geriatric neuropsychology could easily be two or three times the length of the current text. However, to the extent that we have covered in this volume the *essential* elements of geriatric practice, we will have met our goal of providing an informative resource for neuropsychologists working with older adults.

Acknowledgments

The efforts of countless clinicians and researchers who have worked with older adults and studied adult development and aging provide the foundation for the information presented in this book. Although only a fraction of those professionals are referenced in this book, we are grateful for the contributions of all. We are particularly appreciative of our contributing authors, most of whom are recognized as leaders in the areas in which they have contributed. Finally, we offer our heartfelt gratitude to our patients and their families, from whom we have learned so much.

Section I

Introduction

Introduction

Shane S. Bush and Thomas A. Martin

Neuropsychologists play an important role in helping older adults and their loved ones understand and cope with neurologic injury and illness. In recent years, medical, technological, and neuropsychological advances have enhanced our understanding of neurologic dysfunction and the clinical needs of older adults with neuropsychological dysfunction. These advances, occurring when the world population is aging, make this a particularly exciting time for geriatric neuropsychology.

Settings

Older adults undergo neuropsychological evaluation and treatment in a variety of practice settings. For example, elderly individuals may receive neuropsychological services in the same settings as younger adults, including medical, rehabilitation, psychiatric, independent practice, and forensic settings. In addition, older adults receive neuropsychological services in settings such as long-term care and assisted living facilities which focus more specifically on concerns of later life. Regardless of setting, clinical issues may arise that (a) overlap with issues of importance in the assessment and treatment of younger adults and (b) are unique to older adults. For example, the decision to utilize measures to assess response bias is a clinical issue that confronts practitioners working with both older and younger individuals. Depending on the evaluation context, neuropsychologists evaluating older adults, as with younger examinees, may not require a quantitative approach to the determination of symptom validity; however, in some settings neuropsychologists may benefit from, and in fact competent practice may require, quantitative symptom validity assessment (see Chapter 3 in this volume for additional coverage of symptom validity assessment).

Referral questions

With advances in the field of neuroimaging, referrals for neuropsychological evaluations to "localize" or identify areas of brain damage have diminished. Instead, neuropsychologists are frequently asked to help clarify the etiology of cognitive dysfunction, identify the cognitive strengths and weaknesses of a patient, and provide recommendations to promote functioning and quality of life.

Normal aging

Neuropsychologists working with older adults may be asked to determine whether cognitive decline is the result of a pathological process or consistent with "normal aging." "Normal aging" is a broadly used term that may be a source of confusion for health care professionals, including neuropsychologists, and the general public. For instance, "normal" may be used to indicate "healthy"; that is, normal aging is healthy aging, free of medical or neurological symptoms that may commonly occur in older adults. In contrast, "normal" may be used to indicate the norm, that which frequently occurs in a given population. For example, if nearly 50% of individuals 85 years of age or older develop Alzheimer's disease (AD), then a diagnosis of AD in an 85-year-old, given the base rate of AD for that age, may be considered normal, yet it would not be considered healthy aging. Additionally, the different meanings attributed to the term "normal aging" may have important implications for treatment. We have found that some patients, family members, and health care professionals may be less aggressive in their pursuit of treatment and non-institutional living options when the diagnosis is considered to reflect the norm than when it is considered to diverge from healthy aging. We recommend that psychologists who refer to "normal aging" define their use of "normal" or provide an alternate description of aging.

Diagnosis

The assessment of dementia and age-related cognitive decline is a primary activity of many neuropsychologists (APA Presidential Task Force on the Assessment of Age-Consistent Memory Decline and Dementia, 1998). Neuropsychologists performing such assessments often do so in the context of a multidisciplinary diagnostic evaluation. While technologic and scientific advances have improved neurodiagnostic accuracy, the neuropsychological evaluation remains an indispensable procedure for determining neurocognitive strengths and weaknesses, assessing neurocognitive loss, and integrating emotional and personality factors into diagnostic considerations.

Treatment

Treatment of neurologic dysfunction frequently involves providing education and emotional support to patients and their families, and management of behavioral issues that may arise (Sano & Weber, 2003). In addition, the introduction of cholinergic medications in recent years has challenged the notion that the course of cognitive decline cannot be altered. Cholinesterase inhibitors may improve quality of life and cognitive functions (American Academy of Neurology, 2001). In addition, there is some evidence to suggest that memory training may improve cognitive functioning in individuals with dementia (Moore, Sandman, McGrady, & Kesslak, 2001).

Consumer education/prevention

Research from a variety of health care specialties indicates that healthy lifestyle choices may promote neurological wellness, reduce the risk of developing Alzheimer's disease, and improve cognitive functioning in those experiencing early cognitive decline (Arvanitakis, Wilson, Bienias, Evans, & Bennett, 2004; Engelhart et al., 2002; Foley et al. 2001; Fratiglioni, Paillard-Borg, & Winblad, 2004; Fung et al., 2004; Gustafson, Rothenberg, Blennow, Steen, & Skoog, 2003; Kalmijn, van Boxtel, Verschuren, Jolles, & Launer, 2002; Luchsinger, Tang, Siddiqui, Shea, & Mayeux, 2004; Small, 2002; Verghese et al., 2003; Wilson et al., 2002). Directly relevant to neuropsychological treatment, recent research indicates that regularly scheduled cognitive exercise not only reduces the risk of AD (Wilson et al., 2002) but can improve cognitive functioning (Ball et al. 2002; Moore et al., 2001). These preliminary research findings provide neuropsychologists with direction for developing cognitive treatment plans. Consistent with ethical practice in geriatric neuropsychology (Morgan, 2002), clinicians should exercise caution in how they present their treatment plan, emphasizing the potential value of a multidisciplinary approach. While offering patients increased participation in their treatment may increase their sense of autonomy (Juriga & Bush, 2002), generating false hope may have negative emotional consequences. If care is taken to convey an appropriate degree of hope and expectation to patients and families, there seems to be little risk of harming patients by recommending a structured program of cognitive exercise as part of a treatment plan (Bush & Martin, 2004), and even minor gains may be quite meaningful to patients and their families.

Conclusion

As the world population continues to age, there will likely be increased need for neuropsychological expertise in geriatric health care. Neuropsychologists, working with other health care providers and social support services (see Appendix), have much to offer older adults and those involved in their lives.

References

American Academy of Neurology. (2001). Practice parameter: Management of dementia (an evidence-based review): Report of the quality standards subcommittee of the American Academy of Neurology. *Neurology*, *56*, 1154–1161.

APA Presidential Task Force on the Assessment of Age-Consistent Memory Decline and Dementia. (1998). *Guidelines for the evaluation of dementia and age-related cognitive decline*. Washington, DC: American Psychological Association.

Arvanitakis, Z., Wilson, R. S., Bienias, J. L., Evans, D. A., & Bennett, D. A. (2004). Diabetes mellitus and risk of Alzheimer disease and decline in cognitive function. *Archives of Neurology, 61*(5), 661–666.

Ball, K., Berch, D. B., Helmers, K. F., Jobe, J. B., Leveck, M. D., Marsiske, M., et al. (2002). Effects of cognitive training interventions with older adults. *Journal of the American Medical Association, 288*(18), 2271–2281.

Bush, S., & Martin, T. (2004, July 18). *Balancing bioethical principles in computer-based memory treatment*. Poster presentation at the ninth international conference on Alzheimer's Disease and Related Disorders, Philadelphia.

Engelhart, M. J., Geerlings, M. I., Ruitenberg, A., van Swieten, J. C., Hofman, A., Witteman, J. C. M., & Breteler, M. M. B. (2002). Dietary intake of antioxidants and risk of Alzheimer's disease. *Journal of the American Medical Association, 287*(24), 3223–3229.

Foley, D., Monjan, A., Masaki, K., Ross, W., Havlik, R., White, L., et al. (2001). Daytime sleepiness is associated with 3-year incident dementia and cognitive decline in older Japanese-American men. *Journal of the American Geriatrics Society, 49*(12), 1628–1632.

Fratiglioni, L., Paillard-Borg, S., & Winblad, B. (2004). An active and socially integrated lifestyle in late life might protect against dementia. *The Lancet Neurology, 3*(6), 343–353.

Fung, T. T., Stampfer, M. J., Manson, J. E., Rexrode, K. M., Willett, W. C., & Hu, F. B. (2004). Prospective study of major dietary patterns and stroke risk in women. *Stroke, 35*, 2014–2019.

Gustafson, D., Rothenberg, E., Blennow, K., Steen, B., & Skoog, I. (2003). An 18-year follow-up of overweight and risk of Alzheimer disease. *Archives of Internal Medicine, 163*(13), 1524–1528.

Juriga, M., & Bush, S. (2002). Attention to biomedical ethics may improve rehabilitation outcome: A case illustration. *Rehabilitation Psychology, 47*(3), 374–375.

Kalmijn, S., van Boxtel, M. P. J., Verschuren, M. W. M., Jolles, J., & Launer, L. J. (2002). Cigarette smoking and alcohol consumption in relation to cognitive performance in middle age. *American Journal of Epidemiology, 156*, 936–944.

Luchsinger, J., Tang, M., Siddiqui, M., Shea, S., & Mayeux, R. (2004). Alcohol intake and risk of dementia. *Journal of the American Geriatrics Society, 52*(4), 540–546.

Moore, S., Sandman, C. A., McGrady, K., & Kesslak, J. P. (2001). Memory training improves cognitive ability in patients with dementia. *Neuropsychological Rehabilitation, 11*(3/4), 245–261.

Morgan, J. (2002). Ethical issues in the practice of geriatric neuropsychology. In S. S. Bush & M. L. Drexler (Eds.), *Ethical issues in clinical neuropsychology* (pp. 87–101). Lisse, NL: Swets & Zeitlinger Publishers.

Sano, M., & Weber, C. (2003). Psychological evaluation and nonpharmacologic treatment and management of Alzheimer's disease. In P. A. Lichtenberg, D. L. Murman, & A. M. Mellow (Eds.), *Handbook of dementia: Psychological, neurological, and psychiatric perspectives* (pp. 25–47). Hoboken, NJ: John Wiley & Sons.

Small, G. (2002). *The memory bible*. New York: Hyperion.

Verghese, J., Lipton, R. B., Katz, M. J., Hall, C. B., Derby, C. A., Kuslansky, G., et al. (2003). Leisure activities and the risk of dementia in the elderly. *New England Journal of Medicine, 348*(25), 2508–2516.

Wilson, R. S., Mendes de Leon, C. F., Barnes, L. L., Schneider, J. A., Bienias, J. L., Evans, D. A., & Bennett, D. A. (2002). Participation in cognitively stimulating activities and risk of incident Alzheimer disease. *Journal of the American Medical Association, 287*, 742–748.

Section II

Assessment

1   The clinical interview

Jacobus Donders

The clinical interview is typically the first face-to-face contact that the neuro-psychologist has with a newly referred patient. The setting may vary from inpatient to outpatient and from a general medical organization to a special-ized private practice, and these variations will affect the nature of the refer-rals that are typically received and the availability of specific medical and other background records. Requests for neuropsychological evaluations may also come from a wide range of sources, ranging from physicians to family members to lawyers. In each case, however, the clinical interview will allow the neuropsychologist to collect a valuable amount of information about the patient's presenting complaints, background history, and other important characteristics that can help to plan and shape the subsequent assessment process in a way that provides the best care to the patient. Although there is no single, invariant best way to conduct a clinical interview, this chapter will review the major aspects of this process that should probably be addressed on a routine basis, particularly with older adults.

Understanding the referral

There are several things that the neuropsychologist should do before embark-ing on a clinical interview. In order to respond most appropriately and most effectively to a referral, it is essential that one obtain a good understanding of why the patient was referred and what specific questions the physician or other person who made the referral has. A simple script that says, "Please evaluate" does not fit this bill. Under those circumstances, it behooves the neuropsychologist to seek clarification from the referring agent: Is he or she looking for confirmation of an already suspected dementia or is there a ques-tion about a possible confounding issue such as a mood disorder? Was the assessment requested primarily for diagnostic purposes or was there an expectation that it should assist in rehabilitative treatment or assistance with life care planning?

A second step in clarifying the referral is to determine who the client is. For example, in a forensic context where matters like legal competency are being contested, it is possible that the referral comes from an officer of the court who does not represent the patient. It is also possible that although a patient agrees to an evaluation requested by a family member, this does not automatically mean that the patient is comfortable with having the results shared with that same family member. Thus, it is very important to clarify how information will be shared and with whom, and what the limits of confidentiality are. This will all need to be communicated with the patient in a language that he or she can understand, as part of the informed consent process that is inherent to requirements from both the Health Insurance Portability and Accountability Act (HIPAA; http://www.hhs.gov/ocr/hipaa/finalreg.html) and ethical guidelines from the American Psychological Association (APA; http://www.apa.org/ethics/code2002.html).

Review of pertinent medical and other available records is also highly advisable before commencing a clinical interview. This may provide important information about acute and comorbid medical conditions, recent neuroimaging findings, current medications, etc. It may also alert the neuropsychologist to patient characteristics that should be taken into account when conducting the interview, such as knowledge that the patient's primary language is not English, or that he or she has had a negative prior experience with a different neuropsychologist. Many patients also get tired of telling the same story to yet another doctor, so demonstration of some familiarity with their documented history may convey a sense of preparation. When possible, review of medical records should be supplemented by evaluation of educational, employment, and/or military records to complement the picture. The neuropsychologist should be careful, though, to avoid the common mistake of confirmatory bias by focusing in the subsequent interview too narrowly on matters that were already documented in the available records, at the exclusion of other potentially pertinent information. Records sometimes contain inaccuracies, and patients often do not volunteer to anybody who does not ask details about substance abuse or psychiatric problems. Thus, the record review should serve as only the beginning of the exploration of the background of the patient.

Making the first contact

When a neuropsychological evaluation is done on an inpatient basis, usually there are established procedures for arranging patient availability, and most patients are used to having contact with various health professionals during their stay. On an outpatient basis, more extensive preparation and education may be necessary. For example, in light of the fact that some geriatric patients can be expected to be poor historians, it is advisable to request that a significant other or adult child accompany the patient to the evaluation to provide collateral information. Patients may also need to be given specific instructions about time frames for the evaluation and instructions about what to bring (e.g., either a list or all the bottles of the medications that they are currently taking, reading glasses, hearing aid). It is also a good idea to inquire up front about any accommodations that the patient may need such as assistance with toilet transfers after a stroke, or a private room for periodic suctioning or catheterization.

Beginning the interview

Styles of interviewing vary widely across practitioners. Some like to start by reviewing completed questionnaires; others prefer to let the patient tell his or her story first; yet others take a very structured approach in asking specific questions. Regardless of the approach, it is generally a good idea to clarify with the patient first the reason for the referral and what the nature and contingencies (e.g., information sharing, fiscal responsibility) of the neuropsychological evaluation are. Agreement must also be obtained with the patient about who can participate in the interview. Most professional neuropsychological organizations advise against the presence of third parties during the formal psychometric part of neuropsychological evaluations (American Academy of Clinical Neuropsychology, 2001; National Academy of Neuropsychology, 2000), but collateral interviews with family members as part of the history and intake are often very helpful in clarifying the developmental progression of the patient's known, suspected, or disputed problems and any complicating premorbid or comorbid confounding factors. In this context, it is important to get an understanding of what are the goals of the patient and of the family for the evaluation; in other words, what questions should be answered and whether the patient, family and other relevant third parties (e.g., physician) agree on these goals. The neuropsychologist should also discuss with the patient and family the time frame and format for any direct feedback about test results. Establishing the frame of the relationship and the evaluation is essential to the informed consent process (see Chapter 19 in this volume for further discussion of informed consent).

It is often helpful to start the interview with some open-ended questions about the presenting complaints and then gradually move into more specific questions for clarification, probing, and exploration of issues or areas that were not spontaneously addressed by the patient or family (Vanderploeg, 2000). This not only allows patients to tell their story in a way that is most comfortable to them but it also offers the neuropsychologist the opportunity to obtain valuable behavioral observational material, such as the patient's ability to stay on topic, find specific words for verbal expression, maintain an appropriate range and expression of affect, etc. When other family members or third parties are present during the initial interview, it is often advisable to caution them at the beginning that it is crucial to hear directly from the patient first. Some passive patients may otherwise defer too rapidly to others for assistance, whereas at the same time some anxious or impatient third parties may attempt to speak for the patient without this necessarily reflecting the patient's private views. Nonverbal exchanges (e.g., eye contact, speaking in the first vs. the third person) between patient and family members may also reflect on the quality of the support system that is in place outside of the neuropsychologist's office.

History of the presenting problem

After agreement about the ground rules and expectancies for the evaluation, the interview should proceed to focus on the patient's presenting behavioral, cognitive, emotional, physical, and psychosocial complaints and symptoms. It is important to get an understanding of the onset of the problems (e.g., acute or gradual), their progression over time (e.g., relapsing/remitting or stepwise worsening), and their relationship to the patient's premorbid history as well as concurrent external factors (e.g., focal neurological signs, psychosocial stressors). For example, a history of sudden onset of anterograde amnesia in concert with transient sensory or motor symptoms in a person with a prior history of poorly controlled hypertension should raise suspicion of a vascular origin, whereas a progressive loss of remote autobiographical information following a confrontation with an estranged adult child about alleged sexual abuse would be more suggestive of a psychogenic issue.

It is important for the neuropsychologist to note during the query about the presenting problems any inconsistencies or disagreements between reports from patients and family members, and between self-report and overt behavior (Sbordone, 2000). For example, a patient with early frontotemporal dementia may not be aware of personality changes that are of significant concern to her spouse, whereas another patient with moderate depression may overestimate the degree of memory impairment that he has. It may also be necessary to clarify what the patient or family member means by specific complaints. For example, it is not uncommon for individuals to refer to word retrieval difficulties as a "memory" problem. If inconsistencies are noted between patient report and documentation in the medical record, this is typically also an area for further exploration. For example, a patient who denies substance abuse but whose emergency room record demonstrates a blood ETOH level of 0.11 at the time of a fall that caused a moderate traumatic brain injury may not only be in denial but also at increased risk for future injuries.

The timing of following up with further queries or requests for clarification will vary with the clinical presentation of the patient. For example, a person who has difficulty with distractions should probably be allowed first to finish his or her story before being interrupted with detailed questions. It is also advisable to avoid zeroing in on a specific issue too early because it may cause the patient not to address other issues that may be of particular importance. For example, a subjective report about visual hallucinations might tempt the neuropsychologist to start asking questions right away about the motor abnormalities that are often seen with diffuse Lewy body disease, but this might cause one to overlook other possible contributing variables such as a recent change in medication. In general, however, it is often a good idea to ask patients to give specific examples of what they are referring to, preferably by relating it to daily activities. It may be of academic interest to the neuropsychologist whether the patient's memory problem is of an encoding or of a retrieval nature, but the issue of the degree to which this difficulty has caused a safety concern in the person's life (e.g., forgetting to turn off the stove) may be of greater practical relevance.

The history of the development of the primary presenting problems must also be placed in the context of the patient's prior level of functioning, current responsibilities, and ongoing treatment. In this context, it is often helpful to ask the patient and/or family how his or her daily life has changed as the result of the problems, what if anything has been done about it so far, and with what degree of success. For example, an inability to balance a checkbook is not necessarily an indication of an acquired deficit in a patient whose spouse has always handled this responsibility. By the same token, concerns about topographical disorientation will likely be more concerning with a person who insists on driving than with an individual who already resides in an assisted living facility. Or, a person with an emerging memory problem may have already started to use a notebook but consistently has problems relocating it. In such a case, the neuropsychologist should probably use the assessment findings to think of alternative compensatory strategies for the patient.

Other personal history

Although it makes sense to start the interview by addressing the primary complaint of the patient or family, it is crucial to obtain a careful history about the patient's demographic, medical, and psychosocial background and any recent changes therein. There are numerous factors that can confound the results of neuropsychological tests, particularly with an older adult. Some of the most common ones of these are summarized in Table 1.1. Although space limitations prohibit detailed analysis of each single factor, the most significant ones will be discussed here.

There has been considerable controversy in the neuropsychological literature about the pros and cons of demographically adjusted norms for neuropsychological tests but the bulk of the research in this area suggests that variables such as age, education, ethnicity, and, in some cases, gender all have potentially significant influences on performance on such tests in both normal adults (Heaton, Taylor, & Manly, 2003) and clinical samples (Moses, Pritchard, & Adams, 1999; Sherrill-Pattison, Donders, & Thompson, 2000; Vanderploeg, Axelrod, Sherer, Scott, & Adams, 1997). Although an extensive discussion of the exact merits of currently available demographic norms for specific psychometric tests is outside the scope of this chapter, it is nonetheless important for the practitioner to appreciate the demographic differences with which geriatric patients may present. Young old (ages 60+79 years) and older old (those over 80 years of age) cohorts tend to differ significantly in

Table 1.1 Variables to explore in a clinical neuropsychological interview

Demographic information	Age, gender, handedness, ethnicity, acculturation, education (including any special services), English language fluency
Clinical complaint	Reason for referral, subjective complaints, development and progression of symptoms, effects on daily functioning and on family, treatment implemented, compensatory strategies used
Personal history	Birth and early development, family of origin constellation and history, marriage and offspring, primary vocation(s), military service, religious beliefs, personal trauma or abuse, legal history, financial compensation seeking
Medical history	Pre-existing or comorbid medical and psychiatric conditions, current medications, current health concerns, alcohol and other substance abuse, biological family medical and psychiatric history
Psychosocial factors	Spouse health, nuclear family role changes, sexuality, bereavement, recent situational stressors, financial resources, community support, change in residence

medical comorbidities and base rates of cognitive impairment (Hanks & Lichtenberg, 1996). Older patients often tend to have lower levels of education than the current national median, and members of certain ethnic minority groups may also have lesser quality of education and associated literacy levels that put them at a relative disadvantage (Manly, Jacobs, Touradji, Small, & Stern, 2002). The level of acculturation of the patient has implications not only for which tests may be appropriate but also how the interview should be conducted in terms of interpersonal distance, proper ways to query about personal history, etc. (Ferraro, 2002). Whenever possible, patients should also be interviewed in the language that is most common to them.

Obtaining information from the patient and family about employment history is important for a number of reasons. A patient may have chosen a particular line of work in part because of a longstanding pattern of relative cognitive strengths and weaknesses. Some vocations are also associated with specific health risks such as chronic exposure to solvents (Bowler et al., 2001) that may contribute to neurobehavioral difficulties at older age. Of course, information about vocational accomplishments is also crucial in the evaluation of those geriatric patients who still remain active in the workplace.

A careful review of personal and family medical, neurological, and psychiatric history is an additional crucial part of the neuropsychological interview. Many older patients have a variety of systemic physical health problems such as diabetes or hypertension that can seriously affect their neurobehavioral status (Knopman et al., 2001). Comorbid medical conditions and associated frailty have been identified as a major predictor of functional outcome in older rehabilitation patients (Lichtenberg, MacNeill, Lysack, Bank, & Neufeld, 2003; Moore & Lichtenberg, 1996). Pain has been identified as a potential source of distortion of neuropsychological test performance (Martelli, 2001). It is also not uncommon for older patients to be on a variety of medications, some of which can have significant cognitive side effects (Stein & Strickland, 1998). Episodes of depression are common with geriatric patients, especially in those with medical burden and prior psychiatric problems, but these are often not recognized, treated, or spontaneously reported (Brown, McAvay, Raue, Moses, & Bruce, 2003; Bruce et al., 2002; Krishnan et al., 2002).

It is important to review with the patient not only recent medical issues but also early developmental issues and especially lifelong experiences. For example, there is evidence that moderate to severe traumatic brain injury in early adulthood is a risk factor for the later development of dementia of the Alzheimer type (Lye & Shores, 2000; Plassman et al., 2000). In addition, it is often informative to ask specifically about a history of neurodegenerative or psychiatric problems in the biological family because such a presence may put the patient at greater risk for similar problems (Butt & Strauss, 2001; Holmes & Lovestone, 2002).

A careful review of the psychosocial support system that is in place for the geriatric patient is an additional necessary component of the clinical interview. Several studies have suggested that the degree of family support is an important variable in the outcome of stroke in the elderly (Jaracz & Kozubski, 2003; Kriegsman, van Eijk, Penninx, Deeg, & Boeke, 1997). Families may be able to provide crucial transportation, supervision, or physical assistance that may prevent unnecessary institutionalization of persons with significant neurobehavioral impairments. Caregiver burden must also be addressed in this context, as well as potential changes that have occurred in the nature of the relationship between the patient and his or her spouse and children (Tommessen et al., 2002; Wyller et al., 2003). The interview should also address recent unrelated psychosocial stressors and associated patient and family coping styles and resources in this regard.

Neuropsychologists should also be aware of their own biases and expectations when conducting clinical interviews with geriatric patients. For example, although concerns about sexuality are often thought of as relevant for a "younger" generation, these can be significant issues for elderly patients or spouses as well (Aizenberg, Weizman, & Barak, 2002; Eloniemi-Sulkava et al., 2002). Similarly, there is evidence that substance abuse among geriatric patients may be underrecognized (Johnson, Nowers, & West, 2001; Weintraub et al., 2002).

Wrapping up

Sometimes, it is easy to get caught up during interviews in one's own questions, particularly when patient or family responses generate hypotheses for further exploration. On other occasions, patients describe so many complicating issues that it may be difficult to decide where to start or focus. For these reasons, it is often a good idea to ask the patient and family toward the end of the clinical interview to prioritize their concerns. In addition, they should be asked some open-ended questions to elicit any potentially important matters that may not yet have been addressed. For example the neuropsychologist might wish to briefly summarize the main findings from the interview, ask if this is a correct conceptualization, and then inquire if there is anything else that the patient or family would like to add or ask before proceeding with the formal psychometric tests. Practitioners should also be prepared to follow up with an additional interview later on if further medical records or unusual neuropsychological test data become available that raise new questions.

Conclusion

The clinical interview is a dynamic process that may appear to be time consuming but in the end is an indispensable part of a thorough neuropsychological evaluation. A careful history combined with good behavioral observations may go a long way to avoid unnecessary tests or diagnostic misinterpretations. Although there is nothing wrong with "blind" consideration of test results as an academic exercise or as an initial step of the interpretation process, neuropsychological data must always be considered in the context of the referral question and the information obtained during the clinical interview.

References

Aizenberg, D., Weizman, A., & Barak, Y. (2002). Attitudes toward sexuality among nursing home residents. *Sexuality and Disability, 20*, 185–189.

American Academy of Clinical Neuropsychology. (2001). Policy statement on the presence of third party observers in neuropsychological assessments. *The Clinical Neuropsychologist, 15*, 433–439.

Bowler, R. M., Lezak, M., Booty, A., Hartney, C., Megler, D., Levin, J., & Zisman, F. (2001). Neuropsychological dysfunction, mood disturbance, and emotional status of munitions workers. *Applied Neuropsychology, 8*, 74–90.

Brown, E. L., McAvay, G., Raue, P. J., Moses, S., & Bruce, M. L. (2003). Recognition of depression among elderly recipients of home care services. *Psychiatric Services, 54*, 208–213.

Bruce, M. L., McAvay, G. J., Raue, P. J., Brown, E. L., Meyers, B. S., Keohane, D. J., et al. (2002). Major depression in elderly home health care patients. *American Journal of Psychiatry, 159*, 1367–1374.

Butt, Z. A., & Strauss, M. E. (2001). Relationship of family and personal history to the occurrence of depression in persons with Alzheimer's disease. *American Journal of Geriatric Psychiatry, 9*, 249–254.

Eloniemi-Sulkava, U., Notkola, I., Haemaelaeinen, K., Rahkonen, T., Viramo, P., Hentinen, M., et al. (2002). Spouse caregivers' perceptions of influence of dementia on marriage. *International Psychogeriatrics, 14*, 47–58.

Ferraro, R. F. (2002). *Minority and cross-cultural aspects of neuropsychological assessment.* Lisse, The Netherlands: Swets & Zeitlinger.

Hanks, R. A., & Lichtenberg, P. A. (1996). Physical, psychological, and social outcomes in geriatric rehabilitation patients. *Archives of Physical Medicine and Rehabilitation, 77,* 783–792.

Heaton, R. K., Taylor, M. J., & Manly, J. (2003). Demographic effects and use of demographically corrected norms with the WAIS–III and WMS–III. In D. S. Tulsky et al. (Eds.), *Clinical interpretation of the WAIS–III and WMS–III* (pp. 181–210). San Diego, CA: Academic Press.

Holmes, C., & Lovestone, S. (2002). The clinical phenotype of familial and sporadic late onset Alzheimer's disease. *International Journal of Geriatric Psychiatry, 17,* 146–149.

Jaracz, K., & Kozubski, W. (2003). Quality of life in stroke patients. *Acta Neurologica Scandinavica, 107,* 324–329.

Johnson, I., Nowers, M. P., & West, S. H. (2001). Alcohol problems in the elderly: A survey of psychogeriatric admissions. *International Journal of Geriatric Psychiatry, 16,* 235–236.

Knopman, D., Boland, L. L., Mosley, T., Howard, G., Liao, D., Szklo, M., et al. (2001). Cardiovascular risk factors and cognitive decline in middle-aged adults. *Neurology, 56,* 42–48.

Kriegsman, D. M. W., van Eijk, J. T. M., Penninx, B. W. J. H., Deeg, D. J. H., & Boeke, A. J. P. (1997). Does family support buffer the impact of specific chronic diseases on mobility in community-dwelling elderly? *Disability and Rehabilitation, 19,* 71–83.

Krishnan, K. R., Delong, M., Kraemer, H., Carney, R., Spiegel, D., Gordon, C., et al. (2002). Comorbidity of depression with other medical problems in the elderly. *Biological Psychiatry, 52,* 559–588.

Lichtenberg, P. A., MacNeill, S. E., Lysack, C. L., Bank, A. L., & Neufeld, S. W. (2003). Predicting discharge and long-term outcome patterns for frail elders. *Rehabilitation Psychology, 48,* 37–43.

Lye, T. C., & Shores, E. A. (2000). Traumatic brain injury as a risk factor for Alzheimer's disease: A review. *Neuropsychology Review, 10,* 115–129.

Manly, J. J., Jacobs, D. M., Touradji, P., Small, S. A., & Stern, Y. (2002). Reading level attenuates differences in neuropsychological test performance between African American and White elders. *Journal of the International Neuropsychological Society, 8,* 341–348.

Martelli, M. F. (2001). Does pain confound interpretation of neuropsychological test results? *Neurorehabilitation, 16,* 225–230.

Moore, C. A., & Lichtenberg, P. A. (1996). Neuropsychological prediction of independent functioning in a geriatric sample: A double cross-validation study. *Rehabilitation Psychology, 41,* 115–130.

Moses, J. A., Pritchard, D. A., & Adams, R. L. (1999). Normative corrections for the Halstead-Reitan neuropsychological battery. *Archives of Clinical Neuropsychology, 14,* 445–454.

National Academy of Neuropsychology. (2000). Presence of third party observers during neuropsychological testing: Official statement of the National Academy of Neuropsychology. *Archives of Clinical Neuropsychology, 15,* 379–380.

Plassman, B. L., Havlik, R. J., Steffens, D. C., Helms, M. J., Newman, T. N., Drosdick, D., et al. (2000). Documented head injury in early adulthood and risk of Alzheimer's disease and other dementias. *Neurology, 55,* 1158–1166.

Sbordone, R. J. (2000). The assessment interview in clinical neuropsychology. In G. Groth-Marnat (Ed.), *Neuropsychological assessment in clinical practice: A guide to test interpretation and integration* (pp. 94–126). New York: Wiley.

Sherrill-Pattison, S., Donders, J., & Thompson, E. (2000). Influence of demographic variables on neuropsychological test performance after traumatic brain injury. *The Clinical Neuropsychologist, 14*, 496–503.

Stein, R. A., & Strickland, T. L. (1998). A review of the neuropsychological effects of commonly used prescription medications. *Archives of Clinical Neuropsychology, 13*, 259–284.

Tommessen, B., Aarsland, D., Braekhus, A., Oksengaard, A. R., Engedal, K., & Laake, K. (2002). The psychosocial burden on spouses of the elderly with stroke, dementia, and Parkinson's disease. *International Journal of Geriatric Psychiatry, 17*, 78–84.

Vanderploeg, R. D. (2000). Interview and testing: The data collection phase of neuro-psychological evaluations. In R. D. Vanderploeg (Ed.), *Clinician's guide to neuro-psychological assessment* (2nd ed., pp. 3–38). Mahwah, NJ: Lawrence Erlbaum Associates, Inc.

Vanderploeg, R. D., Axelrod, B. N., Sherer, M., Scott, J., & Adams, R. L. (1997). The importance of demographic adjustments on neuropsychological test performance: A reply to Reitan and Wolfson (1995). *The Clinical Neuropsychologist, 11*, 210–217.

Weintraub, E., Weintraub, D., Dixon, L., Delahanty, J., Gandhi, D., Cohen, A., & Hirsch, M. (2002). Geriatric patients on a substance abuse consultation service. *American Journal of Geriatric Psychiatry, 10*, 337–342.

Wyller, T. B., Tommessen, B., Sodring, K. M., Sveen, U., Pettersen, A. M., Bautz-Holter, E., & Laake, K. (2003). Emotional well-being of close relatives of stroke survivors. *Clinical Rehabilitation, 17*, 410–417.

2 Selection and use of screening measures in geriatric neuropsychology

Jean Lengenfelder and John DeLuca

Neuropsychological screening measures are designed to provide a quick, brief assessment of an individual's current neuropsychological functioning. Screening measures may be used to capture an overall global level of functioning or identify specific impairments that may warrant further evaluation. The use of a screen can be a first step in making a distinction between individuals with normal cognitive functioning and those with cognitive dysfunction. Some of the overall advantages of screening measures are as follows: (a) they take little time to administer and can be routinely administered as part of an office visit; (b) minimal examiner training is typically required; (c) with proper training they can be readily administered by a variety of health care professionals; (d) minimized administration time is beneficial for patients who are easily fatigued; and (e) they provide a relatively brief, quantifiable, and standardized method for monitoring neurocognitive functioning.

Some disadvantages of screening measures include: (a) limited sensitivity to mild cognitive impairment, that is, scores in the "normal" range do not necessarily indicate normal cognitive functioning; (b) screening measures are not diagnostic tools and are not meant to identify a definitive diagnosis of pathology; (c) screening measures, like other psychometric instruments, may be biased by educational level, age, or ethnicity; (d) because of the brevity of screening instruments, there is a restricted range in scoring, and ceiling and floor effects present in the scoring may limit the amount of change in an individual's functioning that can be observed; and (e) by their nature of requiring a limited amount of time and training, screening measures compromise sensitivity and specificity.

One benefit of conducting an initial screen is to supply information that medical history alone may not provide. Medical history can be an unreliable source of information as a patient may underreport problems, forget to report specific problems they may be experiencing, or present the details of complaints inaccurately. Also a family member or caregiver may not always be present during a medical evaluation. Therefore, it is important for individuals working with geriatric populations to have a method of identifying any changes in cognition or evidence of pathology in an efficient and cost-effective way.

Another benefit of conducting early routine screens to detect cognitive impairment can be to promote earlier treatment. Despite its prevalence in the geriatric population, dementias like Alzheimer's disease (AD) are reported to be underdiagnosed (Callahan, Hendrie, & Tierney, 1995; Iliffe et al., 1991), with some investigators even suggesting that half of all Alzheimer's cases may not be diagnosed (Ross et al., 1997). Early screening can lead to earlier diagnosis for dementias such as Alzheimer's disease and to subsequent earlier pharmacological treatment methods or behavioral interventions. Earlier diagnosis can also allow individuals and their families to plan and prepare for medical, financial, and legal decisions.

The information gathered in a screen can indicate whether a patient would be able to undergo a comprehensive neuropsychological evaluation or if their level of functioning is too impaired for such an evaluation. Screening information can also direct a neuropsychological assessment to problem areas. Screening measures can provide information in several areas, including (a) mental status, (b) cognitive functioning (global or specific areas such as memory, language, or orientation), (c) behavioral or functional status (e.g., activities of daily living), or (d) psychiatric functioning (e.g., depression, anxiety).

There are numerous screening measures available to physicians, clinicians, and trained health care providers. Many screening instruments have been developed to detect dementia in both community and clinical settings. Overall, the content and methodological construction and validation of available screening instruments is quite variable, and as such there is no one screening measure that is generally considered having the most sensitivity and specificity in detecting impairments in the geriatric population across age, education, and premorbid intelligence. The majority of the instruments that are available and have been well developed are primarily for evaluating cognitive abilities. Instruments evaluating functional or psychiatric symptoms have not been as well developed or researched regarding issues of reliability and validity.

Geriatric neuropsychologists can choose from a variety of brief tests and screening batteries. The purpose of this chapter is to provide a brief overview of some of the mental status/cognitive, psychiatric, and behavioral/functional screening measures that are available. The measures discussed in this chapter are regularly used clinically, have been reported in the literature, or have been designed to be used specifically with geriatric patients. Some of these measures have extensive literatures, and the interested reader is referred to the cited studies for more in-depth review. In the selection of a measure for clinical or research use, neuropsychologists should consider (a) the purpose and context of the evaluation; (b) the administration requirements, psychometric properties, and normative data of the measures; and (c) the characteristics of the individual or population to be assessed.

Screening for mental status/cognitive functioning

Cognitive screening instruments can be classified into two categories, global or specific, based on what information the screen yields. A *global* screen is one that produces one overall total score representing general level of functioning. In comparison, a *specific* screen provides scores in several neuropsychological domains. An example of a global screen would be the widely used Mini-Mental State Exam (MMSE; Folstein, Folstein, & McHugh, 1975), which yields an overall total score, whereas an example of a specific screen would be the Dementia Rating Scale (Mattis, 1988), which, in addition to producing an overall total score, yields scores in neuropsychological domains (i.e., attention, memory, etc.). A criticism of global screens is that they lack sensitivity by only providing an overall score, while the specific screens provide a more detailed description of the nature of cognitive dysfunction (Mysiw, Beegan, & Gatens, 1989). Some of the more utilized instruments are listed alphabetically and described below. Administration times are listed in Table 2.1.

Alzheimer's Disease Assessment Scale

The Alzheimer's Disease Assessment Scale (ADAS) is a global screen that was developed to assess change in cognitive function, specifically those abilities

Table 2.1 Administration time of cognitive screening measures

Test	Estimated Administration Time (minutes)
7 Minute Screen	7–10
ADAS	45
BDS	<10
CAST	15
CCSE	5–15
CDR	40
CDT	2
CERAD	20–40
Cognistat (NCSE)	5–20
DRS-2	30–45
GDS	2–5
Mini-Cog	2–4
MIS	4
MMSE	5–10
MSRQ	<10
RBANS	20–30
SPMSQ	<10

affected in Alzheimer's disease (Rosen, Mohs, & Davis, 1984). It includes both cognitive (ADAS-Cog) and noncognitive (ADAS-Non-Cog) sections and requires 45 minutes to administer in its entirety. The cognitive section is comprised of 11 tasks that assess memory, language, praxis, and orientation and has been used in clinical drug trials for Alzheimer's disease. The cognitive sections are comprised of tasks that include word list recall and recognition, recalling instructions, speech and comprehension, constructional praxis (copying a geometric figure), and ideational praxis (preparing an envelope for mailing). The noncognitive section is comprised of 10 items that assess mood or behavioral changes. Scores are computed for the cognitive and noncognitive sections as well as an overall total score, with higher scores indicating greater impairment.

Blessed Dementia Scale

The Blessed Dementia Scale (BDS; Blessed, Tomlinson, & Roth, 1968) is a screening instrument that assesses orientation, concentration, and memory, as well as changes in activities of daily living, personality, and interests. The BDS is comprised of two parts. The first part is an informant rating scale, often called the Blessed Rating Scale (BRS) or the Blessed Dementia Rating Scale (BDRS), which assesses changes in the patient's everyday activities and habits. A shortened version is used as part of the CERAD battery (Morris et al., 1989). The second part of the BDS is often referred to as the Information-Memory-Concentration Test (IMCT) and consists of tasks assessing memory, orientation, and concentration. This part of the scale is comprised of personal orientation questions, memory for both personal and nonpersonal information, remembering a name and address, reciting the months of the year backwards, and counting from 1 to 20 forward and backward. The BDS takes less than 10 minutes to administer and has been shown to demonstrate adequate sensitivity and specificity in identifying individuals with dementia (Erkinjuntti, Hokkanen, Sulkava, & Palo, 1988).

Clinical Dementia Rating

The Clinical Dementia Rating (CDR; Hughes, Berg, Danziger, Coben, & Martin, 1982) is a structured interview that utilizes both the patient and a significant other as informants. It provides a global rating scale of cognitive performance and degree of dementia in six areas: memory, orientation, judgment and problem solving, community affairs, home and hobbies, and personal care. The scale yields a single score of either 0 for healthy individuals without dementia, 0.5 for questionable dementia, 1 for mild dementia, 2 for moderate dementia, or 3 for severe dementia. The scale is generally completed by a clinician in the course of clinical practice; therefore, much of the information has typically been gathered routinely as part of practice. However, if one were to carry out the interview in its entirety, it would take about 40 minutes. The CDR has demonstrated adequate reliability (Berg, Edwards, Danzinger, & Berg, 1987; Burke et al., 1988; McCulla et al., 1989), although interrater reliability is higher at the two extreme ends of the rating scale (questionable dementia and severe dementia) compared to the ratings for mild and moderate dementia.

Clock Drawing Test

The Clock Drawing Test (CDT) is often used in combination with other cognitive assessment instruments to assess constructional or visuospatial ability. Drawing a clock face, often in conjunction with other items such as a daisy, house, person, or bicycle, has been included in various mental status examinations (Battersby, Bender, Pollack, & Kahn, 1956; Goodglass & Kaplan, 1972, 1983; Strub & Black, 1977, 1985). The CDT takes about 2 minutes to administer and requires patients to draw the face of a clock marking all the hours and then putting in the hands of the clock to indicate a specified time. Using the CDT as a screening measure for dementia and AD is also commonly practiced (Lee, Swanwick, Coen, & Lawlor, 1996; Watson, Arfken, & Birge, 1993), and various scoring systems have been developed (Freedman et al., 1994; Sunderland et al., 1989; Wolf-Klein, Silverstone, Levy, & Brod, 1989). The CDT has demonstrated good reliability and validity. Sensitivity has been reported at 91% and specificity at 95% for patients who were later diagnosed with AD (O'Rourke, Tuokko, Hayden, & Beattie, 1997). The CDT shows good discrimination in identifying individuals with dementia from healthy individuals but has not been able to differentiate between types of dementias (Barr, Benedict, Tune, & Brandt, 1992; Kozura & McCullum, 1994; Libon, Swenson, Barnoski, & Sands, 1993).

Cognistat

Cognistat, previously called the Neurobehavioral Cognitive Status Examination (NCSE; Kiernan, Mueller, Langston, & van Dyke, 1987; Schwamm, van Dyke, Kiernan, Merrin, & Mueller, 1987), is a screening measure that evaluates cognitive functions in five major domains: language, constructional ability, memory, calculation skills, and reasoning/judgment. Language has four subsections: spontaneous speech, comprehension, repetition, and naming. Reasoning has two subsections: similarities and judgment. The measure employs a screen and metric approach. That is, in each domain except memory, an initial screen item is given. If an individual fails the screening item, additional items in that domain are given in order to establish a level of impairment. In addition to the five domains above, more general factors, including level of consciousness, orientation, and attention, are assessed independently. Scores are reported in a cognitive status profile and are defined as either average, mild impairment, moderate impairment, or severe impairment.

Although some early research found the Cognistat to be of value in the assessment of older adults (Fulop, Sachs, Strain, & Fillit, 1992), other studies found the screen and metric approach to result in high misclassification rates (Drane & Osato, 1997; Karzmark, 1997; van Gorp et al., 1999). Factor analytic research with older adults supported a unitary factor structure, despite the Cognistat's multiple neuropsychological domains (Engelhart et al., 1999). Drane, Yuspeh, Huthwaite, Klinger, and Hendry (1998) proposed that combining all subtests to form a single composite score may show the greatest utility in geriatric assessment.

More recent studies have offered geriatric norms to supplement the normative data available in the test manual (Drane et al., 2003; Eisenstein et al., 2002). In the study by Drane et al. (2003), the sample of healthy older adults ranged from 60 to 96 years of age. To improve the reliability and standardization of the measure, the screen and metric approach was abandoned. A composite score was derived in order to convey overall cognitive status. The study demonstrated the importance of matching an examinee's demographic background (age and education) to the normative sample with which test scores are compared. These authors found the Cognistat to be more sensitive than the MMSE to the effects of age on cognition. The Cognistat, administered and scored according to the criteria proposed by Drane et al. (1998), is capable of detecting cognitive difficulties in diagnostic groups commonly encountered in general geriatric rehabilitation (Ruchinskas, Repetz, & Singer, 2001).

Cognitive Assessment Screening Test

The Cognitive Assessment Screening Test (CAST; Drachman & Swearer, 1996) is 28-item self-administered paper-and-pencil test that takes 15 minutes to administer. The test is comprised of three one-page sections: Part A contains 10 easy questions, Part B contains 5 harder questions, and Part C contains 13 self-report questions about the individuals' own perception of memory decline.

Scoring consists of a combination of 28 scored responses from Part A and 12 scored responses from Part B, with scores below 36 associated with cognitive impairment. Parts A and B provide quantitative information regarding cognitive performance, while Part C provides qualitative information about any concerns that the patient may have about any cognitive decline they must be experiencing. The CAST was developed for physicians to identify patients that are suspect for dementia. It has been shown to be sensitive in identifying individuals with dementia, and has been found to have good test–retest reliability (Joan et al., 2002).

Cognitive Capacity Screening Examination

The Cognitive Capacity Screening Examination (CCSE; Jacobs, Bernhard, Delgado, & Strain, 1977) is a 30-item questionnaire that takes 5–15 minutes to administer. Each correct item is scored as 1 point, and total scores below 20 generally indicate cognitive impairment. The CCSE assesses the following areas: orientation, attention and concentration (digit span, serial sevens), language (repetition), memory (short-term verbal recall), and verbal concept formation. The CCSE's greatest asset may be its sensitivity in identifying cognitively impaired from healthy individuals. It has not shown adequate specificity in differentiating different subtypes of dementia (McCartney & Palmateer, 1985). Validation studies have been conducted with healthy controls, psychiatric patients, and medical patients (including neurological patients).

Consortium for the Establishment of a Registry for Alzheimer's Disease Battery

The Consortium for the Establishment of a Registry for Alzheimer's Disease (CERAD) Battery is a collaborative effort of many centers under the direction of the National Institute on Aging, which set out in 1986 to develop a standardized battery of assessment of patients with AD. The battery focuses on three areas of assessment; clinical, neuropsychological, and neuropathological (Morris et al., 1989). The neuropsychological battery of the CERAD was developed using brief, common, and reliable tests that could identify mild to moderate dementia and would be able to be given annually for longitudinal evaluation. The battery was developed to identify the primary deficits associated with AD and differentiate between cognitive changes associated with normal aging and those associated with the onset of AD. The clinical portion of the battery is generally completed with 30–40 minutes, while the neuropsychological portion of the battery takes 20–30 minutes. The neuropsychological battery is comprised of the following seven tests: a 15-item Boston Naming Test, animal naming, constructional praxis (copying circle, diamond, intersecting rectangles, and a cube), MMSE, and a word list memory test (three learning trials of a ten-word list, word list delayed recall, and word list recognition).

Dementia Rating Scale

The Dementia Rating Scale (DRS; Mattis, 1976, 1988) is a cognitive screening measure that requires 30-45 minutes to administer. The DRS was originally developed to provide a brief assessment of dementia and a way to measure cognitive decline over time. The current version, the DRS-2, retained the original 36 DRS tasks and 32 stimuli and added revised normative and scoring information (Jurica, Leitten, & Mattis, 2001). The DRS/DRS-2 provides a total score, which quantifies overall level of cognitive functioning, as well as subscale scores in the areas of attention, initiation/perseveration, construction, conceptualization, and memory. The items are arranged hierarchically in descending order with the most difficult item first so that correct performance on the most difficult item assumes correct performance on the easier items below it. The total score has a maximum of 144, and cutoffs are used to indicate cognitive impairment.

Test–retest reliability has been shown to be .97 for the total score and between .61 and .94 for the subscales. The DRS has been shown to correlate with the MMSE from .78 to .82 (Coblentz et al., 1973). In addition to differentiating healthy adults from individuals with dementia, the DRS has been shown to differentiate between types of dementia, such as Alzheimer's disease, Parkinson's, and Huntington's disease. A shorter version for screening was developed by Colantonio, Becker, and Huff (1993).

Memory Impairment Screen

The Memory Impairment Screen (MIS; Buschke et al., 1999) is a 4-item measure to screen for memory impairment. Since memory impairment is frequently an early sign of dementia, this screen was developed to assess for such impairment. Four words from different categories are learned using category cues, and delayed free and cued retrieval is measured. Scores range from 0 to 8, and a cutoff of 4 or less typically indicates impairment. A second form is available and demonstrates strong alternate reliability. Sensitivity and specificity vary depending on the cutoff score used and severity of dementia. Generally, in moderate dementia sensitivity is .95 for AD and .92 for all dementia. In mild dementia, sensitivity is .79 for AD and .69 for all dementias. The MIS has been compared to the traditional three-word memory tests, and it was found that the MIS demonstrated higher sensitivity (86% vs. 65%) and specificity (97% vs. 85%) when screening for AD (Kuslansky, Buschke, Katz, Sliwinski, & Lipton, 2002).

Memory Self-Report Questionnaire

The Memory Self-Report Questionnaire (MRSQ; Riege, 1982) is a 30-question self-report scale developed to assess memory of healthy older adults. The questions fall into four areas: short-term, interfered, perceptual, and imaginal remembering. Answers are rated on a 4-point scale from "almost never" to "almost always." An abbreviated 14-item version of the scale, the Short Memory Questionnaire (SMQ), has been used to differentiate between AD and healthy individuals. The SMQ has yielded a sensitivity of .94 and a specificity of 1.00 and has been shown to correlate with objective measures of memory such as the CERAD Neuropsychological Battery.

Mini-Cog

The Mini-Cog (Borson, Scanlan, Brush, Vitaliano, & Dokmak, 2000) is comprised of two cognitive tasks—a three-item word memory task and a clock drawing task, with an empirical scoring algorithm—and takes 2–4 minutes to complete. It has demonstrated sensitivity ranging from 76% to 99% and specificity ranging from 89% to 95% (Borson, Scanlon, Chen, & Ganguli, 2003; Scanlan & Borson, 2001). The Mini-Cog was developed to address some of the limitations of other dementia screening measures such as educational and language biases, and the absence of comparisons to widely used procedures such as the MMSE or standardized neuropsychological batteries. It has been validated with the MMSE and a standardized neurocognitive battery (Borson et al., 2003).

Mini-Mental State Examination

The Mini-Mental State Examination (MMSE; Folstein et al., 1975), an 11-item test, is one of the most widely used screening instruments for cognitive impairment. The MMSE contains 30 items and takes 5–10 minutes to administer. Total scores range from 0 to 30. With score less than 24 generally associated with cognitive impairment. MMSE items cover the following domains: orientation, language (naming, repetition, comprehension, reading and writing), memory, praxis (three-step praxis, graphic copy of geometric design), and attention and calculation (serial sevens). A strength of the MMSE is that it covers a variety of cognitive domains, and there is a wealth of longitudinal and cross-sectional research data available. Reliability has been shown to be good at .83 to .99 (Folstein et al., 1975). While the initial reliability and validity of the MMSE was good, there has been a wealth of studies examining subsequent reliability and validity of the measure (for a review, see Tombaugh & McIntyre, 1992). Performance on the MMSE has been shown to be affected by age and education, and normative data based on age and educational level is available (Crum, Anthony, Bassett, & Folstein, 1993). Additionally, it is noteworthy that MMSE performance is strongly mediated by language ability.

The MMSE has recently undergone minor modifications by the authors and has been repackaged for sale by Psychological Assessment Resources. The modifications facilitate administration and scoring, and a pocket norms card provides age- and education-corrected T scores for 14 groups, as well as recommended cutoff scores for classifying severity of cognitive impairment.

Repeatable Battery for the Assessment of Neuropsychological Status

The Repeatable Battery for the Assessment of Neuropsychological Status (RBANS; Randolph, 1998) is a cognitive screening measure that requires 20–30 minutes for administration. It has two parallel forms for repeat administration. Originally developed for screening with dementia populations, the RBANS has been utilized with other populations, including head injury and stroke. The RBANS, comprised of 12 subtests, yields indices for five cognitive domains, including immediate memory, delayed recall, visuospatial/constructional, language, and attention. The 12 subtests comprise list learning, story memory, figure copy, line orientation, digit span, coding, picture naming, semantic fluency, list recall, list recognition, story recall, and figure recall. In addition to being able to differentiate between dementia patients and healthy individuals, the RBANS has also been shown to differentiate between types of dementias, such as Alzheimer's and Huntington's diseases (Randolph, Tierney, Mohr, & Chase, 1998).

The RBANS manual provides age-corrected normative data for 10-year bands from ages 20 to 89 but does not provide education corrections. Due to recommendations for education corrections (Gontkovsky, Mold, & Beatty, 2003; Lineweaver, Zone, Chelune, Herman, & Dow, 2001), Duff et al. (2003) extended the normative information by providing age- and education-corrected scaled scores for the individual subtests, index scores, and total scale scores. Their normative data, based on a large sample of community dwelling older adults, was grouped into overlapping midpoint ranges at 5-year intervals from midpoint ages 70–85. The age range around each midpoint was 10 years. The upper limit of the highest age range (midpoint age 85) was 94 years of age. These expanded norms, requiring modification of the scoring criteria for figure copy and figure recall, increase the clinical utility of the RBANS with older adults. Duff et al. state that the RBANS "is likely to become a popular screening instrument, especially in geriatric neuropsychological evaluations" (p. 352).

Short Portable Mental Status Questionnaire

The Short Portable Mental Status Questionnaire (SPMSQ; Pfeiffer, 1975) is a 10-item instrument assessing memory, orientation, and serial subtraction. The majority of the questions assess personal orientation (e.g., date, address, place, age); two questions ask for the name of the current and previous presidents; and the last is a serial three subtraction task from 20 to the end. Scoring is the total number of errors, with a cutoff of 3 typically indicating cognitive impairment. Sensitive to the effects of ethnicity and education, scoring is adjusted for these factors (Fillenbaum, Heyman, Williams, Prosnitz, & Burchett, 1990). Good test–retest reliability (.82–.85) was demonstrated, and interrater reliability was found to be high (Lesher & Whelihan, 1986; Pfeiffer, 1975). Sensitivity has been reported to be 86% for inpatients and 67% for community dwelling individuals, and specificity has been reported to be 99% for inpatients and 100% for community dwelling individuals (Erkinjuntti, Sulkava, Wikstrom, & Autio, 1987).

The 7 Minute Screen

The 7 Minute Screen (Solomon, 2000) is a paper-and-pencil test that can be administered in an average of 7 minutes. The 7 Minute Screen measures the following areas: orientation, memory, visuospatial abilities, and expressive language. Orientation items involve questions about the day, date, and time. The memory portion asks patients to recall 16 pictures with the aid of category cueing. The visuospatial portion requires patients to draw the face of a clock and set the hands to a specified time. The language portion examines verbal fluency by asking patients to generate as many names of animals as they can in 1 minute. The maximum score on the orientation section is 113, with higher scores indicating more impairment. For the other sections, higher scores indicate greater correct responses, with the following maximum scores: memory section = 16, visuospatial = 7, and language = 45.

The 7 Minute Screen was designed to identify patients who should be further evaluated for AD and was developed with items that would be sensitive to individuals with early AD. The screen has demonstrated sensitivity in correctly identifying 92% patients with AD compared with healthy individuals (Solomon, 2000). The screen has also been found to be sensitive to dementia of various etiology, with Meulen et al. (2004) noting 92.9% sensitivity and 93.5% specificity for AD and 89.4% sensitivity and 93.5% specificity for other types of dementia. Test-retest reliability was found to be between .83 and .93, and interrater reliability was .91 (Solomon, 2000; Solomon, Sullivan, & Pendlebury, 1998).

Screening for depression and other psychiatric symptoms

Routine depression screening can elucidate depression associated with medical conditions often found in geriatric populations, such as diabetes or heart disease. Screening for geriatric depression in a primary care setting is important. In addition to being a primary clinical concern, depression may be an early indication of a cognitive decline or may be masking changes in cognitive status. For example, individuals with cognitive disorders, such as Mild Cognitive Impairment (MCI) or Alzheimer's disease, have a high rate of depression. Studies have reported the presence of depression in 49% of Alzheimer's patients (Lyketsos et al., 1997), and the onset of depression concomitant with MCI has been associated with the progression to later Alzheimer's disease (Visser, Verhey, Ponds, Kester, & Jolles, 2000). Depressive symptomology has also been reported in vascular dementia and Parkinson's disease. While assessment of depression and other psychiatric disorders is covered in depth later in this book (Chapter 12), it is important to mention a few of the more commonly used psychiatric screening instruments here.

Geriatric Depression Scale

The Geriatric Depression Scale (GDS; Yesavage et al., 1983) is a 30-item self-report questionnaire with yes/no answers to evaluate depression in older adults. This is the most frequently used scale to assess depression in the geriatric population and typically takes 2–5 minutes to administer. A score of greater than 11/12 is suspect for depression and yields 84% sensitivity and 95% specificity.

Raising the cutoff score to 14/15 will decrease the sensitivity rate to 80% but increase specificity to 100%. The GDS is not as effective at identifying depression when cognitive impairments are severe enough to impede understanding the questions; for example, when scores on the MMSE are less than 12, the validity of the GDS is questionable (Parmelee, Katz, & Lawton, 1989). There is also shorter version of the GDS available. A 15-item version with cutoff score 6/7 has been shown to be highly correlated with the 30-item scale (Burke, Roccaforte, & Wengel, 1991; Shiekh & Yesavage, 1986). A 5-item version of the GDS also has shown good sensitivity (.94) and specificity (.81) and was found to be as effective as the 15-item version in identifying depression (Rinaldi et al., 2003).

Cornell Scale for Depression in Dementia

The Cornell Scale for Depression in Dementia (CSDD; Alexopoulos, Abrams, Young, & Shamoian, 1988) is a 19-item scale developed for assessing depression in the presence of dementia. Administration takes about 10 minutes with the patient and an additional 20 minutes with a family member or caregiver. The CSDD has been shown to have good reliability and validity for assessing depression in individuals with Alzheimer's disease. Items are rated as "absent," "mild or intermittent," or "severe," and a score of 8 or more is suggestive of depression.

The Neuropsychiatric Inventory

The Neuropsychiatric Inventory (NPI; Cummings, 1997) uses a screening approach to identify behavioral and psychiatric symptoms that occur in dementia patients. It is administered in a structured interview format to a caregiver or significant other and takes 7–10 minutes if no significant psychopathology is endorsed. The NPI assesses 12 symptoms on the basis of frequency and severity: delusions, hallucinations, agitation, dysphoria, anxiety, apathy, irritability, euphoria, disinhibition, aberrant motor behavior, nighttime behavior disturbances, and appetite and eating abnormalities. The NPI yields a total score, a total caregiver distress score, and scores for the individual subtests. Adequate validity and reliability have been reported (Cummings, 1997; Cummings et al., 1994). A brief questionnaire form of the NPI (the NPI-Q) has also been developed and validated with the NPI (Kaufer et al., 2000), and a nursing home version is available.

Screening for behavioral or functional impairment

Early signs of cognitive impairment in the geriatric population may be evidenced in changes in behavior or the ability to function in everyday life. Behavioral changes and symptoms, including delusions, hallucinations, anxiety, and agitation, can occur during the course of AD. Patients with frontotemporal dementia may display changes in personality and behavioral abnormalities including disinhibition, apathy, and euphoria early in the course of their illness. Vascular dementia can include irritability, apathy, or lability. Therefore, screening for changes in behavior and personality may assist with the early diagnosis of a dementia.

Functional impairments can be evidenced in the geriatric population due to dementing illnesses, chronic diseases, medical or physical impairments, or general frailty due to age. Screening for changes in patients' functional abilities is typically done through a caregiver, relative, or significant other. Cognitive impairments impact everyday functioning; for example, early Alzheimer's disease patients may display changes in their ability to manage finances, organize household tasks, or drive. There are numerous functional assessment instruments available, particularly within rehabilitation settings. However, there is great variability in such instruments including lack of normative data, subjective ratings of impairment, assessing broad vs. specific functional deficits, and performance-based evaluation requiring trained personnel, lengthy protocols, or involved scoring procedures.

Dementia Severity Rating Scale

The Dementia Severity Rating Scale (DSRS; Clark & Ewbank, 1996) is an 11-item scale that evaluates current level of functioning and ability to function in the home. It assesses both functional and cognitive areas, including memory, orientation, judgment, social interactions/community affairs, home activities/responsibilities, personal care, language, speech/feeding, recognition, feeding, incontinence, and mobility/walking. A significant other or caregiver rates each area with a score of zero indicating normal abilities and higher scores indicating greater impairment. A total DSRS score is provided, with a cutoff of 4 generally indicating impairment.

Functional Assessment Screening Instrument

The Functional Assessment Screening Instrument (FAS; Pannill, 1991) is a patient-completed screening instrument developed for use in multidisciplinary geriatric assessment and primary care to assess functional and health status and economic and social resources. The nine-question instrument was validated against a structured comprehensive geriatric interview and was used to predict the use of home care services. The FAS demonstrated 91% sensitivity and 64% specificity in identifying functional problems. The screen also demonstrated a sensitivity of 94% and a specificity of 33% in predicting the use of formal services.

Interview for Deterioration in Daily Living Activities in Dementia

The Interview for Deterioration in Daily Living Activities in Dementia (IDDD; Teunisse, Derix, & van Crevel, 1991) is a 33-item structured interview of caregivers that rates functioning in two domains: self-care and complex activities. Self-care items include activities such as bathing, dressing, toileting, and eating. Complex activities include shopping, communicating, telephoning, and writing. The frequency of assistance needed to complete each task is rated on a 3-point scale for each item, rating whether patients required the same frequency of assistance (score = 1), assistance more often (score = 2), or nearly always required assistance (score = 3). Relationships between performance on the IDDD and cognitive impairment and behavioral symptoms have been reported (Teunisse et al., 1991).

Conclusions

The screening measures presented in this chapter represent just a few of the most commonly utilized cognitive, psychiatric, and behavioral/functional options available to neuropsychologists working with older adults. In addition to measures designed specifically as screens, abbreviated versions of larger tests, such as the Wechsler scales, or standardized short forms developed as alternatives to full length measures, such as the California Verbal Learning Test, may be particularly appropriate in geriatric assessments. However, such measures, by design, tend to lack the breadth that is found in some screening measures, such as the Cognistat and the RBANS.

The use of screening measures is an essential aspect of geriatric neuropsychological assessment. It is recommended that clinicians be familiar with a variety of measures and their normative data so that selection of an appropriate measure can be made for any given examinee. Independently established supplements to the normative data available in test manuals can be particularly valuable for expanding the clinical utility of neuropsychological screening measures.

References

Alexopoulos, G. S., Abrams, R. C., Young, R. C., & Shamoian, C. A. (1988). Cornell Scale for Depression in Dementia. *Biological Psychiatry, 23*(3), 271–284.

Barr, A., Benedict, R., Tune, L., & Brandt, J. (1992). Neuropsychological differentiation of Alzheimer's disease from vascular dementia. *International Journal of Geriatric Psychiatry, 7,* 621–627.

Battersby, W. S., Bender, M. B., Pollack, M., & Kahn, L. (1956). Unilateral "spatial agnosia" ("inattention") in patients with cerebral lesions. *Brain, 79,* 68–93.

Berg, G., Edwards, D. F., Danzinger, W. L., & Berg, L. (1987). Longitudinal change in three brief assessments of SDAT. *Journal of the American Geriatrics Society, 35*(3), 205–212.

Blessed, G., Tomlinson, B. E., & Roth, M. (1968). The association between quantitative measures of dementia and of senile changes in the cerebral grey matter of elderly subjects. *British Journal of Psychiatry, 114,* 797–811.

Borson, S., Scanlan, J. M., Brush, M., Vitaliano, P., & Dokmak, A. (2000). The Mini-Cog: A cognitive "vital sign" measure for dementia screening in multi-lingual elderly. *International Journal of Geriatric Psychiatry, 15,* 1021–1027.

Borson, S., Scanlon, J. M., Chen, P., & Ganguli, M. (2003). The Mini-Cog as a screen for dementia: Validation in a population-based sample. *Journal of the American Geriatrics Society, 51*, 1451–1454.

Burke, W. J., Miller, J. P., Rubin, E. H., Morris, J. C., Coben, L. A., Duchek, J., et al. (1988). Reliability of the Washington University Clinical Dementia Rating. *Archives of Neurology, 45*(1), 31–32.

Burke, W. J., Roccaforte, W. H., & Wengel, S. P. (1991). The short form of the Geriatric Depression Scale: A comparison with the 30-item form. *Journal of Geriatric Psychiatry Neurology, 4*, 173–178.

Buschke, H., Kuslansky, G., Katz, M., Stewart, W. F., Sliwinski, M. J., Eckholdt, H. M., et al. (1999). Screening for dementia with the Memory Impairment Screen. *Neurology, 52*, 231–238.

Callahan, C. M., Hendrie, H. C., & Tierney, W. M. (1995). Documentation and evaluation of cognitive impairment in elderly primary care patients. *Annals of Internal Medicine, 122*, 422–429.

Clark, C. M., & Ewbank, D. C. (1996). Performance of the Dementia Severity Rating Scale: A caregiver questionnaire for rating severity in Alzheimer disease. *Alzheimer Disease and Associated Disorders, 10*, 31–39.

Coblentz, J. M., Mattis, S., Zingesser, H., Kasoff, S. S., Wisniewski, H. M., & Katzman, R. (1973). Presenile dementia. *Archives of Neurology, 29*, 299–308.

Colantonio, A., Becker, J. T., & Huff, F. J. (1993). Factor structure of the Mattis Dementia Rating Scale among patients with probable Alzheimer's Disease. *Journal of Clinical Neuropsychology, 7*(3), 313–318.

Crum, R. M., Anthony, J. C., Bassett, S. S., & Folstein, M. F. (1993). Population-based norms for the Mini-Mental State Examination by age and educational level. *Journal of the American Medical Association, 269*, 2386–2391.

Cummings, J. L. (1997). The Neuropsychiatric Inventory: Assessing psychopathology in dementia patients. *Neurology, 48*(Suppl.), S10–16.

Cummings, J. L., Mega, M., Gray, K., Rosenberg-Thompson, S., Carusi, D. A., & Gornbein, J. (1994). The Neuropsychiatric Inventory: Comprehensive assessment of psychopathology in dementia. *Neurology, 44*, 2308–2314.

Drachman, D. A., & Swearer, J. M. (1996). Screening for dementia: Cognitive Assessment Screening Test (CAST). *American Family Physician, 54*(6), 1957–1962.

Drane, D. L., & Osato, S. S. (1997). Using the Neurobehavioral Cognitive Status Examination as a screening measure for older adults. *Archives of Clinical Neuropsychology, 12*, 139–143.

Drane, D. L., Yuspeh, R. L., Huthwaite, J. S., Klingler, L. K., Foster, L. M., Mrazik, M., et al. (2003). Healthy older adult performance on a modified version of the Cognistat (NCSE): Demographic issues and preliminary normative data. *Journal of Clinical and Experimental Neuropsychology, 25*(1), 133–144.

Drane, D. L., Yuspeh, R. L., Huthwaite, J. S., Klinger, L. K., & Hendry, K. M. (1998). Older adult norms for the Cognistat (NCSE). *Archives of Clinical Neuropsychology, 14*, 47–48.

Duff, K., Patton, D., Schoenberg, M. R., Mold, J., Scott, J. G., & Adams, R. L. (2003). Age- and education-corrected independent normative data for the RBANS in a community dwelling elderly sample. *The Clinical Neuropsychologist, 17*(3), 351–366.

Eisenstein, N., Engelhart, C. I., Johnson, V., Wolf, J., Williamson, J., & Losonczy, M. B. (2002). Normative data for healthy elderly persons with the neurobehavioral cognitive status exam (Cognistat). *Applied Neuropsychology, 9*(2), 110–113.

Engelhart, C., Eisenstein, N., Johnson, V., Wolf, J., Williamson, J., Steitz, D., et al. (1999). Factor structure of the Neurobehavioral Cognitive Status Exam (COGNI-STAT) in healthy, and psychiatrically and neurologically impaired, elderly adults. *The Clinical Neuropsychologist, 13*(1), 109–111.

Erkinjuntti, T., Hokkanen, L., Sulkava, R., & Palo, J. (1988). The Blessed Dementia Scale as a Screening Test. *International Journal of Geriatric Psychiatry, 3*(4), 267–273.

Erkinjuntti, T., Sulkava, R., Wikstrom, J., & Autio, L. (1987). Short Portable Mental Status Questionnaire as a screening test for dementia and delirium among the elderly. *Journal of American Geriatric Society, 35*(5), 412–416.

Fillenbaum, G., Heyman, A., Williams, K., Prosnitz, B., & Burchett, B. (1990). Sensitivity and specificity of standardized screens of cognitive impairment and dementia among elderly black and white community residents. *Journal of Clinical Epidemiology, 43*(7), 651–660.

Folstein, M. F., Folstein, S. E., & McHugh, P. R. (1975). Mini-Mental State Examination. *Journal of Psychiatric Research, 12*, 189–198.

Freedman, M., Leach, L., Kaplan, E., Winocur, G., Shulman, K. I., & Delis, D. C. (1994). *Clock drawing: A neuropsychological analysis*. New York: Oxford University Press.

Fulop, G., Sachs, C. J., Strain, J., & Fillit, H. (1992). Usefulness of the Neurobehavioral Cognitive Status Examination in the hospitalized elderly. *International Psychogeriatrics, 4*, 93–102.

Gontkovsky, S. T., Mold, J. W., & Beatty, W. W. (2003). Age and educational influences on RBANS Index scores in a non-demented geriatric sample. *The Clinical Neuropsychologist, 16*, 258–263.

Goodglass, H., & Kaplan, E. (1972). *The assessment of aphasia and related disorders*. Philadelphia: Lea & Febiger.

Goodglass, H., & Kaplan, E. (1983). *Assessment of aphasia and related disorders* (2nd ed.). Philadelphia: Lea & Febiger.

Hughes, C. P., Berg, L., Danziger, W. L., Coben, L. A., & Martin, R. L. (1982). A new clinical scale for the staging of dementia. *British Journal of Psychiatry, 140*, 566–572.

Iliffe, S., Haines, A., Gallivan, S., Booroff, A., Goldenberg, E., & Morgan, P. (1991). Assessment of elderly people in general practice. *British Journal of General Practice, 36*, 662.

Jacobs, J. W., Bernhard, M. R., Delgado, A., & Strain, J. J. (1977). Screening for organic mental syndromes in the medically ill. *Annals of Internal Medicine, 86*, 40–46.

Joan, M., Drachman, D. A., Li, L., Kane, K. J., Dessureau, B., & Tabloski, P. (2002). Screening for dementia in "real world" settings: The Cognitive Assessment Screening Test: CAST. *The Clinical Neuropsychologist, 16*, 128–135.

Jurica, P. J., Leitten, C., & Mattis, S. (2001). *Dementia Rating Scale–2* [DRS-2]. Lutz, FL: Psychological Assessment Resources, Inc.

Karzmark, P. (1997). Operating characteristics of the Neurobehavioral Cognitive Status Exam using neuropsychological assessment as the criterion. *Assessment, 4*, 1–8.

Kaufer, D. I., Cummings, J. L., Ketchel, P., Smith, V., MacMillan, A., Shelley, T., et al. (2000). Validation of the NPI-Q, a brief clinical form of the Neuropsychiatric Inventory. *Journal of Neuropsychiatry and Clinical Neuroscience, 12*(2), 233–239.

Kiernan, R. J., Mueller, J., Langston, J. W., & van Dyke, C. (1987). The Neurobehavioral Cognitive Status Examination: A brief but differentiated approach to cognitive assessment. *Annals of Internal Medicine, 107,* 481–485.

Kozura, E., & McCullum, M. (1994). Qualitative features of clock drawing in normal aging and Alzheimer's disease. *Assessment, 1,* 179–187.

Kuslansky, G., Buschke, H., Katz, M., Sliwinski, M., & Lipton, R. B. (2002). Screening for Alzheimer's disease: The Memory Impairment Screen versus the conventional three-word memory test. *Journal of the American Geriatrics Society, 50*(6), 1086–1091.

Lee, H., Swanwick, G. R., Coen, R. F., & Lawlor, B. A. (1996). Use of the clock drawing task in the diagnosis of mild and very mild Alzheimer's disease. *International Psychogeriatrics, 8*(3), 469–476.

Lesher, E. L., & Whelihan, W. M. (1986). Reliability of mental status instruments administered to nursing home residents. *Journal of Consulting and Clinical Psychology, 54,* 726–727.

Libon, D. J., Swenson, R. A., Barnoski, E. J., & Sands, L. P. (1993). Clock drawing as an assessment tool for dementia. *Archives of Clinical Neuropsychology, 8,* 405–415.

Lineweaver, T. T., Zone, J. A., Chelune, G. J., Herman, B. P., & Dow, C. (2001). Using the RBANS with older adults: Are age-corrections enough? *Journal of the International Neuropsychological Society, 7,* 136.

Lyketsos, C. G., Steele, C., Baker, L., Galik, E., Kopunek, S., Steinberg, M., et al. (1997). Major and minor depression in Alzheimer's disease: Prevalence and impact. *Journal of Neuropsychiatry and Clinical Neurosciences, 9*(4), 556–561.

Mattis, S. (1976). Mental status examination for organic mental syndromes in the elderly patient. In L. Bellak & T. E. Karasu (Eds.), *Geriatric psychiatry* (pp. 77–121). New York: Grune & Stratton.

Mattis, S. (1988). *Dementia Rating Scale: Professional manual.* Odessa, FL: Psychological Assessment Resources.

McCartney, J. R., & Palmateer, L. M. (1985). Assessment of cognitive deficit in geriatric patients: A study of physician behavior. *Journal of American Geriatrics Society, 33*(7), 467–471.

McCulla, M. M., Coats, M., van Fleet, N., Duchek, J., Grant, E., & Morris, J. C. (1989). Reliability of clinical nurse specialists in the staging of dementia. *Archives of Neurology, 46*(11), 1210–1211.

Meulen, E. F., Schmand, B., van Campen, J. P., deKoning, S. J., Ponds, R. W., Scheltens, P., et al. (2004). The Seven Minute Screen: A neurocognitive screening test highly sensitive to various types of dementia. *Journal of Neurology Neurosurgery, and Psychiatry, 75,* 700–705.

Morris, J. C., Heyman, A., Mohs, R. C., Hughes, J. P., van Belle, G., Fillenbaum, G., et al. (1989). The Consortium to Establish a Registry for Alzheimer's Disease (CERAD): Part I. Clinical and neuropsychological assessment of Alzheimer's disease. *Neurology, 39,* 1159–1165.

Mysiw, W. J., Beegan, J. G., & Gatens, P. F. (1989). Prospective cognitive assessment of stroke patients before inpatient rehabilitation: The relationship of the Neurobehavioral Cognitive Status Examination to functional improvement. *American Journal of Physical Medicine and Rehabilitation, 68*(4), 168–171.

O'Rourke, N., Tuokko, H., Hayden, S., & Beattie, B. L. (1997). Early identification of dementia: Predictive validity of the clock test. *Archives of Clinical Neuropsychology, 12,* 257–267.

Pannill, F. C. (1991). A patient-completed screening instrument for functional disability in the elderly. *American Journal of Medicine*, *90*, 320–327.

Parmelee, P. A., Katz, I. R., & Lawton, M. P. (1989). Depression among institutionalized aged: Assessment and prevalence estimation. *Journal of Gerontology*, *44*, 29–34.

Pfeiffer, E. (1975). A short portable mental status questionnaire for the assessment of organic brain deficit in elderly patients. *Journal of the American Geriatric Society*, *23*(10), 433–441.

Randolph, C. (1998). *Repeatable Battery for the Assessment of Neuropsychological Status manual.* San Antonio, TX: Psychological Corporation.

Randolph, C., Tierney, M. C., Mohr, E., & Chase, T. N. (1998). The Repeatable Battery for the Assessment of Neuropsychological Status (RBANS): Preliminary clinical validity. *Journal of Clinical and Experimental Neuropsychology*, *20*, 310–319.

Riege, W. H. (1982). Self-report and tests of memory aging. *Clinical Gerontologist*, *1*, 23–36.

Rinaldi, P., Mecocci, P., Benedetti, C., Ercolani, S., Bregnocchi, M., Menculini, G., et al. (2003). Validation of the five item geriatric depression scale in elderly subjects in three different settings. *Journal of the American Geriatric Society*, *51*(5), 694–698.

Rosen, W. G., Mohs, R. C., & Davis, K. L. (1984). A new rating scale for Alzheimer's disease. *American Journal of Psychiatry*, *141*, 1356–1364.

Ross, G. W., Abbott, R. D., Petrovich, H., Maski, K. H., Murdaugh, C., Trockman, C., et al. (1997). Frequency and characteristics of silent dementia among elderly Japanese-American men. *Journal of the American Medical Association*, *277*, 800–805.

Ruchinskas, R. A., Repetz, N. K., & Singer, H. K. (2001). The use of the Neurobehavioral Cognitive Status Examination with geriatric rehabilitation patients. *Rehabilitation Psychology*, *46*(3), 219–228.

Scanlan, J., & Borson, S. (2001). The Mini-Cog: Receiver operating characteristics with expert and naïve raters. *International Journal of Geriatric Psychiatry*, *16*(2), 216–222.

Schwamm, L. H., van Dyke, C., Kiernan, R. J., Merrin, E. L., & Mueller, J. (1987). The Neurobehavioral Cognitive Status Examination: Comparison with the Cognitive Capacity Screening Examination and the Mini-Mental State Examination in a neurosurgical population. *Annals of Internal Medicine*, *107*, 486–491.

Shiekh, J., & Yesavage, J. (1986). Geriatric Depression Scale: Recent findings in development of a shorter version. In J. Brink (Ed.), *Clinical gerontology: A guide to assessment and intervention.* New York: Haworth Press.

Solomon, P. R. (2000). Recognizing the Alzheimer's disease patient: The 7 Minute Screen. *Revista Neurologica Argentina*, *25*, 13–20.

Solomon, P. R., Sullivan, D. W., & Pendlebury, W. W. (1998). Toward recognition of the Alzheimer's disease patient in primary care practice: The 7 Minute Screen. *Neurology*, *50*(4, Suppl. 4), A162.

Strub, R. L., & F. W. Black (1977). *The mental status examination in neurology.* Philadelphia: F. A. Davis Co.

Strub, R. L., & Black, F. W. (1985). *Mental status examination in neurology* (2nd ed.). Philadelphia: F. A. Davis.

Sunderland, T., Hill, J. L., Mellow, A. M., Lawlor, B. A., Gundersheimer, J., Newhouse, P. A., & Grafman, J. H. (1989). Clock drawing in Alzheimer's disease:

A novel measure of dementia severity. *Journal of the American Geriatric Association, 37,* 725–729.

Teunisse, S., Derix, M., & van Crevel, H. (1991). Assessing the severity of dementia: Patient and caregiver. *Archives of Neurology. 48,* 274–277.

Tombaugh, T. N., & McIntyre, N. J. (1992). The Mini-Mental State Examination: A comprehensive review. *American Journal of Geriatrics Psychiatry, 40*(9), 922–935.

Van Gorp, W., Marcotte, T. D., Sultzer, D., Hinkin, C., Mahler, M., & Cummings, J. (1999). Screening for dementia: Comparison of three commonly used instruments. *Journal of Clinical and Experimental Neuropsychology, 21,* 29–38.

Visser, P. J., Verhey, F. R., Ponds, R. W., Kester, A., & Jolles, J. (2000). Distinction between preclinical Alzheimer's disease and depression. *Journal of the American Geriatrics Society, 48,* 479–484.

Watson, Y. I., Arfken, C. L., & Birge, S. J. (1993). Clock completion: An objective screening test for dementia. *Journal of the American Geriatrics Society, 41,* 1235–1240.

Wolf-Klein, G. P., Silverstone, F. A., Levy, A. P., & Brod, M. S. (1989). Screening for Alzheimer's disease by clock drawing. *Journal of the American Geriatric Association, 37,* 730–734.

Yesavage, J. A., Brink, T. L., Rose, T. L., Lum, O., Huang, V., Adey, M., et al. (1983). Development and validation of a geriatric depression screening scale. *Journal of Psychiatric Research, 17,* 37–49.

3 Neuropsychological batteries for older adults

John L. Woodard and Bradley N. Axelrod

Individuals aged 65 years and older represent a segment of the population that is being increasingly referred for evaluation of cognitive functioning for a variety of reasons. Despite this fact, adequate normative data and comprehensive, clinically useful test batteries for older adults have been limited. The increased rate of age-related medical conditions, dementia, and multiple medication use, together with an increase in frequency of physical and sensory deficits, collectively make neuropsychological evaluation of the elderly challenging. This chapter describes strategies and techniques for neuropsychological evaluation of the older adult, focusing on instruments that comprehensively and reliably assess neuropsychological status.

Individuals over the age of 65 years fall into a group that represents one of the fastest-growing segments of the population in the United States. Older individuals often have significant needs for evaluation of their neuropsychological status given the age-related prevalence of neurodegenerative disorders, traumatic brain injury, stroke, and other conditions that compromise cognitive functioning. Unfortunately, until recently, normative data for older individuals were relatively nonexistent. Newer instruments have focused to varying degrees on including older adults in their normative data. Despite the appearance of better normative data for geriatric populations, older individuals present unique challenges during neuropsychological evaluation given an increased likelihood of fatigue, medication use, and physical and sensory disabilities that may affect their ability to complete a comprehensive cognitive battery. Nevertheless, neuropsychological evaluation of older persons can (a) guide treatment and rehabilitation efforts by identifying patterns of cognitive strengths and weaknesses; (b) identify psychiatric symptoms that may be targeted for management; and (c) help determine the extent to which problematic physical, sensory, and behavioral symptoms may limit cognitive or functional performance.

The focus of this chapter will be to describe and illustrate various methods for evaluating older individuals. This segment of the population poses considerable challenges given the high prevalence of comorbid medical conditions, difficulty obtaining suitable estimates of premorbid functioning, and considerable individual differences with respect to age-related cognitive changes.

What is neuropsychological assessment of the older patient?

Although neuropsychology is commonly associated with the *standardized* assessment of cognitive abilities, the definition of neuropsychology involves the study of brain–behavior relationships (American Psychological Association, Division of Neuropsychology, 1989; Lezak, 1995). Therefore, in addition to a thorough assessment of cognitive abilities, the neuropsychological evaluation includes obtainment of a thorough background history; assessment of possible psychiatric concomitants, such as depression and anxiety; evaluation of symptoms, such as headache, irritability, and balance difficulty; and a review of neurological functions, such as sensory and motor functioning. In short, any aspect of behavior that can be affected by alterations in brain functioning falls under the domain of neuropsychology.

The criterion of where to set the cutoff for describing an individual as younger, older, or middle-aged is inherently subjective. Studies vary with respect to where this criterion is set, but 65 years of age and older appears to be a frequently used criterion for defining the older adult. Nevertheless, both physical and cognitive aging appear to occur on a continuum, with varying degrees of change occurring across the upper end of the age spectrum. These changes in biological and psychological aging begin to accelerate with increasing age. Given these gradual yet progressive changes, it is important to consider the effects of aging as reflecting a continuous process as opposed to a discrete or categorical phenomenon.

In general, normal cognitive and physiological changes associated with advancing age appear to interact adversely with endogenous and exogenous neurological disorders. This phenomenon may be due to the combination of factors including decreased brain volume, increased brain atrophy, neuronal loss, and neuronal shrinkage, an increase in prevalence of comorbid medical conditions (e.g., hypertension, diabetes, cardiovascular disease) and degenerative brain conditions (e.g., Alzheimer's disease, stroke), and sensory and motor changes that occur with aging (e.g., decreased visual acuity, slowed reaction time, decreased auditory acuity). These age-related changes may have an impact on an individual's level of premorbid functioning. Therefore, it is important to consider these normal age-related changes in interpreting the cognitive status of the elderly patient.

Complicating variables with older adults

There are a number of variables that are commonly seen in the elder population that can either be causal or complicating factors of cognitive impairment. These factors should be taken into account when designing intervention strategies, as well as when assessing the severity of impairment or designing rehabilitation plans. These age-related variables include medication use patterns, presence of comorbid medical disease, and physical, sensory, and cognitive impairment.

Medication use patterns

There are a number of surprising statistics associated with medication use in the elderly. For example, 30% of all prescription drugs are taken by people over 65, and 70% of older adults self-medicate with over-the-counter drugs without consulting a physician (Preston, O'Neal, & Talaga, 1997). Persons over age 65 have been estimated to take an average of 3.4–3.8 (Schmader et al., 1998) to as many as 4.6 (Giron et al., 1999) *different* medications per person daily. The most commonly used class of medication in the elderly tends to be cardiovascular and analgesic agents, although patients with dementia are less likely to be taking cardiovascular and analgesic agents and more likely to be taking central nervous system agents when compared to cognitively intact or mildly cognitively impaired persons (Schmader et al., 1998).

Given this extremely high frequency of medication use by older adults, it is perhaps not surprising that 50% of accidental drug-related deaths occur in geriatric patients (Preston et al., 1997). A number of possible age-related factors may contribute to this statistic, such as (a) impaired organ function (e.g., decreased liver metabolism, leading to increased medication levels, and increased sensitivity to side effects); (b) multiple disease states; and (c) sensory impairment (particularly in the visual modality) or cognitive impairment, both of which may lead to confusion of directions and possible overdose. Adverse results of drug use, such as cognitive impairment, falls resulting in hip fracture, and neuroleptic-induced parkinsonism, are proportional to the number of medications taken and occur at double the rate in geriatric patients than in younger age cohorts (Preston et al., 1997). At the other end of the spectrum, medication noncompliance in the elderly is common (usually underdosing) and may be due to factors such as: (a) complicated directions for using the medication, (b) hearing and visual impairment, (c) cognitive and memory deficits, (d) child-resistant packaging, and (e) cost (Preston et al., 1997).

Given these numerous factors, it is clear that medication use is an important variable to consider as a predisposing and complicating factor when evaluating older adults (Cumming et al., 1991). Some medications may either cause or exacerbate cognitive impairment or may produce an acute confusional state. In addition, one must also be familiar with not only the side effects of various medications but also with effects associated with overuse or under use. In these cases, identification and termination of the offending medication(s) can potentially reverse these symptoms. Among the different drug classes, cardiovascular drugs have been reported to be the leading class associated with adverse drug reactions in the elderly, followed by central nervous system agents, nonsteroidal anti-inflammatory drugs, endocrine agents, anti-invectives, gastrointestinal agents, respiratory agents, and blood formation and coagulation agents (Cooper, 1996).

Comorbid chronic health conditions

Age-related chronic health conditions are extremely common in older age. For example, disorders such as arthritis, cancer, diabetes, heart disease, hypertension, stroke, thyroid disease, and pulmonary disease reflect disorders that can produce transient cognitive fluctuation or physical/sensory impairment. In a sample of demented, cognitively impaired without dementia, and cognitively intact community dwelling elder individuals, approximately 27% had been hospitalized on at least one occasion in the prior year (Schmader et al., 1998). For each of the three groups, the most common chronic medical condition was arthritis, followed by hypertension, and heart disease. For the cognitively intact and cognitively impaired groups, diabetes was the fourth most common medical condition, whereas for dementia patients, stroke was fourth most common, followed by diabetes.

Physical, sensory, and cognitive limitations

A number of studies have highlighted the impact of physical, sensory, and cognitive limitations on the ability of older adults to successfully perform activities of daily living (Myers, Young, & Langlois, 1996). In a sample of 50 home-dwelling persons over 85 years of age (Krach, DeVaney, DeTurk, & Zink, 1996), 78% were reported to have difficulty carrying out both basic activities of daily living (BADL) and instrumental activities of daily living (IADL). This study also noted that ability to perform activities of daily living was related most strongly to ratings of both physical and mental functioning, and least strongly to social and economic functioning on the Older American Resources Survey (OARS; Fillenbaum, 1988). In another sample of 84 participants over 90 years of age (Ravaglia et al., 1997), 81% demonstrated either partial or total dependence for performing BADL using the Katz ADL scale (Katz, Downs, Cash, & Grotz, 1970). However, only 7% of women maintained complete ADL independence versus 34% of men. Bathing, dressing, toileting, and transfer were the most difficult BADLs for both men and women, while continence and eating posed the least difficulties. In addition, several studies have shown a relationship between sensory loss and decreased functional ability among elderly participants (Colsher & Wallace, 1993; Oster, 1976; Ravaglia et al., 1997). Functional blindness and reduced visual acuity is also prevalent among older adults (Salive et al., 1992). In short, physical/sensory compromises in older adults may produce decreased strength and mobility, difficulty seeing obstacles and hazards, and reduced ability to use hearing in order to avoid potential hazards, thereby placing older adults at extremely high risk of experiencing an injury, typically a fall (Benson & Lusardi, 1995; Salgado, Lord, Packer, & Ehrlich, 1994; Tinetti, Doucette, Claus, & Marottoli, 1995).

Sensory impairment across multiple domains is particularly problematic. One study (Keller, Morton, Thomas, & Potter, 1999) recently reported that the combination of visual and hearing impairments impacts functional capacity more than single sensory impairments. In addition, multiple domain sensory impairment was noted to influence functional status independently of mental status and comorbid illness (Keller et al., 1999).

In addition to age-related changes in physical and sensory functioning, functional capacity is dependent upon a complex interplay between numerous cognitive abilities in the elderly, and compromises in cognitive functioning can elevate the risk of injury (Myers et al., 1996). For example, the prominent decline in visuospatial ability with increasing age (Flicker, Ferris, Crook, Bartus, & Reisberg, 1986; Howieson, Holm, Kaye, Oken, & Howieson, 1993), as well as age-related changes in executive functioning (Axelrod, Goldman, & Henry, 1992; Carlson et al., 1999; Grigsby, Kaye, Baxter, Shetterly, & Hamman, 1998; Mittenberg, Seidenberg, O'Leary, & DiGiulio, 1989) and memory (Albert, 1988; Baddeley, 1986; Botwinick & Storandt, 1974; Craik, 1986, 1990; Hultsch & Dixon, 1990; Talland, 1965) place older adults at high risk of experiencing an injury (Nyberg & Gustafson, 1997; Rapport, Hanks, Millis, & Deshpande, 1998). Measures of visuospatial ability, executive functioning, and memory have been shown to add unique variance accounted for over and above that of global cognitive status when predicting IADL performance in healthy and demented elderly persons (Benedict, Goldstein, Dobraski, & Tannenhaus, 1997; Loewenstein, Argüelles, Barker, & Duara, 1993; Loewenstein et al., 1992; Mahurin, DeBettignies, & Pirozzolo, 1991; Nadler, Richardson, Malloy, Marran, & Brinson, 1993; Richardson, Nadler, & Malloy, 1995; Vitaliano, Breen, Albert, Russo, & Printz, 1984) and when predicting positive rehabilitation outcomes and discharge destination in cognitively impaired elderly hip fracture patients (Goldstein, Strasser, Woodard, & Roberts, 1997).

As can be gleaned from the above review, assessment of older adults presents a number of unique challenges and considerations. The following section addresses considerations involved in obtaining the greatest possible reliability and validity in assessing the elderly individuals. These considerations include: (a) attending to special needs of the elderly in the testing environment, (b) developing and maintaining rapport, and (c) selection of instruments used in the cognitive evaluation for assessing general severity level. There are also several excellent textbooks that cover these issues in greater detail that should be consulted by the interested reader (La Rue, 1992; Lezak, 1995; Spreen & Strauss, 1998).

Special needs of older adults during neuropsychological assessment

Testing environment

One of the most important factors in neuropsychological assessment of older adults is establishing a testing environment that will encourage optimal performance. Attention to the special needs of this population is perhaps the first step in ensuring a reliable and valid assessment. In addition, selection of measures that are both internally reliable and appropriate to the diagnostic question is also a fundamental step in assessing this patient group.

The testing room itself should be well lit (preferably using full spectrum light, if possible) and adequately ventilated, and a reasonable degree of soundproofing or separation from adjacent rooms that may provide a source of auditory distraction is essential. Although standard stimulus materials should always be used when possible, patients with visual difficulties can potentially benefit from presenting stimulus material that has been enlarged on a photocopier. Small audio amplifiers may also be helpful for individuals with diminished auditory acuity. It is extremely important that the presence of any sensory deficit that may affect performance and deviations from standardized procedures be well documented by the examiner.

Rapport

A fundamental issue in beginning the neuropsychological evaluation in older adults is establishing rapport through a friendly and supportive relationship. Many older individuals may be acutely aware of their cognitive limitations and may be intimidated by the testing session. Other individuals may be less aware of their deficits and may approach the testing session in a defensive fashion. Finally, many patients have not been suitably prepared for what to expect of the neuropsychological evaluation, and many individuals may be frightened, embarrassed, or anxious. It is helpful to begin the evaluation with a face-to-face interview, explaining the purpose of the evaluation at the outset. The patient should be assured that the purpose of the testing is to investigate those areas that are presenting problems for the patient as well as those abilities that are being performed well. Throughout the evaluation, the patient should be congratulated for his/her successes and supported during failures. At times, considerable frustration or fatigue may result, and it may be useful to take periodic breaks. In some cases, breaking the evaluation up into multiple brief testing sessions may minimize fatigue. If this procedure is used, it is helpful to attempt to schedule the patient at the same time of day during each of the testing sessions to minimize diurnal fluctuations in cognitive status. The bottom line is to attempt to obtain the patient's best performance throughout the assessment.

Neuropsychological batteries for older adults

Two principal approaches exist for undertaking neuropsychological assessment with older adults. A fixed battery approach employs a standardized collection of cognitive measures that is given to all examinees, regardless of the nature of the referral question(s). The fixed battery approach is advantageous in the sense that performance across a set of measures can be examined to identify islands of preserved strengths as well as the presence of specific

deficits. Because all measures are given to all examinees, profiles of performance may emerge that can facilitate diagnostic decision making. However,
fixed batteries tend to be long, producing considerable fatigue in the elderly
and raising questions regarding cost-effectiveness. In contrast, a flexible battery approach usually allows some latitude in the selection of the measures
that make up the battery, with the nature of the referral question typically
dictating the domains evaluated. Flexible battery approaches require much
less time to administer than the fixed battery approach, and they enable the
clinician to focus on specific questions of interest in greater depth. A wider
range of instruments is available for selection, and as new measures are developed and supported empirically, they can easily be included in the battery.
However, because the focus of the measure is often relatively narrow, it may
be more difficult to document the patient's range of strengths that may be of
benefit when designing intervention plans or rehabilitation strategies.
General test selection considerations will be reviewed, followed by consideration of popular fixed and flexible battery approaches.

Instrument selection

Only those measures that have demonstrated reliability and validity should be
selected for the evaluation. Unfortunately, most of the measures used in main-
stream neuropsychology have little information regarding reliability and validity in older adults. Normative data are also missing for the upper end of the
age spectrum on many tests. Although some measures, such as the Wechsler
Adult Intelligence Scale–III (WAIS–III; Wechsler, 1997) and Wechsler
Memory Scale–III (WMS–III; Wechsler, 1997), have normative data through
89 years of age, a number of traditional measures have normative data only
through 60 or 70 years of age. In addition, one should focus on selecting only
those measures that address the diagnostic or research/scientific question,
rather than selecting a larger battery that may provide data that are not
diagnostically important. This procedure will make the evaluation as brief as
possible, thereby minimizing the possibility of fatigue.

Recently, a number of researchers have started to implement brief assess-
ment techniques in order to shorten the length of time required to adminis-
ter more lengthy traditional measures (Axelrod, Woodard, Schretlen, &
Benedict, 1996; Axelrod, Henry, & Woodard, 1992; Axelrod, Woodard, &
Henry, 1991; Benedict, Schretlen, Groninger, & Brandt, 1998; Benedict,
Schretlen, Groninger, Dobraski, & Shpritz, 1996; Woodard & Axelrod, 1995;
Woodard et al., 1996; Woodard et al., 1998; Woodard, Goldstein, Roberts, &
McGuire, 1999). While they are not screening measures *per se*, these brief
assessment approaches have the advantage of assessing a construct of inter-
est and minimizing administration time and fatigue. In achieving these goals,
they can be extremely time- and cost-effective.

Most traditional cognitive measures involve a paper-and-pencil format
that is likely to be familiar to most examinees. However, a new generation of

computer-based instruments is gradually being introduced into the assessment community. If such instruments are used, the examiner must be mindful of the fact that many older individuals have had little experience on the computer, particularly when compared to young adults. As a consequence, increased anxiety or confusion may result from the introduction of a computer or sophisticated stimulus recording materials or manipulation. In addition, computer-based assessment approaches suffer from a continued need to establish reliability, validity, and utility, particularly if they are to be used with elderly individuals. At the present time, computer-based tests should be used sparingly, if at all, for clinical purposes with older individuals until their psychometric characteristics can be firmly established.

General level of intellectual functioning

In most neuropsychological evaluations, it is important to obtain a global measure of intellectual functioning. This information is helpful in placing the results of a neuropsychological evaluation in their proper context, and knowledge of global intellectual functioning can facilitate identification of strengths and weaknesses. The WAIS–III is perhaps the most commonly used measure of intellectual functioning. In its current form, normative data exist up to 89 years of age, making possible an accurate comparison between octogenarians and their same age peers. Age scaled scores for each subtests are now used instead of comparisons with a young (20- to 34-year-old) reference group. This procedure insures a fair comparison with same age peers and helps to account for expected age-related cognitive changes.

Research with the normative group has revealed some interesting findings regarding cognitive changes with older age. For instance, although prior neuropsychological research has reported that advanced age tends to reduce Digit Span-Backward more than Digit Span-Forward (Lezak, 1995), on the WAIS–III, the discrepancy between these two measures tends to remain constant across the age span, including adults between the ages of 70 and 89 (Kaufman & Lichtenberger, 1999). Second, gain scores on Full Scale IQ following repeat testing in individuals 55 years of age and older tend to be somewhat diminished (typically 3–4 points) relative to younger persons (typically 5–6 points; Kaufman & Lichtenberger, 1999). Finally, in persons older than 75 years of age, the nature of the Perceptual Organization and Processing Speed Indexes (Factor Scores) are somewhat different than in younger age cohorts. For instance, Block Design, Picture Completion, and Picture Arrangement tend to load more on the Processing Speed factor in persons aged 75–89, while Matrix Reasoning seems to reflect the sole Perceptual Organization measure (Kaufman & Lichtenberger, 1999; Wechsler, 1997). These issues are just a small number of the numerous age-related differences in intellectual functioning that have been identified on the WAIS–III, but they are important to keep in mind when interpreting data from older examinees.

Results from an entire WAIS–III may sometimes be peripheral to the referral question, or the likelihood of fatigue or diminished cooperation from the full WAIS–III may be a particular concern. In these cases, a number of short forms of the WAIS–III may be of interest (Axelrod, Dingell, Ryan, & Ward, 2000; Axelrod, Ryan, & Ward, 2001; Ryan, Lopez, & Werth, 1999). The Wechsler Abbreviated Scale of Intelligence (WASI; Wechsler, 1999) takes approximately 30–45 minutes to administer and may be a potential consideration for use as a benchmark indicator of intellectual functioning. However, some validity concerns have been expressed with this measure (Axelrod, 2002). Other measures for possible use include the Kaufman Adolescent and Adult Intelligence Test (KAIT; Kaufman & Kaufman, 1993, 1997), the Reynolds Intellectual Assessment Scale (Reynolds & Kamphaus, 2003), discussed below, and the Kaufman Brief Intelligence Test (K-BIT; Kaufman & Kaufman, 1990). These measures have normative data through age 90. The KAIT takes approximately 60 minutes to administer for the core battery, and an additional 30 minutes are required to administer the expanded battery. The latter two measures require approximately 30 minutes to administer; a revised K-BIT (the K-BIT–2; Kaufman & Kaufman, 2004) requires only 20 minutes to administer.

Fixed battery approaches

Traditional fixed battery approaches

The Halstead-Reitan Neuropsychological Battery (HRB; Reitan & Wolfson, 1985, 1993) and the Luria-Nebraska Neuropsychological Battery (LNNB; Golden, Hammeke, & Purish, 1980) are the most frequently studied and utilized comprehensive batteries of cognitive assessment. A study of clinical test usage found the HRB and LNNB to be administered by 29% and 8% of reporting psychologists (Butler, Retzlaff, & Vanderploeg, 1991). A study of forensic neuropsychologists reported 28% and 10% use for the HRB and LNNB, respectively (Lees-Haley, Smith, Williams, & Dunn, 1996).

The HRB is composed of a number of subtests, five of which comprise the Halstead Impairment Index summary score. The core battery includes five tests that generate seven scores of interest. Additional tests used in the HRB include measures of language functioning, sensory-perceptual tasks, grip strength, and the Trail Making Test. The WAIS, but not the WAIS–R or WAIS–III, was normed with the HRB and often is included. Descriptions of the core and supplemental tasks appear in Reitan and Wolfson's (1993) manual. Briefly, the Category Test is a complex test of problem solving. The Seashore Rhythm and Speech Sounds Perception Tests evaluate the examinee's ability to identify nonlanguage auditory stimuli, such as rhythmic patterns and nonsense syllables, respectively. Finger Tapping measures one's fine motor speed by assessing how quickly their finger can tap a key in 10 seconds. Finally, the Tactual Performance Test is a measure of kinesthetic learning and memory, with a component of incidental learning. Patients attempt to place 10 blocks of different shapes into a board that has spaces specific to each of the shapes. This task is performed blindfolded, first with the dominant hand, then the nondominant hand, and finally with both hands. After the third trial, the formboard and blocks are removed from view, and the examinee is requested to draw the board with the shapes as they appeared. Three scores (i.e., time to complete the task, shapes recalled correctly on drawing, and shapes located correctly on drawing) are generated.

The HRB in its most pristine presentation is considered insensitive to the effects of age, education, and gender. Reitan and Wolfson explicitly opposed the implementation of demographic adjustments to the raw test scores, arguing for the use of the same impairment cutting scores for all individuals (Reitan & Wolfson, 1995). Their position has been that demographic corrections are unnecessary because the effects of brain damage are greater than the effects of demographic factors such as age and education (Franzen, 2000). In contrast to Reitan and Wolfson, other studies have demonstrated the importance of making allowances for age and education in assessing the utility of test scores (e.g., Shuttleworth-Jordan, 1997; Vanderploeg, Axelrod, Sherer, Scott, & Adams, 1997). With individuals who are older or less educated, appropriate normative comparisons must be made in order to minimize the potential for false positive errors (Leckliter & Matarazzo, 1989). On direct examination, traditional normative cutoff scores were deemed inappropriate for individuals over 75 in one study (Cullum, Thompson, & Heaton, 1989) and over 55 in another study (Elias, Podraza, Pierce, & Robbins, 1990). This need for demographic adjustments is consistent with the demonstrated decline in speed and cognitive efficiency in older normal adults (e.g., Axelrod & Henry, 1992; Bak & Green, 1980; Elias, Robbins, Walter, & Schultz, 1993; Goldstein & Shelly, 1987; Schludermann, Schludermann, Merryman, & Brown, 1983).

In response to the need for demographically-sensitive normative data on the HRB, Heaton et al. developed (Heaton, Grant, & Matthews, 1991) and later revised (Heaton, Miller, Taylor, & Grant, 2004) comprehensive norms for the individual tests as well as the summary scores. The normative data were created via multiple regression analyses in which norms were smoothed over the entire sample rather than having equal numbers of individuals evaluated within each education, gender, and age cell. Strongly criticized for this procedure (Fastenau & Adams, 1996), the method was defended by the authors as being the best method for existing data (Heaton, Grant, Matthews, & Avitable, 1996). Support for these data was subsequently demonstrated in studies in which HRB data were evaluated both with and without demographic correction. Normal adults without brain injury produced fewer false positive scores when the data were assessed using the comprehensive norms than when the traditional cutoff scores were employed (Sweeney, 1999).

The HRB has been used to detect the presence of abnormal cognitive functioning. Its utility in differentiating neurologic conditions in the elderly has been less effective. Gray, Rattan, and Dean (1986) found depressed older adults to perform better on the HRB than elderly individuals diagnosed with dementia or another neurologic condition. However, the HRB was ineffective in differentiating the two neuropathologic groups from each other. Similarly, vascular and progressive dementias could not be distinguished from each other based on summary data, although greater variability across measures for the vascular patients was observed (Erker, Searight, & Peterson, 1995). The HRB was used to effectively predict daily living skills in a sample of geriatric patients with probable dementia (Dunn, Searight, Grisso, Margolis, & Gibbons, 1990). The authors concluded that the global score from the HRB was sufficiently predictive to a global score of functional abilities in this cognitively compromised sample.

Despite the apparent utility of the HRB with appropriate normative data, some arguments have been made against using the HRB with the elderly altogether. The greatest concerns lie in the administration time required, complexity of the tasks, and reliance on motor strength for older individuals (Kaszniak, 1990).

The LNNB was developed as a quantitative assessment of Luria's qualitative approach to neuropsychological evaluation (Golden, Purisch, & Hammeke, 1985), which improved upon the standardized procedures originally offered by Christensen (1979, 1984). Some have argued that the use of Luria's name is misleading to clinicians who believe that the LNNB is based on Luria's method (Spiers, 1981). Regardless, the LNNB is the second most often used standardized neuropsychological test battery.

The LNNB is composed of test items that fall on 11 clinical scales (12 for Form II). Although earlier versions of the battery provided names for the scales, such as Motor Functions, Rhythm, Tactile, and so forth, for the scales, the newest version refers to scales by number (C1–C12). In addition to the clinical scales, five summary scales (Pathognomonic, Right Hemisphere, Left Hemisphere, Profile Elevation, and Impairment) are generated to assess overall impairment as well as tactile-motor impairment. As opposed to having each scale represent a specific construct, the information obtained from the LNNB serves as information to be interpreted collectively across scales and with external information (Franzen, 2000). However, factor analyses of the LNNB have found the items to be effectively grouped in appropriate constructs with the scales (McKay & Golden, 1981; Moses, 1986). One criticism of the LNNB is that it is more reliant on verbal and putative left hemisphere abilities than it is on nonverbal skills (Russell, 1980).

The clinical and summary scales effectively discriminate normal subjects from neurological patients (Golden, Hammeke, & Purisch, 1978). Subsequent studies have demonstrated clinical validity for individuals with psychiatric, substance abuse, and epileptic disorders (Berg & Golden, 1981; Chmielewski & Golden, 1980; Golden, Graber, Moses, & Zatz, 1980). It also appears effective in detecting cognitive changes secondary to AIDS and mild traumatic brain injury (Ayers, Abrans, Newell, & Friedrich, 1987; Newman & Sweet, 1986).

In evaluating alcoholism and aging, Burger, Botwinick, and Storandt (1987) detected age-related changes in performance on the LNNB. In a study of nonpatient community-dwelling individuals ages 60 and older, 92% of the 78 participants performed within normal limits (MacInnes et al., 1983). These data were confirmed when few differences were observed between groups when the sample was divided into young (60–74 years) and old (>74 years). Another study of nonpatient individuals separated the sample into three age groups. In a subsequent study, MacInnes et al. reassessed 59 of the participants 4 years later (MacInnes, Paull, Uhl, & Schima, 1987). They found minimal changes in test scores for these elderly individuals when evaluated longitudinally. In contrast to the previous studies mentioned, the authors found that the oldest group (ages 65 and older) consistently performed worse than middle aged (50–55 years) and younger (17–30 years) adults (Vannieuwkirk & Galbraith, 1985). A more recent study developed normative data for the LNNB adjusting for the demographic variables of age and education (Moses & Pritchard, 1999). However, the authors cautioned that the performance scales may not be accurate for women or for individuals over age 65.

When looking at the existing data regarding the LNNB, it appears to have adequate validity in general. However, its use for a geriatric population likely requires further analyses and study.

New generation battery approaches

The Neuropsychological Assessment Battery (NAB; Stern & White, 2003) and the Reynolds Intellectual Assessment Scales (RIAS; Reynolds & Kamphaus, 2003) are newly introduced neuropsychological batteries that reflect different strategies for assessment of neuropsychological abilities. Because they have just been published, there are few studies in the literature that have implemented these measures. Consequently, the majority of available data regarding their psychometric properties come from their respective manuals. These new generation batteries are unique in the sense that they can be implemented using a fixed or flexible battery approach. In addition, both offer screening procedures as well as full assessment procedures.

The Neuropsychological Assessment Battery

The Neuropsychological Assessment Battery (NAB) is a recently introduced comprehensive neuropsychological battery that uses a modular approach to assessment. The NAB permits one to adopt either a fixed or flexible battery approach. In addition, a separate screening module is available to facilitate the determination of which specific assessment modules should be used. Normative data for the NAB are available for individuals between 18 and 97 years of age. Normative information is broken down separately in one 12-year block (18–29 years), three 10-year blocks (30–39, 40–49, 50–59 years), four 5-year blocks (60–64, 65–69, 70–74, and 75–79 years), and one 17-year block (80–97 years).

The battery consists of specific modules assessing discrete areas of cognitive functioning. These modules include Attention, Language, Memory, Spatial, and Executive Functions. As mentioned earlier, an additional Screening module may be used first to determine which of the cognitive modules would be appropriate to administer. In individuals with a mild degree of cognitive impairment, this strategy has the potential to shorten the evaluation time considerably.

The Attention module consists of an orientation test, a forward and backward digit repetition, a visually presented delayed recognition span measure, a measure incorporating letter cancellation, letter counting, serial addition, and letter cancellation plus serial addition. In addition, an innovative task is also included that requires the individual to view a scene as if he/she was behind a steering wheel and then to subsequently identify new, different, or missing information in additional driving scenes. The Language module assesses oral production, auditory comprehension, naming ability, reading comprehension, narrative writing ability, and ability to pay a bill by writing a check. The Memory module evaluates list learning, story learning, ability to learn shapes, and ability to learn and recall information often encountered in daily living, such as medication information, phone numbers, names, and addresses. The Spatial module evaluates visual discrimination using a visual match-to-target paradigm, design and construction using plastic manipulatives to construct tangrams, ability to draw and recall a moderately complex geometric figure, and ability to answer questions using a city map. The Executive Functions module assesses ability to navigate seven timed paper-and-pencil mazes, respond to judgment questions regarding home safety, health, and medical issues, perform a word generation task, and to perform a classification and categorization task.

A distinct advantage of the NAB is the inclusion of many ecologically valid daily living style tasks. The ability to assess both execution of instrumental activities of daily living (such as check writing and comprehension of health and safety information), together with evaluation of cognitive functioning status can facilitate the ability to diagnose neurodegenerative conditions. In addition, situations that may potentially pose safety risks for the patient can be identified in a standard fashion.

The strengths of the NAB include its ability to be used in either a screening context or for a full battery assessment. In addition, the screening module can be used in conjunction with the full modules to tailor a battery to only those cognitive functions that may be in need of in-depth assessment. The psychometric qualities are excellent, and a considerable amount of time and effort have been devoted toward establishing the battery's reliability and validity. Normative data are available up to age 97, which is a distinct advantage over most other cognitive batteries. As noted above, the inclusion of both cognitive and functional assessment measures is a considerable strength in assessment of the elderly, because impairment in one domain does not necessarily imply impairment in the other domain.

One perceptible weakness of the NAB at this point is its price, which at a cost of $2995 for the complete kit, may be prohibitive for a number of clinicians. The option to purchase the screening module ($795) separately from the standard modules may help to reduce the initial cost outlay. The battery does come with scoring software for no additional cost, and this software generates a report with graphical and numeric depiction of the client's scores. At this time, there are no published studies beyond what is presented in the NAB manual to support the reliability, validity, and utility of NAB scores in different clinical settings. Finally, the upper end of the normative data represents a 17-year block (80–97 years). Given this large age range, cognitive changes among the oldest old may be difficult to detect and quantify appropriately. For instance, assume that two patients achieve the same raw score on a particular measure, but one patient is 81 years of age and the other patient is 91 years of age. Relative to the performance of each patient's same age peers, the 91-year-old patient may be performing at a much higher level than the 81-year-old. However, because performance of the two individuals is compared to the same normative group, these relative performance differences would not be observed.

Reynolds Intellectual Assessment Scales (RIAS)

The RIAS (Reynolds & Kamphaus, 2003) is appropriate for individuals between the ages of 3 and 94 years. Compared with the preceding batteries, the RIAS samples a smaller number of cognitive domains, focusing on intellectual functioning and memory only. Two subtests are used to provide a verbal intelligence index (VIX), which evaluates verbal problem-solving and reasoning skills that rely upon previously learned knowledge and skills. The two subtests are named Verbal Reasoning and Guess What. The Verbal Reasoning subtest consists of analogies that are read to the examinee. The examinee is asked to complete the analogy. The Guess What subtest provides a verbal description of an object or person that is read aloud to the examinee; based on the description, the examinee is asked to guess what the object is. Two additional subtests are used to provide a nonverbal intelligence index (NIX), which assesses spatial ability and reasoning using unfamiliar situations and stimuli. These two subtests are called Odd-Item Out and What's Missing. The Odd-Item Out subtest presents an array of shapes or objects, and the examinee is asked to identify which of the objects in the array does not belong with the other items. The What's Missing subtest is similar to the Picture Completion subtest of the WAIS–III. The examinee is presented with a series of color drawings of objects and is asked to identify what is missing from each drawing. The combination of the four subtests produces a composite intelligence index that taps overall general intellectual functioning. Administration time for the intelligence subtests is stated to take approximately 20–25 minutes. A composite memory index (CMX) can also be obtained from supplemental verbal (measuring verbal recall ability) and nonverbal memory (measuring ability to recall concrete and abstract pictorial stimuli) subtests. The memory assessment requires approximately 10 minutes beyond the time requirements for the intelligence subtests. Raw scores are converted to age-adjusted T scores.

The *RIAS/RIST Professional Manual* (Reynolds & Kamphaus, 2003) reports that the internal consistency coefficients across all six RIAS subtests range from .90 to .95, whereas the internal consistency coefficients for the four indexes range from .94 to .96. Test–retest stability coefficients of the four indexes across a median interval of 21 days range from .83 for the CMX to .91 for VIX. Stability for the six subtests range from .76 for Verbal Memory to .89 for Guess What. Factor analysis supports the two-factor (verbal and nonverbal) solution, and it is stable across age, gender, and ethnic groups. Correlations between the RIAS Index scores and WAIS–III IQ scores are high. The following correlations were reported: VIX–VIQ: .71, NIX–PIQ: .71, CIX–FSIQ: .79. Interestingly, however, the CMX memory factor correlated somewhat more strongly with IQ scores: CMX–VIQ: .76, CMX–PIQ: .76, CMX–FSIQ: .79.

One verbal subtest (the Guess What subtest) and one nonverbal subtest (Odd-Item Out subtest) from the RIAS can also be administered alone in order to perform a brief intellectual screen, referred to as the Reynolds Intellectual Screening Test (RIST). The screen requires approximately 10 minutes of administration time.

One of the strengths of this cognitive assessment battery is its brevity. Often, evaluation of level of intellectual functioning and memory ability are of primary concern in the assessment of older adults. Another advantage is the fact that reading and motor performance and speed do not impact scores on the RIAS/RIST. Often, font size of stimuli to be read can pose problems for older persons with visual difficulties, and the RIAS/RIST eliminates the need for reading. In addition, the well-known tendency of motor speed to decline with age will not influence RIAS/RIST scores. The normative data appear to have been carefully planned. Between the ages of 3 years and 15 years, normative data are presented for 3-month age blocks. Between the ages of 15 years and 20 years, normative data are provided for 1-year age blocks. Between the ages of 20 and 50 years, normative data are provided for 10-year age blocks. Between the ages of 50 and 85 years, normative data are provided for 5-year age blocks. Finally, normative data are provided for persons between the ages of 85 and 94 years, although there is a caution regarding application of the normative data to persons 90 years of age and older due to the small number of normative participants in that age range. The use of 5-year age blocks for persons aged 50 and older will likely be able to characterize level of cognitive functioning relative to one's same age peers quite effectively in older persons.

A potential limitation of the measure may actually be related to one of its strengths—brevity. The limited sample of abilities assessed by the measure can potentially result in a reduced ability to document an examinee's range of potential strengths and weaknesses. In addition, it is somewhat puzzling that the CMX memory index demonstrates somewhat higher correlations with WAIS–III IQ scores than do the intellectual index scores from the RIAS. There are no alternate forms, making the potential for practice effects relatively high. As with the NAB, it is relatively new, so there is limited information that is independent of the manual that has examined the reliability, validity, and utility of RIAS/RIST scores.

Flexible battery approaches

The majority of flexible battery approaches entail selection of at least one measure of general cognitive functioning, together with selection of multiple measures designed to assess functioning in one or more cognitive domains of interest. Typically, performance on domain-specific assessment tools can be compared with relative performance on measure(s) of general cognitive functioning as one way to identify significant performance discrepancies. Comparisons across measures within a domain can also facilitate identification of the nature of performance deficits, if present. For example, a memory evaluation may include both verbal and visuospatial memory measures. The verbal memory measures may include a list learning task using unrelated words, a verbal paired associates task, and a story memory task. Comparison across these measures can facilitate the identification of verbal material that is especially problematic for a given patient. For instance, memory difficulty for material without a context to facilitate recall might be demonstrated by preserved story memory, mildly impaired paired associates learning, and severely impaired word list learning and recall. The visuospatial memory measures may include a measure assessing the patient's ability to draw geometric designs seen moments earlier, a measure evaluating the patient's ability to recognize a series of sequentially presented faces, and a measure that taps the ability to identify the spatial location of objects presented earlier. The relative influence of motor demands on performance can be evaluated across these three measures, in addition to the presence of difficulty recalling a specific type of material (e.g., faces vs. abstract figures, vs. spatial locations). In addition, comparing and contrasting performance across verbal and visuospatial domains can potentially highlight the presence of material specific memory deficits. In short, the flexible battery/domain-specific assessment approaches can provide a wealth of clinically useful data.

The flexible battery approach permits more detailed assessment of the older individual that can be done in a time-efficient manner. Recent techniques have emerged for administering abbreviated batteries and instruments without making enormous sacrifices in terms of reliability and validity. The discussion of instruments that follows is not meant to be a comprehensive overview of all possible measures that can be used for cognitive assessment of the elderly. There are a number of excellent comprehensive resources (Lezak, 1995; Spreen & Strauss, 1998), in addition to the references cited below, for additional details.

Memory

There are a number of possible instruments that can be used for brief assessment of memory functioning. The entire scale or individual subtests of the Wechsler Memory Scale–III (WMS–III; Wechsler, 1997) or Wechsler Memory Scale–Revised (WMS–R; Wechsler, 1987) can be administered to examine aspects of memory for visual or auditory material. In addition, prorating systems are available for the WMS–R or WMS–III that enable one to administer fewer subtests while retaining relatively good ability to predict summary memory indexes (Axelrod, Ryan, & Woodard, 2001; Axelrod & Woodard, 2000; Woodard, 1993; Woodard & Axelrod, 1995, 1996).

A number of auditory-verbal list learning tasks have been put forth in recent years. Some of these instruments use word lists that are drawn from several semantic categories, including the 16-item California Verbal Learning Test (CVLT; Delis, Kramer, Kaplan, & Ober, 1986) and California Verbal Learning Test-II (Delis, Kramer, Kaplan, & Ober, 2000), the 9-item "dementia version" of the CVLT (Kaplan, 1995; Libon et al., 1996; Woodard et al., 1999), and the 12-item Hopkins Verbal Learning Test–Revised (Benedict et al., 1998; Brandt, 1991; Brandt & Benedict, 2001; Shapiro, Benedict, Schretlen, & Brandt, 1999). The 15-item Rey Auditory Verbal Learning Test (Rey, 1958) consists of unrelated items. Because the list words are unrelated, it may often be perceived as more difficult because the examinee must develop an organizational strategy (e.g., subjective organization) in order to facilitate word list recall. A considerable amount of research has been conducted with this measure, particularly in older individuals. An excellent compilation of research and normative data on the Rey AVLT has been presented (Schmidt, 1996). Finally, the Selective Reminding Test (Buschke, 1973; Buschke & Fuld, 1974) is a demanding but helpful procedure for evaluating storage and retention processes in auditory verbal learning. It represents one of the only theoretically based memory tests in clinical use. It was developed using an information processing model of memory, and it has been used extensively for clinical and research purposes.

There are a number of excellent measures that can be used for assessment of memory for visually presented information. For example, the Brief Visuospatial Memory Test–Revised (BVMT–R; Benedict, 1997; Benedict et al., 1996) has normative data available for adults between the ages of 18 and 79 years. This measure has six alternate forms, facilitating serial evaluation and reducing potential practice effects. The BVMT–R assesses learning and recall of six geometric designs presented in a 2 × 3 matrix. Both recall of the design (accuracy) and recall of the design's spatial position (location) are assessed. The six visual stimuli are presented for 10 seconds, and the examinee is then asked to reproduce each design in its correct location after the stimuli are removed from view. There are three study-test trials, followed by a 25-minute delayed recall trial, delayed recognition testing, and a copy trial to rule out visuospatial impairment. Because of its alternate forms, brief administration time, and excellent normative data, this measure provides a way to evaluate initial level of functioning as well as longitudinal changes in visuospatial memory.

The Warrington Recognition Memory Test (RMT; Warrington, 1984) evaluates the ability to recognize printed words and photographs of faces that have been presented moments earlier. The recognition memory for words (RMW) test involves visual presentation of 50 words ranging between 4 and 6 letters at the rate of 3 seconds per word. For each word, the examinee makes a judgment of whether the word is "pleasant" or "not pleasant." After all 50 words have been presented, the examinee is presented with pairs of words and is asked to identify which word in the pair was presented earlier. For the recognition memory for faces (RMF) test, 50 faces are presented to the examinee at the rate of 3 seconds per face. The examinee is asked to judge whether the face is "pleasant" or "not pleasant." After presentation of all 50 faces, a similar forced-choice recognition test is used in which 50 pairs of faces are presented. The examinee is asked to identify which face in the pair was presented earlier. Normative data are presented for individuals between the ages of 18 and 70 years. Age demonstrated a strong negative correlation (−.35) with RMW, while a more modest but significant negative correlation was observed between age and RMF (−.13). The RMT has been shown to differentiate between patients with lateralized cerebral lesions. Patients with right hemisphere lesions showed significant impairment on the RMF but were unimpaired on the RMW. In contrast, left hemisphere lesion patients demonstrated impairment on both recognition memory measures. However, the RMW performance was more impaired and the RMF performance was less impaired than in patients with right hemisphere lesions.

There are a number of other brief measures of memory for visually presented information. For example, include the Benton Visual Retention Test (Sivan, 1992) requires examinees to reproduce a series of geometric designs by drawing. There are three different forms of roughly equivalent difficulty and three different administration procedures (10 second exposure, 5 second exposure, copy) that can be used with this task. The Continuous Visual Memory Test (Trahan & Larrabee, 1988) presents a series of geometric, ambiguous designs in a serial fashion, and examinees are asked to identify whether each of 112 presented designs is "new" or "repeated." A Delayed Recognition task administered 30 minutes after the Acquisition Task assesses the examinee's ability to differentiate the previously presented designs from perceptually similar designs, and a Visual Discrimination task may also be implemented to determine the extent to which an examinee's results are related more to visual perception difficulties or to visual memory difficulties. The task requires approximately 45 minutes (including a 30-minute delay) to administer, and normative data are available for examinees between the ages of 7 and 80+ years of age.

One additional measure deserves consideration for testing memory in older individuals, as well as a variety of other cognitive domains in the elderly. The Fuld Object Memory Evaluation (FOME; Fuld, 1981) was developed for testing learning and memory specifically with elderly persons and has been standardized on both nursing home residents and community-dwelling persons. Ten common objects are presented in a black cloth bag (bottle, ball, key, nail, matchbook, ring, button, playing card, cup, and scissors), and the examinee is asked to identify each of the objects by touch. Left and right hands are systematically alternated in order to provide information regarding right–left discrimination. This measure is unique in that objects are first presented in the tactile modality, followed by visual presentation and verbal naming of the object. Thus, stimulus items are presented in multiple sensory modalities. After identifying all objects by touch and pulling each object out of the bag to see if he/she was right, the objects are replaced in the bag, and the examinee is distracted using a 60-second verbal category generation task (First Names). The examinee is then asked to recall the objects from the bag during a 60-second recall period. Four more recall trials then follow in which the examinee is reminded of the omitted items at the end of each 60-second recall period and distracted using 30-second verbal category generation tasks (foods, things that make people happy, vegetables, things that make people sad). Because it uses a selective reminding paradigm (Buschke & Fuld, 1974), separate measurements may be used to estimate the examinee's storage efficiency (number of items recalled after the distractor task, presumed to be recalled from long-term storage) and retrieval efficiency (number of words recalled on each trial). Retrieval efficiency may further be broken down into repeated retrieval (the number of items recalled on successive trials without reminding), which is presumed to reflect normal memory, and ineffective reminders (the number of failures to recall an item on two successive trials), regarded as a sign of disordered memory.

The use of the FOME in a number of studies of aging, dementia, and therapeutic trials attests to its clinical and research utility. Excellent reliability and normative data are available for use of the FOME with the elderly (Fuld, 1981; Marcopulos, McLain, & Giuliano, 1997). The FOME has been used in a number of studies to predict development of dementia (Fuld, Masur, Blau, Crystal, & Aronson, 1990; Masur, Sliwinski, Lipton, Blau, & Crystal, 1994), and it has shown significant correlations with neuropathological markers of dementia at autopsy (Dickson et al., 1995). It has also shown excellent cross-cultural applicability in both Hispanic (Loewenstein, Duara, Argüelles, & Argüelles, 1995) and Japanese (Fuld, Muramoto, Blau, Westbrook, & Katzman, 1988) populations. It has also been shown to be remarkably insensitive to the effects of education (Marcopulos et al., 1997).

Attention and information processing speed

The Mental Control subtest of the WMS–III investigates aspects of both automatic and effortful attentional deployment. Information processing speed, which typically undergoes decline with advancing age, can be assessed using subtests from the WAIS–III, such as Symbol Search and Digit Symbol-Coding. Each of these subtests takes only 2 minutes to administer. When both of these subtests are administered, a Processing Speed Index score may be computed that creates a composite reflecting performance across both measures collectively, rather than relying on each individual score separately. Digit span forward and backward is also useful for examining relatively automatic (forward) and effortful (backward) processing. Letter-Number Sequencing and Arithmetic subtests from the WAIS–III may be combined to compute the Working Memory Index, which can characterize auditory attentional functioning. The Brief Test of Attention (Schretlen, 1997) investigates auditory attention in an extremely time-efficient manner, taking approximately 8 minutes to administer. Normative data are available through 81 years of age. The Paced Auditory Serial Addition Test (PASAT; Gronwall, 1977; Gronwall & Sampson, 1974) is much more demanding and frustrating, particularly for older, cognitively impaired persons. However, it is extremely sensitive to deficits in attention.

Language

Verbal fluency for generating words beginning with a specific letter under timed conditions (Benton & des Hamsher, 1983) is one frequently used method for assessing verbal output. The individual is asked to generate in 1 minute as many words beginning with the stated letter as possible, with restriction that he/she may not generate a word with a different ending (e.g., eat and eating) or proper nouns. This particular task has been shown to be sensitive to frontal lobe functioning, particularly in the left hemisphere. The task also provides the opportunity for the participant to perseverate on earlier generated words, or commit errors by breaking the rules of the task (e.g., generating a proper noun). Both of these types of errors may be related to impairment in abilities thought to be subserved by the frontal lobe. Verbal letter fluency thus can tap into aspects of executive functioning as well, such as initiation, maintenance, and shifting of cognitive set. Verbal fluency for generating members of specific categories in one minute (e.g., animals) can also be compared to verbal letter fluency to assess the individual's ability to access semantic memory (Monsch et al., 1992).

Ability to name pictured items can be assessed with the Multilingual Aphasia Examination Visual Naming subtest (Benton & des Hamsher, 1983) or with the standard form or an abbreviated form of the Boston Naming Test (Fastenau, Denburg, & Mauer, 1998; Fisher, Tierney, Snow, & Szalai, 1999; Goodglass & Kaplan, 1983; Kaplan, Goodglass, & Weintraub, 1983; Mack, Freed, Williams, & Henderson, 1992; Tombaugh & Hubley, 1997). These measures present standard line drawings of objects presented roughly in decreasing order of frequency of appearance. The Aphasia Screening Test (Halstead & Wepman, 1959) can also serve as a very coarse screening tool for language functioning. Selected subtests from the Boston Diagnostic Aphasia Examination (Goodglass & Kaplan, 1983) may also be used to assess other more detailed aspects of language functioning, such as auditory and written comprehension, repetition, writing, grammar usage, and articulatory agility. Other subtests of the Multilingual Aphasia Examination (Benton & des Hamsher, 1983) can also provide brief measurement of functioning in specific language areas, including language comprehension (e.g., Token Test, Sentence Memory) and expression.

Visuospatial functioning

Nonverbal analytic and synthetic reasoning skills can be tapped by the Matrix Reasoning or Block Design subtests of the WAIS–III. The Matrix Reasoning subtest has the additional advantage of being motor-free and not dependent upon time. Contrasting performance on the Matrix Reasoning subtest versus the Block Design subtest can be informative for examining the effects of performing under timed conditions. The Judgment of Line Orientation (JOLO; Benton & des Hamsher, 1983) is also a motor-free measure of visuospatial reasoning. This measure consists of 30 items that present two lines placed in specific angular orientations along with a standard set of numbered lines against which the individual is asked to compare the two lines. The individual is asked to give the numbers from the standard set of lines that correspond to the same angular orientation as the target lines. Abbreviated versions of the JOLO have been developed using a subset of the same items from the standard version (Woodard et al., 1996, 1998). In addition to assessing conceptual reasoning skills, the Clock Drawing task (Freedman et al., 1994) can also yield information regarding the integrity of visual perceptual abilities. Complex figure copying tasks, such as the Rey-Osterrieth Complex Figure (Osterreith, 1944; Rey, 1941) and the Taylor Complex Figure (Taylor, 1979), assess the strategy involved in copying a detailed figure. Attention to whether the drawing is completed in a piecemeal fashion, starting with individual details, or in a more global fashion, starting with the overall Gestalt of the figure can be helpful in identifying either right hemisphere or left hemisphere damage, respectively. These visuoperceptual and visuoconstructive abilities are particularly important to evaluate in older individuals, given the established relationship between diminished visual ability and risk of falls and hip fractures (Cummings et al., 1995; Elliot et al., 1992).

Executive functioning

Considered to reflect the highest order cognitive abilities, the abilities in this domain are important to evaluate in older individuals. These abilities permit an individual to engage in independent, purposive, and self-serving behavior (Lezak, 1995). Despite their considerable importance in maintaining and improving an individual's capacity for independent living, adequate definitions of exactly what constitutes executive functions have been lacking. Further, strategies for assessing executive functions have also met with variable success.

Lezak (1995) stated that questions about executive functioning ask *how* or *whether* a person goes about doing a task or function, while questions about other cognitive abilities are often phrased in terms of *what* or *how much*. Examples of abilities under the domain of executive functioning includes developing strategies for approaching, planning, or carrying out cognitive tasks, monitoring the quality of performance, emotional regulation, making shifts in attention, capacity to initiate activity, problem solving, and ability to use working memory. Loss of executive functions, despite intact intelligence, memory, and language skills, tends to have a great impact on capacity for independent living.

Assessment of executive functions tends to be extremely challenging in the elderly because these functions are precisely among the abilities that undergo substantial age-related change. Therefore, they can be extremely difficult and challenging for even cognitively intact older individuals, while they may be extremely frustrating and often impossible for cognitively impaired persons. Therefore, the introduction and administration of these measures must be done in a supportive and nonthreatening fashion. Brief measures of executive functioning can be extremely helpful in evaluating an individual's level of functioning across these domains while minimizing frustration and fatigue.

As noted under the Language section, verbal fluency tasks, particularly letter fluency, can be extremely helpful with respect to assessment of initiation, maintenance, and shifting of cognitive set. Typically, three-letter exemplars are used, and the examinee is given 1 minute for each letter. Therefore, this task can be administered in a very brief fashion, while yielding a considerable amount of information. The Stroop Color and Word Test (Golden, 1978) is another measure that can be administered quickly, while yielding considerable information. The examinee is first asked to read a list of color names as quickly as possible for 45 seconds. Next, the examinee is asked to name the color of ink in which a series of Xs is printed, again for 45 seconds. Finally, the examinee is given 45 seconds to rapidly name the color of ink in which color names are printed. However, the color names are all incongruent with the actual ink color. The Stroop Color and Word Test measures capacity for inhibiting a dominant response tendency (i.e., reading the color names rather than the actual ink color).

Assessment of the behavioral regulation of movement has often been informally assessed during the mental status examination. For example, determining whether a patient can perform bilateral alternating movements or learn complex motor sequences can be quickly assessed in a qualitative fashion. However, there are instruments that have been developed to quantify more precisely performance of abilities thought to reflect motor-dependent executive functions. One such instrument is the Behavioral Dyscontrol Scale (BDS), which evaluates the ability to regulate motor control using procedures developed by the Russian neuropsychologist, Alexander Luria (1980). The BDS consists of nine items that are administered in standardized fashion, and the total time required to administer the task ranges from 5 to 15 minutes. It has demonstrated excellent reliability and validity (Grigsby, Kaye, & Robbins, 1992), with interrater reliabilities of .98, test–retest reliabilities of .89 (8-week interval) and .86 (6-month interval), and internal consistency (Cronbach's alpha) of .87. Principal components analysis of the items identified a behavioral intention component (ability to use intention to guide one's behavior), a working memory/behavioral inertia component, and a capacity for inhibition component.

Research using the BDS has shown that it is a strong predictor of functional autonomy and of both impulsivity and apathy among geriatric patients (Kaye, Grigsby, Robbins, & Korzun, 1990). It has also been shown to be superior to the MMSE as a unique predictor of functional autonomy in several studies (Kaye et al., 1990; Suchy, Blint, & Osmon, 1997). Subsequent investigation of this measure in a large community-dwelling sample of 1158 persons between 60 and 99 years of age reported that executive functioning as measured by the BDS was a predictor for self-reported activity of daily living (ADLs) and functionally assessed complex instrumental activities of daily living (IADLs), whereas general mental status predicted functionally assessed ADL performance but not self-report measures of performance (Grigsby et al., 1998). In addition, approximately 10% of participants showed impaired performance on the BDS and intact performance on the MMSE, while an additional 10% of the sample showed intact BDS performance and impaired MMSE score, suggesting a double dissociation between executive functioning and general cognitive ability.

The first item requires the individual to tap twice with the dominant hand and once with the nondominant hand rapidly and repeatedly. The second item reverses the order. A go/no-go task is presented on the third trial in which the examiner takes the individual's hand and asks the examinee to squeeze in response to the word red and do nothing in response to the word green. The fourth item asks the examinee to tap once if the examiner taps twice and to tap twice if the examiner taps once. The fifth and sixth items require the examinee to learn and demonstrate two simple hand position sequences (e.g., repeatedly making a fist with knuckles turned down, extending the fingers and placing the edge of the hand on the table, and turning the outstretched hand palm down on the table). The seventh item involves copying single hand gestures made by the examiner with the examinee positioned across from the examiner. The eighth item involves verbally alternating between counting and reciting the alphabet (e.g., 1-a-2-b-3-c-4-d ...). The final item evaluates the accuracy of the examinee's own assessment of his/her performance. The first eight items are scored on a 0 (failure), 1 (impaired performance), 2 (normal performance) scale, while the last item is scored on a 0 (complete absence of ability to judge one's own performance) to 4 (intact insight) scale. This scoring methodology yields a maximum score of 19, with cognitively normal elderly persons scoring a mean of 12.8 ($SD = 3.9$) (Grigsby et al., 1992). An alternative scoring strategy is available for a higher functioning population in order to avoid possible ceiling effects (Grigsby et al., 1992).

Functional capacity

Functional capacity is defined as the ability to perform basic (e.g., physical self-maintenance) and instrumental activities of daily living. Competency in these skills has been shown to be an important determinant of health care utilization patterns (Krach et al., 1996; Muller, Fahs, & Schechter, 1989; Rock et al., 1996), as well as institutionalization and mortality (Fried et al., 1998; Inouye et al., 1998; Ogawa, Iwasaki, & Yasumura, 1993; Sonn, 1996; Worrall, Chaulk, & Briffett, 1996) in older adults. The assessment of ability to perform basic and instrumental activities of daily living is a frequently neglected assessment domain, but it represents a sphere of functioning that is extremely important to the comprehensive evaluation of older individuals. Not only is documentation of impairment in social or occupational functioning often required for DSM–IV–TR diagnoses, but knowledge of specific capacities and deficits in everyday functioning for a patient can be of substantial assistance in developing effective interventions and support strategies.

A variety of approaches exist for evaluating independence and competency in performing daily living skills. For example, self-report and informant-report questionnaires have been developed to survey the perception of self and others with respect to independence in performing these tasks. However, a large body of research has identified specific patterns of bias associated with self-report and other-report, with self-report tending to overestimate actual ability and other-report tending to underestimate actual ability. The existence of reporter bias associated with these rating scales has led to the development of direct assessment measures of functional status. Examinees are evaluated with respect to their knowledge of and ability to perform specific steps underlying daily living tasks, such as dialing a telephone number or addressing a letter for mailing. Problem-solving based measures of functional status that pose questions regarding what to do in specific situations are helpful for investigating reasoning skills and knowledge about what to do when faced with a variety of life circumstances. Examples of these types of items follow.

Lawton Instrumental Activities of Daily Living Scale

An early attempt at standardizing the assessment of functional capacity was undertaken by Lawton and Brody (1969). They described two scales, one designed to assess Physical Self-Maintenance abilities, the other to assess everyday functional competence. The Physical Self-Maintenance Scale (PSMS) was patterned after a scale developed by Lowenthal (1964). The PSMS evaluates functioning with respect to toileting, feeding, dressing, grooming, physical ambulation, and bathing. The Instrumental Activities of Daily Living (I ADL) scale evaluates independence with respect to the following spheres of instrumental functioning: ability to use a telephone, shopping, food preparation, housekeeping, laundry, transportation use, responsibility for own medications, and ability to handle finances. For each sphere of functioning, the informant (the family, the patient, institutional employees, friends, or combinations of informants) is asked to rate the degree of independence of the patient in that domain. For the PSMS, there are five possible levels of independence, ranging from complete independence to complete dependence. For the I ADL scale, the number of independence categories varies depending on the domain, but the same principle holds: categories range from complete independence to complete dependence.

While the development of these scales represented a significant advance in the assessment of functional capacity, subsequent research has identified potential problems with informant-based functional capacity measures. The principal difficulty with these types of measures involves reporter bias, in which caregivers often underestimate ability, whereas patients often overestimate their abilities (Karagiozis, Gray, Sacco, Shapiro, & Kawas, 1998; Sager et al., 1992). However, a potential strength of rating scales such as the PSMS and the I ADL scale is their relative ease of administration and brevity. However, more objective measurement of functional capacity can be obtained through direct observational methods and problem-solving approaches.

Direct Assessment of Functional Status

The Direct Assessment of Functional Status (DAFS; Loewenstein et al., 1989) was designed as an objective, direct technique for evaluation of a broad array of functional capacities of older persons. The DAFS has a distinct advantage over other methods of assessing functional capacities in that it is not susceptible to reporter bias. The DAFS employs standardized stimulus items and procedural questions evaluating functional capacity in eight domains: (1) Time Orientation (Telling Time and Orientation to Date)—16 points; (2) Communication Abilities (Using the Telephone and Preparing a Letter for Mailing)—14 points; (3) Transportation (Identification of Commonly Encountered Road Signs)—13 points; (4) Pre-Shopping Skills (Registering 6 items to choose from a grocery store)—6 points; (5) Financial Skills (Identify Currency, Counting Currency, Writing a Check, Balancing a Checkbook, Making Change for a Purchase)—22 points; (6) Shopping Skills (Shopping from Memory, Shopping with a Written List)—20 points; (7) Dressing/Grooming Skills—13 points; and (8) Eating Skills—10 points. The first six domains reflect I ADLs and the latter two domains reflect BADLs.

High interrater and test–retest reliabilities, as well as convergent and discriminant validities, have previously been established for the domains assessed by the DAFS (Loewenstein et al., 1989). Further, each of the functional domains assessed by the DAFS has been identified in the literature as important in the assessment of the older adult and have also been tapped by numerous instruments evaluating instrumental activities of daily living in geriatric settings (Kane & Kane, 1981). The description of each functional task is as follows:

- *Reading a clock*: Participants are asked to tell the time at each of four progressively more difficult clock settings using an analog clock.
- *Orientation to date*: Participants are asked the day of the month, the day of the week, the month, and the year.
- *Telephone skills*: The participant is presented with a push button telephone and asked to dial the operator, to dial the number of a person from a list of names and numbers, to dial a single number presented orally, and to dial a single number presented in written form.
- *Preparing a letter for mailing*: The participant is required to address an envelope (the participant is provided with a written name and address), write a correct return address on the envelope, place a stamp on the envelope, fold the letter, insert the letter into the envelope, and seal the envelope.
- *Identifying currency*: The participant is asked to identify specific coin types and bill types from an array of coins and paper currency.
- *Counting currency*: The participant is asked to make change using coins and paper currency over four trials of increasing difficulty.
- *Writing a check*: The participant is asked to make out a check to a party and is given points for writing the correct numeric and written amounts, entering the date, and providing a signature.
- *Balancing a checkbook*: Participants are asked to balance a checkbook at increasing levels of difficulty. These items are simple subtraction problems presented in a checkbook ledger format.
- *Making change for a purchase*: The participant is asked to make change from a five dollar bill for a purchase of a specific amount.
- *Dressing/grooming skills*: The participant is asked to demonstrate steps involved in several grooming and dressing tasks.
- *Eating skills*: The participant is presented with a standardized array of eating utensils. He/she is then asked to demonstrate how to cut and take a bite of a food item, how to eat soup, how to pour from a pitcher, and how to drink the poured beverage.

Independent Living Scales

The Independent Living Scales (ILS) is another instrument designed to directly assess the competence of adults to perform instrumental activities of daily living. This measure involves a number of items that include direct observation of an individual's performance on components of an instrumental activity of daily living (e.g., "show me how you call the fire department"). In addition, the ILS also includes items that are oriented toward problem solving and knowledge of appropriate responses to various life situations (e.g., "If you suddenly began having difficulty breathing, what would you do?"). An advantage of problem-solving oriented functional capacity items is that they are less likely to be affected by physical or sensory limitations.

The ILS consists of five subscales (Memory/Orientation, Managing Money, Managing Home and Transportation, Health and Safety, and Social Adjustment) that may be examined individually and/or combined into an overall score. Items can also be broken into questions that are performance based and questions that are problem-solving based, and scores can be generated for the Problem Solving factor and for the Performance/Information factor. Internal consistency reliability (coefficient alpha) for the subscales ranges from .72 (Social Adjustment) to .87 (Managing Money), according to the *ILS Manual* (Loeb, 1996), whereas the coefficient alphas for the Problem Solving and Performance/Information factors were .86 and .92, respectively. Test–retest data over a mean interval of 14 days ranged from .81 (Social Adjustment) to .92 (Managing Money) for the subscales, .90 for the Problem Solving factor, .94 for the Performance/Information Factor, and .91 for the Full Scale score. Higher scores were observed on the second administration, suggesting a practice effect.

With respect to validity, an exploratory principal components analysis yielded a four-factor solution that best represented the data. The first two factors were retained because they provided information that did not duplicate information provided by the subscales. These factors were labeled Problem Solving and Performance/Information. The second two factors were largely redundant with the Memory/Orientation and Social Adjustment subscales. A concurrent validity study with the WAIS–R revealed strong correlations between the ILS and both subtest and IQ scores from the WAIS–R. The correlation between the ILS Full Scale score and the WAIS–R Full Scale IQ was .73. In addition, the ILS Technical Manual (Loeb, 1996) reports excellent concurrent validity with the Philadelphia Geriatric Center Multilevel Assessment Instrument, criterion-related validity for classifying living status (independent, semi-independent, dependent), and construct validity for identifying cognitively impaired individuals with lower functional abilities.

The ILS has excellent normative data and is relatively easy to administer, typically requiring 45 minutes. The combination of performance-based and problem-solving types of task permits a thorough assessment of what an examinee's capabilities are in a variety of functional domains. As noted earlier, problem-solving-based methods of functional capacity assessment are not as affected by limited physical mobility as direct observational methods. The ability to obtain separate scores for Problem Solving and Performance-based items is a significant advantage in the ILS.

Personality/mood assessment

A variety of self-report measures may be used to screen for neuropsychiatric symptoms, such as anxiety or depression. As with other self-report measures, these instruments may be susceptible to response bias and may be an inaccurate reflection of the patient's true psychiatric state. Therefore, it is extremely important to corroborate responses obtained on self-report measures with observed behavior and reports of family members. It is not uncommon to observe significant neuropsychiatric symptoms, often described by family members as a "personality change." These complaints are extremely important to evaluate, as there are a host of psychiatric and neurologic conditions that are highly associated with injuries that may occur in older persons. For example, in a comprehensive review of the late-occurring effects of TBI (Gualtieri & Cox, 1991), a condition that is frequently seen among elder individuals, TBI was noted to increase the risk of developing depression (by a factor of 5 or 10), seizures (by a factor of 2–5), psychotic disorders (by a factor of 2–5), and dementia (by a factor of 4–5) over general population base rates. In addition severe TBI may elevate these risk rates even further.

Although depression is one of the more common neuropsychiatric conditions among older persons, it is equally important to evaluate for the presence of anxiety symptoms. Instruments such as the MMPI–2 have frequently been used with younger individuals who undergo neuropsychological evaluation. However, it is somewhat more difficult to use with the geriatric population in view of the significant length. Alternatively, brief, domain-focused self-report measures, clinical observation, and family report can sometimes be more effective in identifying the significant neuropsychiatric symptoms in older individuals. The following measures are brief depression and anxiety screening tools that can be used effectively with a geriatric population.

- The *Geriatric Depression Scale* (GDS; Yesavage, Brink, Rose, & Adey, 1986; Yesavage et al., 1983) is a 30-item measure of symptoms related to depression. Each statement on the inventory is responded to in a yes/no format. The score is obtained by summing 20 items that are keyed in the "yes" direction and 10 items that are keyed in the "no" direction. It has been recommended as a screening instrument for depression in the elderly (Yesavage et al., 1986), using a cutoff score of 11–19 to identify a mild level of depressive symptomatology and 20 or greater to identify a moderate to severe level of depressive symptomatology. The yes/no response format of the GDS makes it much easier to comprehend than other depression measures such as the Beck Depression Inventory (Beck, Ward, Mendelson, Mock, & Erbaugh, 1961) or the Zung Self-Rating Scale for Depression (Zung, 1965). In addition, the GDS has been shown to differentiate depressed demented from nondepressed demented elderly patients (Yesavage et al., 1986; Yesavage, Rose, & Lapp, 1981). However, random responding on the instrument as might be seen in patients with moderate dementia can lead to ambiguous scores, making only very low or very high scores interpretable (Woodard & Axelrod, 1999).

- The *Beck Depression Inventory* (Beck, Rush, Shaw, & Emery, 1979) is a 21-item scale listing common symptoms of depression that the respondent may have experienced "in the past week, including today." Each item has four response options listed in increasing severity level that are scored from 0 to 3, yielding a total score ranging from 0 to 63. This scale has been used extensively in research and clinical settings since its development in 1961.

- The *Center for Epidemiological Screening–Depression* (CES–D; Radloff, 1977) was originally developed as a measure of depressive symptoms in community-dwelling adults and has been widely used as a screening instrument in studies of nonclinical populations. The 20 items are rated on a 4-point scale according to the frequency with which symptoms were experienced during the preceding week and are summed to compute a total score. It shows good internal consistency (Cronbach's alpha = .84) for the general population (Corcoran & Fisher, 1987) and correlates strongly ($r = .87$) with the Beck Depression Inventory (Santor, Zuroff, Ramsay, Cervantes, & Palacios, 1995).

- The *Beck Anxiety Inventory* (BAI; Beck, Epstein, Brown, & Steer, 1988) is a 21-item screening test designed to distinguish common symptoms of anxiety from those of depression and to be sensitive to treatment change. It has been extensively validated and has shown excellent test–retest reliability and internal consistency (see Wetherell & Arean, 1997, for a review). Factor analyses have been successful in discriminating between measures of depression and BAI score. The BAI is scored on the basis of self-reported severity of symptoms over the past week, from 0 (not at all) to 3 (severely), yielding a total score between 0 and 63. A two-factor solution typically emerges reflecting cognitive and somatic symptoms.

- The *State–Trait Anxiety Inventory* (STAI; Spielberger, Gorsuch, & Lushene, 1970) consists of 20 items describing anxiety that are scaled 0–4, resulting in a score ranging from 0 to 80. It is designed to measure both state anxiety (more transient, situation-dependent experiencing of anxiety) and trait anxiety (a stable predisposition toward experiencing anxiety). It shows excellent reliability and validity, and the assumptions that it can differentiate state from trait anxiety have been confirmed. It has undergone extensive evaluation and has been used to measure anxiety in more than 2000 studies since it was published in 1970.

- The *Frontal Lobe Personality Scale* (FLOPS; Grace, Stout, & Malloy, 1999; Malloy & Richardson, 1994) is a measure designed to identify behavior and personality changes that may be associated with frontal lobe dysfunction. This scale consists of 32 items that are rated on a 1–5 Likert scale ranging from "almost never" to "almost always." Separate versions are available for the patient, the patient's family, or for staff members to complete.

- The *Brief Psychiatric Rating Scale* (Overall & Gorham, 1962, 1988) is a measure designed to assess the severity of 16 psychiatric symptoms using a behaviorally anchored rating scale. This scale has traditionally been used in assessing psychotic features of psychiatric patients, although it can be helpful in assessing possible psychotic symptoms that may be present. Another scale patterned after the Brief Psychiatric Rating Scale is the *Neurobehavioral Rating Scale* (Levin et al., 1987). This measure is a 28-item observer-rated instrument that contains most of the items from the Brief Psychiatric Rating Scale. This measure has been used extensively with elderly and demented populations and has been reported to have excellent reliability (Sultzer, Berisford, & Gunay, 1995). Principal components analysis of this measure has identified a six-factor solution: Cognition/Insight, Agitation/Disinhibition, Behavioral Retardation, Anxiety/Depression, Verbal Output Disturbance, and Psychosis (Sultzer, Levin, Mahler, High, & Cummings, 1992).

Although the neuropsychological battery can be easily tailored to address a number of different questions, there are some domains that warrant routine investigation, such as executive functioning, memory, anxiety/depression, and attention. A proposed brief assessment battery, presented in Table 3.1, is designed to take approximately 2½ hours, not including a clinical interview with the patient and family members. If abnormalities are detected using this short battery, further assessment can be performed using the measures described above.

Table 3.1 A proposed flexible battery to assess elderly patients

Global intellectual functioning (provides evaluation of verbal reasoning, long-term retrieval of word definitions, visuospatial reasoning and construction)	Wechsler Abbreviated Scale of Intelligence (30 min) Includes Matrix Reasoning, Block Design, Vocabulary, Similarities Alternative: Kaufman Brief Intelligence Test (K–BIT; 30 min)
Auditory attention	WAIS–III Working Memory Index subtests (Digit Span, Letter–Number Sequencing, Arithmetic; 20 min)
Executive functioning	Behavioral Dyscontrol Scale (10 min)
Response inhibition	Stroop Color and Word Test (5 min)
Self-generation of responses	Controlled Oral Word Association Test (5 min)
Learning and memory	Fuld Object Memory Evaluation (includes category fluency; 20 min)
Processing speed	WAIS–III Digit Symbol-Coding and Symbol Search (5 min)
Functional status	Independent Living Scales (ILS; 45 min)
Neuropsychiatric symptoms	Beck Depression Scale and Beck Anxiety Scale (10 min)

Symptom validity testing with older adults

Determination of the validity of the information and data obtained should be part of any neuropsychological evaluation, although the manner in which that is accomplished will vary considerably based on the evaluation setting and the patient population. Iverson (2003) stated, "Any neuropsychological evaluation that does not include careful consideration of the patient's motivation to give their best effort should be considered incomplete" (p. 138). The evaluation of response validity need not consist of specific measures designed to assess effort nor must it focus solely on the question of malingering *per se*. A variety of factors may influence the validity of the information and data obtained from an elderly patient. In addition to litigation, the elderly may put forth suboptimal effort for reasons such as generally opposing an evaluation that has been arranged by family members and that may or may not have the potential to result in a loss of independence.

Although sparse, some research exists on the effects of cognitive functioning (Ashendorf, O'Bryant, & McCaffrey, 2003; Teichner & Wagner, 2004) and emotional state (Ashendorf, Constantinou, & McCaffrey, 2004) on measures or indices of symptom validity in the elderly. With regard to indices from neuropsychological ability measures, currently existing formulas for the Wisconsin Card Sorting Test were found to have limited utility for the detection of malingering with older adults, whereas strategies for detecting symptom invalidity with the California Verbal Learning Test demonstrated clinical utility (Ashendorf et al., 2003).

With regard to symptom validity tests, the Test of Memory Malingering was found to be useful for detecting malingered memory deficits in elderly participants who were cognitively intact or evidenced cognitive impairment in the absence of dementia (Teichner & Wagner, 2004). However, individuals with dementia performed significantly poorer than the other two groups across all trials, and more conservative cutoff points of eight or ten errors did not significantly improve correct classification of individuals with dementia as nonmalingering (Teichner & Wagner, 2004). The findings of Teichner and Wagner differ from those of Tombaugh as reported in the *TOMM Manual* (1996), which indicated that individuals with dementia may perform relatively well on the TOMM. Differences between the results of the studies may be due to different methods of diagnostic classification and different levels of participant impairment (Teichner & Wagner, 2004).

Compared to the impact of neurological status on cognitive symptom validity test results, little research has been conducted on the potential impact of psychological conditions on cognitive symptom validity test results, particularly with elderly individuals. In one study, Ashendorf et al. (2004) found that depression and anxiety levels in an older community-dwelling sample did not negatively affect performance on the TOMM. The usefulness of the MMPI–2 to assess symptom validity with the elderly is limited due to the general limitations of MMPI–2 use with the elderly, as presented earlier in this chapter.

Whereas intentionally poor neuropsychological performance may result in financial or other personal gain in patient groups such as those undergoing litigation, the presence of neuropsychological symptoms in some older adult populations may carry increased likelihood of consequences that such individuals wish to avoid. For example, neuropsychological evaluations that address questions such as the older adult's decision-making capacity, need for a surrogate decision-maker or guardian, functional status, and ability to live independently have direct implications for the examinee's autonomy (Smyer, Schaie, & Kapp, 1996). To avoid a loss of independence, some elderly may present an inaccurately positive picture of themselves. This is also a form of symptom invalidity. In addition, lack of awareness of one's deficits or attribution of cognitive loss to "normal aging" may result in underreporting of symptoms. Overly healthy presentations are typically apparent in the discrepancy between self-report and obtained test results and should be considered in neuropsychological evaluations of the elderly. The clinician, in the unique context of his/her practice, is responsible for determining the appropriate manner in which the validity of the information that has been obtained is assessed.

In some geriatric settings, the assessment of response validity may be best accomplished by examining consistency of responses with observed behavior, with patient self-report, and with the report of collateral sources; consistency of responses with known patterns of cognitive dysfunction; and indicators embedded within ability measures, such as forced choice components of memory tests. The existence of some studies of symptom validity testing with elderly participants offers preliminary guidance for clinicians; however, replication studies are needed. Determination of how to best assess the validity of the information and data obtained during neuropsychological evaluation, like all other areas assessed, rests with the examiner.

Summary

This chapter has focused on a description of a number of measures that can be used to evaluate cognitive and functional status in older individuals. There are advantages and disadvantages of fixed and flexible neuropsychological batteries. Although several fixed batteries, such as the HRB and the LNNB, have been used for several decades and have a considerable amount of research behind them, newer generation fixed batteries, such as the NAB and RIAS, offer a number of advantages including better normative data, shorter administration times, and innovative strategies for assessing cognitive and functional abilities. Various components of flexible batteries that are suitable for use with older participants have also been explored. These instruments can be used in order to tailor an evaluation to a specific referral question.

Neuropsychological evaluation of the older patient can present a number of challenges that must be taken into consideration. As has been discussed, it may be difficult to identify specific measures that have adequate normative data for persons over 65 years of age. However, new generation instruments that have recently been developed are attending more to extending the upper age limits in their normative data. In addition, older individuals may come to the evaluation with factors that may contribute to cognitive impairment, including the presence of comorbid chronic diseases, use of multiple medications that may individually or collectively affect cognition, and the presence of physical and/or sensory limitations. The presence of fatigue that may develop during the assessment is also a major consideration in obtaining accurate assessment data. Again, newer generation cognitive measures have focused on development of screening measures or brief administration times in order to mitigate this potential difficulty. It is important to take these factors into account during the clinical interview and integrate their presence into the overall clinical picture.

Making a determination regarding the validity of the information and data obtained is an essential aspect of the neuropsychological evaluation. Depending on the examination context, the patient population, and the availability of supporting research, the examiner must select the best methods for making such determination.

Despite the potential challenges that may be presented, it is clear that there is a tremendous amount of information to be gained from neuropsychological evaluation of the older patient. Cognitive strengths and limitations can be identified and can be used in order to develop effective rehabilitation strategies and treatment interventions that capitalize on the patient's strengths while minimizing limitations. Several brief measures of mood status have also been described that can contribute toward determination of the impact of mood factors on cognition. With the development of better measures of functional capacity, these instruments can identify potential areas of problematic daily living skills that may limit or jeopardize continued independent living status. This information can be used to develop alternative strategies to enable the patient carry out these activities of daily living. Moreover, the interplay between specific cognitive abilities and ability to execute daily living tasks can be delineated and used in order to maximize the patient's independence, quality of life, and safety.

References

Albert, M. S. (1988). Cognitive function. In M. S. Albert & M. B. Moss (Eds.), *Geriatric neuropsychology* (pp. 33–53). New York: Guilford.

American Psychological Association, Division of Neuropsychology. (1989). Definition of a clinical neuropsychologist. *The Clinical Neuropsychologist, 3*(1), 22.

Ashendorf, L., Constantinou, M., & McCaffrey, R. J. (2004). The effect of depression and anxiety on the TOMM in community-dwelling older adults. *Archives of Clinical Neuropsychology, 19*, 125–130.

Ashendorf, L., O'Bryant, S. E., & McCaffrey, R. J. (2003). Specificity of malingering detection strategies in older adults using the CVLT and WCST. *The Clinical Neuropsychologist, 17*(2), 255–262.

Axelrod, B., Woodard, J., Schretlen, D., & Benedict, R. (1996). Corrected estimates of WAIS–R short form reliability and standard error of measurement. *Psychological Assessment, 8*, 222–223.

Axelrod, B. N. (2002). Validity of the Wechsler abbreviated scale of intelligence and other very short forms of estimating intellectual functioning. *Assessment, 9*(1), 17–23.

Axelrod, B. N., Dingell, J. D., Ryan, J. J., & Ward, L. C. (2000). Estimation of Wechsler Adult Intelligence Scale-III index scores with the 7-subtest short form in a clinical sample. *Assessment, 7*(2), 157–161.

Axelrod, B. N., Goldman, R. S., & Henry, R. R. (1992). Sensitivity of the Mini-Mental State Examination to frontal lobe dysfunction in normal aging. *Journal of Clinical Psychology, 48*(1), 68–71.

Axelrod, B. N., & Henry, R. R. (1992). Age-related performance on the Wisconsin Card Sorting, Similarities, and Controlled Oral Word Association tests. *The Clinical Neuropsychologist, 6*, 14–24.

Axelrod, B. N., Henry, R. R., & Woodard, J. L. (1992). Analysis of an abbreviated form of the Wisconsin Card Sorting Test. *The Clinical Neuropsychologist, 6*(1), 27–31.

Axelrod, B. N., Ryan, J. J., & Ward, L. C. (2001). Evaluation of seven-subtest short forms of the Wechsler Adult Intelligence Scale-III in a referred sample. *Archives of Clinical Neuropsychology, 16*(1), 1–8.

Axelrod, B. N., Ryan, J. J., & Woodard, J. L. (2001). Cross-validation of prediction equations for Wechsler Memory Scale-III Indexes. *Assessment, 8*(4), 367–372.

Axelrod, B. N., & Woodard, J. L. (2000). Parsimonious prediction of Wechsler Memory Scale-III memory indices. *Psychological Assessment, 12*(4), 431–435.

Axelrod, B. N., Woodard, J. L., & Henry, R. R. (1991). A comparison of the standard and abbreviated forms of the Wisconsin Card Sorting Test. *Journal of Clinical and Experimental Neuropsychology, 13*, 89.

Ayers, M. R., Abrans, D. I., Newell, T. G., & Friedrich, F. (1987). Performance of individuals with AIDS on the Luria-Nebraska Neuropsychological Battery. *International Journal of Clinical Neuropsychology, 9*, 101–105.

Baddeley, A. D. (1986). *Working memory*. Oxford, UK: Oxford University Press.

Bak, J. S., & Green, R. L. (1980). Changes in neuropsychological functioning in an aging population. *Journal of Consulting and Clinical Psychology, 48*, 395–399.

Beck, A., Ward, C., Mendelson, M., Mock, J., & Erbaugh, J. (1961). An inventory for measuring depression. *Archives of General Psychiatry, 4*, 561–571.

Beck, A. T., Epstein, N., Brown, G., & Steer, R. A. (1988). An inventory for measuring clinical anxiety: Psychometric properties. *Journal of Consulting and Clinical Psychology, 56*, 893–897.

Beck, A. T., Rush, A. J., Shaw, B. F., & Emery, G. (1979). *Cognitive therapy of depression*. New York: Guilford Press.

Benedict, R. H., Goldstein, M. Z., Dobraski, M., & Tannenhaus, J. (1997). Neuropsychological predictors of adaptive kitchen behavior in geriatric psychiatry inpatients. *Journal of Geriatric Psychiatry and Neurology, 10*(4), 146–153.

Benedict, R. H. B. (1997). *Brief Visuospatial Memory Test–Revised professional manual*. Odessa, FL: Psychological Assessment Resources.

Benedict, R. H. B., Schretlen, D., Groninger, L., & Brandt, J. (1998). The Hopkins Verbal Learning Test–Revised: Normative data and analysis of inter-form and test–retest reliability. *The Clinical Neuropsychologist, 12*(1), 43–55.

Benedict, R. H. B., Schretlen, D., Groninger, L., Dobraski, M., & Shpritz, B. (1996). Revision of the Brief Visuospatial Memory Test: Studies of normal performance, reliability, and validity. *Psychological Assessment, 8*, 145–153.

Benson, C., & Lusardi, P. (1995). Neurologic antecedents to patient falls. *Journal of Neuroscience Nursing, 27*(6), 331–337.

Benton, A. L., & des Hamsher, K. (1983). *Multilingual Aphasia Examination.* Iowa City: AJA Associates, Inc.

Berg, R. A., & Golden, C. J. (1981). Identification of neuropsychological deficits in epilepsy using the Luria-Nebraska Neuropsychological Battery. *Journal of Consulting and Clinical Psychology, 49*, 745–747.

Botwinick, J., & Storandt, M. (1974). *Memory related functions and age.* Springfield, IL: Charles C. Thomas.

Brandt, J. (1991). The Hopkins Verbal Learning Test: Development of a new memory test with six equivalent forms. *The Clinical Neuropsychologist, 5*(2), 125–142.

Brandt, J., & Benedict, R. H. B. (2001). *Hopkins Verbal Learning Test–Revised professional manual.* Lutz, FL: Psychological Assessment Resources.

Burger, M. C., Botwinick, J., & Storandt, M. (1987). Aging, alcoholism, and performance on the Luria-Nebraska Neuropsychological Battery. *Journal of Gerontology, 42*(1), 69–72.

Buschke, H. (1973). Selective reminding for analysis of memory and learning. *Journal of Verbal Learning and Verbal Behavior, 12*, 543–550.

Buschke, H., & Fuld, P. A. (1974). Evaluating storage, retention and retrieval in disordered memory and learning. *Neurology, 24*, 1019–1025.

Butler, M., Retzlaff, P., & Vanderploeg, R. (1991). Neuropsychological test usage. *Professional Psychology: Research and Practice, 22*, 510–512.

Carlson, M. C., Fried, L. P., Xue, Q. L., Bandeen-Roche, K., Zeger, S. L., & Brandt, J. (1999). Association between executive attention and physical functional performance in community-dwelling older women. *Journal of Gerontology. Series B, Psychological Sciences and Social Sciences, 54*(5), S262–270.

Chmielewski, C., & Golden, C. J. (1980). Alcoholism and brain damage: An investigation using the Luria-Nebraska Neuropsychological Battery. *International Journal of Neuroscience, 10*(2–3), 99–105.

Christensen, A. (1979). *Luria's neuropsychological investigation* (2nd ed.). Copenhagen, Denmark: Munksgaard.

Christensen, A. L. (1984). The Luria method of examination of the brain impaired patient. In P. F. Logue & J. M. Schear (Eds.), *Clinical neuropsychology: A multidisciplinary approach* (pp. 5–28). Springfield, IL: C. C. Thomas.

Colsher, P. L., & Wallace, R. B. (1993). Geriatric assessment and driver functioning. *Clinics in Geriatric Medicine, 9*(2), 365–375.

Cooper, J. W. (1996). Probable adverse drug reactions in a rural geriatric nursing home population: A four-year study. *Journal of the American Geriatrics Society, 44*(2), 194–197.

Corcoran, K., & Fisher, J. (1987). *Measures for clinical practice: A source book.* New York: Free Press.

Craik, F. I. M. (1986). A functional account of age differences in memory. In F. Kliz & H. Hagendorf (Eds.), *Human memory and cognitive capabilities: Mechanisms and performances* (pp. 409–422). Amsterdam: Elsevier.

Craik, F. I. M. (1990). Changes in memory with normal aging: A functional view. *Advances in Neurology, 51*, 201–205.

Cullum, C. M., Thompson, L. L., & Heaton, R. K. (1989). The use of the Halstead-Reitan Test Battery with older adults. *Clinics in Geriatric Medicine*, 5(3), 595–610.

Cumming, R. G., Miller, J. P., Kelsey, J. L., Davis, P., Arfken, C. L., Birge, S. J., et al. (1991). Medications and multiple falls in elderly people: The St Louis OASIS study. *Age and Ageing*, 20(6), 455–461.

Cummings, S. R., Nevitt, M. C., Browner, W. S., Stone, K., Fox, K. M., Ensrud, K. E., et al. (1995). Risk factors for hip fracture in white women: Study of Osteoporotic Fractures Research Group. *New England Journal of Medicine*, 332(12), 767–773.

Delis, D. C., Kramer, J., Kaplan, E., & Ober, B. A. (1986). *The California Verbal Learning Test*. San Antonio, TX: Psychological Corporation.

Delis, D. C., Kramer, J. H., Kaplan, E., & Ober, B. A. (2000). *CVLT–II: California Verbal Learning Test second edition adult version manual*. San Antonio, TX: Psychological Corporation.

Dickson, D. W., Crystal, H. A., Bevona, C., Honer, W., Vincent, I., & Davies, P. (1995). Correlations of synaptic and pathological markers with cognition of the elderly. *Neurobiological Aging*, 16(3), 285–298; discussion 298–304.

Dunn, E. J., Searight, H. R., Grisso, T., Margolis, R. B., & Gibbons, J. L. (1990). The relation of the Halstead-Reitan neuropsychological battery to functional daily living skills in geriatric patients. *Archives of Clinical Neuropsychology*, 5(2), 103–117.

Elias, M. F., Podraza, A. M., Pierce, T. W., & Robbins, M. A. (1990). Determining neuropsychological cut scores for older, healthy adults. *Experimental Aging Research*, 16(4), 209–220.

Elias, M. F., Robbins, M. A., Walter, L. J., & Schultz, N. R., Jr. (1993). The influence of gender and age on Halstead-Reitan neuropsychological test performance. *Journal of Gerontology*, 48(6), P278–281.

Elliot, J. R., Hanger, H. C., Gilchrist, N. L., Frampton, C., Turner, J. G., Sainsbury, R., et al. (1992). A comparison of elderly patients with proximal femoral fractures and a normal elderly population: A case control study. *New Zealand Medical Journal*, 105(944), 420–422.

Erker, G. J., Searight, H. R., & Peterson, P. (1995). Patterns of neuropsychological functioning among patients with multi-infarct and Alzheimer's dementia: A comparative analysis. *International Psychogeriatrics*, 7(3), 393–406.

Fastenau, P. S., & Adams, K. M. (1996). Heaton, Grant and Matthews' Comprehensive Norms: An overzealous attempt or a good start? *Journal of Clinical and Experimental Neuropsychology*, 18, 444–448.

Fastenau, P. S., Denburg, N. L., & Mauer, B. A. (1998). Parallel short forms for the Boston Naming Test: Psychometric properties and norms for older adults. *Journal of Clinical and Experimental Neuropsychology*, 20(6), 828–834.

Fillenbaum, G. G. (1988). *Multidimensional functional assessment of older adults*. Hillsdale, NJ: Lawrence Erlbaum Associates, Inc.

Fisher, N. J., Tierney, M. C., Snow, W. G., & Szalai, J. P. (1999). Odd/even short forms of the Boston Naming Test: Preliminary geriatric norms. *The Clinical Neuropsychologist*, 13(3), 359–364.

Flicker, C., Ferris, S. H., Crook, T., Bartus, R. T., & Reisberg, B. (1986). Cognitive decline in advanced age: Future directions for the psychometric differentiation of normal and pathological age changes in cognitive function. *Developmental Neuropsychology*, 2(4), 309–322.

Franzen, M. D. (2000). *Reliability and validity in neuropsychological assessment* (2nd ed.). New York: Kluwer Academic/Plenum Publishers.

Freedman, M., Leach, L., Kaplan, E., Winocur, G., Shulman, K. I., & Delis, D. C. (1994). *Clock drawing: A neuropsychological analysis.* New York: Oxford University Press.

Fried, L. P., Kronmal, R. A., Newman, A. B., Bild, D. E., Mittelmark, M. B., Polak, J. F., et al. (1998). Risk factors for 5-year mortality in older adults: The Cardiovascular Health Study [see comments]. *Journal of the American Medical Association, 279*(8), 585–592.

Fuld, P. A. (1981). *The Fuld Object-Memory Evaluation.* Chicago: Stoelting Instrument Company.

Fuld, P. A., Masur, D. M., Blau, A. D., Crystal, H., & Aronson, M. K. (1990). Object-memory evaluation for prospective detection of dementia in normal-functioning elderly: Predictive and normative data. *Journal of Clinical and Experimental Neuropsychology, 12*, 520–528.

Fuld, P. A., Muramoto, O., Blau, A., Westbrook, L., & Katzman, R. (1988). Cross-cultural and multi-ethnic dementia evaluation by mental status and memory testing. *Cortex, 24*(4), 511–519.

Giron, M. S. T., Claesson, C., Thorslund, M., Oke, T., Winblad, B., & Fastbom, J. (1999). Drug use patterns in a very elderly population: A seven-year review. *Clinical Drug Investigation, 17*(5), 389–398.

Golden, C., Hammeke, T., & Purish, A. (1980). *Luria-Nebraska Neuropsychological Battery: A manual for clinical and experimental uses.* Los Angeles: University of Nebraska Press.

Golden, C. J., Graber, B., Moses, J. A., & Zatz, L. M. (1980). Differentiation of chronic schizophrenics with and without ventricular enlargement by the Luria-Nebraska Neuropsychological Battery. *International Journal of Neuroscience, 11*(2), 131–138.

Golden, C. J., Hammeke, T. A., & Purisch, A. D. (1978). Diagnostic validity of a standardized neuropsychological battery derived form Luria's neuropsychological tests. *Journal of Consulting and Clinical Psychology, 46*, 1258–1265.

Golden, C. J., Purisch, A. D., & Hammeke, T. A. (1985). *Luria-Nebraska Neuropsychological Battery: Forms I and II.* Los Angeles: Western Psychological Services.

Golden, J. C. (1978). *Stroop Color and Word Test.* Chicago: Stoelting.

Goldstein, F. C., Strasser, D. C., Woodard, J. L., & Roberts, V. J. (1997). Functional outcome of cognitively impaired hip fracture patients on a geriatric rehabilitation unit [see comments]. *Journal of the American Geriatrics Society, 45*(1), 35–42.

Goldstein, G., & Shelly, C. (1987). The classification of neuropsychological deficit. *Journal of Psychopathological and Behavioral Assessment, 9*, 183–202.

Goodglass, H., & Kaplan, E. (1983). *The assessment of aphasia and related disorders.* Philadelphia: Lea & Febiger.

Grace, J., Stout, J. C., & Malloy, P. F. (1999). Assessing frontal lobe behavioral syndromes with the frontal lobe personality scale. *Assessment, 6*(3), 269–284.

Gray, J. W., Rattan, A. I., & Dean, R. S. (1986). Differential diagnosis of dementia and depression in the elderly using neuropsychological methods. *Archives of Clinical Neuropsychology, 1*, 341–350.

Grigsby, J., Kaye, K., Baxter, J., Shetterly, S. M., & Hamman, R. F. (1998). Executive cognitive abilities and functional status among community-dwelling older persons in the San Luis Valley Health and Aging Study. *Journal of the American Geriatrics Society*, *46*(5), 590–596.

Grigsby, J., Kaye, K., & Robbins, L. J. (1992). Reliabilities, norms and factor structure of the Behavioral Dyscontrol Scale. *Perceptual and Motor Skills*, *74*(3, Pt. 1), 883–892.

Gronwall, D. M. (1977). Paced auditory serial-addition task: A measure of recovery from concussion. *Perceptual and Motor Skills*, *44*(2), 367–373.

Gronwall, D. M. A., & Sampson, H. (1974). *The psychological effects of concussion*. Auckland, New Zealand: Auckland University Press/Oxford University Press.

Gualtieri, T., & Cox, D. R. (1991). The delayed neurobehavioural sequelae of traumatic brain injury. *Brain Injury*, *5*(3), 219–232.

Halstead, W. C., & Wepman, J. M. (1959). The Halstead-Wepman Aphasia Screening Test. *Journal of Speech and Hearing Disorders*, *14*, 9–15.

Heaton, R. K., Grant, I., & Matthews, C. G. (1991). *Comprehensive norms for an expanded Halstead-Reitan Battery: Demographic corrections, research findings, and clinical applications*. Odessa, FL: Psychological Assessment Resources.

Heaton, R. K., Grant, I., Matthews, C. G., & Avitable, N. (1996). Demographic corrections with comprehensive norms: An overzealous attempt or a good start? *Journal of Clinical and Experimental Neuropsychology*, *18*, 449–458.

Heaton, R. K., Miller, S. W., Taylor, M. J., & Grant, I. (2004). *Comprehensive norms for an expanded Halstead-Reitan Battery: Demographically adjusted neuropsychological norms for African American and Caucasian American adults*. Odessa, FL: Psychological Assessment Resources.

Howieson, D. B., Holm, L. A., Kaye, J. A., Oken, B. S., & Howieson, J. (1993). Neurologic function in the optimally healthy oldest old: Neuropsychological evaluation. *Neurology*, *43*, 1882–1886.

Hultsch, D. F., & Dixon, R. A. (1990). Learning and memory in aging. In J. E. Birren & K. W. Shaie (Eds.), *Handbook of the psychology of aging* (pp. 259–274). New York: Academic Press.

Inouye, S. K., Peduzzi, P. N., Robison, J. T., Hughes, J. S., Horwitz, R. I., & Concato, J. (1998). Importance of functional measures in predicting mortality among older hospitalized patients. *Journal of the American Medical Association*, *279*(15), 1187–1193.

Iverson, G. L. (2003). Detecting malingering in civil forensic evaluations. In A. M. Horton, Jr., & L. C. Hartlage (Eds.), *Handbook of forensic neuropsychology* (pp. 137–177). New York: Springer Publishing Company.

Kane, R. A., & Kane, R. L. (1981). *Assessing the elderly: A practical guide to measurement*. Lexington, MA: Lexington Books.

Kaplan, E. (1995). California Verbal Learning Test (dementia version). In M. D. Lezak (Ed.), *Neuropsychological assessment* (p. 448, personal communication). New York: Oxford University Press.

Kaplan, E. F., Goodglass, H., & Weintraub, S. (1983). *The Boston Naming Test* (2nd ed.). Philadelphia: Lea & Febiger.

Karagiozis, H., Gray, S., Sacco, J., Shapiro, M., & Kawas, C. (1998). The Direct Assessment of Functional Abilities (DAFA): A comparison to an indirect measure of instrumental activities of daily living. *The Gerontologist*, *38*(1), 113–121.

Kaszniak, A. W. (1990). Psychological assessment of the aging individual. In J. E. Birren & K. W. Schaie (Eds.), *Handbook of the psychology of aging* (3rd ed., pp. 427–445). New York: Oxford University Press.

Katz, S., Downs, T. D., Cash, H. R., & Grotz, R. C. (1970). Progress in development of the index of ADL. *The Gerontologist, 10*(1), 20–30.

Kaufman, A. S., & Kaufman, N. L. (1990). *Manual for the Kaufman Brief Intelligence Test (K-BIT)*. Circle Pines, MN: American Guidance Service.

Kaufman, A. S., & Kaufman, N. L. (1993). *Kaufman Adolescent and Adult Intelligence Test (KAIT) manual*. Circle Pines, MN: American Guidance Service.

Kaufman, A. S., & Kaufman, N. L. (1997). The Kaufman Adolescent and Adult Intelligence Test (KAIT). In D. P. Flanagan, J. L. Genshaft, & P. L. Harrison (Eds.), *Contemporary intellectual assessment: Theories, tests, and issues* (pp. 209–229). New York: Guilford.

Kaufman, A. S., & Kaufman, N. L. (2004). *Kaufman Brief Intelligence Test* (2nd ed.) [KBIT–2]. Circle Pines, MN: AGS Publishing.

Kaufman, A. S., & Lichtenberger, E. O. (1999). *Essentials of WAIS–III assessment*. New York: John Wiley & Sons.

Kaye, K., Grigsby, J., Robbins, L. J., & Korzun, B. (1990). Prediction of independent functioning and behavior problems in geriatric patients. *Journal of the American Geriatrics Society, 38*(12), 1304–1310.

Keller, B. K., Morton, J. L., Thomas, V. S., & Potter, J. F. (1999). The effect of visual and hearing impairments on functional status. *Journal of the American Geriatrics Society, 47*(11), 1319–1325.

Krach, P., DeVaney, S., DeTurk, C., & Zink, M. H. (1996). Functional status of the oldest-old in a home setting. *Journal of Advanced Nursing, 24*(3), 456–464.

La Rue, A. (1992). *Aging and neuropsychological assessment*. New York: Plenum.

Lawton, M. P., & Brody, E. M. (1969). Assessment of older people: Self-maintaining and instrumental activities of daily living. *The Gerontologist, 9*(3), 179–186.

Leckliter, I. N., & Matarazzo, J. D. (1989). The influence of age, education, IQ, gender, and alcohol abuse on Halstead-Reitan Neuropsychological Test Battery performance. *Journal of Clinical Psychology, 45*(4), 484–512.

Lees-Haley, P. R., Smith, H. H., Williams, W. W., & Dunn, J. T. (1996). Forensic neuropsychological test usage: An empirical survey. *Archives of Clinical Neuropsychology, 11*(1), 45–51.

Levin, H. S., High, W. M., Goethe, K. E., Sisson, R. A., Overall, J. E., Rhoades, H. M., et al. (1987). The neurobehavioural rating scale: Assessment of the behavioural sequelae of head injury by the clinician. *Journal of Neurology, Neurosurgery and Psychiatry, 50*(2), 183–193.

Lezak, M. D. (1995). *Neuropsychological assessment* (3rd ed.). New York: Oxford University Press.

Libon, D. J., Mattson, R. E., Blosser, G., Kaplan, E., Malamut, B. L., Sands, L. P., et al. (1996). A nine-word dementia version of the California Verbal Learning Test. *The Clinical Neuropsychologist, 10*, 237–244.

Loeb, P. A. (1996). *Independent Living Scales (ILS) manual*. San Antonio, TX: Psychological Corporation.

Loewenstein, D. A., Amigo, E., Duara, R., Guterman, A., Hurwitz, D., Berkowitz, N., et al. (1989). A new scale for the assessment of functional status in Alzheimer's disease and related disorders. *Journal of Gerontology, 4*, 114–121.

Loewenstein, D. A., Argüelles, T., Barker, W. W., & Duara, R. (1993). A comparative analysis of neuropsychological test performance of Spanish-speaking and English-speaking patients with Alzheimer's disease. *Journal of Gerontology, 48*, P142–149.

Loewenstein, D. A., Duara, R., Argüelles, T., & Argüelles, S. (1995). Use of the Fuld Object-Memory Evaluation in the detection of mild dementia among Spanish- and English-speaking groups. *American Journal of Geriatric Psychiatry, 3*(4), 300–307.

Loewenstein, D. A., Rubert, M. P., Berkowitz-Zimmer, N., Guterman, A., Morgan, R., & Hayden, S. (1992). Neuropsychological test performance and prediction of functional capacities in dementia. *Behavior, Health, and Aging, 2*, 149–158.

Lowenthal, M. F. (1964). *Lives in distress.* New York: Basic Books.

Luria, A. R. (1980). *Higher cortical functions in man.* New York: Basic Books.

MacInnes, W. D., Gillen, R. W., Golden, C. J., Graber, B., Cole, J. K., Uhl, H. S., et al. (1983). Aging and performance on the Luria-Nebraska neuropsychological battery. *International Journal of Neuroscience, 19*(1–4), 179–189.

MacInnes, W. D., Paull, D., Uhl, H. S., & Schima, E. (1987). Longitudinal neuropsychological changes in a "normal" elderly group. *Archives of Clinical Neuropsychology, 2*(3), 273–282.

Mack, W. J., Freed, D. M., Williams, B. W., & Henderson, V. W. (1992). Boston Naming Test: Shortened versions for use in Alzheimer's disease. *Journal of Gerontology, 4*, 154–158.

Mahurin, R. K., DeBettignies, B. H., & Pirozzolo, F. J. (1991). Structured assessment of independent living skills: Preliminary report of a performance measure of functional abilities in dementia. *Journal of Gerontology, 46*, 58–66.

Malloy, P. F., & Richardson, E. D. (1994). Assessment of frontal lobe functions. *Journal of Neuropsychiatry and Clinical Neurosciences, 6*, 399–410.

Marcopulos, B. A., McLain, C. A., & Giuliano, A. J. (1997). Cognitive impairment or inadequate norms? A study of healthy, rural, older adults with limited education. *The Clinical Neuropsychologist, 11*(2), 111–131.

Masur, D. M., Sliwinski, M., Lipton, R. B., Blau, A. D., & Crystal, H. A. (1994). Neuropsychological prediction of dementia and the absence of dementia in healthy elderly persons. *Neurology, 44*, 1427–1432.

McKay, S. E., & Golden, C. J. (1981). The assessment of specific neuropsychological skills using scales derived from factor analysis of the Luria-Nebraska Neuropsychological battery. *International Journal of Neuroscience, 14*(3–4), 189–204.

Mittenberg, W., Seidenberg, M., O'Leary, D. S., & DiGiulio, D. V. (1989). Changes in cerebral functioning associated with normal aging. *Journal of Clinical and Experimental Neuropsychology, 11*(6), 918–932.

Monsch, A. U., Bondi, M. W., Butters, N., Salmon, D. P., Katzman, R., & Thal, L. J. (1992). Comparisons of verbal fluency tasks in the detection of dementia of the Alzheimer's type. *Archives of Neurology, 49*, 1253–1258.

Moses, J. A. (1986). Factor analysis of the Luria-Nebraska Neuropsychological Battery by sensorimotor, speech, and conceptual item bands. *International Journal of Clinical Neuropsychology, 8*, 26–35.

Moses, J. A., Jr., & Pritchard, D. A. (1999). Performance scales for the Luria-Nebraska Neuropsychological Battery–Form I. *Archives of Clinical Neuropsychology, 14*(3), 285–302.

Muller, C., Fahs, M. C., & Schechter, M. (1989). Primary medical care for elderly patients. Part I: Service mix as seen by an expert panel. *Journal of Community Health, 14*(2), 79–87.

Myers, A. H., Young, Y., & Langlois, J. A. (1996). Prevention of falls in the elderly. *Bone, 18*(1, Suppl.), 87S–101S.

Nadler, J. D., Richardson, E. D., Malloy, P. F., Marran, M. E., & Brinson, M. E. H. (1993). The ability of the Dementia Rating Scale to predict everyday functioning. *Archives of Clinical Neuropsychology, 8*, 449–460.

Newman, P. J., & Sweet, J. J. (1986). The effects of clinical depression on the Luria-Nebraska Neuropsychological Battery. *International Journal of Clinical Neuropsychology, 8*, 109–114.

Nyberg, L., & Gustafson, Y. (1997). Fall prediction index for patients in stroke rehabilitation. *Stroke, 28*(4), 716–721.

Ogawa, Y., Iwasaki, K., & Yasumura, S. (1993). [A longitudinal study on health status and factors relating to it in elderly residents of a community]. *Nippon Koshu Eisei Zasshi, 40*(9), 859–871.

Oster, C. (1976). Sensory deprivation in geriatric patients. *Journal of the American Geriatrics Society, 24*(10), 461–464.

Osterreith, P. (1944). Le test de copie d'une figure complexe. *Archives de Psychologie, 30*, 206–356.

Overall, J. E., & Gorham, D. R. (1962). The Brief Psychiatric Rating Scale. *Psychological Reports, 10*, 799–812.

Overall, J. E., & Gorham, D. R. (1988). Introduction—The Brief Psychiatric Rating Scale (BPRS): Recent developments in ascertainment and scaling. *Psychopharmacology Bulletin, 24*, 97–99.

Preston, J. D., O'Neal, J. H., & Talaga, M. C. (1997). *Handbook of clinical psychopharmacology for therapists* (2nd ed.). Oakland, CA: New Harbinger Publications.

Radloff, L. (1977). The CES-D scale: A new self report depression scale for research in the general population. *Applied Psychological Measures, 1*, 385–401.

Rapport, L. J., Hanks, R. A., Millis, S. R., & Deshpande, S. A. (1998). Executive functioning and predictors of falls in the rehabilitation setting. *Archives of Physical Medicine and Rehabilitation, 79*(6), 629–633.

Ravaglia, G., Forti, P., Maioli, F., Boschi, F., Cicognani, A., Bernardi, M., et al. (1997). Determinants of functional status in healthy Italian nonagenarians and centenarians: A comprehensive functional assessment by the instruments of geriatric practice. *Journal of the American Geriatrics Society, 45*(10), 1196–1202.

Reitan, R. M., & Wolfson, D. (1985). *The Halstead-Reitan Neuropsychological Test.* Tucson, AZ: Neuropsychology Press.

Reitan, R. M., & Wolfson, D. (1993). *The Halstead-Reitan Neuropsychological Test Battery: Theory and clinical interpretation.* Tucson, AZ: Neuropsychology Press.

Reitan, R. M., & Wolfson, D. (1995). Influence of age and education on neuropsychological test results. *The Clinical Neuropsychologist, 9*, 151–158.

Rey, A. (1941). L'examen psychologique dans les cas d'encéphalopathie traumatique. *Archives de Psychologie, 28*, 286–340.

Rey, A. (1958). *L'examen clinique en psychologie.* Paris: Presses Universitaires de France.

Reynolds, C. R., & Kamphaus, R. W. (2003). *Reynolds Intellectual Assessment Scale* [RIAS]/*Reynolds Intellectual Screening Test* [RIST]. Lutz, FL: Psychological Assessment Resources.

Richardson, E. D., Nadler, J. D., & Malloy, P. F. (1995). Neuropsychologic prediction of performance measures of daily living skills in geriatric patients. *Neuropsychology, 9*, 565–572.

Rock, B. D., Goldstein, M., Harris, M., Kaminsky, P., Quitkin, E., Auerbach, C., et al. (1996). Research changes a health care delivery system: A biopsychosocial approach to predicting resource utilization in hospital care of the frail elderly. *Social Work and Health Care*, *22*(3), 21–37.

Russell, E. W. (1980). *Theoretical bases of Luria-Nebraska and Halstead-Reitan batteries*. Paper presented at the annual meeting of the American Psychological Association, Montreal, PQ, Canada.

Ryan, J. J., Lopez, S. J., & Werth, T. R. (1999). Development and preliminary validation of a Satz-Mogel short form of the WAIS–III in a sample of persons with substance abuse disorders. *International Journal of Neuroscience*, *98*(1–2), 131–140.

Sager, M. A., Dunham, N. C., Schwantes, A., Mecum, L., Halverson, K., & Harlowe, D. (1992). Measurement of activities of daily living in hospitalized elderly: A comparison of self-report and performance-based methods. *Journal of the American Geriatrics Society*, *40*(5), 457–462.

Salgado, R., Lord, S. R., Packer, J., & Ehrlich, F. (1994). Factors associated with falling in elderly hospital patients. *Gerontology*, *40*(6), 325–331.

Salive, M. E., Guralnik, J., Christen, W., Glynn, R. J., Colsher, P., & Ostfeld, A. M. (1992). Functional blindness and visual impairment in older adults from three communities. *Ophthalmology*, *99*(12), 1840–1847.

Santor, D. A., Zuroff, D. C., Ramsay, J. O., Cervantes, P., & Palacios, J. (1995). Examining scale discriminability in the BDI and CES-D as a function of depressive severity. *Psychological Assessment*, *7*, 131–139.

Schludermann, E. H., Schludermann, S. M., Merryman, P. W., & Brown, B. W. (1983). Halstead's studies in the neuropsychology of aging. *Archives of Gerontology and Geriatrics*, *2*(1–2), 49–172.

Schmader, K. E., Hanlon, J. T., Fillenbaum, G. G., Huber, M., Pieper, C., & Horner, R. (1998). Medication use patterns among demented, cognitively impaired and cognitively intact community-dwelling elderly people. *Age and Ageing*, *27*(4), 493–501.

Schmidt, M. (1996). *Rey Auditory and Verbal Learning Test: A handbook*. Los Angeles: Western Psychological Services.

Schretlen, D. (1997). *Brief Test of Attention professional manual*. Odessa, FL: Psychological Assessment Resources.

Shapiro, A. M., Benedict, R. H., Schretlen, D., & Brandt, J. (1999). Construct and concurrent validity of the Hopkins Verbal Learning Test–revised. *The Clinical Neuropsychologist*, *13*(3), 348–358.

Shuttleworth-Jordan, A. B. (1997). Age and education effects on brain-damaged subjects: "Negative" findings revisited. *The Clinical Neuropsychologist*, *11*, 205–209.

Sivan, A. B. (1992). *Benton Visual Retention Test* (5th ed.). San Antonio, TX: Psychological Corporation.

Smyer, M., Schaie, K.W., & Kapp, M. B. (Eds.). (1996). *Older adults' decision-making and the law*. New York: Springer Publishing Co.

Sonn, U. (1996). Longitudinal studies of dependence in daily life activities among elderly persons. *Scandinavian Journal of Rehabilitation Medicine*, *34*(Suppl.), 1–35.

Spielberger, C. D., Gorsuch, R. C., & Lushene, R. E. (1970). *Manual for the State–Trait Anxiety Inventory*. Palo Alto, CA: Consulting Psychologists Press.

Spiers, P. A. (1981). Have they come to praise Luria or to bury him?: The Luria-Nebraska Battery controversy. *Journal of Consulting and Clinical Psychology*, *49*(3), 331–341.

Spreen, O., & Strauss, E. (1998). *A compendium of neuropsychological tests: Administration, norms, and commentary* (2nd ed.). New York: Oxford University Press.

Stern, R. A., & White, T. (2003). *Neuropsychological Assessment Battery (NAB)*. Lutz, FL: Psychological Assessment Resources.

Suchy, Y., Blint, A., & Osmon, D. C. (1997). Behavioral Dyscontrol Scale: Criterion and predictive validity in an inpatient rehabilitation unit population. *The Clinical Neuropsychologist*, *11*(3), 258–265.

Sultzer, D. L., Berisford, M. A., & Gunay, I. (1995). The Neurobehavioral Rating Scale: Reliability in patients with dementia. *Journal of Psychiatric Research*, *29*(3), 185–191.

Sultzer, D. L., Levin, H. S., Mahler, M. E., High, W. M., & Cummings, J. L. (1992). Assessment of cognitive, psychiatric, and behavioral disturbances in patients with dementia: The Neurobehavioral Rating Scale. *Journal of the American Geriatrics Society*, *40*(6), 549–555.

Sweeney, J. E. (1999). Raw, demographically altered, and composite Halstead-Reitan Battery data in the evaluation of adult victims of nonimpact acceleration forces in motor vehicle accidents. *Applied Neuropsychology*, *6*(2), 79–87.

Talland, G. A. (1965). Three estimates of work span and their stability over the adult years. *Quarterly Journal of Experimental Psychology*, *17*, 301–307.

Taylor, L. B. (1979). Psychological assessment of neurosurgical patients. In T. Rasmussen & R. Marino (Eds.), *Functional neurosurgery* (pp. 165–180). New York: Raven Press.

Teichner, G., & Wagner, M. T. (2004). The test of memory malingering (TOMM): Normative data from cognitively intact, cognitively impaired, and elderly patients with dementia. *Archives of Clinical Neuropsychology*, *19*, 455–464.

Tinetti, M. E., Doucette, J., Claus, E., & Marottoli, R. (1995). Risk factors for serious injury during falls by older persons in the community. *Journal of the American Geriatrics Society*, *43*(11), 1214–1221.

Tombaugh, T. N. (1996). *Test of Memory Malingering (TOMM)*. New York: Multi-Health Systems, Inc.

Tombaugh, T. N., & Hubley, A. M. (1997). The 60-item Boston Naming Test: Norms for cognitively intact adults aged 25 to 88 years. *Journal of Clinical and Experimental Neuropsychology*, *19*(6), 922–932.

Trahan, D. E., & Larrabee, G. J. (1988). *Continuous Visual Memory Test*. Odessa, FL: Psychological Assessment Resources.

Vanderploeg, R. D., Axelrod, B. N., Sherer, M., Scott, J. G., & Adams, R. L. (1997). The importance of demographic adjustments on neuropsychological test performance: A response to Reitan and Wolfson (1995). *The Clinical Neuropsychologist*, *11*, 210–217.

Vannieuwkirk, R. R., & Galbraith, G. G. (1985). The relationship of age to performance on the Luria-Nebraska Neuropsychological Battery. *Journal of Clinical Psychology*, *41*(4), 527–532.

Vitaliano, P. P., Breen, A. R., Albert, M. S., Russo, J., & Printz, P. N. (1984). Memory, attention, and functional status in community residing Alzheimer type dementia patients and optimally healthy aged individuals. *Journal of Gerontology*, *39*, 58–64.

Warrington, E. K. (1984). *Recognition Memory Test*. Los Angeles: Western Psychological Services.

Wechsler, D. (1987). *Wechsler Memory Scale–Revised*. San Antonio, TX: Psychological Corporation.

Wechsler, D. (1997). *WAIS–III/WMS–III technical manual*. San Antonio, TX: Psychological Corporation.

Wechsler, D. (1999). *Wechsler Abbreviated Scale of Intelligence manual*. San Antonio, TX: Psychological Corporation.

Wetherell, J. L., & Arean, P. A. (1997). Psychometric evaluation of the Beck Anxiety Inventory with older medical patients. *Psychological Assessment*, *9*, 136–144.

Woodard, J. L. (1993). A prorating system for the Wechsler Memory Scale–Revised. *The Clinical Neuropsychologist*, *7*(2), 219–223.

Woodard, J. L., & Axelrod, B. N. (1995). Parsimonious prediction of Wechsler Memory Scale–Revised memory indices. *Psychological Assessment*, *7*(4), 445–449.

Woodard, J. L., & Axelrod, B. N. (1996). "Parsimonious prediction of Wechsler Memory Scale–Revised memory indices": Correction. *Psychological Assessment*, *8*(4), 382.

Woodard, J. L., & Axelrod, B. N. (1999). Interpretative guidelines for neuropsychiatric measures with dichotomously scored items. *International Journal of Geriatric Psychiatry*, *14*(5), 385–388.

Woodard, J. L., Benedict, R. H., Roberts, V. J., Goldstein, F. C., Kinner, K. M., Capruso, D. X., et al. (1996). Short-form alternatives to the Judgment of Line Orientation Test. *Journal of Clinical and Experimental Neuropsychology*, *18*(6), 898–904.

Woodard, J. L., Benedict, R. H., Salthouse, T. A., Toth, J. P., Zgaljardic, D. J., & Hancock, H. E. (1998). Normative data for equivalent, parallel forms of the Judgment of Line Orientation Test. *Journal of Clinical and Experimental Neuropsychology*, *20*(4), 457–462.

Woodard, J. L., Goldstein, F. C., Roberts, V. J., & McGuire, C. (1999). Convergent and Discriminant Validity of the CVLT (dementia version). *Journal of Clinical and Experimental Neuropsychology*, *21*(4), 553–558.

Worrall, G., Chaulk, P., & Briffett, E. (1996). Predicting outcomes of community-based continuing care: Four-year prospective study of functional assessment versus clinical judgment. *Canadian Family Physician*, *42*, 2360–2367.

Yesavage, J. A., Brink, T. L., Rose, T. L., & Adey, M. (1986). The Geriatric Depression Rating Scale: Comparison with other self-report and psychiatric rating scales. In L. Poon (Ed.), *Handbook for clinical memory assessment of older adults* (pp. 153–167). Washington, DC: American Psychological Association.

Yesavage, J. A., Brink, T. L., Rose, T. L., Lum, O., Huang, V., Adey, M., et al. (1983). Development and validation of a geriatric depression screening scale: A preliminary report. *Journal of Psychiatric Research*, *17*, 37–49.

Yesavage, J. A., Rose, T. L., & Lapp, D. (1981). *Validity of the Geriatric Depression Scale in subjects with senile dementia*. Palo Alto, CA: Clinical Diagnostic and Rehabilitation Unit, Veterans Administration Medical Center.

Zung, W. W. K. (1965). A self-rating depression scale. *Archives of General Psychiatry*, *12*, 63–70.

4 Applications of technology to assessment and intervention with older adults

Philip Schatz

According to the US Census Bureau, there were 33.6 million residents over the age of 65 in 2002, and by the year 2010, this number is projected to increase to over 40 million. By the year 2030, the number of adults over the age of 65 is expected to increase to 86 million, representing 21% of the US population (US Census Bureau, 2004). Since the introduction of the personal computer in the early 1980s, the percentage of US households with a computer has risen dramatically, from only 8.2% in 1984 to 42% in 1998 and 52% in 2000 (Newburger, 2001). In 2000, more than half (55%) of all adults 18 years old and over lived in a household with at least one computer; 25% of "householders" 65 years of age and older had a home computer, 18% had Internet access, and 13% reported using the Internet at home. Given that nearly one-fifth of older adults are "wired" or technologically aware, the efficacy of technological applications to older adults should not be hindered merely due to age effects. This chapter will focus on three areas in which technology has been or can be applied to older adults: Internet use, assessment, and technology-based devices or environments.

Applications of Internet use with older adults

Negative stereotypes of the elderly have typically focused on their inability and unwillingness to learn new computer technologies (Ryan, Szechtman, & Bodkin, 1992), with age biases focusing on older adults being less likely than both younger and middle-aged adults to engage in or complete a computer course. Researchers have even pointed to decreased ATM use among the elderly as a sign of technological rejection; however, their willingness to use less interactive forms of technology, such as supermarket checkout scanners, may reflect technological adoption in some contexts (Zeithaml & Gilly, 1987). Of course, not all research has supported these stereotypes. Jay and Willis (1992) found that negative attitudes towards computers among the elderly are more attributable to lack of computer experience than to age. In fact, older adults were found to underestimate their computer knowledge and abilities, thus leading to difficulty in mastering new computer technologies (Marquie, Jourdan-Boddaert, & Huet, 2002). White et al. (2002) found that 74% of older adults who had completed an Internet training program were using the Internet on a weekly basis, and use of the Internet among these older adults was associated with decreased loneliness and depression. In this study, they found that Internet training significantly increased the number of confidants reported by older adults. Similarly, Bradley and Poppen (2003) showed that participation in their "Computers for the Homebound and Isolated Individuals Project" (CHIP) allowed elderly individuals to form a sort of virtual community. They found that elderly participants, disabled individuals, and even caregivers felt a sense of camaraderie and friendship, with 1-year follow-up data supporting the program with increased satisfaction in the amount of contact with others.

Older adults have been found to show no differences in attitudes towards computer use, as compared to younger respondents (Czaja & Sharit, 1998). However, when questioned about their feelings towards working with computers, older adults do report decreased comfort, feelings of dehumanization, and decreased control. These self-reported feelings do not generalize to all forms of interacting with computers; van Gerven, Paas, van Merrienboer, Hendriks, and Schmidt (2003) found that older adults were equally likely to benefit from multimedia-based instructional techniques as younger adults. Japanese sociologists have identified the Internet as an essential part of the communication infrastructure. Kumagai (2001) described the importance of "community networks" to provide citizens with better access to local services, and pointed to the importance of a medial literacy education for the elderly to allow for use of this new avenue of communication.

Given these findings, clinical neuropsychologists should include technological abilities and perceptions as part of their initial interview with older clients. Providing links to Internet-based resources may assist in providing these clients with feedback and education regarding the nature of the services provided, more information regarding their diagnosis or condition, and contacts to support groups or social services. "Wired" older adults can use Internet-based communications as part of an interactive peer community. Such interactions, if only for a select subsample of older adults, could serve to increase socialization and esteem, and decrease feelings of loneliness and isolation.

Applications of technology to assessment of older adults

Computer-based assessment has received considerable attention in the recent literature, as well as in the computerization of paper-based test measures (for a more comprehensive review, see Schatz & Browndyke, 2002). Computer-based assessment measures have certain benefits in the form of accurate recording of reaction time and response latencies, automated analysis of response patterns (Wilson & McMillan, 1991), and have been shown to provide precise control over the presentation of test stimuli, thereby potentially increasing psychometric reliability. Because computerized tests can allow customized controls of visual and auditory stimulus characteristics and other features such as color, animation, and sound, nearly all aspects of the assessment process, including the instructions, can be "fine-tuned" for the participant. Given these benefits, programs that can adaptively control the order, number, presentation rate, and complexity of items, as well as other aspects of auditory and visual stimuli, may provide benefits that cannot be achieved with conventional testing (Kane & Reeves, 1997; Mead & Drasgow, 1993). For the practitioner, the option to use an established, reliable, and valid measure, with standardized instructions and means of presentation, may be desirable or advantageous, especially when working with a specific patient population or suspected diagnosis for which the test was developed. This section will focus on specific applications of computer-based assessment to elderly adults in the areas of driving assessment and technological adaptations to neuropsychological assessment.

Driving assessment

As the population has increased in age, there has also been rising awareness of the need for driver evaluations of the elderly, which has even been described as a growing public health concern (Johansson & Lundberg, 1997). A review of driving behavior indicated that there are a growing number of older adults (aged 65 and older) who maintain a valid driver's license, and this group of individuals is driving for longer distances than in the past (NHTSA, 1994). Elderly drivers are nearly three times more likely to be involved in a motor vehicle collision (MVC) per driven mile when compared to middle-aged drivers (Williams & Carsten, 1989), and the likelihood of being involved in a fatal MVC increases with age. Drivers 65 to 69 years of age are twice as likely to be involved in fatal multivehicle crashes as drivers aged 40–49 years, and drivers 85 years of age and older are 11 times more likely than drivers aged 40–49 years to be involved in fatal crashes (NHTSA, 1994).

Investigation of the circumstances surrounding MVCs reveals that elderly drivers are more likely to be at fault for the collision (McGwin & Brown, 1999), are more vulnerable to significant injury during MVCs (Evans, 1988), and are more likely to die from MVC-related injuries (Verhaegen, 1995). As a group, the elderly are not at a higher risk for MVC involvement, primarily because elderly drivers do not operate motor vehicles with the same frequency as middle aged or younger adults (Daigneault, Joly, & Frigon, 2002). However, when factoring their increased risk for heart disease and stroke and use of medication, crash rates and at-risk ratios do increase with normal aging (McGwin, Sims, Pulley, & Roseman, 2000). Recent surveys of elderly drivers revealed that self-restriction of driving activities occurred primarily due to problems with eyesight and concern for risk of accidents (Ragland, Satariano, & MacLeod, 2004), with female drivers more likely to self-restrict their driving activities (Bauer, Adler, Kuskowski, & Rottunda, 2003).

The primary factor attributed to increased accidents per miles driven among the elderly is impairment in visual function. Research shows that elderly drivers show more visual search errors than younger drivers (Ho, Scialfa, Caird, & Graw, 2001), and elderly drivers with either decreased mental status or deficits in visual attention experience three to four times more accidents that normal controls (Owsley, Ball, Sloane, Roenker, & Bruni, 1991). Other researchers identified those older drivers with prior traffic convictions (Gebers & Peck, 1992) and older drivers with prior accident involvement (Daigneault et al., 2002) as being at higher risk for MVCs.

Driving evaluations have taken many forms, including on-road assessments, off-road screening measures, and driving simulation machines. On-road evaluations have long been identified as useful tools for assessing driving ability. With respect to the elderly, lane changing, low-speed maneuvers, failure to maintain position, speed, and safety margins were key determinants between pass/fail decisions (DiStefano & Macdonald, 2003). Elderly drivers have been shown to make fewer steering and eye-movement adjustments, resulting in greater drifting than younger drivers (Perryman & Fitten, 1996). Researchers have attempted to use neuropsychological tests to predict on-road driving ability in both brain injured and elderly populations, with limited success (van Zomeren, Brouwer, & Minderhoud, 1987; Withaar, Brouwer, & van Zomeren, 2000). Intelligent Vehicle Highway Systems have been identified as a potential solution to provide older adults with greater time to perceive and react to upcoming stimuli, but these systems also have the potential to create disadvantageous situations that require even faster reactions (Lerner, 1994).

As an alternative to on-road assessments, driving simulators have allowed driving evaluators to assess driver readiness while remaining safely off-road. Simulators have been found to be valid measures for assessing declines in visual attention in elderly drivers (Lee, Lee, & Cameron, 2003) and identifying at-risk drivers (Lee, Lee, Cameron, & Li-Tsang, 2003). Reaction time (RT) has long been considered to be a major factor in the determination of fitness to drive and Benton (1977) showed significant RT declines with normal aging. Indeed, research has found that RT measures can provide an estimation of the reaction speed minimally required in executing critical driving tasks (Stokx & Gaillard, 1986). Computer-based assessment measures have been developed for the assessment of cognitive functions, and some have been used to assess cognitive functioning in elderly samples. Erlanger et al. (2002) used their Cognitive Stability Index (CSI) with a sample of 284 individuals, including 55 individuals 70 years of age or older. They presented age-based normative data and Reliable Change Indices, and their results showed that elderly individuals are able to complete computer-based assessment measures without specific modifications.

Recent applications of technology have centered on using virtual reality (VR) as a tool in cognitive rehabilitation (Rizzo & Buckwalter, 1997), functional assessments (Schultheis, Himelstein, & Rizzo, 2002), and simulated driving assessment (Schultheis & Mourant, 2001). Lengenfelder, Schultheis, Al-Shihabi, Mourant, and DeLuca (2002) used VR to investigate the influence of divided attention on driving and identified VR as an innovative medium for direct evaluation of basic cognitive functions not previously available through traditional neuropsychological measures. Wald, Liu, Hirsekorn, and Taylar (2000) piloted a VR tool for assessing driving performance of persons with brain injury, as compared to on-road, cognitive, visual-perceptual, and driving video test results, and identified VR as a useful adjunctive tool in driving assessment. Soon after, Wald and Liu (2001) established moderate psychometric relationships between their VR program and the Trail Making Test. While not directly related to driving ability, Brooks, Rose, Potter, Jayawardena, and Morling (2004) employed age-matched controls in their assessment of prospective memory in stroke patients using VR technology. The controls averaged 68 years of age, and the stroke group 71 years of age. The researchers not only reported no difficulties with the VR environment, but found the VR-based environment to be more sensitive with respect to prospective memory impairment. To date, no study has utilized VR technology to assess driving ability in the elderly, but there appear to be no technological limitations in this population.

Technological adaptations in neuropsychological assessment

Traditional neuropsychological test measures take their form in paper-based formats and were not developed for the purpose of technological customization or adaptation. "Fixed" neuropsychological test batteries have specific guidelines for presentation (e.g., Reitan & Wolfson, 1993), making such adaptation impractical. However, traditional neuropsychological test measures have been successfully adapted for presentation by computer (Space, 1981), including the Wechsler Adult Intelligence Scale (Elwood & Griffin, 1972), and many researchers have found computerized versions of tests to be psychometrically equivalent, when compared to traditional versions (Campbell et al., 1999; Elwood & Griffin, 1972). In the computer-based form, however, assessment measures have features that may be either absent or less accurate than when administered through traditional pencil-and-paper-based forms. These features include timing of responses and latencies, automated analysis of response patterns, transfer of results to a database for further analysis, and ease of normative data collection in a group setting (Wilson & McMillan, 1991). Thus, on general performance test measures, the speed and accuracy of differentiating visual stimuli may be superior to examiner based testing, representing advantages over conventional testing (Kane & Kay, 1992; Mead & Drasgow, 1993).

One cannot look to the dementia literature for examples of technological adaptation of neuropsychological test measures for older adults, as this is not a population traditionally known for computer use or comfort. One model for technological adaptations to neuropsychological test measures comes from the Amyotrophic Lateral Sclerosis (ALS) literature. It has been difficult to assess cognitive functioning in individuals with extreme motor deficits that prevent efferent movement or speech. Researchers have posited numerous cognitive deficits in ALS patients, including poor functioning in response generation, verbal fluency, and working memory (Abrahams et al., 2000; Hanagasi et al., 2002).

While the literature is scarce with studies focusing on technological modifications to neuropsychological test measures for use with older adults, initial efforts appear to have focused on identifying cognitive abilities in the absence of response modalities. Kotchoubey, Lang, Winter, and Birbaumer (2003) used event-related brain potentials to document intact language comprehension, showing that some ALS patients possess normal information processing capacity even in a locked-in state. Kubler et al. (1999) developed a "thought translation device" for ALS patients with no motor activity. This device translated cortical potentials to track and control a computer cursor, and initial findings showed that after several months of training "locked-in" individuals were able to achieve 70–80% accuracy. Ayala et al. (2003) piloted the "SliP" test (Screening the Locked-in Patient) designed to measure cognitive functioning in six categories: orientation, language, attention, memory, visual spatial, and executive functioning. When taking the SliP test, participants responded with a simple click as the computer used a strobing technique highlighting the various choices, in order to compensate for the motor deficits of locked-in patients. In their pilot study the test was found to validly differentiate between groups of older adults, age-matched dementia patients, and younger adults.

Neuropsychologists wishing to apply technology to adapt traditional measures, or develop novel measures, for use with older adults can utilize findings from the ALS literature. The following recommendations are offered.

1. Response modalities should be able to be customized by the examiner, in order to account for decreased response times, motor weakness, or even paralysis.
2. Motor-based responses collected through a computer mouse should allow for customization of the time required to differentiate between a single click and a double click.
3. Custom hand- or foot-based response collection devices should be adapted for single-click responses in the absence of the ability to manipulate a computer mouse. Eye-gaze response systems should also be considered in those cases where motor impairment is significant.
4. Instructions for competing tasks should be able to be presented in one or more modalities (e.g., visual, verbal) in order to compensate for sensory deficits or receptive language deficits.
5. Tasks requiring examinees to click on a particular item on a computer screen should incorporate a "strobe" effect wherein each item is "lit" for a set period of time, with the examiner being able to set custom time intervals to suit the needs of the examinee.

6. Voice activation of task commencement and cessation can be used to measure reaction times and response latencies in the presence of motor impairment.

Technological adaptations and interventions

Falls account for 10% of all unintentional injuries (Centers for Disease Control, 2004), and over two-thirds of these falls occur in individuals 65 years of age and older. Assistive devices and home modifications have been shown to be effective in halting decline in functional status for physically frail older adults living at home (Mann, Ottenbacher, Fraas, Tomita, & Granger, 1999). Acceptance of assistive devices and technologies appears to be synonymous with acceptance of functional limitations. Lilja, Bergh, Johansson, and Nygard (2003) found that elderly individuals who accepted rehabilitation were more able, better equipped, and better supported with assistive technology than those individuals who declined rehabilitation. The term "assistive technologies" has traditionally been used to describe a variety of devices (e.g., canes, walkers, bath benches) and home modifications (e.g., ramps, lower cabinets), but not actual "technological" devices.

Prior to the 1980s, general cognitive factors such as memory, attention, orientation, and activities of daily living (ADL) were "retrained" or rehabilitated through tutorials or practice exercises (Gianutsos, 1980). With the advent of the microcomputer, select tasks or exercises were soon digitized, and many cognitive skills retraining programs became the foundation of computer-based cognitive rehabilitation. Despite contributing little in the form of tangible outcome, by the mid-1980s over two-thirds of all rehabilitation programs used microcomputers for the purpose of cognitive rehabilitation (Bracy, Lynch, Sbordone, & Berrol, 1985). At that time, much of the cognitive rehabilitation/retraining software was criticized for being primitive, unstable, having poor interface, and being inconsistent with neuropsychological principles (Lynch, 1988). In response to this criticism, Chute, Conn, DiPasquale, and Hoag (1988) presented a software-based prosthetic support to compensate for memory and communication deficits. Applications of this "ProsthesisWare" to the elderly included cognitive retraining, as well as an augmentive device for cognitive or motor deficiencies (Chute & Bliss, 1994).

In the 20 years that have followed the introduction of home computer-based prosthetics, much has changed. The introduction of the Internet made it possible for individual homes to be part of a much larger, even global, network. Such technological advances make it possible for caregivers to monitor individuals through software-based programs, with little modification required beyond the purchase of a computer, software, and peripheral devices. "Telemonitoring" integrates Internet technology in the home to monitor specific door openings, sense floor vibrations consistent with falls, and record more complex physiological data using biosensors

(Rialle, Lamy, Noury, & Bajolle, 2003; Rialle, Noury, & Herve, 2001). The collection of such devices in a home creates a "smart house," which makes it possible to provide health care services for people with special needs who wish to remain independent and living in their own home (Rialle, Duchene, Noury, Bajolle, & Demongeot, 2002). Allen (1996) recognized the specific benefit of smart house technology for the elderly, as it provides a holistic tool to facilitate independent living. However, he spoke of the importance of design and implementation, with a particular emphasis on ensuring a proper balance between the technological assistance and individual control or autonomy. While the potential for smart-home technology has been recognized, it is not yet clear how it will be implemented, and smart homes have been referred to as a technology in search of an application (Eriksson & Timpka, 2002).

Summary

Older adults comprise an ever-increasing percentage of our population and will continue to require neuropsychological services in the form of assessment and intervention. Older adults are not, by default, tech-savvy, but are also not technophobic. Clinicians should consider the role that the Internet can play in providing alternative forms of communication and peer interaction, especially for those older adults who are isolated and without nearby family or support systems. Clinicians providing services to older adults may consider providing training on Internet-based activities, as such training programs have been shown to decrease feelings of isolation and loneliness.

Neuropsychological test measures have not been widely adapted specifically for use with older adults. While technological adaptation may seem paradoxical with this population, research has shown that driving assessment, virtual reality, and computerized neuropsychological assessment measures have all been successfully used to measure cognitive functioning in older adults. Clinicians and researchers working to develop and customize assessment measures have a wealth of literature to guide their efforts, as well as specific recommendations for adapting computer-based measures.

References

Abrahams, S., Leigh, P. N., Harvey, A., Vythelingum, G. N., Grise, D., & Goldstein, L. H. (2000). Verbal fluency and executive dysfunction in amyotrophic lateral sclerosis (ALS). *Neuropsychologia, 38*(6), 734–747.

Allen, B. (1996). An integrated approach to Smart House technology for people with disabilities. *Medical Engineering and Physics, 18*(3), 203–206.

Ayala, J., Jefferson, A., Cosentino, S., Kelley, R., Lippa, C., Koffler, S., et al. (2003). Validation of a computerized cognitive assessment tool: Assessing the locked in patient. *Archives of Clinical Neuropsychology, 18*(7), 773.

Bauer, M. J., Adler, G., Kuskowski, M. A., & Rottunda, S. (2003). The influence of age and gender on the driving patterns of older adults. *Journal of Women and Aging, 15*(4), 3–16.

Benton, A. L. (1977). Interactive effects of age and brain disease on reaction time. *Archives of Neurology, 34*, 369–370.

Bracy, O., Lynch, W., Sbordone, R., & Berrol, S. (1985). Cognitive retraining through computers: Fact or fad? *Cognitive Rehabilitation*, March/April, 10–23.

Bradley, N., & Poppen, W. (2003). Assistive technology, computers and Internet may decrease sense of isolation for homebound elderly and disabled persons. *Technology and Disability, 15*, 19–25.

Brooks, B. M., Rose, F. D., Potter, J., Jayawardena, S., & Morling, A. (2004). Assessing stroke patients' prospective memory using virtual reality. *Brain Injury, 18*(4), 391–401.

Campbell, K. A., Rohlman, D. S., Storzbach, D., Binder, L. M., Anger, W. K., Kovera, C. A., et al. (1999). Test–retest reliability of psychological and neurobehavioral tests self-administered by computer. *Assessment, 6*, 21–32.

Centers for Disease Control. (2004). Deaths: Injuries, 2001: DHHS Publication No. (PHS) 2004-1120. *Center for Disease Control, National Vital Statistics Reports, 52*(21), 1–87.

Chute, D. L., & Bliss, M. E. (1994). ProsthesisWare: Concepts and caveats for micro-computer-based aids to everyday living. *Experimental Aging Research, 20*(3), 229–238.

Chute, D. L., Conn, G., DiPasquale, M. C., & Hoag, M. (1988). ProsthesisWare: A new class of software supporting the activities of daily living. *Neuropsychology, 2*, 41–57.

Czaja, S. J., & Sharit, J. (1998). Age differences in attitudes toward computers. *Journal of Gerontology. Series B, Psychological Sciences and Social Sciences, 53*(5), P329–340.

Daigneault, G., Joly, P., & Frigon, J. Y. (2002). Previous convictions or accidents and the risk of subsequent accidents of older drivers. *Accident: Analysis and Prevention, 34*(2), 257–261.

DiStefano, M., & Macdonald, W. (2003). Assessment of older drivers: Relationships among on-road errors, medical conditions and test outcome. *Journal of Safety Research, 34*(4), 415–429.

Elwood, D. L., & Griffin, R. (1972). Individual intelligence testing without the examiner. *Journal of Consulting and Clinical Psychology, 38*(1), 9–14.

Eriksson, H., & Timpka, T. (2002). The potential of smart homes for injury prevention among the elderly. *Injury Control and Safety Promotion, 9*(2), 127–131.

Erlanger, D. M., Kaushik, T., Broshek, D., Freeman, J., Feldman, D., & Festa, J. (2002). Development and validation of a web-based screening tool for monitoring cognitive status. *Journal of Head Trauma Rehabilitation, 17*(5), 458–476.

Evans, L. (1988). Older driver involvement in fatal and severe traffic crashes. *Journal of Gerontology, 43*(6), S186–193.

Gebers, M. A., & Peck, R. C. (1992). The identification of high-risk older drivers through age-mediated point systems. *Journal of Safety Research, 23*, 81–93.

Gianutsos, R. (1980). What is cognitive rehabilitation? *Journal of Rehabilitation, 46*(3), 36–40.

Hanagasi, H. A., Gurvit, I. H., Ermutlu, N., Kaptanoglu, G., Karamursel, S., Idrisoglu, H. A., et al. (2002). Cognitive impairment in amyotrophic lateral sclerosis: Evidence from neuropsychological investigation and event-related potentials. *Brain Research: Cognitive Brain Research, 14*(2), 234–244.

Ho, G., Scialfa, C. T., Caird, J. K., & Graw, T. (2001). Visual search for traffic signs: The effects of clutter, luminance, and aging. *Human Factors, 43*(2), 194–207.

Jay, G. M., & Willis, S. L. (1992). Influence of direct computer experience on older adults' attitudes toward computers. *Journal of Gerontology, 47*(4), P250–257.

Johansson, K., & Lundberg, C. (1997). The 1994 International Consensus Conference on Dementia and Driving: A brief report. Swedish National Road Administration. *Alzheimer Disease and Associated Disorders, 11*(Suppl. 1), 62–69.

Kane, R. L., & Kay, G. G. (1992). Computerized assessment in neuropsychology: A review of tests and test batteries. *Neuropsychology Review, 3*(1), 1–117.

Kane, R. L., & Reeves, D. L. (1997). Computerized test batteries. In A. M. Horton, Jr., D. Wedding, & J. Webster (Eds.), *The neuropsychology handbook: Vol. 1. Foundations and assessment* (2nd ed., pp. 423–467). New York: Springer Publishing Co.

Kotchoubey, B., Lang, S., Winter, S., & Birbaumer, N. (2003). Cognitive processing in completely paralyzed patients with amyotrophic lateral sclerosis. *European Journal of Neurology, 10*(5), 551–558.

Kubler, A., Kotchoubey, B., Hinterberger, T., Ghanayim, N., Perelmouter, J., Schauer, M., et al. (1999). The thought translation device: A neurophysiological approach to communication in total motor paralysis. *Experimental Brain Research, 124*(2), 223–232.

Kumagai, F. (2001). Possibilities for using the Internet in Japanese education in the information age society. *International Journal of Japanese Sociology, 10*, 29–44.

Lee, H. C., Lee, A. H., & Cameron, D. (2003). Validation of a driving simulator by measuring the visual attention skill of older adult drivers. *American Journal of Occupational Therapy, 57*(3), 324–328.

Lee, H. C., Lee, A. H., Cameron, D., & Li-Tsang, C. (2003). Using a driving simulator to identify older drivers at inflated risk of motor vehicle crashes. *Journal of Safety Research, 34*(4), 453–459.

Lengenfelder, J., Schultheis, M. T., Al-Shihabi, T., Mourant, R., & DeLuca, J. (2002). Divided attention and driving: A pilot study using virtual reality technology. *Journal of Head Trauma Rehabilitation, 17*(1), 26–37.

Lerner, N. (1994). Giving the older driver enough perception-reaction time. *Experimental Aging Research, 20*(1), 25–33.

Lilja, M., Bergh, A., Johansson, L., & Nygard, L. (2003). Attitudes towards rehabilitation needs and support from assistive technology and the social environment among elderly people with disability. *Occupational Therapy International, 10*(1), 75–93.

Lynch, W. (1988). Computers in neuropsychological assessment. *Journal of Head Trauma Rehabilitation, 3*, 92–94.

Mann, W. C., Ottenbacher, K. J., Fraas, L., Tomita, M., & Granger, C. V. (1999). Effectiveness of assistive technology and environmental interventions in maintaining independence and reducing home care costs for the frail elderly: A randomized controlled trial. *Archives of Family Medicine, 8*(3), 210–217.

Marquie, J. C., Jourdan-Boddaert, L., & Huet, N. (2002). Do older adults underestimate their actual computer knowledge? *Behavior and Information Technology, 2*(4), 273–280.

McGwin, G., Jr., & Brown, D. B. (1999). Characteristics of traffic crashes among young, middle-aged, and older drivers. *Accident: Analysis and Prevention, 31*(3), 181–198.

McGwin, G., Jr., Sims, R. V., Pulley, L., & Roseman, J. M. (2000). Relations among chronic medical conditions, medications, and automobile crashes in the elderly: A population-based case-control study. *American Journal of Epidemiology, 152*(5), 424–431.

Mead, A. D., & Drasgow, F. (1993). Equivalence of computerized and paper-and-pencil cognitive ability tests: A meta-analysis. *Psychological Bulletin, 114*(3), 449–458.

Newburger, E. C. (2001). *Current population reports: Home computers and Internet use in the United States, August 2000.* Washington, DC: US Department of Commerce, US Census Bureau.

NHTSA. (1994). *National Center for Statistics and Analysis: Traffic safety facts 1994: Older population.* Washington, DC: US Department of Transportation.

Owsley, C., Ball, K., Sloane, M. E., Roenker, D. L., & Bruni, J. R. (1991). Visual/cognitive correlates of vehicle accidents in older drivers. *Psychology and Aging, 6*(3), 403–415.

Perryman, K. M., & Fitten, L. J. (1996). Effects of normal aging on the performance of motor-vehicle operational skills. *Journal of Geriatric Psychiatry and Neurology, 9*(3), 136–141.

Ragland, D. R., Satariano, W. A., & MacLeod, K. E. (2004). Reasons given by older people for limitation or avoidance of driving. *Gerontologist, 44*(2), 237–244.

Reitan, R., & Wolfson, D. (1993). *The Halstead-Reitan Neuropsychological Test Battery: Theory and clinical interpretation.* Tucson, AZ: Neuropsychology Press.

Rialle, V., Duchene, F., Noury, N., Bajolle, L., & Demongeot, J. (2002). Health "Smart" home: Information technology for patients at home. *Telemedicine Journal and E-Health, 8*(4), 395–409.

Rialle, V., Lamy, J. B., Noury, N., & Bajolle, L. (2003). Telemonitoring of patients at home: A software agent approach. *Computer Methods and Programs in Biomedicine, 72*(3), 257–268.

Rialle, V., Noury, N., & Herve, T. (2001). An experimental health smart home and its distributed Internet-based information and communication system: First steps of a research project. *Medinfo, 10*(Pt. 2), 1479–1483.

Rizzo, A. A., & Buckwalter, J. G. (1997). Virtual reality and cognitive assessment and rehabilitation: The state of the art. *Studies in Health and Technology Informatics, 44*, 123–145.

Ryan, E. B., Szechtman, B., & Bodkin, J. (1992). Attitudes toward younger and older adults learning to use computers. *Journal of Gerontology, 47*(2), P96–101.

Schatz, P., & Browndyke, J. N. (2002). Applications of computer-based neuropsychological assessment. *Journal of Head Trauma Rehabilitation, 17*(5), 395–410.

Schultheis, M. T., Himelstein, J., & Rizzo, A. A. (2002). Virtual reality and neuropsychology: Upgrading the current tools. *Journal of Head Trauma Rehabilitation, 17*(5), 378–394.

Schultheis, M. T., & Mourant, R. R. (2001). Virtual reality and driving: The road to better assessment of cognitively impaired populations. *Presence: Teleoperators and Virtual Environments, 10*(4), 436–444.

Space, L. G. (1981). The computer as psychometrician. *Behavior Research Methods and Instrumentation, 13*(4), 595–606.

Stokx, L. C., & Gaillard, A. W. (1986). Task and driving performance of patients with a severe concussion of the brain. *Journal of Clinical and Experimental Neuropsychology, 8*(4), 421–436.

US Census Bureau. (2004). *US interim projections by age, sex, race, and Hispanic origin*. Retrieved 18 March, 2004, from http://www.census.gov/ipc/www/usinterim-proj/

Van Gerven, P. W., Paas, F., van Merrienboer, J. J., Hendriks, M., & Schmidt, H. G. (2003). The efficiency of multimedia learning into old age. *British Journal of Educational Psychology, 73*(Pt. 4), 489–505.

Van Zomeren, A. H., Brouwer, W. H., & Minderhoud, J. M. (1987). Acquired brain damage and driving: A review. *Archives of Physical Medicine and Rehabilitation, 68*(10), 697–705.

Verhaegen, P. (1995). Liability of older drivers in collisions. *Ergonomics, 38*, 499–507.

Wald, J., & Liu, L. (2001). Psychometric properties of the driVR: A virtual reality driving assessment. *Studies in Health Technology and Informatics, 81*, 564–566.

Wald, J., Liu, L., Hirsekorn, L., & Taylar, S. (2000). The use of virtual reality in the assessment of driving performance in persons with brain injury. *Studies in Health Technology and Informatics, 70*, 365–367.

White, H., McConnell, E., Clipp, E., Branch, L. G., Sloane, R., Pieper, C., et al. (2002). A randomized controlled trial of the psychosocial impact of providing Internet training and access to older adults. *Aging and Mental Health, 6*(3), 213–221.

Williams, A. F., & Carsten, O. (1989). Driver age and crash involvement. *American Journal of Public Health, 79*, 326–327.

Wilson, S. L., & McMillan, T. M. (1991). Microcomputers in psychometric and neuropsychological assessment. In A. Ager (Ed.), *Microcomputers and clinical psychology: Issues, applications and future developments* (pp. 79–94). Chichester, UK: John Wiley & Sons Ltd.

Withaar, F. K., Brouwer, W. H., & van Zomeren, A. H. (2000). Fitness to drive in older drivers with cognitive impairment. *Journal of the International Neuropsychological Society, 6*(4), 480–490.

Zeithaml, V. A., & Gilly, M. C. (1987). Characteristics affecting the acceptance of retailing technologies: A comparison of elderly and nonelderly consumers. *Journal of Retailing, 67*(1), 49–68.

5 Test accommodations in geriatric neuropsychology

Bruce Caplan and Judith A. Shechter

Accurate and informative psychological and neuropsychological assessment of older individuals presents a unique set of challenges not typically encountered with other age groups (Morris, 2004). It is the premise of this chapter that these factors, along with certain ethical and professional mandates, support the thoughtful and judicious use of certain modifications of standardized assessment procedures in the service of obtaining clinically useful and ecologically relevant information.

We have previously (Caplan & Shechter, 1995) argued the case for nonstandard neuropsychological assessment with persons with disabilities, marshalling support from the literature and providing examples of productive modifications of testing materials and procedures. While "elderly" does not equate to "disabled,"[1] we believe many points in that chapter apply to assessment of the elderly, most fundamentally that "considerations of validity, utility, fairness[2], professional ethics, and law support the use of nonstandard modified test procedures" (p. 368). Furthermore, the practice of "testing the limits" (a subcategory of nonstandard evaluation procedures) has a long and honorable history.

In that earlier work, we cited a representative sample of writings from experienced clinicians who explicitly opined that "appropriate minor adjustments in testing procedures" (Heaton & Heaton, 1981, p. 526) are quite permissible. Hibbard and Gordon (1992) promoted the use of procedural modifications with persons who have sustained strokes in order to elicit their optimal (not typical) performance, a goal with which both Heaton and Heaton and Wilson (1986) agree. In the same spirit, but pertaining to assessment of children, Wilson wrote of the need to modify test procedures to elicit worthwhile data. She firmly stated her position that simply adhering to standard procedures is too limiting, especially if all one finds is that the examinee "cannot do" the task. She urged a more flexible approach aimed at "obtaining all information possible about the functioning capacities of the child and to facilitate the production of maximum performance" (p. 158). We believe this tenet applies to assessment of older persons as well, and in this we are joined by numerous other authors (e.g., Albert, 1988; Braden, 2003; Lezak, 1986, 1995; Mendoza, 2001; Morris, 2004; Rockey, 1997).

In this chapter, we first note some components of professional documents that concern the need for and role of nonstandard procedures. We then consider some of the constraints that can affect assessment of the elderly and that we believe permit, if not dictate, procedural modifications. Finally, we describe some empirical investigations of particular manipulations that provide clinicians with a scientific basis (admittedly a rudimentary one) for employing an "elastic" style.

Before proceeding, we should address an important definitional matter. Behuniak (2002) notes that some authors draw distinctions between the terms "modification" and "accommodation" while others use them interchangeably. He adheres to the former stance, as do Lee, Reynolds, and Willson (2003) who cite Hollenbeck's (2002) detailed parsing of the two terms. According to the latter, four conditions are required for a test alteration to represent an "accommodation": (a) the measured construct(s) must be unchanged, (b) the change in content and/or procedure must derive directly from the need of the particular examinee, (c) the effect of the alteration on the score of the examinee with a disability must exceed the gain among their peers without the disability,[3] and (d) inferences derived from the adapted measure must equate with those derived from standard administration.

Hollenbeck (2002) argues that test alterations that meet these four conditions represent "accommodations." To the extent that any or all of these conditions are not achieved, the alteration moves along a continuum toward "modification." We endorse this perspective and guidelines, with the proviso that the last of these refers to inferences about the *central, salient constructs*, not the "irrelevant" ones that the accommodation is designed to eliminate.

Pertinent professional standards and guidelines

Several major professional documents speak to the matter of nonstandard test administration. In the recent (2004) guidelines to working with older adults, the American Psychological Association (APA) urged psychologists to "develop skill in tailoring assessments to accommodate older adults' specific characteristics and contexts" (Guideline 11). Two years earlier, the revised *Ethics Code* (APA, 2002) stated: "Psychologists administer, *adapt*, score, interpret, or use assessment techniques, interviews, tests, or instruments in a manner and for purposes that are appropriate in light of the research on or evidence of the usefulness and proper application of the techniques" (Standard 9.02, emphasis added).

It is a pervasive professional principle that practice should be based on research, and we fully support this notion. However, in the absence of empirical studies, psychologists, confronted with pressing clinical imperatives, must sometimes employ their best clinical judgment in judiciously altering procedures when circumstances dictate. As Braden (2003) pointed out, "clinicians must make decisions based on their assessments of the client, and the purposes of assessment. Research cannot completely address the constellation of unique client characteristics, setting, demands, and assessment contexts and purposes clinicians confront" (p. 454).

The Code also contained the caveat that in interpreting test results, "psychologists take into account the purpose of the assessment as well as the various test factors, test-taking abilities, and other characteristics of the person being assessed, such as situational, personal, linguistic, and cultural differences" (APA, 2002, Standard 9.06). This Standard would seem to encompass the elderly and/or those with disabilities. However, it is less specific than Standard 2.04 of the previous version of the Code, which clearly named "age" and "disability" as factors to be considered when interpreting test data (APA, 1992). A related publication from APA (Canter, Bennett, Jones, & Nagy, 1994) urged psychologists to "identify those situations that mandate the use of special procedures or that, because of other factors, require adjustments in the administration of psychological procedures or interpretation of results" (p. 72). Interested readers might consult Hanson, Kerkhoff, and Bush (2005, chap. 3) for an informative discussion of ethical issues surrounding the use of nonstandard procedures in rehabilitation.

The *Standards for Educational and Psychological Testing* (American Educational Research Association, American Psychological Association, & National Council on Measurement in Education, 1999) clearly state that assessment of persons with disabilities may necessitate alteration of standard procedures (Standard 5.1). The subsequent "comment" notes that decisions to employ modifications "should be tempered by the consideration that departures from standard procedures may jeopardize the validity of test score interpretations" (p. 63).

In a short chapter in the *Standards* (American Educational Research Association et al., 1999) dealing with evaluation of persons with disabilities, a distinction is made between "accommodations" and "modifications." The former is said to be "the general term for any action taken in response to a determination that an individual's disability requires a departure from established testing protocol" (p. 101). Accommodation can encompass modification of the testing process (e.g., how instructions are conveyed; permissible response modality; timing) or content (e.g., enlarged stimuli; spatial rearrangement). "No connotation that modification implies a change in the construct(s) being measured is intended" (p.101). It is notable that the preceding sentence mentions *multiple* constructs, while virtually all of the remainder of the chapter seems to assume that tests measure *single* constructs. We disagree with the latter notion, as we view the vast majority of tests as multifactorial in nature. As a corollary, we conceive of the essential purpose of nonstandard testing as the removal of "construct-irrelevant variance" (Messick, 1995).[4] This involves alterations of procedure, materials, etc. that eliminate or minimize the impact of the disability on one (presumably less important) of several factors assessed by a given test.[5] Certainly, in neuropsychological evaluation, peripheral problems such as sensory and motor impairments produce variance that is usually extraneous to the purpose of assessment of higher cognitive function.

Other portions of this chapter of the *Standards* (American Educational Research Association et al., 1999) are quite relevant to our position. It is asserted that, if certain factors such as reading ability or fatigue "are incidental to the construct intended to be measured by the test, modifications of tests and test administration procedures may be necessary for an accurate assessment" (p. 101). Furthermore, test users should be familiar with research relevant to assessment of persons with disabilities (Standard 10.2). Also, examiners "should take steps to ensure that the test score inferences accurately reflect the intended constructs rather than any disabilities and their associated characteristics extraneous to the intent of the measurement" (Standard 10.1).

When there is evidence of score comparability on standard and modified administrations (and this is unlikely to be the case in the great majority of circumstances), or "if a modification is provided for which there is no reasonable basis for believing that the modification would affect score comparability" (a more ambiguous situation), the score need not be "flagged" in the written report (American Educational Research Association et al., 1999, Standard 10.11 and comment). If evidence is lacking of score comparability, Standard 10.11 states: "specific information about the nature of the modification should be provided, if permitted by law, to assist test users properly to interpret and act on test scores." The subsequent "comment" warns that the report should contain no reference to the existence or nature of the test taker's disability. As worded, this standard seems to us to be a "catch-22" situation, imposing a considerable burden on the psychologist to describe and justify the modification that directly stemmed from the disability without naming the disability. Mehrens and Ekstrom (2002) provide a useful discussion of this and related conflicts between and among various standards, practices, and legal constraints. They conclude that accommodations and modifications ought to be explicitly documented in reports (unless federal laws would thereby be violated), but that "flagging" itself, as well as variations in policies and procedures dictated by various organizations, should be minimized. We support this view, and await the day that users of test data no longer automatically view "flagged" scores with skepticism.

Several standards urge that test developers and users conduct research to demonstrate the value and validity of test modifications. While the desirability of this endeavor cannot be questioned, we believe that it is likely to remain "aspirational," largely for economic reasons. As acknowledged by Geisinger et al. (2002), the fundamental flaw with most studies that have investigated the effects of nonstandard administration is the small number of subjects tested. It seems unlikely that test companies or Federal agencies will offer much support to study the utility of tests with limited applicability.[6] In addition, Mehrens and Ekstrom (2002) pointed out that the Americans with Disabilities Act has created another obstacle to large-scale research by requiring that accommodations be made on an individual basis. An adequate research design would require a large number of persons with the same kind and extent of disability undergoing the same "accommodated testing."

For those examiners who encounter situations where test modifications may be indicated, Braden (2003) provides a decision-tree model to follow, and Smith (2002) offers a related, partially overlapping step-by-step approach. Behuniak (2002) provided an overview of the sorts of test accommodations that are most often requested by individuals with disabilities; these include changes to the physical testing environment, duration of testing, presentation of test directions, and permissible response modalities. He recognized the potential effect on test validity of any given alteration of content or procedure, noting that validity may be affected in either positive or negative ways. While lengthening time limits on a reading test might be an acceptable variation, the same modification would subvert the purpose of a test of typing speed.

Lee et al. (2003) reviewed the literature on the effects of various types of test modifications. They concluded that even relatively minor changes may "lead to significant alterations in individuals' test performance in some instances, but not in all cases. Perhaps more problematic is the great difficulty in predicting on any rational basis just what changes in administration procedures will have just what specific effects" (p. 72). These authors urged great caution on the part of those who employ modified tests, and they emphasized the risks clinicians may run in the legal arena under the Daubert[7] standard if they use such procedures without empirical backing. We agree that deviations from standard procedures in assessing persons with disabilities may well change their scores, but that is precisely the point, to obtain a "purer" measure of the person's skill on the central factors that the test was intended to evaluate.

Despite the conclusion of Lee et al. (2003), some studies do inspire confidence that modifications may achieve their intended purpose without sabotaging information obtained via standard procedures. Gaudette and Smith (1998) employed the nonstandard "tell the story" procedure with the WAIS–R Picture Arrangement subtest; this variation is one of the series of modifications to the WAIS–R developed by Kaplan, Fein, Morris, and Delis (1991) based on Kaplan's process-oriented approach to assessment. Gaudette and Smith found no effect on quantitative outcome of this qualitative procedure; thus, clinicians may still interpret obtained scores with reference to the large normative database, while at the same time gaining access to potentially rich "process" information. Furthermore, Willingham et al. (1988) compared standard and nonstandard administrations of college and graduate school admissions tests for persons with four types of disability, reaching the overall conclusion that, except for modifications of test timing, "the nonstandard versions of the SAT and GRE administered to handicapped examinees are generally comparable to the standard tests in most important respects" (p. xiii).

Before proceeding further, we should state that the perspectives and techniques discussed here constitute evaluation "extras," gravy on the meat of standard testing. By no means do we suggest that standardized procedures be jettisoned, nor do we wish to elevate flexibility in testing to the contortionist level. Rather, we wish to urge examiners to go "beyond the information given" and exploit the tools at hand to extract all possible potentially informative data about the subject of investigation. Furthermore, we endorse the caveats offered by others that this endeavor must be undertaken with caution and with full disclosure of the underlying rationale, modifications/accommodations provided, and results. Our position dovetails with that of Lezak (1986), who argued for the importance of combining "clinical" and "psychometric" approaches especially in the evaluation of elderly persons; the latter permits quantified assessment of neuropsychological changes while the former fosters more flexible inquiry into performance-limiting factors, often yielding information upon which treatment recommendations are based. We also concur with Braden's (2003) implication that assessment is a blend of science and art with acceptable roles for both empirical data and clinical judgment.

Factors that may warrant nonstandard modification in the assessment of older adults

We now discuss several relevant influences on test performance that are relatively common among the aging and that require flexibility on the part of the examiner. We also offer suggestions for limiting their impact.

Unfamiliarity with the testing process

Having missed the present-day proliferation of school-based testing programs, most elderly persons were probably not subjected to routine standardized assessment during their educational careers; furthermore, on the whole, they are likely to have had less schooling (Albert, 1988). Hence, simply the process of undergoing such evaluation may be foreign and disconcerting, if not outright intimidating. There are useful strategies to aid in establishing rapport and placing the examinee at ease. First, provide clear explanation about the nature and purpose of the evaluation, how the findings are to be used and how they may be helpful to the examinee. Also, forewarn them about the range of difficulty of test items—that is, that there will be a blend of easy and hard items—so that some failures are expected and will not be devastating when they occur. Start with a more manageable task or two, and follow more challenging measures with ones that provide a "breather."

Diminished sensation

There are well-documented age-related sensory changes that may impede the assessment process (Kline & Scialfa, 1996). For example, persons with diminished visual acuity may encounter difficulty on certain IQ subtests (especially on the Performance scale) for this reason alone, although simple visual discrimination may not be among the primary skills that the examiner intended to be assessed with that measure.[8] Even though the stimulus materials have been enlarged in the third revision of the WAIS, a low score on

Picture Arrangement obtained by a person with poor vision may tell the examiner nothing of value about the examinee's sequencing skill, understanding of nonverbal social cues, etc. Worse yet, a careless clinician who did not detect the individual's visual impairment might draw incorrect inferences from the impaired performance and, worse still, offer unfounded recommendations for treatment, activity restriction, or loss of privileges.

Given the high incidence of impaired sensation among the elderly, it is incumbent upon examiners to make certain that patients are advised well in advance to come to the session with any necessary eyeglasses or hearing aids. Inquiry should be made about any history of cataracts, glaucoma, or diplopia. For those with visual difficulties (Fozard, 1990), examiners need to ensure adequate illumination of the testing environment, as well as clarity and legibility of test materials. For patients with hemianopia, the examiner should remember to place materials in the good visual field.

It may be useful for examiners to lower the tone of their voice, as high frequency hearing loss is quite common among older persons. Also, as suggested by Green (2000), maintaining eye contact, reading instructions in a natural way, and repeating or paraphrasing instructions when needed all foster good understanding of test directions. Green also makes the valuable observation that the test-giver is already familiar with the instructions and may therefore speak more rapidly than the test-taker can process. We have often found it useful to ask patients to repeat to us what they understand they are supposed to do for a given task; this provides the opportunity for any necessary corrective. For those with severely impaired hearing, Lezak (1995, p. 133) suggests that examiners might write out instructions that are normally spoken. Of course, this presupposes that the patient's reading skills are adequate to the task.

Fatigability

The elderly examinee may fatigue sooner than a younger person, although this can be a consequence of illness rather than the aging process alone (e.g., Ingles, Eskes, & Phillips, 1999; Lou, Kerns, Oken, Sexton, & Nutt, 2000). Test results obtained from a weary examinee can be of questionable reliability and validity. It may be useful to ask about the individual's typical waking (and napping) time and take that into account when scheduling the evaluation. During testing, clinicians must be alert for subtle signs of fatigue and offer rest breaks on a regular basis, perhaps even enforcing an occasional interlude. In some instances it may be necessary to discontinue the session and reschedule for another day.

Behavioral slowing

From simple reaction time (which actually begins to lengthen around age 30) to execution of more complex actions, the elderly typically respond more slowly than younger persons. This is reflected in age norms for any number of tests, according to which the same raw score yields a higher percentile for the older person. Also contributing to this phenomenon is the heightened degree of cautiousness (Schaie, 1974) that is common in older people, which may produce additional delays in responding. Some generosity in enforcing time limits may be advisable, especially if the examinee is nearing completion of an item when the allotted time expires. Interrupting at such times may only serve to create frustration and diminished cooperation. Scores can be calculated and reported for both time-limited and unlimited performances, with requisite consideration of the meaning of the difference between the two.

Comorbid conditions

Older persons often carry multiple medical diagnoses, and some of these (e.g., hypertension, diabetes, heart disease) may have psychological and/or neuropsychological consequences beyond those of the condition with respect to which the examination was requested (Tuokko & Hadjistavropoulos, 1998). Consider a 78-year-old man with probable Parkinson's disease (PD) who is sent by his neurologist for neuropsychological evaluation. The presence of a comorbid condition such as alcohol abuse may modify the obtained test pattern from what one would expect on the basis of PD alone. Ruchinskas and Curylo (2003) allude to several studies demonstrating cognitive deficits in association with conditions that would not, at first glance, seem likely to have such consequences—for example, hip fracture and peripheral vascular disease.

Medication effects

A corollary of the above point is the larger number of medications often required by the elderly as well as their enhanced sensitivity to medication effects (Tuokko & Hadjistavropoulos, 1998). While drugs may promote better health, their effects—both positive and negative—must be considered in interpretation of test data.

Research on specific modifications

Some two decades ago, Golden and Robbins (1985) observed that few psychometrically adequate tests were available that had been normed on persons with disabilities. The statement remains true, although some modest headway has been made in a few areas. We now describe a few encouraging developments that have the potential for enlarging the clinical armamentarium of the geriatric neuropsychologist, conferring greater flexibility in the testing process. Interested readers should consult Caplan and Shechter (1995) for discussion of earlier work in this area.

Impaired motor function

It is common for elderly persons to have motor limitations resulting from joint disease such as arthritis or from a hemiparesis caused by stroke. If the condition affects the dominant hand and arm, clinicians, aware of dominant–nondominant differences on tasks such as finger tapping and grip strength (Heaton, Miller, Taylor, & Grant, 2004), may automatically eliminate from consideration those tests that demand motor responses. However, some have found that the nondominant hand can perform certain tasks virtually as quickly and efficiently as the dominant one. In such cases, tests can be retained that might otherwise have been excluded, and a more complete evaluation can be obtained.

For example, instructions for administering the Trail Making Test (TMT) do not specify the use of the dominant hand (Reitan & Wolfson, 1985), although it is safe to say that this is typically inferred by the subject and encouraged by the examiner. Existing normative data bases presumably contain scores for dominant hand (DH) performance. However, there is some evidence suggesting that the nondominant hand (NDH) performs equally well. Horowitz and Caplan (1998) reported data from 60 healthy undergraduate students and 30 general rehabilitation patients without neurological conditions. Intermanual differences were statistically and clinically insignificant. LoSasso, Rapport, Axelrod, and Reeder (1998) also studied both intermanual and alternate form equivalence in 980 undergraduates and found a very small difference (1.9 seconds) between DH and NDH across the four tests. They concluded that "patients with dominant hand paralysis may be tested using the nondominant hand with some degree of confidence in the results" and that doing so "does not yield a clinically meaningful difference in score" (p. 109).

Toyokura, Sawatari, Nishimura, and Ishida (2003) demonstrated cross-cultural validity of this modification of the TMT administration. They developed Japanese versions of the TMT using kana letters in place of English letters for part B. They also created mirror-image forms on the assumption that these would elicit NDH performance more comparable to that of the dominant hand with the standard forms. They also examined the impact of order of hand use by requiring half of their neurologically intact participants to use the right hand during the first session and the others to use the left hand; 1 week later, all participants were retested using the opposite hand. These investigators found evidence of a learning curve—that is, superior performance by the second hand tested, regardless of side—but overall DH–NDH differences were nonsignificant for time to completion of parts A and B as well as for derived scores (A/B; A+B; A–B). Their hypothesis concerning the mirror-image version was not confirmed. It should be noted that their data cannot be directly applied to the standard TMT, as the figures accompanying the article show that Toyokura et al. relocated the stimuli across the test sheets. However, the general point about equivalent performance between the two hands still holds.

A series of investigations by Bush highlights the potential impact of demographic factors and medical condition on "manual interchangeability".

Using a clock drawing task with a 15-point maximum score, Bush (2000a) found miniscule intermanual differences (DH mean = 14.61, *SD* = 0.69; NDH mean = 14.39, *SD* = 0.87) among a well-educated (mean = 16 years) young adult (mean age = 29 years) sample. Although the test of the difference between the hands barely missed statistical significance, the absolute differences were clearly quite small. Furthermore 95% of the participants obtained NDH scores that were within normal limits.

A subsequent study (Bush, 2000b) examined clock-drawing performances in an older (mean age = 79.6 years), less well-educated (mean = 12.1 years) sample of 19 subacute rehabilitation patients with no history of neurological or psychiatric condition, visual impairment, or upper extremity deficit. A much wider range of scores was obtained, as well as lower overall performance (DH mean = 11.95, *SD* = 1.93; NDH mean = 9.11, *SD* = 4.15). Two-thirds of participants scored in the normal range with the NDH.

Using the Rey Complex Figure Test, Bush and Martin (2004) found comparable performances with the two hands in 58 adults (mean age = 36.3 years; mean education = 14.4 years) residing in the community who reported negative neurological and psychiatric histories and had no visual or upper extremity motor impairment. Average DH score was 33.01 (*SD* = 2.39) of a possible 36 and NDH average was 32.49 (*SD* = 2.38). Interestingly, fully one-quarter of participants obtained a higher NDH than DH score. As Bush (2000b) suggested, through larger scale studies it may be possible to establish correction factors for particular tests in order to "equate" NDH and DH levels.

Visual deficits

As mentioned above, visual impairment is quite common among elderly individuals. In addition to changes such as cataracts and glaucoma that are primarily age related, certain conditions such as diabetes may be accompanied by decreased visual acuity. Clearly, this limits the scope of neuropsychological evaluation (Price, Mount, & Coles, 1987). The examiner can legitimately employ, for example, such language-based tasks as WAIS–III Verbal subtests, verbal memory measures, and generative fluency tests, as well as the Cognitive Test for the Blind, which has recently been shown to have a high correlation with the Verbal portion of the WAIS–R (Nelson, Dial, & Joyce, 2002). However, some spheres, such as components of executive function, would seem to be incapable of valid assessment, as most measures felt to evaluate these aspects of executive skills (e.g., Category Test; Wisconsin Card Sorting Test; Trail Making Test, part B) require adequate vision.

Recently, however, Beauvais, Woods, Delaney, and Fein (2004) reported initial data on the construct validity of a tactile version of the Wisconsin Card Sorting Test (TWCST). These researchers developed three "key" cards, on each of which were one to three circles, triangles, or squares constructed from one or the other side of a Velcro swatch (i.e., the "rough" or "wooly" side). There were 54 response cards, each of which contained a varying number of shapes and textures, and each response card shared at least one feature with a key card. A stimulus board was built with "frames" that held the three key cards. Instructions were modified from those for the original WCST in the obvious, required ways—for example, by having participants palpate the board and each key card in order to learn their positions. Participants were then given the larger deck, made their sorts, and received feedback from the examiner as in standard WCST procedure. Scores were derived for virtually all of the same variables as are calculated from the standard test. Consistent with their hypotheses, Beauvais et al. found that the TWCST differentiated persons with both visual and neurological impairment from healthy controls as well as neurologically intact persons with visual impairment. Although the groups were small, the effect sizes were large, suggesting robust findings.

In some instances, examiners may find that using enlarged stimuli minimizes the impact of diminished visual discrimination ability, allowing more accurate assessment of other subskills; a large-print version of the Wide Range Achievement Test—Revised (Jastak & Wilkinson, 1984) is commercially available. As mentioned above, however, this does not always promote improved performance (e.g., Storandt & Futterman, 1982). Ferraro, Barth, Morton, and Whetham (1997) administered one of three versions of the Boston Naming Test to younger (mean age = 27.5 years) and older (men age = 68.7 years) healthy adults. At each age, small groups (N = 10) of subjects saw standard BNT stimuli or pictures that had been either reduced or enlarged by a factor of 1.5. Younger subjects performed slightly better with the enlarged materials while older participants had a higher mean score with the smaller pictures, contrary to what one might expect; however, the differences were small and nonsignificant. Ferraro et al. assert that the fact that performances under the various conditions were statistically comparable allows examiners to use the larger stimuli without worrying about altering score interpretation. They point to potential advantages of using larger materials with older persons, including reducing anxiety that may accompany the testing process and complying with the preference of many older individuals for larger type newspapers and magazines.

Expressive language difficulty

Obstacles to testing expressive language may result from cultural differences, educational limitations, or neurological conditions, such as stroke or traumatic brain injury, that can produce aphasia or dysarthria. While one useful goal of testing may be to establish the presence and degree of linguistic limitations, many tests that demand a verbal response are intended to assess primarily nonlinguistic factors. Such tasks may be performed poorly by those with language deficits for that reason alone, sabotaging efforts to assess the other (more central) skills evaluated by the test.

As an example of this point, consider the Hooper Visual Organization Test (HVOT; Hooper, 1958), which consists of a series of fragmented object drawings that the participant must mentally synthesize and identify. The HVOT has proved clinically useful in evaluating persons with a variety of neurological conditions (Fitz, Conrad, & Sarff, 1992; York & Cermak, 1995), but caution has been urged (Lezak, 1995) in the interpretation of data from persons with naming difficulties. In an attempt to minimize the impact of anomia on HVOT performance, Schultheis, Caplan, Ricker and Woessner (2000) developed a multiple-choice version (MC-HVOT) by adding four printed response alternatives below each picture. Participants could respond by pointing to their selection or saying the number of their choice. Anomic subjects demonstrated significant improvement under the multiple-choice format. The authors concluded that use of the MC-HVOT version "purifies" assessment of visual analysis and synthesis in persons with naming difficulty.

Fatigue

As previously discussed, fatigability is another common consequence of aging and associated comorbid illnesses, and this can clearly affect test performance, even within administration of a single test. The Paced Auditory Serial Addition Test (PASAT) demands sustained attention and working memory, as participants must monitor strings of digits that are read aloud to them and sequentially add each pair of numbers. Much, albeit not all, evidence suggests that PASAT performance declines with age (Spreen & Strauss, 1998). Some examiners may not even consider using the PASAT with elderly clients, fearing that it will overtax and perhaps even confuse them, leading to increased resistance to testing. As a means of both reducing the attentional load and simplifying the task, while retaining certain essential elements, Greenberg (personal communication, 2004) developed the Tens Test. Like the PASAT, this task consists of strings of auditorally presented digits which the individual must monitor. Unlike the PASAT, which demands a response on every trial and simultaneous maintenance of information in working memory, the Tens Test merely requires an affirmative response only when two consecutive numbers add to 10. The individual can respond manually, if desired, thereby also eliminating the need for spoken language. Total administration time is just over 6 minutes, roughly one-third the duration of the PASAT. This test remains under development, but has promise as a useful addition to the geriatric neuropsychologist's tool box.

Test batteries

The modifications discussed thus far involve individual tests that were altered in the service of permitting more valid assessment of discrete cognitive skills. The following discussion concerns two batteries that were modified with the needs of elderly and/or disabled individuals in mind. The Primary Mental Abilities Test has a long history in psychology, representing the seminal work of Thurstone and Thurstone (1962). Recognizing the limitations of the PMA in the evaluation of the elderly, Schaie et al. developed the Schaie-Thurstone Adult Mental Abilities Test (STAMAT; Schaie, 1985) which incorporated some "user-friendly" principles.

First, all materials were photo-enlarged. Second, in lieu of answer sheets separated from the stimulus materials, the STAMAT uses disposable book-lets that allow respondents to write their answers directly on the test sheets. Next, parallel forms were created of two subtests (Spatial Relations and Inductive Reasoning) using meaningful materials; for example, the "rotation" test employs real objects such as tools and appliances, rather than geometric shapes. Finally, Schaie (1985) wrote that instructions were framed in such a way as to indicate clearly when guessing should be encouraged (to counteract the older person's presumably greater caution and/or fear of being wrong) and when incorrect responses will be penalized.

In order to permit IQ testing of persons with speech impairment or upper extremity motor dysfunction, Berninger, Gans, St. James, and Connors (1988) developed adaptations of 9 of the 11 subtests that comprise the Wechsler Adult Intelligence Scale–Revised (1981). They created sets of response alternatives for each Verbal subtest item and for Picture Completion, mounting these on lam-inated displays. Examinees could respond by pointing, naming the letter asso-ciated with their choice, or indicating by any available output mechanism (e.g., nodding, eye blink) when the examiner pointed to the answer they wished to select. Presaging the subsequent edition of the Wechsler scale, the Picture Arrangement and Picture Completion stimuli were enlarged; for the former, the examiner could elicit instructions from the examinee concerning their desired sequencing of the cards. Finally, for the two constructional subtests, examinees could direct the examiner to position the components on a magnetic board.

Conclusion

Assessment of the geriatric patient demands a high level of scientist-practi-tioner skill. In addition to the requisite familiarity with the facts about phys-iological and cognitive aging, awareness of the impact of social and environmental factors, and demonstrable interpersonal sensitivity, we believe the clinician benefits by being something of an artist-innovator.

A central feature of this perspective is that tests are viewed as one means to the end of "evaluation." We share with others cited above the conviction that the purpose of the evaluation dictates how testing is conducted. If the aim is to detect brain damage or dysfunction, there may be little need for other than pure, standard administration of a test battery. If, however, what is sought is infor-mation about specific types of competence (e.g., cognitive "power" divorced from the need for speeded performance), performance-limiting and perform-ance-enhancing factors and their implications for management, capacity to function safely, or a host of other possible referral questions, then what we have termed an "elastic" approach to the use of tests is often more fruitful.

Nonetheless, certain caveats apply. Test accommodations should only be undertaken with considerable thought and analysis and after search for alternate means of assessing the desired construct(s). If one elects to "test the limits" of a standardized instrument, this should be done only after completion of conventional administration so that existing normative data can be employed, in addition to whatever information the amended test permits one to extract. Except where specific legal constraints exist, full disclosure of changes of procedure or content to the users of test results is essential.

Notes

1 However, recent data show that the incidence of disability increases from 19% for persons between the ages of 15 and 64 to 52.5% for persons 65 and over (data from the United States Census Bureau, as cited in Ekstrom & Smith, 2002).

2 "Fairness" is a relatively recent concept in psychometrics. It refers to the degree to which a test yields valid results for all groups (Geisinger, Boodoo, & Noble, 2002). As Foote (2002) pointed out, unfair assessment may breach ethical standards and put the examiner in violation of laws such as the Americans with Disabilities Act.

3 But see Braden (2003) for a conflicting view of "differential boost."

4 Braden (2003) concurs with this primary purpose of test accommodations, but also notes that the source of "assessment invalidity" identified by Messick (1995)—namely, construct underrepresentation—can occur when tests are modified. He gives the example of measuring intelligence in individuals who are deaf solely with the Performance subtests of the Wechsler scales. While eliminating Verbal subtests decreases construct-irrelevant variance, it also diminishes the assessment of intelligence to the extent that "intelligence" encompasses language-based skills.

5 Of interest here is the distinction drawn by Phillips (1993, 1994) between "target" skills (those that are central to the purposes of the assessment) and "access" skills (those that permit the individual to gain access to and participate in assessment such as being able to sit at the testing table at the required angle).

6 One finds a parallel with the difficulties in obtaining research funding encountered by those who study low-incidence diseases.

7 Under Daubert v. Merrill Dow Pharmaceuticals, Inc. (1993), admissible testimony must be derived from concepts that have been tested by the scientific method and subjected to peer review.

8 It should be noted, however, that Storandt and Futterman (1982) found that stimulus size did not affect the performance of either younger or older adults on the Picture Completion or Picture Arrangement subtests. Of course, this does not mean that some older (or younger) persons would not benefit from photoenlarged stimuli.

References

Albert, M. (1988). Assessment of cognitive dysfunction. In M. S. Albert & M. B. Moss (Eds.), *Geriatric neuropsychology* (pp. 57–81). New York: Guilford Press.

American Educational Research Association, American Psychological Association, & National Council on Measurement in Education. (1999). *Standards for educational and psychological testing*. Washington, DC: American Educational Research Association.

American Psychological Association. (1992). Ethical principles of psychologists and code of conduct. *American Psychologist, 47*, 1597–1611.

American Psychological Association. (2002). Ethical principles of psychologists and code of conduct. *American Psychologist, 57*(12), 1060–1073.

American Psychological Association. (2004). Guidelines for psychological practice with older adults. *American Psychologist, 59*(4), 236–260.

Beauvais, J. E., Woods, S. P., Delaney, R. C., & Fein, D. (2004). The development of a tactile Wisconsin Card Sorting Test. *Rehabilitation Psychology, 49*(4), 282–287 .

Behuniak, P. (2002). Types of commonly requested accommodations. In R. B. Ekstrom & D. K. Smith (Eds.), *Assessing individuals with disabilities in educational, employment, and counseling settings* (pp. 45–58). Washington, DC: American Psychological Association.

Berninger, V., Gans, B., St. James, P., & Connors, T. (1988). Modified WAIS–R for patients with speech and/or hand dysfunction. *Archives of Physical Medicine and Rehabilitation, 69*, 250–255.

Braden, J. P. (2003). Accommodating clients with disabilities on the WAIS–III and WMS. In D. S. Tulsky, D. H. Saklofske, G. J. Chelune, R. K. Heaton, R. J. Ivnik, R. Bornstein, et al. (Eds.), *Clinical interpretation of the WAIS–III and WMS–III* (pp. 451–486). San Diego, CA: Academic Press.

Bush, S. (2000a). Intermanual differences in performing a visuoconstructional task. *Archives of Physical Medicine and Rehabilitation, 81*, 1151–1152.

Bush, S. (2000b). Intermanual visuoconstructional differences in rehabilitation patients. *Journal of Cognitive Rehabilitation, 18*, 10–13.

Bush, S., & Martin, T. A. (2004). Intermanual differences on the Rey Complex Figure Test. *Rehabilitation Psychology, 49*(1), 76–78.

Canter, M. B., Bennett, B. E., Jones, S. E., & Nagy, T. F. (1994). *Ethics for psychologists*. Washington, DC: American Psychological Association.

Caplan, B., & Shechter, J. (1995). Nonstandard neuropsychological assessment: History, rationale, and examples. In L. Cushman & M. Scherer (Eds.), *Psychological assessment in medical rehabilitation* (pp. 359–381). Washington, DC: American Psychological Association.

Daubert v. Merrill Dow Pharmaceuticals, Inc., 509 US S. Ct. (1993).

Ekstrom, R. B., & Smith, D. K. (2002). Introduction. In R. B. Ekstrom & D. K. Smith (Eds.), *Assessing individuals with disabilities in educational, employment, and counseling settings* (pp. 3–8). Washington, DC: American Psychological Association.

Ferraro, F. R., Barth, J., Morton, M., & Whetham, T. (1997). Stimulus size effects in Boston Naming Test performance in younger and older adults. *Applied Neuropsychology, 4*, 249–251.

Fitz, A., Conrad, D., & Sarff, P. (1992). Hooper visual organization test performance in lateralized brain injury. *Archives of Clinical Neuropsychology, 7*, 243–250.

Foote, W. E. (2002). The clinical assessment of people with disabilities. In R. B. Ekstrom & D. K. Smith (Eds.), *Assessing individuals with disabilities in educational, employment, and counseling settings* (pp. 103–120). Washington, DC: American Psychological Association.

Fozard, J. (1990). Vision and hearing in aging. In J. Birren & K. Schaie (Eds.), *Handbook of the psychology of aging* (3rd ed., pp. 150–170). New York: Guilford Press.

Gaudette, M. D., & Smith, J. A. (1998). Process-oriented administration of the picture arrangement test does not affect the quantitative outcome. *Applied Neuropsychology, 5*(3), 154–158.

Geisinger, K. F., Boodoo, G., & Noble, J. P. (2002). The psychometrics of testing individuals with disabilities. In R. B. Ekstrom & D. K. Smith (Eds.), *Assessing individuals with disabilities in educational, employment, and counseling settings* (pp. 33–42). Washington, DC: American Psychological Association.

Golden, C. J., & Robbins, D. E. (1985). Considerations in cases of visual, auditory, or motor impairment. In D. P. Swiercinsky (Ed.), *Testing adults: A reference guide for special psychodiagnostic assessments* (pp. 89–100). Kansas City, MO: Test Corporation of America.

Green, J. (2000). *Neuropsychological evaluation of the older adult: A clinician's guidebook*. San Diego, CA: Academic Press.

Hanson, S., Kerkhoff, T., & Bush, S. (2005). *Health care ethics for psychologists*. Washington, DC: American Psychological Association.

Heaton, S., & Heaton, R. (1981). Testing the impaired patient. In S. B. Filskov & T. J. Boll (Eds.), *Handbook of clinical neuropsychology* (pp. 526–544). New York: Wiley.

Heaton, R., Miller, S. W., Taylor, M. J., & Grant, I. (2004). *Revised comprehensive norms for an expanded Halstead-Reitan battery*. Lutz, FL: Psychological Assessment Resources.

Hibbard, M. R., & Gordon, W. A. (1992). The comprehensive psychological assessment of individuals with stroke. *Neurorehabilitation, 2*, 9–20.

Hollenbeck, K. (2002). Determining what test alterations are valid accommodations or modifications for large-scale assessment. In G. Tindal & T. M. Haladyna (Eds.), *Large-scale assessment programs for all students* (pp. 395–425). Mahwah, NJ: Lawrence Erlbaum Associates, Inc.

Hooper, H. (1958). *The Hooper visual organization test manual*. Los Angeles: Western Psychological Services.

Horowitz, T., & Caplan, B. (1998). Dominant and nondominant hand performance on the Trail Making Test. *Archives of Clinical Neuropsychology, 13*, 71–72.

Ingles, J., Eskes, G., & Phillips, S. (1999). Fatigue after stroke. *Archives of Physical Medicine and Rehabilitation, 80*, 173–178.

Jastak, S., & Wilkinson, D. (1984). *Wide Range Achievement Test–revised administration manual*. Wilmington, DE: Jastak Associates.

Kaplan, E., Fein, D., Morris, R., & Delis, D. C. (1991). *WAIS–R as a neuropsychological instrument*. San Antonio, TX: Psychological Corporation.

Kline, D., & Scialfa, C. (1996). Visual and auditory aging. In J. Birren & K. Schaie (Eds.), *Handbook of the psychology of aging* (4th ed., pp. 181–203). San Diego, CA: Academic Press.

Lee, D., Reynolds, C. R., & Willson, V. L. (2003). Standardized test administration: Why bother? *Journal of Forensic Neuropsychology, 3*(3), 55–81.

Lezak, M. (1986). Neuropsychological assessment. In L. Teri & P. M. Lewinsohn (Eds.), *Geropsychological assessment and treatment* (pp. 3–37). New York: Springer Publishing Company.

Lezak, M. (1995). *Neuropsychological assessment* (3rd ed.). New York: Oxford University Press.

LoSasso, G. L., Rapport, L. J., Axelrod, B. N., & Reeder, K. P. (1998). Intermanual and alternate-form equivalence on the Trail Making Tests. *Journal of Clinical and Experimental Neuropsychology, 20*, 107–110.

Lou, J., Kerns, G., Oken, B., Sexton, G., & Nutt, J. (2000). Exacerbated physical fatigue and mental fatigue in Parkinson's disease. *Movement Disorders, 16*, 190–196.

Mehrens, W. A., & Ekstrom, R. B. (2002). Score reporting issues in the assessment of people with disabilities: Policies and practices. In R. B. Ekstrom & D. K. Smith (Eds.), *Assessing individuals with disabilities in educational, employment, and counseling settings* (pp. 87–100). Washington, DC: American Psychological Association.

Mendoza, J. (2001). Reporting the results of the neuropsychological evaluation. In C. G. Armengol, E. Kaplan, & E. J. Moes (Eds.), *The consumer-oriented neuropsychological report* (pp. 95–122). Lutz, FL: Psychological Assessment Resources.

Messick, S. A. (1995). Validity of psychological assessment: Validation of inferences from persons' responses and performances as scientific inquiry into score meaning. *American Psychologist, 50*(9), 741–749.

Morris, R. G. (2004). Neuropsychology of older adults. In L. H. Goldstein & J. E. McNeil (Eds.), *Clinical neuropsychology: A practical guide to assessment and management for clinicians* (pp. 301–318). Chichester, UK: John Wiley & Sons.

Nelson, P. A., Dial, J. G., & Joyce, A. (2002). Validation of the cognitive test for the blind as a measure of intellectual functioning. *Rehabilitation Psychology, 47*(2), 184–193.

Phillips, S. E. (1993). Testing condition accommodations for disabled students. *West's Education Law Quarterly, 2*(2), 366–389.

Phillips, S. E. (1994). High-stakes testing accommodations: Validity versus disabled rights. *Applied Measurement in Education, 7*(2), 93–120.

Price, J. R., Mount, G. R., & Coles, E. A. (1987). Evaluating the visually impaired: Neuropsychological techniques. *Journal of Visual Impairment and Blindness, 81*, 28–30.

Reitan, R., & Wolfson, D. (1985). *The Halstead-Reitan neuropsychological test battery: Theory and clinical interpretation.* Tucson, AZ: Neuropsychology Press.

Rockey, L. A. (1997). Memory assessment of the older adult. In P. D. Nussbaum (Ed.), *Handbook of neuropsychology and aging* (pp. 385–393). New York: Plenum Press.

Ruchinskas, R. A., & Curylo, K. J. (2003). Cognitive screening in geriatric rehabilitation. *Rehabilitation Psychology, 48*(1), 14–22.

Schaie, K. W. (1974). Translations in gerontology from lab to life: Intellectual functioning. *American Psychologist, 29*, 802–807.

Schaie, K. W. (1985). *Manual for the Schaie-Thurstone test of adult mental abilities.* Mountain View, CA: Consulting Psychologists' Press. Available from the author, Penn State Gerontology Center, 105 Henderson S, Penn State University, University Park, PA 16802.

Schultheis, M. T., Caplan, B., Ricker, J. H., & Woessner, R. (2000). Fractioning the Hooper: A multiple-choice response format. *The Clinical Neuropsychologist, 14*(2), 196–210.

Smith, D. (2002). The decision-making process for developing testing accommodations. In R. B. Ekstrom & D. K. Smith (Eds.), *Assessing individuals with disabilities in educational, employment, and counseling settings* (pp. 71–86). Washington, DC: American Psychological Association.

Spreen, O., & Strauss, E. (1998). *A compendium of neuropsychological tests.* New York: Oxford University Press.

Storandt, M., & Futterman, A. (1982). Stimulus size and performance on two subtests of the Wechsler Adult Intelligence Scale by younger and older adults. *Journal of Gerontology, 37*(5), 602–603.

Thurstone, L. L., & Thurstone, T. G. (1962). *Primary Mental Abilities Test, Revised.* Chicago: Science Research Associates.

Toyokura, M., Sawatari, M., Nishimura, Y., & Ishida, A. (2003). Nondominant hand performance of the Japanese Trail Making Test and its mirror version. *Archives of Physical Medicine and Rehabilitation, 84,* 691–693.

Tuokko, H., & Hadjistavropoulos, T. (1998). *An assessment guide to geriatric neuropsychology.* Mahwah, NJ: Lawrence Erlbaum Associates, Inc.

Wechsler, D. (1981). *Wechsler Adult Intelligence Scale–revised.* New York: Psychological Corporation.

Willingham, W. W., Ragosta, M., Bennett, R. E., Braun, H., Rock, D. A., & Powers, D. (1988). *Testing handicapped people.* Boston: Allyn & Bacon.

Wilson, B. C. (1986). An approach to neuropsychological assessment of the preschool child with developmental deficits. In S. B. Filskov & T. J. Boll (Eds.), *Handbook of clinical neuropsychology* (Vol. 2, pp. 121–171). New York: Wiley.

York, C., & Cermak, S. (1995). Visual perception and praxis in adults after stroke. *American Journal of Occupational Therapy, 49,* 543–550.

6 Cultural considerations in the neuropsychological assessment of older adults

Desiree A. Byrd and Jennifer J. Manly

One of the most common applications of neuropsychology is the assessment of cognitive dysfunction in older adults. The United States Census Bureau approximates that the demographic composition of Americans over the age of 65 will experience a profound shift in the coming decades. It is estimated that by 2030 ethnic minority elders will comprise one-quarter of the geriatric population (US Bureau of the Census, 1996; US Bureau of the Census and National Institute on Aging, 1993). The projected change in the ethnic composition of the geriatric population requires that neuropsychologists be prepared to accurately meet the assessment needs of this population.

It is well established that neuropsychological test scores are sensitive to an array of factors other than brain damage, among them: age, education, gender, and socioeconomic status (Bornstein, 1985; Heaton, Ryan, Grant, & Matthews, 1996; Heaton, Taylor, & Manly, 2003; Neisser et al., 1996; Nichols & Anderson, 1974; Prigatano & Parsons, 1976). Consideration of these factors help neuropsychologists detect brain damage more accurately and thus provide more valid assessment services (Heaton et al., 1996; Lichtenberg, Ross, & Christensen, 1994). However, it has not been until recently that the impact of ethnicity has been rigorously explored in neuropsychology (Byrd, Touradji, & Manly, 2004; Ferraro, 2002; Fletcher-Janzen, Strickland, & Reynolds, 2000; Geisinger, 1994; Loewenstein, Arguelles, Arguelles, & Linn-Fuentes, 1994; Manly, Byrd, Touradji, Sanchez, & Stern, 2004). The knowledge base of cross-cultural neuropsychology has been primarily acquired through research with geriatric populations (Ferarro, 2002; Fillenbaum, Heyman, Williams, Prosnitz, & Burchett, 1990; Lichtenberg, Ross, Youngblade, & Vangel, 1998; Manly, Jacobs et al., 1998; Manly, Jacobs, Touradji, Small, & Stern, 2002; Marcopulos, McLain, & Giuliano, 1997; Unverzagt, Hall, Torke, & Rediger, 1996). A review of published studies examining Hispanic neuropsychological performance indicated that 76% of the studies were completed with older adults (Gasquoine, 2001). Therefore, geriatric cross-cultural neuropsychology is the most established subsection of this emerging specialty area.

One consistent finding across cross-cultural studies of cognition in American ethnic groups is the existence of significant performance differences between neurologically healthy minority and Caucasian elders that persist after statistical corrections and matching for age, years of education, and gender (Arnold, Montgomery, Castaneda, & Longoria, 1994; Gladsjo et al., 1999; Jacobs et al., 1997; Longobardi, Cummings, & Anderson-Hanley, 2000; Loewenstein, Duara, Arguelles, & Arguelles, 1995; Manly, Jacobs et al., 1998; Stricks, Pittman, Jacobs, Sano, & Stern, 1998). These differences, which are reflective of differential, though normal performance variations, often result in disproportionate misdiagnoses of cognitive disorders among minority elders (Bohnstedt, Fox, & Kohatsu, 1994; Gurland, Wilder, Cross, Teresi, & Barrett, 1992; Manly, Miller et al., 1998; Mungas, Marshall, Weldon, Haan, & Reed, 1996; Patton et al., 2003; Welsh et al., 1995). Given the many dangers associated with misunderstood ethnicity-related cognitive test differences, social, educational, and ethical concerns demand an increased understanding of the neuropsychological functioning of culturally diverse elders.

The goals of this chapter are to: (1) inform neuropsychologists of the multiple ways that culture can influence geriatric neuropsychological assessment, (2) review sources of culture-based performance differences, (3) offer guidelines for conducting clinical assessments with culturally diverse elders, and (4) highlight useful directions for future neuropsychological research with minority elders.

Definition of culture

Culture is a complex, multi-dimensional, fluid construct that is commonly conceptualized as learned and shared beliefs, traditions, and values among a group of people (Bentacourt & Lopez, 1993; Okazaki & Sue, 1995; Phinney, 1996). Though the concept of culture is often considered synonymous with the notion of race, culture is not defined by biological characteristics such as skin tone or traditional "racial" classifications. There can be significant cultural variation within groups that share physical characteristics or racial categories. An illustration of the separability of culture from race is revealed in a study by Touradji, Manly, Jacobs, and Stern (2001) in which the cognitive test performance of United States versus foreign-born Caucasian elders was compared. Significant differences were reported between the groups. Foreign-born Caucasians earned lower scores on measures of verbal abstraction, naming, and verbal fluency, than the United States-born Caucasians. Results such as these highlight the importance of differentiating culture, which includes language use, from "race" in neuropsychological research and practice.

Culture and geriatric assessment

The neuropsychological assessment process is completed in several stages: referral, interview, test selection, test administration, interpretation, and recommendations/feedback. Below, we review the impact of cultural background on several of these stages.

Referral

All neuropsychological assessments start with a patient referral to the clinician. This initial phase of assessment is important for planning the testing session. The demographic information contained in the referral can help the clinician select measures and arrange for consultation (as needed). Some clinics, physicians, and senior centers may become frequent referral sources for patients from particular cultural groups. It is worthwhile to note when this occurs as such referral sources may also be able to provide valuable education for the specific ethnic group regarding cultural conceptualizations of dementia, attitudes toward psychology and testing, and caregiving patterns. In addition, these types of referral sources may be a starting point for the recruitment of bilingual psychometricians.

Cultural background also influences the point in the disease process at which elders from different ethnic groups are referred for dementia diagnostic exams. For example, there is evidence for delayed diagnosis among minority populations. African-American elders with dementia have been reported to first present to physicians with greater symptom severity, suggesting increased tolerance of symptoms among these patients and their families (Shadlen & Larson, 1999). Watari and Gatz (2004) reported that among Korean Americans with dementia, problematic behavioral symptoms such as wandering, rather than cognitive symptoms, were more likely to prompt the initial medical visit. The reasons for diagnostic delay in minority elders are multifactorial. Minority elders and their family members may hold alternative views of aging and dementia, and lack information about the disease (Hinton, 2002). Studies have also reported higher tolerance and normalization of dementia symptoms in these populations (Elliot, Di Minno, Lam, & Tu, 1996; Shadlen & Larson, 1999). Further, minority elders may not prioritize cognitive impairments in the face of other pressing concerns (i.e., economic challenges, other medical illness; Daker-White, Beattie, Gilliard, & Means, 2002). In an empirical study of the multiple barriers to dementia treatment for ethnic minorities, Ortiz and Fitten (2000) reported that personal beliefs (i.e., forgetfulness is a normal consequence of aging), lower socioeconomic status, and limited English proficiency were the primary factors that interfered with rapid diagnosis and treatment of dementia in minority elders.

Interview

The interview stage of assessment is primarily utilized to collect critical information regarding the client's social, medical, educational, occupational, and functional background. The interview is also used to establish rapport with the client and explain the assessment procedure. Rapport building may be more difficult with minority elders due to the increased likelihood of unfamiliarity with formal assessment procedures and culture-based notions regarding psychology and testing (i.e., suspiciousness; Millet,

Sullivan, Schwebel, & Myers, 1996; Poreh, 2002). Such notions may incline minority elders to be somewhat wary of the assessment process and require that the neuropsychologist make special effort to clarify procedures. Since many minority and immigrant older adults may have limited assessment experience, the neuropsychologist should not assume that they are aware of the purpose of the assessment, limits of confidentiality, expected testing behaviors (e.g., question answer format, speeded performance, etc.), or possible implications of the test results (Echemendia & Julian, 2001; Perez-Arce, 1999).

In light of the lack of data on the ecological validity of neuropsychological tests in ethnic minorities and the inherent difficulty in establishing accurate estimates of premorbid levels of functioning in these groups, the interview offers a valuable opportunity to obtain detailed information regarding functional status. The interview (with the client and appropriate collaterals) may provide the clinician with the most accurate sense of the patient's actual functional level. The interview can also elucidate cultural norms for functional expectations of elders, which may vary by gender (Loewenstein, Ardila, Rosselli, & Hayden, 1992; McCurry et al., 2002). For example, in patriarchal cultural groups, it may be normal for older adult men to not cook or complete housework while older adult women may not be expected to drive or make financial decisions. Without knowledge of the cultural guidelines that determine the expression of these behaviors, such normal variations risk misinterpretation as functional impairment. Additionally, in ethnic minority families, there is greater nonspousal care of dementia patients (Shadlen & Larson, 1999). This difference in caregiver–patient relationship must be considered when interview information is collected from collateral sources as it can influence the perception and evaluation of functional abilities. In summary, interviews with minority geriatric clients will be enhanced by sensitivity to cultural variations in interaction style, thorough explanations of procedures, and expanded inquiry regarding functional status.

Selection of assessment measures

The clinician's choice of assessment measures is especially pertinent when evaluating culturally diverse elders. The overall utility of the evaluation is heavily dependent on the measures used for the assessment. Many neuropsychologists prefer to utilize a standard battery for the benefit of familiarity, standardization across patients, and the ability to gain internal, client-referenced normative standards. However, if the selected battery does not include measures that have been validated in ethnic minority populations or that contain appropriate normative data, the clinician risks an invalid assessment. Evaluations with ethnic minority elders may require the clinician to alter their standard battery, especially if the client has limited education and/or minimal English language proficiency. The crucial process of selecting assessment measures for use with ethnic minority elders will require the clinician to remain abreast of developments in the cross-cultural neuropsychological literature as normative data for minority elders are continuously published.

Screening measures

Cognitive screening measures, such as the Mini-Mental State Examination (MMSE; Folstein, Folstein, & McHugh, 1975) are often used to diagnose and monitor neurocognitive disorders such as dementia. These measures yield a single score that is intended to reflect gross cognitive status. Screening measures are extremely popular in clinical and research settings due to the low cost, ease of administration, brief administration time, and absence of required specialized administration training. Screening measures such as the MMSE have been translated into numerous languages and used in a number of international studies (Ostrosky-Solis, Lopez-Arango, & Ardila, 2000; Small, Viitanen, & Backman, 1997; Werner, Heinik, Mendel, Reicher, & Bleich, 1999).

While screening measures are not a critical component of neuropsychological batteries, these types of tests pervade the scientific literature on studies of "cognition" and its relationship to functional status, rehabilitation, caregiver stress, disease progression, and treatment efficacy. Such measures are also used in research settings to categorize patients into dementia severity groups. Despite their widespread use in geriatric populations, numerous studies reveal their diminished sensitivity and specificity in minority and low education elderly (Gurland et al., 1992; Lampley-Dallas, 2001; Mungas, Wallace, & Reed, 1998; Taussig, Mack, & Henderson, 1996; Teresi et al. 1995). For example, Fillenbaum et al. (1990) reported that the specificity of the MMSE for detecting dementia was significantly lower for African-Americans (59%) than Caucasians (94%). Because of the significant influence of cultural background on cognitive screening tests, we suggest that clinicians from all fields employ more sensitive and extensive neuropsychological test batteries for the assessment and staging of dementia in minority elders.

Batteries and domain specific tests

An impressive amount of neuropsychological test development and normative data collection has taken place with minority elders in the past decade. These tests and supplemental normative data can guide test selection for neuropsychologists providing clinical or research services to minority elders. A summary of references to 20 tests from five cognitive domains (general ability, attention, memory, language, and visuospatial skills) that have been adapted or developed for use with Spanish speakers appears in a chapter by Ardila, Rodriguez-Menendez, and Rosselli (2002). In addition to these individual tests, several neuropsychological test batteries have been developed specifically for Spanish speakers, including the NEUROPSI (Ostrosky,

Ardila, & Roselli, 1999), the Batería Neuropsicológica en Español (Artiola I Fortuny, Hermosillo, Heaton, & Pardee, 1999), and the Neuropsychological Screening Battery for Hispanics (NeSBHIS; Pontón et al., 1996).

Numerous studies have provided African-American and Hispanic normative data for domain specific tests, screening measures, and dementia test batteries. These include data from New York City (Stricks et al., 1998), Detroit (Lichtenberg et al., 1998), the CERAD study (Fillenbaum et al., 1990), Indianapolis (Unverzagt et al., 1996), rural Virginia (Marcopulos et al., 1997), Los Angeles (Gonzalez, Mungas, Reed, Marshall, & Haan, 2001; Mungas, Reed, Marshall, & Gonzalez, 2000), and Jacksonville (Lucas et al., 2005). Neuropsychologists who serve African-American clients can also consult the recently published age-, education-, and gender-corrected normative dataset that includes data for African-American seniors (Heaton, Miller, Taylor, & Grant, 2004). This large-scale normative project based in southern California is the first of its kind to offer such accessible normative data for a comprehensive battery of neuropsychological tests that includes an expanded Halstead-Reitan battery, the Wechsler Adult Intelligence Scale, the California Verbal Learning Test, and the Wisconsin Card Sorting Test.

Translation of English-language tests

Clinicians and researchers sometimes erroneously assume that instruments are equivalent across populations as long as the test is administered in the native language of the individual. However, literal translation may not produce items with comparable word frequency and/or salience in each culture, resulting in different difficulty levels (Loewenstein et al., 1994; Sano et al., 1997; Teng, 1996). In addition, idiosyncrasies of different languages may introduce problems in equating certain tests. For example, when asked to name as many animals as possible in one minute, Hispanics produce fewer exemplars than do Vietnamese. This discrepancy can be explained by the fact that most animal names in Spanish are multisyllabic, while most animal names in Vietnamese are monosyllabic (Kempler, Teng, Dick, Taussig, & Davis, 1998).

Translators of cognitive measures must use extreme caution and proper methods to adapt measures into another language. Artiola I Fortuny and Mullaney (1997) describe several examples of Spanish versions of tests that include syntactic, lexical, and spelling errors. These authors also suggest that investigators consult only those who possess native fluency and in-depth knowledge of the culture before attempting to translate a measure. The accuracy of translated and adapted instruments should be checked following established guidelines (Artiola I Fortuny & Mullaney, 1997; Brislin, 1970, 1980; Loewenstein et al., 1994; van de Vijver & Hambleton, 1996). Researchers and clinicians must also develop standards to determine in which language bilinguals should be assessed.

Translation of measures is not simply a linguistic issue; measures must be culturally equivalent as well. That is, it must be determined whether the use of a particular test format to assess the cognitive skill of interest is equally valid within every culture in which the test will be administered (Teng, 1996; Teng et al., 1994).

Investigators must be aware that the published norms for tests administered in English are not necessarily valid when the tests are administered in another language (Demsky, Mittenberg, Quintar, Katell, & Golden, 1998). Further, they should not assume that test norms can be applied to distinct populations simply because they share a language. For example, there is evidence that several instruments developed in Spanish-speaking countries may not be functionally or linguistically equivalent when used among Spanish-speakers in the US (Artiola I Fortuny, Heaton, & Hermosillo, 1998). Similarly, tests and norms developed among a particular group of immigrants to the US (e.g., Cuban Americans) may not be valid among other groups in the US who share a language (e.g., Dominican or Puerto-Rican Americans; Loewenstein et al., 1994). Therefore, users of non-English tests should note the nationality of the normative sample to ascertain the appropriateness for use with specific patients.

Most normative data used by neuropsychologists are limited by a number of factors (e.g., geographic restrictions, small sample sizes, limited age ranges, lack of conormed measures, etc.). The normative datasets discussed above are no exception. However, they represent an important development in cross-cultural neuropsychology and can serve as an invaluable resource for neuropsychologists working with minority older adults.

Finally, the selection of measures to be used in research batteries for comparative cultural purposes should include a measure of literacy. Recent work by our research team demonstrates the importance of these brief measures for predicting test performance across ethnic groups on a number of cognitive tests (see "Quality of Education" section below). Likewise, the inclusion of measures of acculturation (including years in the United States for immigrants) can be used to help researchers better estimate actual ability level.

Test administration

The administration of neuropsychological tests follows standardized procedures. However, several cultural considerations can enhance this stage of assessment with minority clients. The application of the "process approach" to testing (e.g., examining the nature of errors, providing multiple-choice response options, allowing additional time to complete items, etc.) after the completion of standard assessments might yield useful information regarding the true cognitive potential of culturally diverse elders (Milberg, Hebben, & Kaplan, 1996; White & Rose, 1997). Additionally, neuropsychologists who utilize psychometrists to administer tests should sensitize them to the subtle nuances of cross-cultural interactions with older adult clients that might influence test administration (e.g., expected formality, level of comfort, and confidence with testing, eye contact, etc.).

Test administration and non-English speaking elders

A significant portion of minority elders may have limited English proficiency. Assessment of these elders is an especially difficult task given the language dependence of neuropsychological evaluations. Nonetheless, non-English speaking elders will inevitably present with assessment needs. The solution first considered by clinicians may be to enlist the assistance of interpreters. However, the use of untrained and uncertified interpreters is fraught with problems that can invalidate the assessment (e.g., unfamiliarity with neuropsychological terms, insufficient proficiency in one or both languages, compromised standardization, interference with timed tests) and should generally be avoided (Ardila, Rosselli, & Puente, 1994; Artiola I Fortuny & Mullaney, 1998; Echemendia & Julian, 2002; LaCalle, 1987; Puente & Ardila, 2000; Wong, Strickland, Fletcher-Janzen, Ardila, & Reynolds, 2000). Another consideration for the assessment of the non-English speaking elder might be the direct translation of test instructions and stimuli. However, when this procedure is applied without the collection of appropriate normative data, sensitivity and specificity can be severely reduced (Demsky et al., 1998). A final consideration might be the reliance on nonverbal measures, but this technique alone is also insufficient. Culture-related influences on testing supersede those related strictly to language, as demonstrated in a study by Jacobs et al. (1997) in which neurologically healthy Spanish-speaking elders earned significantly lower scores on tests of visuoconstruction and visuoperception than Caucasian elders, even after the differences in years of education had been statically controlled. Additionally, tests that rely on visual, rather than verbal, stimuli require verbal instructions and may involve the verbalization of completion strategies that are vulnerable to the language threats mentioned above.

Neuropsychologists who are asked to assess patients who speak an unfamiliar language should first seek referrals to colleagues who share the language of the client. This process can be facilitated through communication with professional organizations (e.g., the Ethnic Minority Affairs Committee of American Psychological Association's Division 40, the National Academy of Neuropsychology, the International Neuropsychological Society, and the Hispanic Neuropsychological Society). When a language-appropriate referral is not available due to geographic restrictions or, more commonly, the limited availability of bilingual practitioners, the use of interpreters may be unavoidable. In such cases, the identification of interpreters with professional training (e.g., trained psychometrists, court interpreters; Artiola I Fortuny & Mullaney, 1998; De Jongh, 1991) is optimal. While the need for interpreters has increased dramatically, empirical research and standard guidelines for their use have not mirrored the growth. Studies of the use of interpreters in mental health highlight the inherent difficulties with this process and suggest a starting point for the development of training guidelines (Hwa-Froelich & Westby, 2003; Raval & Smith, 2003). Increasing the linguistic diversity of testers and improving the availability of trained translators are thus worthwhile goals for investigators; when this is not feasible, the possibility of misinterpretation must be taken into consideration when interpreting results.

For bilingual clients, the literature suggests that, at least for Spanish-speaking bilinguals, the most valid performance estimates are gained through assessments in their dominant language and that the choice of assessment language should be made by the client (Artiola I Fortuny & Mullaney, 1998; Harris, Cullum, & Puente, 1995). As suggested by Ardila et al. (2002), reports from assessments completed with bilingual clients should certainly include notation of the language used for testing, whether an interpreter was used, the degree of the patient's bilingualism, and the degree of caution related to the possible penalizing effect of bilingualism.

Some cultural groups may possess strict provisions regarding the appropriateness of females being interviewed/tested outside of the presence of the male members of their family. In these situations, it may be necessary to provide the family with an extended discussion of the need for individualized testing and/or allow a family member to remain in the room during testing with explicit restrictions (i.e., seated outside of the range of view of the testee, no communication with testee, etc.) and include notation of the testing arrangement in the report.

Interpretation

The interpretation of neuropsychological test results is the most decisive aspect of the assessment process. In the assessment of ethnic minority older adult clients, the difficult task of interpretation of low test scores involves the determination of whether the results are due to language differences, limited education (if applicable), cultural background, or true cognitive dysfunction. Neuropsychologists working with culturally diverse elders should be aware of the ways in which the client's cultural background can influence the interpretation of test results.

The most detrimental consequence of not carefully considering cultural background is the misdiagnosis and mismanagement of neurocognitive disorders. It is possible that the test performance of a neurologically healthy minority elder will be influenced significantly enough by their cultural experience that their scores will be classified in the impaired range when, in fact, no disease process is present. Numerous studies have documented the disproportionate rates of misdiagnoses in functionally normal, neurologically healthy Hispanics and African-Americans when standard cutoff scores and normative data adjusting for years of education are used (Bohnstedt et al., 1994; Callahan, Hendrie, & Tierney, 1995; Gurland et al., 1992; Heaton et al., 2003; Manly, Jacobs et al., 1998; Mungas et al., 1996; Patton et al., 2003; Welsh et al., 1995; Wilder, Cross, Chen, & Gurland, 1995). Fillenbaum et al. demonstrated that misdiagnosis rates for dementia were higher for African-Americans than Caucasians when performance on five screening measures was compared against neurologists' diagnosis (1990). When misdiagnoses occur in clinical settings, the potential ramifications for the patient and family are daunting and can include: unnecessary pharmacologic intervention and diagnostic referrals, restriction of driving privileges, psychological distress, and improper residential placement. The implications of systematic misdiagnoses that occur in the context of research settings are equally harmful. Failure to consider culture in the interpretation of ethnic group performance differences can lead scientists to make erroneous conclusions regarding ethnicity and geriatric cognitive disorders, as well as misclassification of participants in randomized clinical trials aimed at slowing the progression of dementia or preventing the onset of cognitive dysfunction.

The vast health disparities among ethnic minority older adults highlight the need for neuropsychologists to consider a host of medical illnesses among the risk factors for certain cognitive disorders (Manton & Stollard, 1997; Smedley, Stith, & Nelson, 2003). Non-neurological medical diseases that can affect cognition could also be a source of cultural differences on cognitive test performance. For example, disproportionately high rates of hypertension, adult onset diabetes, and stroke place African-American older adults at increased risk for vascular dementia (Gorelick et al., 1994; Smith, Sayre, & Perry, 1996).

Functional status/ecological validity

The simultaneous assessment of functional and cognitive ability level is an important component of diagnosing dementias. Further, functional status is a core consideration in rating the severity of dementia and other neurological disorders as well as gauging the effectiveness of various treatments. As with the assessment of cognitive functioning, culture also influences the measurement of functional status, and the cultural validity of existing functional measures is not well established. Several studies report significant differences between minority and Caucasian elders on a number of functional measures (Carrasquillo, Lantigua, & Shea, 2000; Kelley-Moore & Ferraro, 2004). While the ability of neuropsychological tests to predict functional status has been reported to be in the moderate range, the extent to which this relationship is comparable in minority elders is yet to be determined (Sbordone, 1996).

To help ensure that the diagnostic decisions for ethnic minority older adults are valid, we suggest that neuropsychologists make special effort to support the diagnosis with confirmatory data from functional evaluations, reports from collateral sources, and the results of medical testing. Additionally, when a progressive disease such as dementia is suspected, neuropsychologists can consider offering provisional diagnoses until the disorder is confirmed through longitudinal assessments in which the patient's initial test scores serve as a baseline to which future assessments (6–12 months) are compared. We also suggest that clinicians utilize demographically appropriate normative data, such as those referenced in the Test Selection section, for the interpretation of test results from minority older adult clients. Finally, it is recommended that neuropsychologists explicitly discuss the influence of cultural factors on the interview, test administration, and interpretation of results in the final report.

Dementia

Culture is an important consideration for the diagnosis and management of dementia. Several population-based studies have reported significant cultural variations in the prevalence and incidence of dementia, with higher rates observed in African-American and Hispanic populations, relative to Caucasians (Fillenbaum et al., 1998; Gurland et al., 1999; Harwood & Ownby, 2000; Husaini et al., 2003; Perkins et al., 1997; Rosenstein, 1998; Tang et al., 2001; Unverzagt et al., 2001). The exact sources of these disparities are unknown and likely to be numerous. Available research identifies differential rates of cardiovascular risk factors (i.e., hypertension, diabetes), methodological and statistical limitations of studies, genetic factors, social influences, and ethnic discrepancies in the sensitivity and specificity of measures used to detect dementia, as major contributing factors (Fillenbaum et al., 1998; Gorelick et al., 1994; Harwood et al., 1999; Harwood, Barker, Ownby, & Duara, 2000; Kaufman et al., 1997; Manly, Jacobs, & Mayeux, 1999; Whitfield, Brandon, & Wiggins, 2002). Despite disproportionate diagnostic rates, the course and progression of dementia have been reported to be similar in African-American and Caucasian patients (Fillenbaum et al., 1998).

Culture-based variations also exist in help-seeking behaviors, assigned meanings to cognitive decline and dementia (Dilworth-Anderson & Gibson, 2002), rates at which comprehensive diagnostic evaluations are performed (Harwood et al., 1999), barriers to care for dementia patients (Ortiz & Fitten, 2000), familial patterns of caregiving (Harwood et al., 1998; Janevic & Connell, 2001), service utilization (Ho, Weitzman, Cui, & Levkoff, 2000), and the recognition and management of dementia (Harwood et al., 1999, 2000).

Sources of cultural effects on neuropsychological test performance

As suggested by Helms (1992), specification of experiential, attitudinal, or behavioral variables that distinguish those belonging to different ethnic groups, and that also vary among individuals within an ethnic group, may allow investigators to understand better the underlying reasons for the relationship between ethnic background and cognitive test performance. There is tremendous diversity in geographic, economic, and educational experiences, as well as level of exposure to White American culture among ethnic minorities. Current racial and ethnic classifications ignore this diversity. Yet it is these cultural and experiential factors that may account for the differences between ethnic groups on cognitive tests. Why not define and measure cultural experience instead of using classifications that ignore it? The following sections will describe investigations of within-group cultural and educational factors on neuropsychological test performance among ethnic minorities. This investigational approach may illuminate factors which can not only explain ethnic group differences on cognitive tests, but can inform us in the future development of measures designed to assess cognitive abilities salient within ethnic minority cultures. In addition, the effects of these cultural and educational factors on cognitive test performance must be well understood before test developers attempt to design "culture fair" measures.

Cultural experience

Level of acculturation was the first variable that our research team used to operationalize within-group cultural variability. Previous studies have identified ideologies, beliefs, expectations, and attitudes as important components of acculturation, as well as cognitive and behavioral characteristics such as language and cognitive style (Berry, 1976; Moyerman & Forman, 1992; Negy & Woods, 1992; Padilla, 1980). Acculturation has traditionally been measured among immigrant groups such as Hispanic and Asian Americans; however, Landrine and Klonoff (1994) reported the development of a reliable and valid measure of African-American acculturation. This scale assesses traditional childhood experiences, religious beliefs and practices, preferences for African-American music, media, and people, and the preparation and consumption of traditional foods. When acculturation is measured, the association of cultural experience with cognitive test performance can be assessed, and hypotheses regarding test performance among individuals with lifestyles that are very dissimilar to the majority culture can be tested.

Previous research on Hispanic groups has shown a relationship between acculturation and performance on selected tests of the Halstead-Reitan Battery among college students (Arnold et al., 1994), as well as a relationship between years in the US (a strong correlate of acculturation level) and perseverative errors on the Wisconsin Card Sorting Test (Artiola I Fortuny et al., 1998). Three studies have explored the relationship of African-American acculturation to cognitive test performance. Manly, Miller et al. (1998) found that among neurologically intact African-Americans aged 20–65, those who were less acculturated (more traditional) obtained lower scores on the WAIS–R Information subtest and the Boston Naming Test than more acculturated African-Americans. Among older African-Americans living in Jacksonville, FL, acculturation accounted for a significant amount of variance in WAIS–R Verbal IQ, Boston Naming Test, and delayed recall of stories from the Wechsler Memory Scale–Revised (Lucas, 1998). A recent study found that among African-American patients with traumatic brain injury, those who were less acculturated obtained lower scores on a neuropsychological test battery overall and specifically on the Grooved Pegboard and WAIS–R Block Design, and achieved a lower number of categories on the Wisconsin Card Sorting Test

(Kennepohl, 2002). A preliminary study among older, nondemented African-American residents of Northern Manhattan revealed that those who were more traditional (less acculturated), obtained lower scores on measures of figure memory, naming, repetition, and figure matching (Manly, Jacobs et al., 1998).

Taken together, investigations of acculturation level suggest that there are cultural differences within people of the same ethnicity that relate to neuropsychological measures of verbal and nonverbal skills, and that accounting for cultural experience may help to improve the accuracy of certain neuropsychological tests. Acculturation level probably reflects other cognitive and noncognitive factors that have a direct influence on test performance. For example, acculturation level may reflect the salience that a particular task has in everyday life. Specifically, those with ethnically traditional lifestyles may engage in fewer activities that are similar to those required for successful neuropsychological test performance. Acculturation may also reflect the emphasis that was placed on a particular task during development. Traditional ethnic minorities may not be as "testwise" or as proficient in the implicit and explicit requirements of cognitive measures. Acculturation may also reflect motivation or attitude toward testing. If individuals are suspicious of the value or intent of a task, they may not deliver their maximum performance. We assume that internalized competition will cause everyone to try their hardest, but competition on formal cognitive tests may be more valued in White American culture, and thus vary with level of acculturation among ethnic minorities.

Quality of education/literacy/years of education

Schooling is another aspect of cultural experience that has been proven to have significant effects on neuropsychological test performance, regardless of ethnicity (Adams, Boake, & Crain, 1982; Heaton, Grant, & Matthews, 1986; Lezak, 1995). However, in the United States there can be a great deal of discordance between years of education and quality of education; this is especially true among ethnic minorities and immigrants. Factors such as whether African-Americans attended school before or after the United States Supreme Court's 1954 Brown v. Board of Education decision banning segregation in public schools, unequal distribution of educational funds, variable teacher education, shorter length of school year, and lower attendance due to required work had a profound effect on the quality of education received by African-Americans (Anderson, 1988; Margo, 1990). Previous studies have demonstrated that African-Americans had reading skills which were significantly below their self-reported education level (Albert & Teresi, 1999; Baker, Johnson, Velli, & Wiley, 1996; Manly et al., 2002). Therefore, disparate school experiences, and resulting different bases of problem-solving strategies, knowledge, familiarity, and practice with test-like materials could explain why some African-Americans obtain lower scores on cognitive measures even after controlling for years of education. Because quality of education differs so dramatically between ethnic minorities and Caucasians and also within ethnic minority groups (depending on whether they were educated in segregated or integrated schools, or in other countries, for example), statistical control for years of education may be an inadequate method for equating ethnic groups on educational experience (Kaufman, Cooper, & McGee, 1997; Loewenstein et al., 1994).

Our research group recently reported a study that sought to determine if discrepancies in quality of education could explain differences in cognitive test score between African-American and Caucasian elders matched on years of education (Manly et al., 2002). A comprehensive neuropsychological battery was administered to a sample of nondemented African-American and Caucasian participants in an epidemiological study of normal aging and dementia in the Northern Manhattan community. The Reading Recognition subtest from the Wide Range Achievement Test–Version 3 (WRAT–3) was used as an estimate of quality of education. African-American elders obtained significantly lower scores than Caucasians on measures of word list learning and memory, figure memory, abstract reasoning, fluency, and visuospatial skill even though the groups were matched on years of education. However, after adjusting the test scores for WRAT–3 reading score, the overall effect of race was greatly reduced and racial differences on all tests (except fluency and a drawing measure) became nonsignificant. This finding suggests that years of education is an inadequate measure of the educational experience among multicultural elders and that adjusting for quality of education may improve the specificity of certain neuropsychological measures across racial groups.

These results suggest that reading level is sensitive to aspects of educational experience important for successful performance on measures across several cognitive domains that are not captured by years of education. Future work must clarify whether reading level is an accurate measure of quality of education and whether reading level-based norms provide more accurate detection of cognitive deficit than ethnicity-based norms.

Stereotype threat

Level of comfort and confidence during the testing session may also vary among ethnic minorities and contribute to performance on cognitive tests. The concept of stereotype threat has been described as a factor that may attenuate the performance of African-Americans on cognitive tests. Stereotype threat describes the effect of attention diverting from the task at hand to the concern that one's performance will confirm a negative stereotype about one's group. Steele and Aronson (1995) demonstrated that when a test consisting of difficult verbal GRE exam items was described as measuring intellectual ability, African-American undergraduates performed worse than SAT score-matched Caucasians. However, when the same test was described as a "laboratory problem-solving task" that was unrelated to intellectual ability, scores of African-Americans matched those of Caucasian students. Researchers have also shown that when gender differences in math ability were highlighted, stereotype threat undermined performance of women on math tests (Spencer, Steele, & Quinn, 1999) and the performance of White males when comparisons to Asians were invoked (Aronson et al., 1999). The role of stereotype threat in neuropsychological test performance of African-Americans has not been investigated to date. In addition, it is likely that the salience of negative stereotypes differs among African-Americans, and there-fore, stereotype threat will likely affect some test takers more than others. Investigations of the experiential, social, and cultural variables that affect vul-nerability to stereotype threat remain to be investigated.

Unknowns

The complete range of cognitive skills and learning strategies of ethnic minority elders may not be adequately tapped by standard cognitive tasks. Traditional cognitive measures are based within a dominant culture that emphasizes individualism, detail, and speeded performance, whereas tradi-tional ethnic minorities are more likely to ascribe to a belief system that is spiritually-based, holistic, and emphasizes interpersonal relationships (Asante, 1990; Boykin, Jagers, Ellison, & Albury, 1997; Shade, 1991). Therefore, culturally influenced variability in information analysis (e.g., holis-tic vs. detail oriented, functional vs. descriptive) may explain the observed ethnic group differences on several measures.

Perhaps traditional neuropsychological tests simply do not elicit the full poten-tial of all members of ethnic minority groups. Assessment of these yet unmeas-ured strengths could be the best way to detect subtle neurocognitive dysfunction among ethnic minorities. Evidence that supports this possibility is derived from studies that demonstrate that when test stimuli are more culturally pertinent to the experiences of African-Americans, performance improves (Hayles, 1991). Prior research indicates that African-Americans obtain higher scaled scores on meas-ures of divergent thinking or creativity than on traditional measures of general information or verbal abstraction (Price-Williams & Ramirez, 1977; Torrance, 1971). In addition, some research shows that in contrast to reports of lower African-American performance on memory tests with verbal and figural stimuli, African-Americans obtain higher scores on measures of facial recognition (both White and Black faces) than Whites (Barkowitz & Brigham, 1982; Golby, Gabrieli, Chiao, & Eberhardt, 2001), suggesting increased salience or experience with human face processing among African-Americans. These studies point to several alternative ways in which neuropsychological measures can be used to assess cognitive abilities that are salient within African-American culture.

Continued challenges

Recent and projected shifts in the demographics of the older adult popula-tion have increased the awareness of the importance of cross-cultural considerations in geriatric neuropsychology. As a result, cross-cultural neuropsychology has evolved as a burgeoning subspecialty. Scientists conducting research in this area face major challenges in the advancement of the field. For example, most of the literature in this area has focused on African-Americans and Hispanics. Research with other ethnic groups is necessary for a comprehensive understanding of the influence of culture on test performance and the diagnosis and progression of cognitive disorders. To this end, several studies have been completed. In a study of Japanese-American men aged 71–93 years living in Hawaii, the age-standardized prevalence of dementia was 7.6%, which was higher than rates for Japanese men living in Japan (4–6%), and similar to European populations (White et al., 1996). The authors suggested that environmental or cultural exposures associated with migration from Japan to Hawaii influenced the development of Alzheimer's disease in these Japanese-Americans.

Available studies suggest that most minority groups display similar patterns of earning overall scores that are significantly lower than Caucasian groups. Authors such as McCurry and colleagues (2001) and Shadlen and colleagues (2001) report that, similar to other American ethnic minority groups, Japanese-American elders earned consistently lower scores on most subtests of their batteries relative to the normative (Caucasian) sample. Such results highlight the need for research on the sources of similarities among non-Caucasian groups rather than the exclusive focus on the documentation of differences between Caucasians and specific ethnic minority groups. Perhaps through such efforts, insight into the importance of not sharing the same culture as the testmaker may emerge.

Cultural considerations in geroneuropsychology will benefit from increased exploration of the methodological properties of neuropsychological measures in minority populations. Additional studies are sorely needed to determine the functional equivalence and construct, predictive, and ecological validity of neuropsychological measures in culturally diverse elders (Skinner, Teresi, Holmes, Stahl, & Stewart, 2002; Teresi & Holmes, 2001).

Conclusions

As the American geriatric population becomes increasingly diverse, neuro-psychologists must rise to the challenge of valid assessment of ethnic minority older adults. Adequately addressing these issues is a complex task that will not be resolved by any simple or single resolution. Rather, it will require the concerted effort of neuropsychologists from multiple geographic locations who employ a variety of approaches and measures. In spite of the challenges, neuropsychological work with ethnic minority older adults does not have to be an overwhelming task. Work with culturally diverse elders has the potential to add a wealth of information to geroneuropsychology. In fact, increased understanding of cognitive processes and their interaction with treatment interventions and functional abilities in these heterogeneous groups is sure to broaden, and possibly change, the ways in which we think about the brain and how it expresses itself through the richness of the human experience. We encourage neuropsychologists to embrace the diversification of the recipients of our services. With the proper educational and empirical foundation, neuropsychology can meet the assessment needs of the growing ethnic minority older adult population.

References

Adams, R. L., Boake, C., & Crain, C. (1982). Bias in a neuropsychological test classification related to age, education and ethnicity. *Journal of Consulting and Clinical Psychology*, *50*, 143–145.

Albert, S. M., & Teresi, J. A. (1999). Reading ability, education, and cognitive status assessment among older adults in Harlem, New York City. *American Journal of Public Health*, *89*, 95–97.

Anderson, J. D. (1988). *The education of Blacks in the South, 1860–1935*. Chapel Hill, NC: University of North Carolina Press.

Ardila, A., Rodriguez-Menendez, G., & Rosselli, M. (2002). Current issues in neuropsychological assessment with Hispanics/Latinos. In F. R. Ferraro (Ed.), *Minority and cross-cultural aspects of neuropsychological assessment* (pp. 161–179). Lisse, The Netherlands: Swets & Zeitlinger.

Ardila, A., Rosselli, M., & Puente, A. (1994). *Neuropsychological assessment of the Spanish speaker*. New York: Plenum.

Arnold, B. R., Montgomery, G. T., Castaneda, I., & Longoria, R. (1994). Acculturation and performance of Hispanics on selected Halstead-Reitan neuropsychological tests. *Assessment*, *1*, 239–248.

Aronson, J., Lustina, M. J., Good, C., Keough, K., Steele, C. M., & Brown, J. (1999). When White men can't do math: Necessary and sufficient factors in stereotype threat. *Journal of Experimental and Social Psychology*, *35*, 29–46.

Artiola I Fortuny, L., Heaton, R. K., & Hermosillo, D. (1998). Neuropsychological comparisons of Spanish-speaking participants from the US-Mexico border region versus Spain. *Journal of the International Neuropsychological Society*, *4*, 363–379.

Artiola I Fortuny, L., Hermosillo, H., Heaton, R. K., & Pardee, D. (1999). *Bateria Neuropsicologica en Espanol*. Odessa, FL: Psychological Assessment Resources.

Artiola I Fortuny, L., & Mullaney, H. (1997). Neuropsychology with Spanish speakers: Language use and proficiency issues for test development. *Journal of Clinical and Experimental Neuropsychology*, *19*, 615–622.

Artiola I Fortuny, L., & Mullaney, H. A. (1998). Assessing patients whose language you do not know: Can the absurd be ethical? *The Clinical Neuropsychologist*, *12*, 113–126.

Asante, M. K., &. Asante, K. W. (1990). *African culture and the rhythms of unity*. Trenton, NJ: Africa World Press.

Baker, F. M., Johnson, J. T., Velli, S. A., & Wiley, C. (1996). Congruence between education and reading levels of older persons. *Psychiatric Services*, *47*, 194–196.

Barkowitz, P., & Brigham, J. C. (1982). Recognition of faces: Own-race, incentive, and time-delay. *Journal of Applied Social Psychology*, *12*, 225–268.

Bentacourt, H., & Lopez, E. R. (1993). The study of culture, ethnicity, and race in American psychology. *American Psychologist*, *48*, 629–637.

Berry, J. W. (1976). *Human ecology and cognitive style*. New York: Sage-Halstead.

Bohnstedt, M., Fox, P. J., & Kohatsu, N. D. (1994). Correlates of Mini-Mental Status Examination scores among elderly demented patients: The influence of race-ethnicity. *Journal of Clinical Epidemiology*, *47*, 1381–1387.

Bornstein, R. A. (1985). Normative data on selected neuropsychological measures from a nonclinical sample. *Journal of Clinical Psychology*, *41*, 651–659.

Boykin, W., Jagers, R. J., Ellison, C. M., & Albury, A. (1997). Communalism: Conceptualization and measurement of an Afrocultural social orientation. *Journal of Black Studies*, *27*, 409–418.

Brislin, R. W. (1970). Back-translation for cross-cultural research. *Journal of Cross-Cultural Psychology*, *1*, 185–216.

Brislin, R. W. (1980). Translation and content-analysis of oral and written material. In H. C. Triandis & J. W. Berry (Eds.), *Handbook of cross-cultural psychology: Vol. 2. Methodology* (pp. 389–444). Boston: Allyn & Bacon.

Byrd, D. A., Touradji, P., & Manly, J. J. (2004). Cancellation test performance in an ethnically diverse elderly sample. *Journal of the International Neuropsychology Society*, *10*, 401–411.

Callahan, C., Hendrie, H. C., & Tierney, W. M. (1995). Documentation and evaluation of cognitive impairment in elderly primary care patients. *Annals of Internal Medicine*, *122*, 422–429.

Carrasquillo, O., Lantigua, R. A., & Shea, S. (2000). Differences in functional status of Hispanic versus non-Hispanic White elders: Data from the Medical Expenditure Panel Survey. *Journal of Aging and Health*, *12*, 342–361.

Daker-White, G., Beattie, A. M, Gilliard, J., & Means, R. (2002). Minority ethnic groups in dementia care: A review of service needs, service provision and models of good practice. *Aging and Mental Health*, 6, 101–108.

De Jongh, E. M. (1991). Foreign language interpreters in the courtroom: The case for linguistic and cultural proficiency. *Modern Language Journal*, *75*, 285–295.

Demsky, Y. I., Mittenberg, W., Quintar, B., Katell, A. D., & Golden, C. J. (1998). Bias in the use of standard American norms with Spanish translations of the Wechsler Memory Scale–Revised. *Assessment*, *5*, 115–121.

Dilworth-Anderson, P., & Gibson, B. E. (2002). The cultural influence of values, norms, meanings, and perceptions in understanding dementia in ethnic minorities. *Alzheimer Disease and Associated Disorders*, *16*, S56–S63.

Echemendia, R. J., & Julian, L. (2002). Neuropsychological assessment of Latino children. In F. R. Ferraro (Ed.), *Minority and cross-cultural aspects of neuropsychological assessment* (pp. 182–203). Lisse, The Netherlands: Swets & Zeitlinger.

Elliott, K. S., Di Minno, M., Lam, D., & Tu, A. M. (1996). Working with Chinese families in the context of dementia. In G. Yeo & D. Gallagher-Thompson (Eds.), *Ethnicity and the dementias* (pp. 89–108). Washington, DC: Taylor & Francis.

Ferraro, F. R. (Ed.). (2002). *Minority and cross-cultural aspects of neuropsychological assessment.* Lisse, The Netherlands: Swets & Zeitlinger.

Fillenbaum, G., Heyman, A., Huber, M., Woodbury, M. A., Leiss, J., Schmader, K. E., et al. (1998). The prevalence and three-year incidence of dementia in older Black and White community residents. *Journal of Clinical Epidemiology*, *51*(7), 587–595.

Fillenbaum, G., Heyman, A., Williams, K., Prosnitz, B., & Burchett, B. (1990). Sensitivity and specificity of standardized screens of cognitive impairment and dementia among elderly black and white community residents. *Journal of Clinical Epidemiology*, *43*, 651–660.

Fletcher-Janzen, E., Strickland, T. L., & Reynolds, C. (Eds.). (2000). *Handbook of cross-cultural neuropsychology*. New York: Kluwer Academic/Plenum Publishers.

Folstein, M. F., Folstein, S. E., & McHugh, P. R. (1975). "Mini-mental State": A practical method for grading the cognitive state of patients for the clinician. *Journal of Psychiatric Research, 12*, 189–198.

Gasquoine, P. G. (2001). Research in clinical neuropsychology with Hispanic American participants: A review. *The Clinical Neuropsychologist, 15*, 2–12.

Geisinger, K. F. (1994). Cross-cultural normative assessment: Translation and adaptation issues influencing the normative interpretation of assessment instruments. *Psychological Assessment, 6*, 507–524.

Gladsjo, J. A., Evans, J. D., Schuman, C. C., Peavy, G. M., Miller, S. W., & Heaton, R. K. (1999). Norms for letter and category fluency: Demographic corrections for age, education, and ethnicity. *Assessment, 6*, 147–178.

Golby, A. J., Gabrieli, J. D., Chiao, J. Y., & Eberhardt, J. L. (2001). Differential responses in the fusiform region to same-race and other-race faces. *Nature Neuroscience, 4*, 845–850.

Gonzalez, H. M., Mungas, D., Reed, B. R., Marshall, S., & Haan, M. N. (2001). A new verbal learning and memory test for English- and Spanish-speaking older people. *Journal of the International Neuropsychological Society, 7*, 544–555.

Gorelick, P. B., Freels, S., Harris, Y., Dollear, T., Billingsley, M., & Brown, N. (1994). Epidemiology of vascular and Alzheimer's dementia among African Americans in Chicago, IL: Baseline frequency and comparison of risk factors. *Neurology, 44*, 1391–1396.

Gurland, B. J., Wilder, D. E., Cross, P., Teresi, J., & Barrett, V. W. (1992). Screening scales for dementia: Toward reconciliation of conflicting cross-cultural findings. *International Journal of Geriatric Psychiatry, 7*, 105–113.

Gurland, B. J., Wilder, D. E., Lantigua, R., Stern, Y., Chen, J., Killeffer, E. H., & Mayeux, R. (1999). Rates of dementia in three ethnoracial groups. *International Journal of Geriatric Psychiatry, 14*, 481–493.

Harris, J. G., Cullum, C. M., & Puente, A. E. (1995). Effects of bilingualism on verbal learning and memory in Hispanic adults. *Journal of the International Neuropsychological Society, 1*, 10–16.

Harwood, D. G., Barker, W. W., Cantillon, M., Loewenstein, D. A., Ownby, R., & Duara, R. (1998). Depressive symptomatology in first degree family caregivers of Alzheimer disease patients: A cross-ethnic comparison. *Alzheimer Disease and Associated Disorders, 12*(4), 340–346.

Harwood, D. G., Barker, W. W., Loewenstein, D. A., Ownby, R. L., St.George-Hyslop, P., Mullan, M., & Duara, R. (1999). A cross-ethnic analysis of risk factors for AD in white Hispanics and white non-Hispanics. *Neurology, 52*, 551–556.

Harwood, D. G., Barker, W. W., Ownby, R. L., & Duara, R. (2000). Clinical characteristics of community-dwelling black Alzheimer's disease patients. *Journal of the National Medical Association, 92*, 424–429.

Harwood, D. G., & Ownby, R. L. (2000). Ethnicity and dementia. *Current Psychiatry Reports, 2*, 40–45.

Hayles, V. R. (1991). African American strengths: A survey of empirical findings. In R. L. Jones (Ed.), *Black psychology* (pp. 379–400). Berkeley, CA: Cobb & Henry Publishers.

Heaton, R. K., Grant, I., & Matthews, C. G. (1986). Differences in neuropsychological test performance associated with age, education, and sex. In I. Grant & K. M.

Adams (Eds.), *Neuropsychological assessment of neuropsychiatric disorders* (pp. 100–120). New York: Oxford University Press.

Heaton, R. K., Miller, S. W., Taylor, M. J., & Grant, I. (2004). *Revised comprehensive norms for an expanded Halstead-Reitan Battery: Demographically adjusted neuro-psychological norms for African American and Caucasian adults.* Odessa, FL: Psychological Assessment Resources.

Heaton, R. K., Ryan, L., Grant, I., & Matthews, C. G. (1996). Demographic influences on neuropsychological test performance. In I. Grant & K. M. Adams (Eds.), *Neuropsychological assessment of neuropsychiatric disorders* (pp. 141–163). New York: Oxford University Press.

Heaton, R. K., Taylor, M., & Manly, J. (2003). Demographic effects and demographically corrected norms with the WAIS–III and WMS–III. In D. Tulsky, R. K. Heaton, G. Chelune, I. Ivnik, R. A. Bornstein, A. Prifitera, & M. Ledbetter (Eds.), *Clinical interpretations of the WAIS–III and WMS–III* (pp. 183–210). San Diego, CA: Academic Press.

Helms, J. E. (1992). Why is there no study of cultural equivalence in standardized cognitive ability testing? *American Psychologist, 47,* 1083–1101.

Hinton, L. (2002). Improving care for ethnic minority elderly and their family caregivers across the spectrum of dementia severity. *Alzheimer Disease and Associated Disorders, 16,* S50–S55.

Ho, C. J., Weitzman, P. F., Cui, X., & Levkoff, S. E. (2000). Stress and service use among minority caregivers to elders with dementia. *Journal of Gerontological Social Work, 33,* 67–88.

Husaini, B. A., Sherkat, D. E., Moonis, M., Levine, R., Holzer, C., & Cain, V. A. (2003). Racial differences in the diagnosis of dementia and its effects on the use and costs of health care services. *Psychiatric Services, 54,* 92–96.

Hwa-Froelich, D. A., & Westby, C. E. (2003). Considerations when working with interpreters. *Communication Disorders Quarterly, 24,* 78–85.

Jacobs, D. M., Sano, M., Albert, S., Schofield, P., Dooneief, G., & Stern, Y. (1997). Cross-cultural neuropsychological assessment: A comparison of randomly selected, demographically matched cohorts of English- and Spanish-speaking older adults. *Journal of Clinical and Experimental Neuropsychology, 19,* 331–339.

Janevic, M. R., & Connell, C. (2001). Racial, ethnic, and cultural differences in the dementia caregiving experience: Recent findings. *The Gerontologist, 4,* 334–347.

Kaufman, J. S., Cooper, R. S., & McGee, D. L. (1997). Socioeconomic status and health in blacks and whites: The problem of residual confounding and the resilience of race. *Epidemiology, 8,* 621–628.

Kelley-Moore, J. A., & Ferraro, K. F. (2004). The black/white disability gap: Persistent inequality in later life? *Journals of Gerontology: Series B, Psychological Sciences and Social Sciences, 59,* S34–43.

Kempler, D., Teng, E. L., Dick, M., Taussig, I. M., & Davis, D. S. (1998). The effects of age, education, and ethnicity on verbal fluency. *Journal of the International Neuropsychological Society, 4,* 531–538.

Kennepohl, S. (2002). African American acculturation and neuropsychological test performance following traumatic brain injury: An exploratory study. *Dissertation Abstracts International: Section B: The Physical Sciences and Engineering, 63*(4-B). (UMI No. 2002-95020-240).

LaCalle, J. J. (1987). Forensic psychological evaluations through an interpreter: Legal and ethical issues. *American Journal of Forensic Psychology, 5,* 29–43.

Lampley-Dallas, V. T. (2001). Neuropsychological screening tests in African Americans. *Journal of the National Medical Association, 93*(9), 323–328.

Landrine, H., & Klonoff, E. A. (1994). Cultural diversity in causal attributions for illness: The role of the supernatural. *Journal of Behavioral Medicine, 17*(2), 181–193.

Lezak, M. D. (1995). *Neuropsychological assessment* (3rd ed.). New York: Oxford University Press.

Lichtenberg, P. A., Ross, T., & Christensen, B. (1994). Preliminary normative data on the Boston Naming Test for an older urban population. *The Clinical Neuropsychologist, 8,* 109–111.

Lichtenberg, P. A., Ross, T., Youngblade, L., & Vangel, S. J. (1998). Normative Studies Research Project test battery: Detection of dementia in African American and European American urban elderly patients. *The Clinical Neuropsychologist, 12*(2), 146–154.

Loewenstein, D. A., Ardila, A., Rosselli, M., & Hayden, S. (1992). A comparative analysis of functional status among Spanish- and English-speaking patients with dementia. *Journal of Gerontology, 47*(6), P389–P394.

Loewenstein, D. A., Arguelles, T., Arguelles, S., & Linn-Fuentes, P. (1994). Potential cultural bias in the neuropsychological assessment of the older adult. *Journal of Clinical and Experimental Neuropsychology, 16,* 623–629.

Loewenstein, D. A., Duara, R., Arguelles, T., & Arguelles, S. (1995). Use of the Fuld Object-Memory Evaluation in the detection of mild dementia among Spanish- and English-speaking groups. *American Journal of Geriatric Psychiatry, 3,* 300–307.

Longobardi, P., Cummings, J., & Anderson-Hanley, C. (2000). Multicultural perspectives on the neuropsychological and neuropsychiatric assessment and treatment of the elderly. In E. Fletcher-Janzen, T. L. Strickland, & C. R. Reynolds (Eds.), *Handbook of cross-cultural neuropsychology* (pp. 123–142). New York: Kluwer Academic/Plenum Publishers.

Lucas, J. A. (1998). Acculturation and neuropsychological test performance in elderly African Americans. *Journal of the International Neuropsychological Society, 4,* 77.

Lucas, J. A., Ivnik, R. J., Smith, G. E., Ferman, T. J., Willis, F. B., Petersen, R. C., et al. (2005). Mayo's Older African Americans Normative Studies: Norms for Boston Naming Test, Controlled Oral Word Association, Category Fluency, Animal Naming, Token Test, Wrat–3 Reading, Trail Making Test, Stroop Test, and Judgment of Line Orientation. *The Clinical Neuropsychologist, 19*(2), 243–269.

Manly, J. J., Byrd, D., Touradji, P., Sanchez, D., & Stern, Y. (2004). Literacy and cognitive change among ethnically diverse elders. *International Journal of Psychology, 39,* 47–60.

Manly, J. J., Jacobs, D. M., & Mayeux, R. (1999). Alzheimer disease among different ethnic and racial groups. In R. D. Terry, R. Katzman, S. S. Sisodia, & K. L. Bick (Eds.), *Alzheimer's disease* (2nd ed., pp. 117–132). Philadelphia: Lippincott, Williams & Wilkins.

Manly, J. J., Jacobs, D. M., Sano, M., Bell, K., Merchant, C.A., Small, S.A., & Stern, Y. (1998). African American acculturation and neuropsychological test performance among nondemented community elders. *Journal of the International Neuropsychological Society, 4,* 77.

Manly, J. J., Jacobs, D. M., Touradji, P., Small, S. A., & Stern, Y. (2002). Reading level attenuates differences in neuropsychological test performance between African American and White elders. *Journal of the International Neuropsychological Society, 8,* 341–348.

Manly, J. J., Miller, S. W., Heaton, R. K., Byrd, D., Reilly, J., Velasquez, R. J., et al. (1998). The effect of African-American acculturation on neuropsychological test performance in normal and HIV positive individuals. *Journal of the International Neuropsychological Society, 4,* 291–302.

Manton, K. G., & Stollard, E. (1997). Health and disability differences among racial and ethnic groups. In L. G. Martin & B. J. Soldo (Eds.), *Racial and ethnic differences in the health of older Americans* (pp. 43–105). Washington, DC: American Psychological Association.

Marcopulos, B. A., McLain, C. A., & Giuliano, A. J. (1997). Cognitive impairment or inadequate norms: A study of healthy, rural, older adults with limited education. *The Clinical Neuropsychologist, 11,* 111–131.

Margo, R. A. (1990). *Race and schooling in the South, 1880–1950: An economic history.* Chicago: University of Chicago Press.

McCurry, S. M., Gibbons, L. E., Bond, G. E., Rice, M. M., Graves, A., Kukull, W. A., et al. (2002). Older adults and functional decline: A cross-cultural comparison. *International Psychogeriatrics, 14*(2), 161–179.

McCurry, S. M., Gibbons, L. E., Uomoto, J. M., Thompson, M. L., Graves, A. B., Edland, S. D., et al. (2001). Neuropsychological test performance in a cognitively intact sample of older Japanese American adults. *Archives of Clinical Neuropsychology, 16,* 447–459.

Milberg, W. P., Hebben, N., & Kaplan, E., (1996). The Boston process approach to neuropsychological assessment. In I. Grant & K. Adams (Eds.), *Neuropsychological assessment of neuropsychiatric disorders* (2nd ed., pp. 58–80). New York: Oxford University Press.

Millet, P. E., Sullivan, B. F., Schwebel, A. I., & Myers, L. J. (1996). Black Americans' and White Americans' views of the etiology and treatment of mental health problems. *Community Mental Health Journal, 32,* 235–242.

Moyerman, D. R., & Forman, B. D. (1992). Acculturation and adjustment: A meta-analytic study. *Hispanic Journal of Behavioral Sciences, 14,* 163–200.

Mungas, D., Marshall, S. C., Weldon, M., Haan, M., & Reed, B. R. (1996). Age and education correction of Mini-Mental State Examination for English and Spanish-speaking elderly. *Neurology, 46,* 700–706.

Mungas, D., Reed, B. R., Marshall, S. C., & Gonzalez, H. M. (2000). Development of psychometrically matched English and Spanish language neuropsychological tests for older persons. *Neuropsychology, 14,* 209–223.

Mungas, D., Wallace, R., & Reed, B. R. (1998). Dimensions of cognitive ability in dementia: Differential sensitivity to degree of impairment in Alzheimer's disease. *The Clinical Neuropsychologist, 12*(2), 129–142.

Negy, C., & Woods, D. J. (1992). The importance of acculturation in understanding research with Hispanic-Americans. *Hispanic Journal of Behavioral Sciences, 14,* 224–247.

Neisser, U., Boodoo, G., Bouchard, T. J., Boykin, A. W., Brody, N., Ceci, S. J., et al. (1996). Intelligence: Knowns and unknowns. *The American Psychologist, 5,* 77–101.

Nichols, P. L., & Anderson, V. E. (1974). Intellectual performance, race, and socioeconomic status. *Social Biology, 20,* 367–374.

Okazaki, S., & Sue, S. (1995). Methodological issues in assessment research with ethnic minorities. *Psychological Assessment, 7*(3), 367–375.

Ortiz, F., & Fitten, L. J. (2000). Barriers to healthcare access for cognitively impaired older Hispanics. *Alzheimer Disease and Associated Disorders, 14*(3), 141–150.

Ostrosky-Solis, F., Ardila, A., & Rosselli, M. (1999). NEUROPSI: A brief neuropsy-chological test battery in Spanish with norms by age and educational level. *Journal of the International Neuropsychological Society*, *5*, 413–433.

Ostrosky-Solis, F., Lopez-Arango, G., & Ardila, A. (2000). Sensitivity and specificity of the Mini-Mental State Examination in a Spanish-speaking population. *Applied Neuropsychology*, *7*, 25–31.

Padilla, A. M. (1980). *Acculturation: Theory, models, and some new findings.* Boulder, CO: Westview Press for the American Association for the Advancement of Science.

Patton, D., Duff, K., Schoenberg, M., Mold, J., Scott, J., & Adams, R. (2003). Performance of cognitively normal African Americans on the RBANS in community dwelling older adults. *The Clinical Neuropsychologist*, *17*, 515–530.

Perez-Arce, P. (1999). The influence of culture on cognition. *Archives of Clinical Neuropsychology*, *14*(7), 581–592.

Perkins, P., Annegers, J. F., Doody, R. S., Cooke, N., Aday, L., & Vernon, S. W. (1997). Incidence and prevalence of dementia in a multiethnic cohort of municipal retirees. *Neurology*, *49*, 44–50.

Phinney, J. S. (1996). When we talk about American ethnic groups, what do we mean? *The American Psychologist*, *51*, 918–927.

Pontón, M. O., Satz, P., Herrera, L., Ortiz, F., Urrutia, C. P., Young, R., et al. (1996). Normative data stratified by age and education for the Neuropsychological Screening Battery for Hispanics (NeSBHIS): Initial report. *Journal of the International Neuropsychological Society*, *2*, 96–104.

Poreh, A. (2002). Neuropsychological and psychological issues associated with cross-cultural and minority assessment. In R. F. Ferraro (Ed.), *Minority and cross-cultural aspects of neuropsychological assessment: Studies on neuropsychology, development, and cognition* (pp. 329–343). Lisse, The Netherlands: Swets & Zeitlinger.

Price-Williams, D. R., & Ramirez, M. (1977). Divergent thinking, cultural deficiencies and civilizations. *Journal of Social Psychology*, *103*, 3–11.

Prigatano, G. P., & Parsons, O. A. (1976). Relationship of age and education to Halstead test performance in different patient populations. *Journal of Clinical and Consulting Psychology*, *44*, 527–533.

Puente, A., & Ardila, A. (2000). Neuropsychological assessment of Hispanics. In E. Fletcher-Janzen, T. L. Strickland, & C. R. Reynolds (Eds.), *Handbook of cross-cultural neuropsychology* (pp. 87–104). New York: Kluwer Academic/Plenum Publishers.

Raval, H., & Smith, J. A. (2003). Therapists' experiences of working with language interpreters. *International Journal of Mental Health*, *32*, 6–31.

Rosenstein, D. L. (1998). Differential diagnosis of the major progressive dementias and depression in middle and late adulthood: A summary of the literature of the early 1990's. *Neuropsychology Review*, *8*, 109–168.

Sano, M., Mackell, J. A., Ponton, M., Ferreira, P., Wilson, J., Pawluczyk, S., et al. (1997). The Spanish Instrument Protocol: Design and implementation of a study to evaluate treatment efficacy instruments for Spanish-speaking patients with Alzheimer's disease. The Alzheimer's Disease Cooperative Study. *Alzheimer's Disease and Associated Disorders*, *11*(Suppl. 2), 57–64.

Sbordone, R. J. (1996). Ecological validity: Some critical issues for the neuropsychologist. In R. J. Sbordone & C. J. Long (Eds.), *Ecological validity of neuropsychological testing* (pp. 15–41). Boca Raton, FL: St. Lucie Press.

Shade, B. J. (1991). African American patterns of cognition. In R. L. Jones (Ed.), *Black psychology* (pp. 231–247). Berkeley, CA: Cobb & Henry Publishers.

Shadlen, M. F., & Larson, E. B. (1999). Unique features of Alzheimer's disease in ethnic minority populations. In T. P. Miles (Ed.), *Full-color aging: Facts, goals, and recommendations for America's diverse elders* (pp. 33–52). Washington, DC: Gerontological Society of America.

Shadlen, M. F., Larson, E. B., Gibbons, L. E., Rice, M. M., McCormick, W. C., Bowen, J., et al. (2001). Ethnicity and cognitive performance among older African Americans, Japanese Americans, and Caucasians: The role of education. *Journal of the American Geriatrics Society, 49*, 1371–1378.

Skinner, J. H., Teresi, J. A., Holmes, D., Stahl, S., & Stewart, A. L. (Eds.). (2002). *Multicultural measurement in older populations.* New York: Springer Publishing Co.

Small, B. J., Viitanen, M., & Backman, L. (1997). Mini-Mental State Examination item scores as predictors of Alzheimer's disease: Incidence data from the Kungsholmen Project, Stockholm. *Journals of Gerontology. Series A, Biological Sciences and Medical Sciences, 52*, M299–M304.

Smedley, B. D., Stith, A. Y., & Nelson, A. R. (Eds.). (2003). *Unequal treatment: Confronting racial and ethnic disparities in health care.* Washington, DC: National Academies Press.

Smith, M. A., Sayre, L. M., & Perry, G. (1996). Diabetes mellitus and Alzheimer's disease: Glycation as a biochemical link. *Diabetologia, 39*, 247.

Spencer, S. J., Steele, C. M., & Quinn, D. M. (1999). Stereotype threat and women's math performance. *Journal of Experimental and Social Psychology, 35*, 4–28.

Steele, C. M., & Aronson, J. (1995). Stereotype threat and the intellectual test performance of African Americans. *Journal of Personality and Social Psychology, 69*, 797–811.

Stricks, L., Pittman, J., Jacobs, D., Sano, M., & Stern, Y. (1998). Normative data for a brief neuropsychological battery administered to English- and Spanish-speaking community-dwelling elders. *Journal of the International Neuropsychological Society, 4*, 311–318.

Tang, M. X., Cross, P., Andrews, H., Jacobs, D. M., Small, S., Bell, K., et al. (2001). Incidence of Alzheimer's disease in African-Americans, Caribbean Hispanics and Caucasians in northern Manhattan. *Neurology, 56*, 49–56.

Taussig, I. M., Mack, W. J., & Henderson, V. W. (1996). Concurrent validity of Spanish-language versions of the Mini-Mental State Examination, Mental Status Questionnaire, Information-Memory-Concentration Test, and Orientation-Memory-Concentration Test: Alzheimer's disease patients and nondemented elderly comparison subjects. *Journal of the International Neuropsychological Society, 2*, 286–298.

Teng, E. L. (1996). Cross-cultural testing and the Cognitive Abilities Screening Instrument. In G. Yeo & D. Gallagher-Thompson (Eds.), *Ethnicity and the dementias* (pp. 77–85). Washington, DC: Taylor & Francis.

Teng, E. L., Hasegawa, K., Homma, A., Imai, Y., Larson, E., Graves, A., et al. (1994). The Cognitive Abilities Screening Instrument (CASI): A practical test for cross-cultural epidemiological studies of dementia. *International Psychogeriatrics, 6*, 45–58.

Teresi, J. A., Golden, R. R., Cross, P., Gurland, B., Kleinman, M., & Wilder, D. (1995). Item bias in cognitive screening measures: Comparisons of elderly white,

Afro-American, Hispanic and high and low education subgroups. *Journal of Clinical Epidemiology, 48*, 473–483.

Teresi, J. A., & Holmes, D. (2001). Some methodological guidelines for cross-cultural comparisons. *Journal of Mental Health and Aging, 7*, 13–19.

Torrance, E. P. (1971). Are the Torrance Tests of Creative Thinking biased against or in favor of "disadvantaged" groups? *Gifted Child Quarterly, 15*, 75–80.

Touradji, P., Manly, J. J., Jacobs, D. M., & Stern, Y. (2001). Neuropsychological test performance: A study of non-Hispanic White elderly. *Journal of Clinical and Experimental Neuropsychology, 23*, 643–649.

United States Bureau of the Census. (1996). *Current populations reports, special studies, P23–190, 65+ in the United States.* Washington, DC: US Government Printing Office.

United States Bureau of the Census and National Institute on Aging. (1993). *Racial and ethnic diversity of America's elderly.* Washington, DC: US Government Printing Office.

Unverzagt, F. W., Gao, S., Baiyewu, O., Ogunniyi, A. O., Gureje, O., Perkins, A., et al. (2001). Prevalence of cognitive impairment: Data from the Indianapolis Study of Health and Aging. *Neurology, 57*, 1655–1662.

Unverzagt, F. W., Hall, K. S., Torke, A. M., & Rediger, J. D. (1996). Effects of age, education and gender on CERAD neuropsychological test performance in an African American sample. *The Clinical Neuropsychologist, 10*, 180–190.

Van de Vijver, F., & Hambleton, R. K. (1996). Translating tests: Some practical guidelines. *The European Psychologist, 1*, 89–99.

Watari, K. F., & Gatz, M. (2004). Pathways to care for Alzheimer's disease among Korean Americans. *Cultural Diversity and Ethnic Minority Psychology, 10*, 23–38.

Welsh, K. A., Fillenbaum, G., Wilkinson, W., Heyman, A., Mohs, R. C., Stern, Y., et al. (1995). Neuropsychological test performance in African-American and white patients with Alzheimer's disease. *Neurology, 45*, 2207–2211.

Werner, P., Heinik, J., Mendel, A., Reicher, B., & Bleich, A. (1999). Examining the reliability and validity of the Hebrew version of the Mini Mental State Examination. *Aging—Clinical and Experimental Research, 11*, 329–334.

White, L., Petrovitch, H., Ross, G. W., Masaki, K. H., Abbott, R. D., Teng, E. L., et al. (1996). Prevalence of dementia in older Japanese-American men in Hawaii: The Honolulu-Asia Aging Study. *Journal of the American Medical Association, 276*, 955–960.

White, R., & Rose, F. (1997). The Boston process approach: A brief history and current practice. In G. Goldstein & T. M. Incagnoli (Eds.), *Contemporary approaches to neuropsychological assessment: Critical issues in neuropsychology* (pp. 171–211). New York: Plenum Press.

Whitfield, K. E., Brandon, D. T., & Wiggins, S. (2002). Sociocultural influences in genetic designs of aging: Unexplored perspectives. *Experimental Aging Research, 28*, 391–405.

Wilder, D., Cross, P., Chen, J., & Gurland, B. (1995). Operating characteristics of brief screens for dementia in a multicultural population. *American Journal of Geriatric Psychiatry, 3*, 96–107.

Wong, T. M., Strickland, T. L., Fletcher-Janzen, E., Ardila, A., & Reynolds, C. R. (2000). Theoretical and practical issues in the neuropsychological assessment and treatment of culturally dissimilar patients. In E. Fletcher-Janzen, T. L. Strickland, & C. R. Reynolds (Eds.), *Handbook of cross-cultural neuropsychology* (pp. 3–18). New York: Kluwer Academic/Plenum Publishers.

7 Structural and functional neuroimaging findings in normal and pathological aging

James T. Becker, Howard Aizenstein, and Meryl A. Butters

Over the past two decades new brain imaging techniques have become increasingly important components of the neuropsychologist's armamentarium. With the advent of computer-assisted tomography, and later magnetic resonance imaging (MRI), we left behind the pneumoencephalogram and other painful, and often risky, procedures. This revolution of neuroimaging now allows the scientist access to high resolution images of the brain that can be acquired quickly and without great risk to the patient or research subject. Functional neuroimaging techniques, such as positron emission tomography (PET), functional MRI (fMRI), and magnetoencephalography now permit the examination of brain activation during the performance of specific cognitive tasks, as well as localizing and quantifying various neurotransmitters, brain metabolites, and pathological deposits. All of these advances occur in concert with advances in data analysis techniques that have led to new (or newly adapted) methods for dealing with large datasets with unusual statistical assumptions.

One area of neuropsychology where these techniques have had a profound impact has been the area of the degenerative diseases of the elderly. Studies have addressed the relationship between the patterns of cognitive impairment and the underlying brain regional atrophy or dysfunction that might be responsible for such functional abnormalities. Further, structural and functional imaging data have been used to examine the risk of impending dementia, or the likelihood of developing Mild Cognitive Impairment. Another area of neuropsychology where neuroimaging is beginning to make significant inroads has been the area of geriatric depression. Studies have identified structural and functional brain changes that characterize depression in later life and that distinguish clinically significant subgroups of elderly depressed individuals. The purpose of this chapter is to describe some of these neuroimaging techniques, and to summarize some of the major findings in both dementia and late-life depression.

Structural neuroimaging

The most common method for analyzing brain structure involves the use of MRI technology. Although the methods vary, the goal is to determine, on either a regional or a brain-wise basis, the nature and extent of differences in volume (and in some cases shape) between subjects with the condition of interest and the appropriate controls. Generally, the analysis of brain structure falls into one of three categories: visual ratings of atrophy and white matter hyperintensities (e.g., the Cardiovascular Health Study; Bernick et al., 2001; Heckbert et al., 1997); manual tracing of either specific individual brain regions (e.g., Jack et al., 1997, 1999) or of the entire brain (e.g., Jernigan, Archibald et al., 1991; Jernigan, Salmon, Butters, & Hesselink, 1991); or automated (or semiautomated) analysis on a brain-wise basis (e.g., Voxel-Based Morphometry; Ashburner & Friston, 2000). Each of these techniques makes different assumptions about the principles underlying the analysis of brain structure, and thus each yields complementary information, and each has its own relative merits.

Structural imaging analysis of dementia

Structural neuroimaging studies are a standard component of any evaluation of an individual with a suspected neurodegenerative dementia (Knopman et al., 2001). Not only is the study useful for identifying causal factors of a neurobehavioral abnormality (e.g., cerebrovascular disease, tumor), but the pattern of brain atrophy can be informative for the differential diagnosis. Detailed analyses of the patterns of regional brain atrophy using the techniques of Voxel-Based Morphometry[1] (VBM) have revealed the prototypical pattern of gray matter loss in patients meeting the criterion for probable Alzheimer's disease (McKhann et al., 1984).

For example, in a VBM study of 20 probable Alzheimer's disease patients enrolled in University of Pittsburgh Alzheimer's Disease Research Center, the typical pattern of less gray matter in Alzheimer's disease (AD) can be demonstrated. In this study subjects were scanned using a Signa 1.5 Tesla scanner (GE Medical Systems, Milwaukee). All subjects underwent a volumetric spoiled gradient recalled (SPGR) MRI scan (TE = 5 ms, TR = 25 ms, 1.5 mm slice thickness, 0 mm gap, 40° flip angle). The SPGR sequence maximizes contrast between gray and white matter, and in order to minimize partial-volume averaging at the gray-white matter interface, the data were acquired in the coronal plane.

All MRI data were processed using Statistical Parametric Mapping (Wellcome Department of Cognitive Neurology, University College London) running in MATLAB (Mathworks, Sherborn, MA). The SPGR images were first reoriented into the axial plane, then spatially normalized into the same stereotactic space through registration with a T1-weighted template image (Montreal Neurological Institute template); the normalized images were saved with $1 \times 1 \times 1$ mm voxels. These normalized images were then segmented into gray matter, white matter, and "other" using a modified mixture model cluster analysis technique. This algorithm assigns each voxel a value reflective of a tissue type based on prior probability images and voxel intensity. The segmented images were smoothed using an 8 mm isotropic Gaussian kernel, and the general linear model was applied to localize brain regional differences in gray matter.

The results of a simple VBM analysis are shown in Figure 7.1 (see color plate section). The data are rendered onto the standard young, normal control subject brain available in SPM. The colored areas indicate the individual voxels whose gray matter volume was significantly less among the AD patients than among the controls. As would be expected, the medial temporal lobe and temporal and parietal cortices show the greatest degree of brain-regional atrophy.

Brain-regional differences in structure in AD with and without psychosis

These structural images can also be used to examine the relationship between brain atrophy and the presence of a specific neurobehavioral sign or symptom. For example, a similar VBM analysis was completed on probable AD patients, to determine whether there was a neuroanatomical difference as a function of the presence of psychosis. Psychotic symptoms in AD (AD with psychosis, AD+P) are identified with a heritable phenotype (Steet, Nimgaonkar, Devlin, Lopez, & DeKosky, 2002; Steet et al., 1998), and functional imaging studies have reported that AD+P is associated with dysfunction in the prefrontal-temporal (Lopez, Smith, Becker, Meltzer, & DeKosky, 2001), cingulate, ventral striatal-thalamic, and parietal regions (Mega et al., 2000). Postmortem magnetic resonance spectroscopy studies indicate that AD+P is associated with reduced neuronal and synaptic markers in the neocortical regions. Thus, Prasad, Davis, Becker, Keshavan, and Sweet (2003) completed a VBM analysis to elucidate the brain regions that could be structurally abnormal in AD+P, compared to AD without psychotic features.

The MRI scans from 18 patients with psychotic features (i.e., delusions and/or hallucinations) were compared with those of 22 AD patients without psychosis and 16 normal controls. The psychotic symptoms were assessed by geriatric psychiatrists using the CERAD Behavioral Rating Scale (Hughes, Berg, & Danzinger, 1982). Among the AD+P patients were 13 with misidentification syndromes, and 5 with paranoid delusions. The groups were equivalent in terms of age, gender, number of years of education, and duration of AD.

Figure 7.2 (see color plate section) shows the areas of brain regional atrophy; of particular importance was the finding that the AD+P patients had greater atrophy in the basal ganglia as well as the amygdala, which raises the possibility that dopamine systems may be more impaired in AD+P than in AD without psychosis.

Brain regional differences in good/poor naming in AD

In a further analysis of these kinds of structure:function relationships, we examined the visual naming defect in AD. The temporal lobes are particularly vulnerable to the disease process, especially the mesial temporal structures of the hippocampus and parahippocampal gyrus (Juottonen et al., 1998;

Krasuski et al., 1998). In an effort to establish a relationship between semantic memory function and the structural integrity of the temporal lobe in AD, we correlated the size of specific temporal lobe regions with performance on the simple naming task included in the Alzheimer's Disease Assessment Scale (ADAS). Using the procedure described by Convit et al. (1995) we measured the volumes of the middle and inferior temporal lobes, the fusiform and parahippocampal gyri, and the hippocampus proper (bilaterally) among right-handed AD patients. The data suggest that there is a relatively specific association between atrophy in the left middle temporal gyrus and naming ability among right-handed patients (see Figure 7.3) (Miller et al., 2000). A multiple linear regression analysis of the behavioral and morphometry data revealed that, after controlling for age, education, and sex, there was a significant association between middle temporal cortex volume and the number of errors on the ADAS naming test, $t(19) = -3.45, p = .005$.

Structural imaging analysis of mild cognitive impairment

The transitional state between normal aging and AD has become a focus of research due to the development of effective pharmacotherapy aimed at altering the natural history of the disease. Mild cognitive impairment (MCI) is considered such a transitional state (Bowen et al., 1997; Lopez, Jagust, DeKosky et al., 2003; Morris et al., 2001; Petersen et al., 1999) and thus warrants identification as a potential target for therapeutic intervention. MCI includes those individuals who have: (1) subjective memory complaint, (2) objective evidence of abnormal memory functioning for age, (3) otherwise normal general cognitive function, (4) the absence of dementia, and (5) no alteration in activities of daily living.

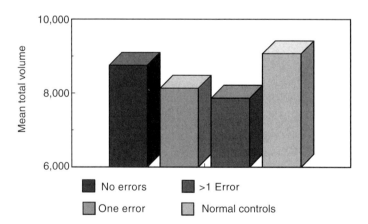

Figure 7.3   The relationship between middle temporal gyrus volume and performance on the naming subtest of the ADAS. The volumes were calculated using the method of Convit et al. (1995).

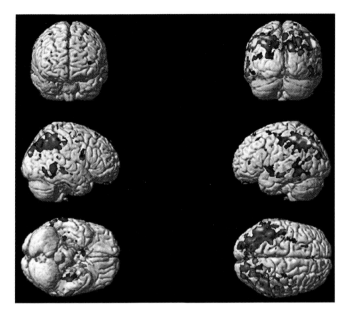

Figure 7.1   The results of the VBM analysis comparing probable AD patients with healthy, elderly controls. The voxels that had significantly decreased volume in the patients compared to the controls is rendered onto the surface of an individual, control subject's brain.

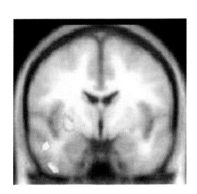

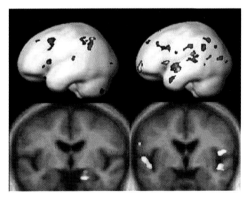

Figure 7.2   Coronal image from SPM showing area of decreased gray matter volume in AD patients with psychosis (compared to healthy control subjects).

Figure 7.4   Results of VBM analysis comparing gray matter volumes in MCI-A (left column) and MCI-MCD (right column) to normal control subjects. The top row shows the regions of cortical atrophy projected onto an average brain image. The bottom row shows the regional atrophy projected onto a coronal section through an average MCI patient brain.

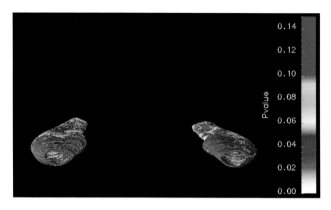

Figure 7.5 Three-dimensional mesh images of the hippocampus showing areas of atrophy in AD patients.

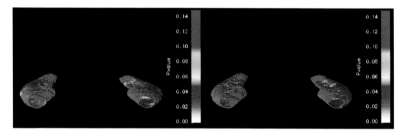

Figure 7.6 Three-dimensional mesh images of the hippocampus showing areas of atrophy in MCI patients. The left-hand image shows the areas of atrophy in the amnesic MCI cases, while the right-hand image shows the atrophy in the MCI-MCD cases. Although the MCI-A cases had significantly smaller hippocampi than did the controls, the MCI-MCD cases did not.

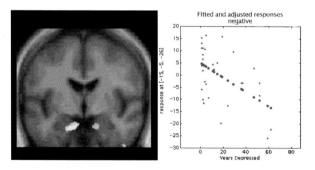

Figure 7.7 The relationship between hippocampal atrophy and depression. The figure on the left shows the correlation (overlaid onto a coronal section through the hippocampus) between brain volume and years since first depressive episode. The right-hand figure shows the same relationship, but plotted as a function of time.

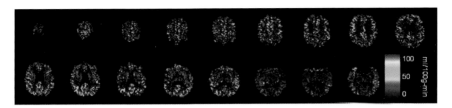

Figure 7.8 Multislice CASL perfusion maps in elderly volunteer at 1.5 T. Alternating label and control images were acquired using a 3.7 s RF irradiation period, a 0.7 s transit delay, and a 1 s multislice acquisition using echo planar imaging (EPI: 64 × 64, 20 cm field of view, 21 ms echo time, 90° flip angle, 5 mm thick, 0 spacing) (courtesy of H. Michael Gach, University of Pittsburgh).

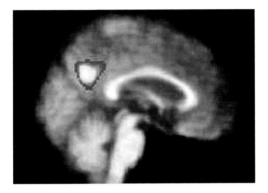

Figure 7.10 Regional CBF in the posterior ingulate cortex among AD patients with a better response to cholinesterase inhibition.

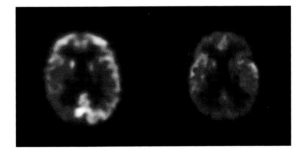

Figure 7.11 FDG scans of brain metabolism in AD and DLB. The left-hand image shows an AD patient with decreased glucose metabolic activity in the right parietal cortex, and preservation of occipital metabolism. The right-hand image shows the metabolism of a DLB patient with more severe (and bilateral) metabolic reductions, most prominent in the parietal and the occipital cortices (courtesy of N. Bohnen, University of Pittsburgh).

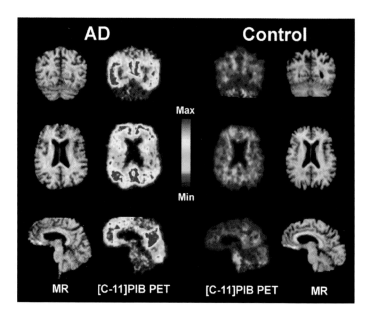

Figure 7.12 Example of visualization of beta-amyloid using the Pittsburgh Compound-B, and brain metabolism as shown by FDG (courtesy of W. Klunk, University of Pittsburgh).

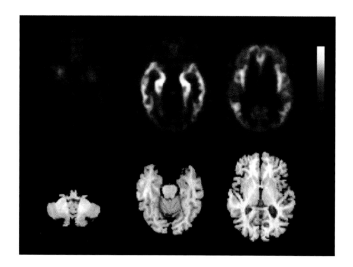

Figure 7.13 Coregistered PET and MR images of a healthy 74-year-old man, showing the distribution of 5-HT1A receptors, including midbrain region of the raphe and hippocampus (top row, middle image). Lack of binding in the cerebellum, where there are negligible 5-HT1A receptors, is also demonstrated (top row, left image) (courtesy of C. C. Meltzer, University of Pittsburgh).

A number of brain structural abnormalities have been identified among MCI patients with abnormal memory; there is significant reduction in the volume of the hippocampus (De Santi et al., 2001; Soininen et al., 1994; Wolf et al., 2001), medial occipitotemporal lobe (Convit et al., 2000), parahippocampal gyrus, entorhinal cortex, superior temporal gyrus, and anterior cingulate gyrus (Killiany et al., 2000; Visser et al., 1999). These morphological abnormalities are particularly severe among those MCI patients who progress to AD compared to those who do not (Killiany et al., 2000; Visser et al., 1999; Visser, Verhey, Hofman, Scheltens, & Jolles, 2002). Although many individuals diagnosed with MCI go on to develop AD, others do not, and the relationship between MCI and AD remains a topic of active study.

Although the most common definition of MCI relies heavily on the presence of memory dysfunction, a growing number of studies have concluded that performance in other cognitive domains is not entirely normal (Hanninen et al., 1995, 1997; Lopez, Jagust, DeKosky et al., 2003; Petersen et al., 1999). In addition to memory impairment, patients with MCI can have verbal fluency, attention, and executive function deficits. Some MCI patients can have altered neuropsychological test performance in multiple cognitive areas, which may or may not include memory, and have mild or no significant deterioration of activities of daily living. Indeed, recent population studies have shown that the MCI-amnestic type (MCI-A) is less frequent than the MCI with a broader range of cognitive deficits (Lopez, Jagust, DeKosky et al., 2003; Lopez, Jagust, Dulberg et al., 2003).

Using a VBM analysis, Bell-McGinty, Lopez et al. (2002) compared and contrasted the cortical volumes of the two types of MCI patients: MCI-A ($n = 9$) or MCI-Multiple Cognitive Domain (MCI-MCD; $n = 28$). All of the MCI patients had subjective complaints of cognitive impairment with little alteration of activities of daily living, and a history of normal intellectual function before symptom onset. The subgroups differed in terms of the nature and extent of objectively measured cognitive impairment. MCI-A patients met diagnostic criteria for an idiopathic amnestic disorder; they had an isolated memory deficit with performance at least two standard deviation units below the level expected on measures of memory and learning, with otherwise normal cognitive functions. MCI-MCD patients performed abnormally ($-1 \geq z \geq -2$) on at least one measure in two or more cognitive domains, which may or may not have included memory.

The MCI subjects, as a group, had significantly decreased volume in the hippocampus and middle temporal gyrus, bilaterally (see Figure 7.4 in color plate section). In addition, the left inferior parietal, left middle frontal, and right superior frontal volumes were also reduced in MCI relative to control subjects. The MCI-A subjects had significantly reduced volume of the mesial temporal lobe on the right, including the hippocampus, entorhinal cortex, and cingulate (see Figure 7.4) compared to control subjects. In addition, reduced volume was observed in the left inferior parietal, inferior and middle frontal, and superior temporal gyri. Subjects diagnosed with MCI-MCD had significant bilateral volume loss of the hippocampus, middle and superior temporal, and inferior frontal gyri compared to controls. In addition, the left inferior parietal gyrus and the right superior frontal gyrus were significantly decreased in MCI-MCD relative to controls.

Among all MCI patients who progressed to AD during follow-up, there was greater atrophy in the left entorhinal cortex, bilateral superior temporal gyri, and right inferior frontal gyrus relative to those who did not progress. Using the peak coordinates from these four regions identified, we extracted the adjusted values (using age as a covariate) from within SPM99. Partial correlation analyses, controlling for age, showed significant positive correlations between the MMSE score and the volumes of the left entorhinal cortex, $r = .35$, $df = 34$, $p = .04$, and right inferior frontal gyrus, $r = .36$, $df = 34$, $p = .03$.

These data demonstrate that there are distinct brain structural abnormalities in the two subgroups of MCI patients. Specifically, MCI-A patients have structural abnormalities of the hippocampus and entorhinal cortex, as would be expected, but there are additional structural abnormalities in the medial temporal lobes (cingulate), and neocortex (inferior parietal, inferior and middle frontal, and superior temporal gyri on the left). Moreover, MCI-MCD subjects, who have a wider range of cognitive deficits, showed more diffuse and extensive volume loss in the neocortical heteromodal association areas (Mesulam, 1985) (bilateral middle and superior temporal and inferior frontal gyri, right superior frontal gyrus, and the left inferior parietal gyrus), with less involvement of the medial temporal lobe structures, compared to those diagnosed with MCI-A.

These data also confirm that structural abnormalities in specific cortical regions precede the development of dementia in MCI patients; those who later developed AD had significantly decreased volume of the left entorhinal cortex, bilateral superior temporal gyri, and right inferior frontal gyrus compared to those MCI subjects who did not progress. The degree of cognitive impairment, a marker of how close the patient is to a diagnosis of AD, was significantly related to the degree of volume loss in both the frontal and entorhinal areas.

Another method of analysis of brain structure uses three-dimensional reconstructions of hippocampus to determine not only total regional volume, but also shape and size of abnormalities (Narr et al., 2004). Investigators at the University of Pittsburgh ADRC, in collaboration with colleagues at the Laboratory of Neuroimaging at the University of California—Los Angeles (http://www.loni.ucla.edu/) have recently completed an analysis comparing hippocampal volumes among AD patients ($n = 20$), MCI-MCD ($n = 20$), MCI-A ($n = 6$), and age- and education-equivalent control subjects ($n = 20$) (Davis et al., 2004). Figures 7.5 and 7.6 (see color plate section) show the results of the analysis of the three dimensional mesh images of the hippocampi. As would be expected, the AD patients had significantly atrophic hippocampi compared to the controls. Furthermore, the MCI patients differed in their pattern of atrophy depending on whether they were of the amnestic or the multiple cognitive domain type. Specifically, the MCI-A cases showed significant atrophy along the inferior regions of the hippocampus, bilaterally, compared to the controls. However, there was no significant difference between the MCI-A and AD groups. By contrast, the MCI-MCD patients showed significant differences from the AD patients, but *no* significant differences from the controls.

These data are consistent with the VBM analysis in that they show that the two forms of MCI have different patterns of brain regional atrophy. Furthermore, the fact that the MCI-A group is more like the AD patients than the controls is consistent with the hypothesis that these patients have more AD-like pathology (at least in the temporal lobe) than the MCI-MCD patients. Thus, while the rate of conversion from MCI to AD may be the same in both groups (i.e., 12–15% per year), the focus of the neuropathological abnormalities differs between the groups.

Structural imaging analysis of depression in later life

Geriatric depression is a major public health problem, affecting approximately 15% of individuals over the age of 65. For these individuals, current treatments have only limited efficacy, with approximately 20–40% of elderly individuals with depression having a limited or delayed response to first-line antidepressant treatment (Lebowitz et al., 1997). A prominent theory for the delayed treatment response is that geriatric depression differs from depression in younger individuals by the presence of cerebrovascular and/or neurodegenerative changes associated with dysfunction in frontostriatal circuits.

Convergent evidence from structural neuroimaging, cognitive testing, and other methodologies supports the frontostriatal hypothesis of later life depression (LLD). Structural MRI studies (Alexopoulos, Kiosses, Choi, Murphy, & Lim, 2002; Krishnan, Hays, & Blazer, 1997) have shown that elderly depressed individuals have higher incidence of subcortical white matter and deep gray matter changes consistent with small vessel ischemic disease. LLD patients are impaired on tests of executive function as well as those of psychomotor speed, also suggestive of frontostriatal dysfunction.

Older depressed subjects have decreased parenchymal tissue density (by CT scan) as well as central and cortical atrophy (reviewed by Morris & Rapoport, 1990), and MRI studies have generally replicated these findings (Ballmaier, Sowell et al., 2004; Pantel et al., 1997; Rabins, Pearlson, Aylward, Kumar, & Dowell, 1991). LLD is also associated with changes in reduced frontal lobe volume in general (Kumar, Bilker, Jin, & Udupa, 2000), and in particular, the orbitofrontal cortex (Ballmaier, Toga et al., 2004; Lai, Payne, Byrum, Steffens, & Krishnan, 2000; Lee et al., 2003) as well as the gyrus rectus and anterior cingulate (Ballmaier, Toga et al., 2004). There also are basal ganglia lesions (Rabins et al., 1991; Steffens & Krishnan, 1998; Tupler et al., 2002), especially in the caudate, lenticular nuclei (Krishnan et al., 1996), and the putamen (Steffens & Krishnan, 1998; Tupler et al., 2002), that may be worse among late-onset patients. Finally, there is an association between chronic, treatment-resistant depression in groups of mixed ages and right, frontostriatal atrophy

(Shah, Glabus, Goodwin, & Ebmeier, 2002) and reduced volume of the left temporal cortex including the hippocampus (Shah, Ebmeier, Glabus, & Goodwin, 1998).

The hippocampus appears to be especially sensitive to the effects of major depression. Reduced hippocampal volume is particularly, but not exclusively, related to later age-of-onset (Steffens et al., 2000), and hippocampal volume is inversely related to conversion to dementia (Steffens et al., 2002). Further, significantly greater atrophy in the hippocampus was found among those LLD patients who were APOE e4 positive compared to those without the e4 allele.

The lifetime duration of depression (measured either as years since first episode or total number of days spent depressed) is very closely associated with hippocampal volume (Bell-McGinty, Butters et al., 2002; Sheline, Wang, Gado, Csernansky, & Vannier, 1996). Figure 7.7 (see color plate section) (Bell-McGinty, Butters et al., 2002) shows the correlation between mesial temporal regions and time since first depressive episode across the patients' lifespan. This indicates that these regions are particularly vulnerable to the chronic effects of major affective disorder, even when such disorders are optimally controlled.

One potential explanation for this association is that over time, repeated stress during recurrent depressive episodes results in injury to the hippocampus (Lupien et al., 1998, 1999). Possible mechanisms underlying the neuronal injury include glucocorticoid neurotoxicity, decreased brain-derived growth factor, decreased neurogenesis and loss of plasticity (for a review, see Sheline, 2003).

LLD is a heterogeneous disorder, and it is possible that the decreased hippocampal volume could be the result of more than one underlying process. For example, individuals with early onset, recurrent, depression may have hippocampal volume loss due to the repeated stress associated with recurrent depression. It is also possible that many individuals with later onset depression are in the prodromal stage of AD, their hippocampi having already sustained substantial neuronal loss due to cumulative AD neuropathology.

Functional neuroimaging

Altered cerebral blood flow in MCI and AD as measured by arterial spin labeling

Quantitative measure of cerebral blood flow (CBF) has previously been possible only with invasive procedures such as PET (see Table 7.1). However, recent advances in fMRI have permitted the measurement of "absolute" CBF using arterial spin labeling (ASL). Briefly, this technique uses nonionizing radiofrequency radiation to invert, or tag, proton spins in arterial water before they enter the tissue region of interest. CBF maps are derived from the difference images acquired with (label) and without (control) RF tagging, after normalization based on tracer kinetics and inversion efficiencies.

Table 7.1 CBF changes in dementia

Modality	Temporal			Parietal				Frontal			Occipital	Cingulate		Insular Cortex	Precuneus	Putamen
	Global	Association Cortex	Medial	Tempro-parietal	Global	Association Cortex	Medial	Global	Association Cortex	Medial		Posterior	Anterior			
MRI	−	−	+/−	−	−	−	−		−	−		−				
SPECT			−	−	−			−		−		−	+/−	−	−	−
PET					−			−			−					
Xe	−				−			−			−					

Hypoperfusion (−), hyperperfusion (+).
Sources: Alsop & Casement (2004); Alsop, Detre, & Grossman (2000); Brown et al. (1996); Glydensted & Oste-gaard (2004); Johnson & Jahng (2004); Johnson & Moran (2004); Kataki (2004); Nagata & Maruya (2000); Wang & Chu (2004).

Current multislice continuous ASL (CASL) techniques allow whole brain coverage using clinical imaging systems (Alsop & Detre, 1998) (see Figure 7.8 in color plate section). Perfusion measurements using ASL in humans have high correlation with alternative techniques ^{15}O PET and dynamic susceptibility contrast (DSC) MRI (Weber & Gunther, 2003; Ye & Berman, 2000).

However, there remain several technical issues associated with ASL that are currently being addressed by researchers in the field. First, the ASL difference signals are approximately 1% of the image signal, resulting in low perfusion signal-to-noise ratio (SNR) compared to relative CBF techniques. Higher magnetic fields (3 and 7 Tesla) offer both improved SNR and longer tracer life (Duong & Yacoub, 2002; Talagala & Chuang, 2004; Talagala & Ye, 2002; Zaharchuk & Ledden, 1999). Second, the specifics of blood and tissue exchange and transit times in ASL are still being characterized, particularly in the elderly who have a higher incidence of cerebrovascular disease and different arterial hemodynamics compared to younger or healthier populations (Parkes & Rashid, 2004). Nevertheless, the kinetics of the CASL endogenous tracer is much simpler than exogenous tracer techniques because of the former's localized bolus (Buxton et al., 1998; Thomas & Lythgoe, 2000). Third, aging and dementia are correlated with structural atrophy and morphometric variability (Chetelat & Baron, 2003), which affect measurement and localization of CBF. Computer-based methods for brain segmentation, coregistration, and perfusion analysis are most successful and accurate when using reference templates developed from elderly brains (Dai & Davis, 2004).

Gach et al. (2005) have further refined the technique to provide more reliable data, and have implemented it in elderly normal subjects, and patients with either MCI or AD. Using data obtained from an ongoing longitudinal study of MCI in a community-based epidemiological sample, they compared the blood flow of normal elderly controls, with that of AD patients. The results suggest that the relationship between blood flow and disease is more complex than previously thought. In particular, the CBF of subjects with vascular disease or hypertension (both patients and controls) is lower than that of healthier subjects. And, further, there is a suggestion that at least a subset of AD patients may be able to maintain a compensatory response, resulting in an *increase* in CBF.

BOLD finger tapping in aging

Given that there are alterations in cerebral blood flow in dementia, and that older individuals have altered hemodynamics, it is important to understand how these factors affect the blood oxygen level dependent (BOLD) response, which is the basis for fMRI. Several studies have demonstrated that the BOLD hemodynamic response function (HRF) in the precentral gyrus has a similar amplitude in young and elderly subjects (Buckner, Snyder, Sanders, Raichle, & Morris, 2000; D'Esposito, Zarahn, Aguirre, & Rypma, 1999; Huettel, Singerman, & McCarthy, 2001). However, when other brain regions are considered, different

HRF peaks are found between the young and elderly; for example, Buckner et al. (2000) reported that the HRF in the visual cortex has a greater amplitude in younger subjects than in the elderly in response to the finger tapping visual stimulus. Previous resting CBF studies (e.g., Marchal et al., 1992) and block-design fMRI studies of visual stimulation (e.g., Ross et al., 1997) have also found decreased signal in elderly subjects. In contrast to these results, Huettel et al. (2001) found similar BOLD amplitude peaks in the young and elderly subjects in the visual cortex on a visual checkerboard experiment.

Aizenstein et al. (2004) compared the mean HRFs of young and old subjects using a simple finger-tapping task. The subjects simply pressed keys (using both index fingers) when a visual stimulus was presented on a screen in the bore of the magnet. The results indicated that the HRF (represented as a time series in 2-second bins; see Figure 7.9) was abnormal in the elderly subjects compared to controls.

Of particular importance in this study was the method for determining the locus of functional activation. Functional imaging studies comparing elderly and young subjects are confounded by differences in brain anatomy between elderly and young subjects. Elderly brains have greater anatomic variability and often show decreased regional size. Thus, standard methods for aligning the functional imaging data into a common anatomic space may be biased. One method for addressing this concern is to use a single-subject region of interest (ROI) based analysis, focusing on regions for which there are initial hypotheses, and also limiting errors due to poor registration by selecting the ROI separately for each subject. For the HRF data described above, the time series were selected from brain regions defined using the template-based ROI, which had been projected onto the individual subject's own functional imaging dataset using a nonlinear warp and segmentation.

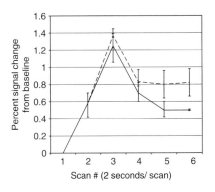 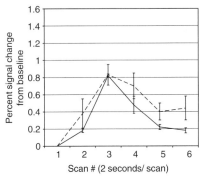

Figure 7.9 Alterations in the HRF in normal aging. The time series for visual (left side) and motor (right side) ROIs are shown here. Solid line represents mean young ($n = 9$) percentage signal change from baseline, dotted line is elderly ($n = 9$) percentage signal change. Error bars represent $+/-$ 1 *SEM.*

Functional imaging in AD and related dementias

Functional brain imaging using PET has been instrumental in identifying the neurobiological basis of important aspects of AD and related dementias. For example, CBF is a significant predictor of risk to convert to AD (Silverman et al., 2001), and degree of metabolic abnormality is a good index of disease stage (and a tool for understanding cognitive reserve; Stern, Alexander, Prohovnik, & Mayeux, 1992).

One very important contribution of functional imaging has been the study of treatment response in AD. Lopez, Becker et al. (2003) studied a group of AD patients prior to the initiation of anticholinesterase therapy, and again after 8–10 weeks of treatment. In line with other work, the posterior cingulate was found to have significantly decreased metabolism prior to treatment. However, what was more important was that the degree of cingulate abnormality was inversely related to treatment response. That is, those patients who showed a better response to cholinesterase inhibition had higher levels of blood flow in the cingulate prior to treatment (see Figure 7.10 in color plate section; Lopez, Becker et al., 2003).

Functional imaging data also help with the differential diagnosis of dementia syndromes. Although the clinical criteria for dementia with Lewy Bodies (DLB; McKeith, Fairbairn, & Perry, 1992) have low sensitivity and specificity in the context of AD (Lopez et al., 1998; Lopez, Hamilton et al., 2000; Lopez, Wisniewski et al., 2000), some patients with clinical DLB have characteristic abnormalities on PET imaging. Figure 7.11 (see color plate section) shows FDG (fluorodeoxyglucose) PET data in transaxial slices for individual AD and DLB patients (N. Bohnen, personal communication). The AD patient shows decreased glucose metabolic activity in the right parietal cortex with preservation of occipital metabolism; the asymmetric reduction indicates the patient has only mild disease. By contrast, the FDG scan of the DLB patient shows overall more severe (and bilateral) metabolic reductions, most prominent in the parietal cortex but also including the occipital cortex. It is this occipital hypometabolism that is the hallmark FDG marker for DLB.

Visualization of amyloid deposition in AD

One of the most exciting recent advances in functional neuroimaging, which also demonstrates how the traditional boundaries between structural and functional analysis have become blurred, is the recent development by Klunk et al. (2004) and Mathis et al. (2002) of a radio-labeled compound that permits localization of amyloid within the brain; the *Pittsburgh Compound B* (PIB) is an ^{11}C labeled form of thioflavine dye that can cross the blood–brain barrier. The compound identifies structural abnormalities (deposits of amyloid) which are the result of an alteration in brain function. As shown in Figure 7.12 (see color plate section), there is a significant increase in amyloid deposition in AD patients compared to controls, as well as the commonly observed decreases in glucose metabolism. The development of this compound, and the research that it will permit, is important as the need for earlier detection of disease (or disease risk) increases. Furthermore, as compounds are developed to delay, prevent, or reverse the pathology, it will be critical to be able to quantify the degree of change in this pathological marker of AD.

Functional imaging in LLD

Structural imaging findings in late-life depression have supported a vascular depression hypothesis (Alexopoulos et al., 1997; Krishnan et al., 1997), which suggests that cerebrovascular disease is a prominent factor in the depression of the elderly. This is supported by observations that individuals with LLD have been found to have a number of MRI abnormalities that are consistent with cerebrovascular disease, including increased white matter hyperintensities in periventricular areas and in the subcortical regions, and an increased incidence of subcortical lacunes.

More recently, the vascular depression hypothesis of late-life depressions has evolved into a frontostriatal dysfunction hypothesis (Alexopoulos, 2002), that cerebrovascular and/or neurodegenerative changes in geriatric depression are associated with dysfunction in frontal and striatal cognitive circuits. While a variety of neuropsychological and structural imaging data suggest that dysfunction of the subcortical-frontal neural circuitry may be an important factor in LLD-related cognitive impairments, these findings have been reinforced by *in vivo* functional neuroimaging studies. LLD subjects have reduced CBF bilaterally in the dorsal anterior cingulate and the hippocampus (as measured by $[^{15}O]H_2O$ PET compared to controls during a word generation task; de Asis et al., 2001), and decreased CBF in the frontal lobe (demonstrated with the xenon inhalation technique; Sackeim et al., 1990). Among depressed elderly, there are consistent decreases in blood flow and metabolism in the frontal cortex as measured by PET (Baxter et al., 1989; Bench, Friston, Brown, Frackowiak, & Dolan, 1993; Dolan et al., 1992; Kumar, 1993; Kumar et al., 1993; Sackeim, Prohovnik, Moeller, Mayeux, & Stern, 1993), compared to younger depressed subjects.

The functional imaging data also support the view that there are distinct subtypes of LLD (Nobler, Pelton, & Sackeim, 1999). In LLD, the caudate nucleus, the dorsolateral prefrontal cortex (DLPFC), and the hippocampus all have decreased activation. However, there is some discrepancy regarding the functional integrity of the anterior cingulate cortex (ACC). Some studies have found increased blood flow and activation in this region, specifically in the region anterior to the corpus collosum (Mayberg et al., 1997; Smith et al., 1999), while others have found decreases of activation in similar regions (Bench, Frackowiak, & Dolan, 1995).

One possible resolution of this paradox is suggested by Drevets (1998). Specifically, the changes in ACC activity might arise due to impairment somewhere else in the circuit, and that the changes in the ACC reflect a diaschisis and the interconnectivity of the neural system. According to this view, decreased ACC activity would be secondary to decreased engagement of the ACC, whereas increased ACC activity might then be due to increased work of the cingulate. Alternatively, the ACC changes during resting functional imaging studies might be secondary to a local impairment within the ACC. In this case, the decreased activity may be a direct reflection of an impaired ACC, and the increased activation could be a compensatory response. This mechanism of decreased efficiency is also thought to be the general mechanism responsible for increases in activation found in functional imaging studies in dementia (Bookheimer et al., 2000; Grady et al., 1993).

As is the case for AD, functional neuroimaging provides an approach to identifying the neurobiologic predictors of treatment response. Increased ACC activity prior to antidepressant treatment predicts favorable treatment response among those with mid-life depression (Mayberg et al., 1997; Wu et al., 1999), and in late-life depression, ACC activity at baseline decreased with treatment response.

Similarly, Meltzer et al. have shown associations between serotonin and treatment response. Figure 7.13 (see color plate section) shows co-registered [11C-carbonyl] WAY100635 PET images, summed over the 15–60 minute postinjection interval, and the structural MR images of a healthy 74-year-old man (Meltzer et al., 2001). The PET images reflect the distribution of 5-HT1A receptors, including midbrain region of the raphe and hippocampus (top row, middle image). Lack of binding in the cerebellum, where there are negligible 5-HT1A receptors, is also demonstrated (top row, left image). Figure 7.14 shows scatter plots depicting a positive correlation between the binding potential of the serotonin 1a receptor in the dorsal raphe nucleus and pretreatment levels of depression (as measured by the Hamilton Depression Rating Scale), $r = .60$, $p = .014$, and a trend level correlation between DRN BP and time to remission, $r = .52$, $p = .067$ (Meltzer et al., 2004).

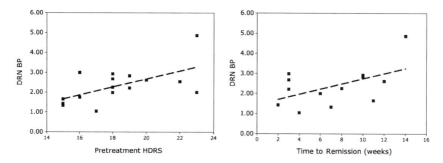

Figure 7.14   Scatter plots depict a positive correlation between the patient serotonin binding potential and pretreatment Hamilton Depression Rating score (left-hand graph), and the correlation with time to remission (right-hand graph) (courtesy of C. C. Meltzer, University of Pittsburgh).

Summary and conclusions

The continued development of acquisition and analysis tools for the study of brain structure and function is one of the most exciting areas of neuropsychology. Current methods of structural brain imaging analysis reveal that there are specific alterations in brain structure prior to the development of dementia syndromes. Furthermore, the nature and extent of the neurobehavioral dysfunction is related to the locus of the brain atrophy. In the case of LLD, regional brain atrophy occurs as a consequence of chronic affective disorder, and is also related to the risk of subsequent dementia. Brain functional studies reveal that both AD and LLD are accompanied by changes in regional metabolism and blood flow—perhaps due to overlapping etiologies. Measurement of cortical function and regional neurotransmitter levels provides evidence of treatment response in dementia and depression.

Thus, the neuropsychologist is no longer limited in the use of the tools through which they can view the functional integrity of the central nervous system (CNS). The combination of the direct knowledge of brain structural and functional integrity, combined with first rate evaluation of cognitive functions (the visible expression of CNS integrity) provides a powerful means to understand evolving syndromes in older patient populations.

Acknowledgements

Preparation of this chapter was supported in parts by funds from the National Institute on Aging (AG05133), and the National Institute of Mental Health (MH07033 and MH01684). The authors are grateful to their colleagues in the University of Pittsburgh Alzheimer's Research Center, in particular C. C. Meltzer, W. Klunk, M. Gach, and N. Bohnen, for their assistance in the preparation of this chapter.

Note

1 Voxel-based morphometry analyses permit comprehensive, global assessment of brain structures without a priori identification of regions of interest. This approach is not biased to one brain region and permits identification of potential unsuspected brain structure abnormalities. This approach also may be more sensitive to within-structure neuroanatomical differences relative to the more traditional volumetric analyses that measure volumes of entire structures. Furthermore, this approach detects regional areas of decreased brain tissue volume that are consistent across patients.

References

Aizenstein, H. J., Clark, K. A., Butters, M. A., Cochran, J. L., Stenger, V. A., Meltzer, C. C., et al. (2004). The BOLD hemodynamic response in healthy aging. *Journal of Cognitive Neuroscience, 16*(5), 786–793.

Alexopoulos, G. S. (2002). Frontostriatal and limbic dysfunction in late-life depression. *American Journal of Geriatric Psychiatry, 10*(6), 687–695.

Alexopoulos, G. S., Kiosses, D. N., Choi, S. J., Murphy, C. F., & Lim, K. O. (2002). Frontal white matter microstructure and treatment response of late-life depression: A preliminary study. *American Journal of Psychiatry, 159*(11), 1929–1932.

Alexopoulos, G. S., Meyers, B. S., Young, R. C., Campbell, S., Silbersweig, D., & Charlson, M. (1997). "Vascular depression" hypothesis. *Archives of General Psychiatry, 54*(10), 915–922.

Alsop, D. C., & Casement, M. (2004). *Perfusion MRI reveals elevated function of temporal and inferior frontal regions in early AD.* Paper presented at the ninth international conference on Alzheimer's Disease and Related Disorders, Philadelphia, PA.

Alsop, D. C., & Detre, J. A. (1998). Multisection cerebral blood flow MR imaging with continuous arterial spin labeling. *Radiology, 208*, 410–416.

Alsop, D. C., Detre, J. A., & Grossman, M. (2000). Assessment of cerebral blood flow in Alzheimer's disease by spin-labeled magnetic resonance imaging. *Annals of Neurology, 47*(1), 93–100.

Ashburner, J., & Friston, K. J. (2000). Voxel-based morphometry: The methods. *Neurology, 11*, 805–821.

Ballmaier, M., Sowell, E. R., Thompson, P. M., Kumar, A., Narr, K. L., Lavretsky, H., et al. (2004). Mapping brain size and cortical gray matter changes in elderly depression. *Biological Psychiatry, 55*(4), 382–389.

Ballmaier, M., Toga, A. W., Blanton, R. E., Sowell, E. R., Lavretsky, H., Peterson, J., et al. (2004). Anterior ingulate, gyrus rectus, and orbitofrontal abnormalities in elderly depressed patients: An MRI-based parcellation of the prefrontal cortex. *American Journal of Psychiatry, 161*, 99–108.

Baxter, L. R., Schwartz, J. M., Phelps, M. E., Mazziotta, J. C., Guze, B. H., Selin, C. E., et al. (1989). Reduction of prefrontal cortex glucose metabolism common to three types of depression. *Archives of General Psychiatry, 46*(3), 243–250.

Bell-McGinty, S., Butters, M. A., Meltzer, C. C., Greer, P. J., Reynolds, C. F., & Becker, J. T. (2002). Brain morphometric abnormalities in geriatric depression: Long-term neurobiological effects of illness duration. *American Journal of Psychiatry, 159*, 1424–1427.

Bell-McGinty, S., Lopez, O. L., Meltzer, C. C., Scanlon, J. M., Whyte, E. M., DeKosky, S. T., & Becker, J. T. (2002). Brain morphologic abnormalities in mild cognitive impairment [Abstract]. *Neurology, 58*(Suppl. 3), A215.

Bench, C. J., Frackowiak, R. S., & Dolan, R. J. (1995). Changes in regional cerebral blood flow on recovery from depression. *Psychological Medicine, 25*(2), 247–261.

Bench, C. J., Friston, K. J., Brown, R. G., Frackowiak, R. S., & Dolan, R. J. (1993). Regional cerebral blood flow in depression measured by positron emission tomography: The relationship with clinical dimensions. *Psychological Medicine, 23*(3), 579–590.

Bernick, C., Kuller, L., Dulberg, C., Longstreth, W. T., Manolio, T., Beauchamp, N., & Price, T. (2001). Silent MRI infarcts and the risk of future stroke: The cardiovascular health study. *Neurology, 57*(7), 1222–1229.

Bookheimer, S. Y., Strojwas, M. H., Cohen, M. S., Saunders, A. M., Pericak-Vance, M. A., Mazziotta, J. C., & Small, G. W. (2000). Patterns of brain activation in people at risk for Alzheimer's disease [see comments]. *New England Journal of Medicine, 343*(7), 450–456.

Bowen, J., Teri, L., Kukull, W., McCormick, W., McCurry, S. M., & Larson, E. B. (1997). Progression to dementia in patients with isolated memory loss. *Lancet, 349*(9054), 763–765.

Brown, D. R., Hunter, R., Wyper, D. J., Patterson, J., Kelly, R. C., Montaldo, D., & McCulloch, J. (1996). Longitudinal changes in cognitive function and regional cerebral function in Alzheimer's disease: A SPECT blood flow study. *Journal of Psychiatric Research, 30*(2), 109–126.

Buckner, R. L., Snyder, A. Z., Sanders, A. L., Raichle, M. E., & Morris, J. C. (2000). Functional brain imaging of young, nondemented, and demented older adults. *Journal of Cognitive Neuroscience, 12*(Suppl. 2), 24–34.

Buxton, R. B., Frank, L. R., Wong, E. C., Seiwert, B., Warach, S., & Edelman, R. R. (1998). A general kinetic model for quantitative perfusion imaging with arterial spin labeling. *Magnetic Resonance in Medicine, 40*, 383–396.

Chetelat, G., & Baron, J. C. (2003). Early diagnosis of Alzheimer's disease: Contribution of structural neuroimaging. *NeuroImage, 18*(2), 525–541.

Convit, A., de Asis, J., de Leon, M. J., Tarshish, C. Y., de Santi, S., & Rusinek, H. (2000). Atrophy of the medial occipitotemporal, inferior, and middle temporal gyri in non-demented elderly predict decline to Alzheimer's disease. *Neurobiology of Aging, 21*(1), 19–26.

Convit, A., deLeon, M. J., Hoptman, M. J., Tarshish, C., DeSanti, S., & Rusinek, H. (1995). Age related changes in brain: I. Magnetic resonance imaging measures of temporal lobe volumes in normal subjects. *Psychiatric Quarterly, 66*, 343–355.

Dai, W. S., & Davis, S. W. (2004). *Segmentation comparison between the MNI and the University of Pittsburgh elderly template.* Paper presented at the ninth international conference on Alzheimer's Disease and Related Disorders, Philadelphia, PA.

Davis, S. W., Hayashi, K. M., Meltzer, C. C., Thompson, P. M., Tga, A. W., Lopez, O. L., & Becker, J. T. (2004). *Mapping hippocampal volume changes in Alzheimer's disease and mild cognitive impairment.* Paper presented at the annual meeting of the Society for Neuroscience, San Diego, CA.

De Asis, J. M., Stern, E., Alexopolous, G. S., Pan, H., van Gorp, W., Blumberg, H., et al. (2001). Hippocampal and anterior ingulate activation deficits in patients with geriatric depression. *American Journal of Psychiatry, 158*(8), 1321–1323.

De Santi, S., de Leon, M. J., Rusinek, H., Convit, A., Tarshish, C. Y., Roche, A., et al. (2001). Hippocampal formation, glucose metabolism, and volume losses in MCI and AD. *Neurobiology of Aging, 22*, 529–539.

D'Esposito, M., Zarahn, E., Aguirre, G. K., & Rypma, B. (1999). The effect of normal aging on the coupling of neural activity to the bold hemodynamic response. *NeuroImage, 10*(1), 6–14.

Dolan, R. J., Bench, C. J., Brown, R. G., Scott, L. C., Friston, K. J., & Frackowisk, R. S. (1992). Regional cerebral blood flow abnormalities in depressed patients with cognitive impairment. *Journal of Neurology, Neurosurgery and Psychiatry, 55*, 768–773.

Drevets, W. C. (1998). Functional neuroimaging studies of depression: The anatomy of melancholia. *Annual Review of Medicine, 49*, 341–361.

Duong, T. Q., & Yacoub, E. (2002). High resolution, spin echo BOLD, and CBF fMRI at 4 and 7 T. *Magnetic Resonance in Medicine, 48*, 589–593.

Gach, M., Dai, W., Lopez, O. L., Carmichael, O., Lakkavaram, V., Becker, J. T., & Kuller, L. H. (2005). Differences in regional cerebral blood flow in mild cognitive impairment and early Alzheimer's disease measured with continuous spin labeled MRI. *Neurology, 64*(Suppl. 1), A166.

Glydensted, L., & Ostergaard, L. (2004). *Perfusion weighted magnetic resonance imaging (PW-MRI) in Alzheimer's Disease (AD) and mild cognitive impairment (MCI); initial experience.* Paper presented at the ninth international conference on Alzheimer's Disease and Related Disorders, Philadelphia, PA.

Grady, C. L., Haxby, J. V., Horwitz, B., Gillette, J., Salerno, J. A., Gonzalez-Aviles, A., et al. (1993). Activation of cerebral blood flow during a visuoperceptual task in patients with Alzheimer-type dementia. *Neurobiology of Aging, 14*, 35–44.

Hanninen, M. A., Hallikainen, M., Koivisto, K., Partanen, K., Laakso, M. P., Riekkinen, P. J., & Soininen, H. (1997). Decline of frontal lobe functions in subjects with age-associated memory impairment. *Neurology, 48*, 148–153.

Hanninen, T., Hallikainen, M., Koivisto, K., Helkala, E. L., Reinikainen, K. J., Soininen, H., et al. (1995). A follow-up study of age-associated memory impairment: Neuropsychological predictors of dementia. *Journal of the American Geriatrics Society, 43*(9), 1007–1015.

Heckbert, S. R., Longstreth, W. T., Psaty, B. M., Murros, K. E., Smith, N. L., Newman, A. B., et al. (1997). The association of antihypertensive agents with MRI white matter findings and with Modified Mini-Mental State Examination in older adults. *Journal of the American Geriatrics Society, 45*(12), 1423–1433.

Huettel, S. A., Singerman, J. D., & McCarthy, G. (2001). The effects of aging upon the hemodynamic response measured by functional MRI. *NeuroImage, 13*(1), 161–175.

Hughes, C. P., Berg, L., & Danzinger, W. L. (1982). A new clinical scale for the staging of dementia. *British Journal of Psychiatry, 140*, 566–572.

Jack, C. R., Petersen, R. C., Xu, Y. C., O'Brien, P. C., Smith, G. E., Ivnik, R. J., et al. (1999). Prediction of AD with MRI-based hippocampal volume in mild cognitive impairment. *Neurology, 52*(7), 1397–1403.

Jack, C. R., Petersen, R. C., Xu, Y. C., Waring, S. C., O'Brien, P. C., Tangalos, E. G., et al. (1997). Medial temporal atrophy on MRI in normal aging and very mild Alzheimer's disease. *Neurology, 49*, 786–794.

Jernigan, T. L., Archibald, S. L., Berhow, M. T., Sowell, E. R., Foster, D. S., & Hesselink, J. R. (1991). Cerebral structure on MRI, part I: Localization of age-related changes. *Biological Psychiatry, 29*(1), 55–67.

Jernigan, T. L., Salmon, D. P., Butters, N., & Hesselink, J. R. (1991). Cerebral structure on MRI: II. Specific changes in Alzheimer's and Huntington's diseases. *Biological Psychiatry, 29*, 68–81.

Johnson, K. A., & Moran, E. K. (2004). *Prediction of clinical stability vs. progression in questionable AD using perfusion SPECT.* Paper presented at the ninth international conference on Alzheimer's Disease and Related Disorders, Philadelphia, PA.

Johnson, N. A., & Jahng, G. H. (2004). *Patterns of cerebral hypoperfusion in Alzheimer's disease and mild cognitive impairment measured with arterial spin labeled MRI.* Paper presented at the ninth international conference on Alzheimer's Disease and Related Disorders, Philadelphia, PA.

Juottonen, K., Laasko, M. P., Insausti, R., Lehtovirta, M., Pitkanen, A., Partanen, K., & Soininen, H. (1998). Volumes of the entorhinal and perirhinal cortices in Alzheimer's disease. *Neurobiology and Aging, 19*(1), 15–22.

Kataki, M. (2004). *SPECT findings in Alzheimer's disease (AD) and correlation with disease severity*. Paper presented at the ninth international conference on Alzheimer's Disease and Related Disorders, Philadelphia, PA.

Killiany, R. J., Gomez-Isla, T., Moss, M., Kikinis, R., Sandor, T., Jolesz, F., et al. (2000). Use of structural magnetic resonance imaging to predict who will get Alzheimer's disease. *Annals of Neurology, 47*, 430–439.

Klunk, W. E., Engler, H., Nordberg, A., Wang, Y., Blomqvist, G., Holt, D. P., et al (2004). Imaging brain amyloid in Alzheimer's disease with Pittsburgh Compond-B. *Annals of Neurology, 55*, 306–319.

Knopman, D. S., DeKosky, S. T., Cummings, J. L., Chui, H., Corey-Bloom, J., Relkin, N., et al. (2001). Practice parameter: Diagnosis of dementia (an evidence-based review). Report of the Quality Standards Subcommittee of the American Academy of Neurology. *Neurology, 56*, 1143–1153.

Krasuski, J. S., Alexander, G. E., Horwitz, B., Daly, E. M., Murphy, D. G., Rapoport, S. I., & Schapiro, M. B. (1998). Volumes of medial temporal lobe structures in patients with Alzheimer's disease and mild cognitive impairment (and in healthy controls). *Biological Psychiatry, 43*(1), 60–68.

Krishnan, K. R., Hays, J. C., & Blazer, D. G. (1997). MRI-defined vascular depression. *American Journal of Psychiatry, 154*(4), 497–501.

Krishnan, K. R., Tupler, L. A., Ritchie, J. C., McDonald, W. M., Knight, D. L., Nemeroff, C. B., & Carroll, B. J. (1996). Apolipoprotein E-epsilon 4 frequency in geriatric depression. *Biological Psychiatry, 40*(1), 69–71.

Kumar, A. (1993). Functional brain imaging in late-life depression and dementia. *Journal of Clinical Psychiatry, 54S*, S21–S25.

Kumar, A., Bilker, W., Jin, Z., & Udupa, J. (2000). Atrophy and high intensity lesions: Complementary neurobiological mechanisms in late-life major depression. *Neuropsychopharmacology, 22*(3), 264–274.

Kumar, A., Newberg, A., Alavi, A., Berlin, J., Smith, R., & Reivich, M. (1993). Regional cerebral glucose metabolism in late-life depression and Alzheimer disease: A preliminary positron emission tomography study. *Proceedings of the National Academy of Sciences, USA, 90*(15), 7019–7023.

Lai, T.-J., Payne, M. E., Byrum, C. E., Steffens, D. C., & Krishnan, K. R. R. (2000). Reduction of orbital frontal cortex volume in geriatric depression. *Biological Psychiatry, 48*, 971–975.

Lebowitz, B. D., Pearson, J. L., Schneider, L. S., Reynolds, C. F., III, Alexopoulos, G. S., Bruce, M. L., et al. (1997). Diagnosis and treatment of depression in late life. Consensus statement update. *Journal of the American Medical Association, 278*(14), 1186–1190.

Lee, S. H., Payne, M. E., Steffens, D. C., McQuoid, D. R., Lai, T. J., Provenzale, J. M., & Krishnan, K. R. (2003). Subcortical lesion severity and orbitofrontal cortex volume in geriatric depression. *Biological Psychiatry, 54*(5), 529–533.

Lopez, O. L., Becker, J. T., Meltzer, C. C., Scanlon, J., Greer, P., & DeKosky, S. T. (2003). CNS mechanisms of dementia treatment. *Neurology, S1*, A413.

Lopez, O. L., Hamilton, R., Becker, J. T., Wisniewski, S. R., Kaufer, D. I., & DeKosky, S. T. (1998). *Clinical features and predictors of progression in patients with Alzheimer's disease and with the Lewy Body variant of Alzheimer's disease*. Paper presented at the 50th annual meeting of the American Academy of Neurology, Minneapolis, MN.

Lopez, O. L., Hamilton, R. L., Becker, J. T., Wisniewski, S., Kaufer, D. I., & DeKosky, S. T. (2000). Severity of cognitive impairment and the clinical diagnosis of Alzheimer's disease with Lewy bodies. *Neurology*, *54*, 1780–1787.

Lopez, O. L., Jagust, W. J., DeKosky, S. T., Becker, J. T., Fitzpatrick, A., Dulberg, C., et al. (2003). Prevalence and classification of mild cognitive impairment in the Cardiovascular Health Study: Part 1. *Archives of Neurology*, *60*, 1385–1389.

Lopez, O. L., Jagust, W. J., Dulberg, C., Becker, J. T., DeKosky, S. T., Fitzpatrick, A., et al. (2003). Risk factors for mild cognitive impairment in the Cardiovascular Health Study Cognition Study: Part 2. *Archives of Neurology*, *60*, 1394–1399.

Lopez, O. L., Smith, G., Becker, J. T., Meltzer, C. C., & DeKosky, S. T. (2001). The psychotic phenomenon in probable Alzheimer's disease: A positron emission tomographic study. *Journal of Neuropsychiatry and Clinical Neurosciences*, *13*, 50–55.

Lopez, O. L., Wisniewski, S., Hamilton, R. L., Becker, J. T., Kaufer, D. I., & DeKosky, S. T. (2000). Predictors of progression in patients with Alzheimer's disease and Lewy bodies. *Neurology*, *54*, 1774–1779.

Lupien, S. J., de Leon, M., de Santi, S., Convit, A., Tarshish, C., Nair, N. P., et al. (1998). Cortisol levels during human aging predict hippocampal atrophy and memory deficits. [see comment] [erratum in *Nature Neuroscience*, 1998, *1*(4), 329]. *Nature Neuroscience*, *1*(1), 69–73.

Lupien, S. J., Nair, N. P., Briere, S., Maheu, F., Tu, M. T., Lemay, M., et al. (1999). Increased cortisol levels and impaired cognition in human aging: Implication for depression and dementia in later life. *Reviews in the Neurosciences*, *10*(2), 117–139.

Marchal, G., Rioux, P., Petit-Taboue, M. C., Sette, G., Travere, J. M., Le Poec, C., et al. (1992). Regional cerebral oxygen consumption, blood flow, and blood volume in healthy human aging. *Archives of Neurology*, *49*(10), 1013–1020.

Mathis, C. A., Bacskai, B. J., Kajdasz, S. T., McLellan, M. E., Frosch, M. P., Hyman, B. T., et al. (2002). A lipophilic thioflavin-T derivative for positron emission tomography (PET) imaging of amyloid in brain. *Bioorganic and Medicinal Chemical Letters*, *12*(3), 295–298.

Mayberg, H. S., Brannan, S. K., Mahurin, R. K., Jerabek, P. A., Brickman, J. S., Tekell, J. L., et al. (1997). Cingulate function in depression: A potential predictor of treatment response [see comments]. *Neuroreport*, *8*(4), 1057–1061.

McKeith, I. G., Fairbairn, A. F., & Perry, R. H. (1992). Clinical diagnostic criteria for Lewy body dementia. *Dementia*, *3*, 251–252.

McKhann, G., Drachman, D. A., Folstein, M. F., Katzman, R., Price, D. L., & Stadlan, E. (1984). Clinical diagnosis of Alzheimer's disease: Report of the NINCDS-ADRDA Work Group under the auspices of the Department of Health and Human Services Task Force on Alzheimer's disease. *Neurology*, *34*, 939–944.

Mega, M. S., Lee, L., Dinov, I. D., Mishkin, F., Toga, A. W., & Cummings, J. L. (2000). Cerebral correlates of psychotic symptoms in Alzheimer's disease. *Journal of Neurology, Neurosurgery, and Psychiatry*, *69*(2), 148–149.

Meltzer, C. C., Drevets, W. C., Price, J. C., Mathis, C. A., Lopresti, B., Greer, P. J., et al. (2001). Gender-specific aging effects on the serotonin 1A receptor. *Brain Research*, *895*(1–2), 9–17.

Meltzer, C. C., Price, J. C., Mathis, C. A., Butters, M. A., Ziolko, S. K., Masumdar, S., et al. (2004). Serotonin 1A receptor binding and treatment response in late-life depression. *Neuropsychopharmacology*, *29*(12), 2258–2265.

Mesulam, M.-M. (1985). *Principles of behavioral neurology.* Philadelphia: F. A. Davis & Company.

Miller, S., Yufik, T., DeKosky, L., Meltzer, C. C., Nebes, R. D., Dekosky, S. T., & Becker, J. T. (2000). Identification of temporal lobe structures associated with visual naming using voxel-based analysis of MRI scans in probable Alzheimer's disease. *NeuroImage, 11*(5, S1), S393.

Morris, J. C., Storandt, M., Miller, J. P., McKeel, D. W., Price, J. L., Rubin, E. H., & Berg, L. (2001). Mild cognitive impairment represents early-stage Alzheimer disease. *Archives of Neurology, 58*, 397–405.

Morris, P., & Rapoport, S. I. (1990). Neuroimaging and affective disorder in late life: A review. *Canadian Journal of Psychiatry, 35*(4), 347–354.

Nagata, K., & Maruya, H. (2000). Can PET data differentiate Alzheimer's disease from vascular dementia? *Annals of the New York Academy of Sciences, 903*, 252–261.

Narr, K. L., Thompson, P. M., Szeszko, P., Robinson, D., Jang, S., Woods, R. P., et al. (2004). Regional specificity of hippocampal volume reductions in first-episode schizophrenia. *NeuroImage, 21*(4), 1563–1575.

Nobler, M. S., Pelton, G. H., & Sackeim, H. A. (1999). Cerebral blood flow and metabolism in late-life depression and dementia. *Journal of Geriatric Psychiatry and Neurology, 12*(3), 118–127.

Pantel, J., Schroder, J., Schad, L. R., Friedlinger, M., Knopp, M. V., Schmitt, R., et al. (1997). Quantitative magnetic resonance imaging and neuropsychological functions in dementia of the Alzheimer type. *Psychological Medicine, 27*, 221–229.

Parkes, L. M., & Rashid, W. (2004). Normal cerebral perfusion measurements using arterial spin labeling: Reproducibility, stability, and age and gender effects. *Magnetic Resonance in Medicine, 51*(4), 736–743.

Petersen, R. C., Smith, G. E., Waring, S. C., Ivnik, R. J., Tangalos, E. G., & Kokmen, E. (1999). Mild cognitive impairment: Clinical characterization and outcome. *Archives of Neurology, 56*, 303–308.

Prasad, K. M. R., Davis, S., Becker, J. T., Keshavan, M. S., & Sweet, R. A. (2003). *Neurobiological substrates of Alzheimer's disease with psychosis: An exploratory study of structural MRI using a voxel-based morphometric approach.* Paper presented at the annual meeting of the Society for Neuroscience.

Rabins, P. V., Pearlson, G. D., Aylward, E., Kumar, A. J., & Dowell, K. (1991). Cortical magnetic resonance imaging changes in elderly inpatients with major depression. *American Journal of Psychiatry, 148*(5), 617–620.

Ross, M. H., Yurgelun-Todd, D. A., Renshaw, P. F., Maas, L. C., Mendelson, J. H., Mello, N. K., et al. (1997). Age-related reduction in functional MRI response to photic stimulation. *Neurology, 48*(1), 173–176.

Sackeim, H. A., Prohovnik, I., Moeller, J. R., Brown, R. P., Apter, S., Prudic, J., et al. (1990). Regional cerebral blood flow in mood disorders. I. Comparison of major depressives and normal controls at rest. *Archives of General Psychiatry, 47*(1), 60–70.

Sackeim, H. A., Prohovnik, I., Moeller, J. R., Mayeux, R., & Stern, Y. (1993). Regional cerebral blood flow in mood disorders. II. Comparison of major depression and Alzheimer's disease. *Journal of Nuclear Medicine, 34*, 1090–1101.

Shah, P. J., Ebmeier, K. P., Glabus, M. F., & Goodwin, G. M. (1998). Cortical grey matter reductions associated with treatment-resistant chronic unipolar depression. Controlled magnetic resonance imaging study. *British Journal of Psychiatry, 172*(6), 527–532.

Shah, P. J., Glabus, M. F., Goodwin, G. M., & Ebmeier, K. P. (2002). Chronic, treatment-resistant depression and right fronto-striatal atrophy. *British Journal of Psychiatry, 180*, 434–440.

Sheline, Y. I. (2003). Neuroimaging studies of mood disorder effects on the brain. *Biological Psychiatry, 54*(3), 338–352.

Sheline, Y. I., Wang, P. W., Gado, M. H., Csernansky, J. G., & Vannier, M. W. (1996). Hippocampal atrophy in recurrent major depression. *Proceedings of the National Academy of Sciences, USA, 93*, 3908–3913.

Silverman, D. H., Small, G. W., Chang, C. Y., Lu, C. S., DeAburto, K., Chen, W., et al. (2001). Positron emission tomography in evaluation of dementia: Regional brain metabolism and long-term outcome. *Journal of the American Medical Association, 286*(17), 2120–2127.

Smith, G. S., Reynolds, C. F., III, Pollock, B., Derbyshire, S., Nofzinger, E., Dew, M. A., et al. (1999). Cerebral glucose metabolic response to combined total sleep deprivation and antidepressant treatment in geriatric depression. *American Journal of Psychiatry, 156*(5), 683–689.

Soininen, H. S., Partanen, K., Pitkanen, A., Vainio, P., Hanninen, T., Hallikanen, M., et al. (1994). Volumetric MRI analysis of the amygdala and the hippocampus in subjects with age-associated memory impairment: Correlation to visual and verbal memory. *Neurology, 44*, 1660–1668.

Steet, R. A., Nimgaonkar, V. L., Devlin, B., Lopez, O. L., & DeKosky, S. T. (2002). Increased familial risk of the psychotic phenotype of Alzheimer's disease. *Neurology, 58*(6), 907–911.

Steet, R. A., Nimgaonkar, V. L., Kamboh, M. I., Lopez, O. L., Zhang, F., & DeKosky, S. T. (1998). Dopamine receptor genetic variation, psychosis, and aggression in Alzheimer's disease. *Archives of Neurology, 55*, 1335–1340.

Steffens, D. C., Byrum, C. E., McQuoid, D. R., Greenberg, D. L., Payne, M. E., Blitchington, T. F., et al. (2000). Hippocampal volume in geriatric depression. *Biological Psychiatry, 48*(4), 301–309.

Steffens, D. C., & Krishnan, K. R. (1998). Structural neuroimaging and mood disorders: Recent findings, implications for classification, and future directions. *Biological Psychiatry, 43*(10), 705–712.

Steffens, D. C., Payne, M. E., Greenberg, D. L., Byrum, C. E., Welsh-Bohmer, K. A., Wagner, H. R., & MacFall, J. R. (2002). Hippocampal volume and incident dementia in geriatric depression. *American Journal of Geriatric Psychiatry, 10*(1), 62–71.

Stern, Y., Alexander, G. E., Prohovnik, I., & Mayeux, R. (1992). Inverse relationship between education and parietotemporal perfusion deficit in Alzheimer's disease. *Annals of Neurology, 32*(3), 371–375.

Talagala, S. L., & Chuang, K. H. (2004). *Whole brain perfusion MRI at 3T using a 16 second receiver coil array*. Workshop on Quantitative Cerebral Perfusion Imaging using MRI: A Technical Perspective, conducted at ISMRM, Venice.

Talagala, S. L., & Ye, F. Q. (2002). *Whole brain 3D perfusion MRI at 3T using CASL with a separate labeling coil*. Paper presented at the 10th scientific meeting of the International Society for Magnetic Resonance in Medicine, Honolulu, Hawaii.

Thomas, D. L., & Lythgoe, M. F. (2000). The measurement of diffusion and perfusion in biological systems using magnetic resonance imaging. *Physics in Medicine and Biology, 45*, R97–R138.

Tupler, L. A., Krishnan, K. R., McDonald, W. M., Dombeck, C. B., D'Souza, S., & Steffens, D. C. (2002). Anatomic location and laterality of MRI signal hyperintensities in late-life depression. *Journal of Psychosomatic Research, 53*(2), 665–676.

Visser, P. J., Scheltens, P., Verhey, F. R. J., Schmand, B., Launer, L. J., Jolles, J., & Jonker, C. (1999). Medial temporal lobe atrophy and memory dysfunction as predictors for dementia in subjects with mild cognitive impairment. *Journal of Neurology, 246*, 477–485.

Visser, P. J., Verhey, F. R. J., Hofman, P. A. M., Scheltens, P., & Jolles, J. (2002). Medial temporal lobe atrophy predicts Alzheimer's disease in patients with minor cognitive impairment. *Journal of Neurology, Neurosurgery, and Psychiatry, 72*, 491–497.

Wang, H., & Chu, Y. (2004). *Regional cerebral hypoperfusion of medial temporal lobe in mild cognitive impairment.* Paper presented at the ninth international conference on Alzheimer's Disease and Related Disorders, Philadelphia, PA.

Weber, M. A., & Gunther, M. (2003). Comparison of arterial spin labeling techniques and dynamic susceptibility-weighted contrast-enhanced MRI in perfusion imaging of normal brain tissue. *Investigative Radiology, 38*(11), 712–718.

Wolf, H., Grunwald, M., Kruggel, F., Riedel-Heller, S. G., Angerhfer, S., Hojjatoleslami, A., et al. (2001). Hippocampal volume discriminates between normal cognition: Questionable and mild dementia in the elderly. *Neurobiology of Aging, 22*(2), 177–186.

Wu, J., Buchsbaum, M. S., Gillin, J. C., Tang, C., Cadwell, S., Wiegand, M., et al. (1999). Prediction of antidepressant effects of sleep deprivation by metabolic rates in the ventral anterior cingulate and medial prefrontal cortex [erratum in *American Journal of Psychiatry,* 1999, *156*(10), 1666]. *American Journal of Psychiatry, 156*(8), 1149–1158.

Ye, F. Q., & Berman, K. F. (2000). $H_2^{15}O$ PET validation of steady-state arterial spin tagging cerebral blood flow measurements in humans. *Magnetic Resonance in Medicine, 44*, 450–456.

Zaharchuk, G., & Ledden, P. J. (1999). Multislice perfusion and perfusion territory imaging in humans with separate label and image coils. *Magnetic Resonance in Medicine, 41*, 1095–1098.

Section III

Neuropsychological disorders

8 Neuropsychology of Alzheimer's disease and other dementias

Ronald F. Zec and Nicole R. Burkett

Almost a century ago, Alois Alzheimer reported the clinicopathological findings of a 55-year-old woman, Auguste D, who displayed a progressive dementing disorder associated with numerous neurofibrillary tangles and amyloid plaques in the brain. Alzheimer first reported the case at a meeting in 1906 and a brief note from this meeting was published in 1907 (Alzheimer, 1907, 1977). Recently rediscovered brain sections confirm that Auguste D had a large number of neurofibrillary tangles and amyloid plaques in the cerebral cortex (Graeber, Kosel, Grasbon-Frodl, Moller, & Mehraein, 1998). In 1976, Katzman, in an editorial titled "The Prevalence and Malignancy of Alzheimer Disease: A Major Killer," estimated that the senile form of Alzheimer's disease was the fourth or fifth most common cause of death in the United States.

Neuropsychological assessment plays a critical role in the clinical evaluation of patients suspected of having a dementing disorder, including those enrolled in research studies. Neuropsychological testing provides an objective, quantitative measurement of the severity, extent, and pattern of a patient's impairments across different cognitive domains. This data is critical to the early detection of a dementing disorder, provides a baseline against which to chart the course of the disorder, can aid in differential diagnosis, and provides valuable information to guide case management. Neuropsychological assessment and cognitive neuroscience also play an important role in the study of the nature and evolution of the cognitive impairment in Alzheimer's disease, and in the study of clinicopathological correlations and efficacy of treatment interventions.

Chapter overview

In this chapter, the neuropsychology of Alzheimer's disease (AD) will be reviewed, including the role of neuropsychological assessment in early detection, differential diagnosis, and measuring progression of dementia. The effects of early AD on memory and other cognitive functions are reviewed. Recommendations are made regarding the use of neuropsychological assessment in the early detection of Alzheimer dementia. Treatments are also reviewed.

The major sections in this chapter comprise: Epidemiology, Neuropathology of AD, Neuropathologic Criteria for the Diagnosis of AD, The Use of Neuropsychological Assessment in the Diagnosis of AD, Early Detection of Alzheimer Dementia, Brief Mental Status Tests and Neuropsychological Batteries for Evaluation of Dementia, Attention, General Cognitive Slowing in Aging and AD, Executive Functioning and Problem Solving, Awareness of DeWcit, Memory Impairment in AD, Language, Visuospatial Functioning, Mild Cognitive Impairment, DiVerential Diagnosis of AD and Other Dementing Disorders, Treatment and Case Management, and Conclusions.

Epidemiology

Hebert, Beckett, Scherr, and Evans (2001) projected that the annual incidence rates of AD in the US will likely more than double from 377,000 new onset cases in 1995 to 959,000 in 2050. Evans et al. (2003) reported that the incidence of AD in a biracial urban community over a mean of 4.1 years was 1.45% per year among persons 65–74 years old, 4.73% among those 75–84 years old, and 9.11% among those 85 years and older. The prevalence of dementia in persons over the age of 65 is 8–10% in the US and may be 15% or more if very mild dementia is included, and approaches 50% in those over age 85 (Mendez & Cummings, 2003). Hy and Keller (2000) pooled the AD prevalence rates for whites from 21 studies of Europeans and North Americans and applied it to the US 1996 population and obtained an estimated prevalence of 1.7–1.9 million cases in the US. Hebert, Scherr, Bienias, Bennett, and Evans (2003) reported higher prevalence rates based on a population-based study in Chicago, i.e., there were 4.5 million people with AD in the US in 2000, and the prevalence was predicted to increase almost three-fold to 13.2 million by 2050.

Despite some disagreement in terms of estimates of prevalence of AD across different studies (Hy & Keller, 2000), there is general agreement about the following points (Albert & Drachman, 2000). The prevalence and incidence rates of AD double every 5 years after the age of 65. Prevalence estimates indicate that at least 1 in 4 and as many as 1 in 2 people aged 85 and older have AD, which is the most rapidly increasing age group in the population. A 50% decrease in the prevalence of clinically diagnosable cases of dementia due to AD could be achieved by delaying the onset of symptoms by 5 years because other illness would result in death before the emergence of dementia (Brookmeyer, Gray, & Kawas, 1998).

Neuropathology of Alzheimer's disease

> The lesions of Alzheimer's disease consist of synapse and neuron loss associated with progressive deposition of amyloid as diffuse and neuritic plaques and accumulating tau abnormalities in the form of neurofibrillary tangles and neuropil threads.
>
> (Hansen & Terry, 1997: 71)

Alzheimer brains in the later stages of the disorder (Braak stages V and VI) are atrophic (shrinkage of gyri and widening of sulci) on gross inspection with the most prominent atrophy in the temporoparietal and anterior frontal cortical regions, with relative sparing of the primary motor, somatosensory, and occipital cortices (Cummings & Benson, 1992). Ventricular dilatation is also present and there is a decrease in overall brain weight. Neurofibrillary tangles (NFTs) and neuritic plaques (NPs) have been the defining neuro-pathological characteristics of AD since first described by Alois Alzheimer in 1907. However, in addition to NFTs and NPs, histologic examination reveals other dramatic changes in cortical neurons, including amyloid deposits, neuro-pil threads (NTs), granulovacuolar degeneration (found primarily in hippocampal pyramidal neurons), gliosis, synaptic loss, and neuronal loss (Braak & Braak, 1993). Amyloid angiopathy is also found in almost all Alzheimer brains.

NFTs are intraneuronal pathological changes that consist mainly of a mass of insoluble cytoskeletal proteins (e.g., the abnormal phosphorylated tau protein) within nerve cell bodies and axons. A considerable amount of the neuronal loss in AD is due to the formation of NFTs and NTs (Braak & Braak, 1993). NTs appear in the dendrites of tangle-bearing pyramidal neurons and represent a substantial percentage of the total amount of neurofibrillary changes.

Senile plaques (SPs) are complex neuropil (i.e., extracellular) lesions consisting of a deposition of the abnormal beta amyloid protein. Braak and Braak (1993, 1994) have argued that the term "senile plaque" is an imprecise term referring to neuritic plaques and/or amyloid deposits (i.e., diffuse plaques). Typically separate analyses are now reported on neuritic plaques versus diffuse plaques (i.e., pure amyloid deposits lacking neurites) (e.g., Schmitt et al., 2000). Amyloid plaque is another term that has been used to refer to both neuritic plaques and diffuse plaques (Price & Morris, 1999). Neuritic plaques are amyloid plaques that contain dystrophic argyophilic neurites (which are thickened and darkly stained) and/or contain a dense beta-amyloid core (Price & Morris, 1999). Diffuse plaques are amyloid deposits without any thickened, dark-staining neurites and without a dense central core (Price & Morris, 1999).

The density of pure amyloid deposits is considerably higher than NPs in the AD brain, and many nondemented elderly have large numbers of amyloid deposits in the cortex (Braak & Braak, 1994). Some researchers had speculated that diffuse plaques might be the forerunner of NPs (Davies & Mann, 1993), but the distribution of amyloid deposits and NPs differs markedly, and thus the association between the two is unclear (Braak & Braak, 1994). Neither the density of amyloid deposits nor NPs correlate with dementia severity (Braak & Braak, 1994), but the presence of NPs is relatively specific for AD. The density of NFTs, on the other hand, does correlate with the severity of cognitive impairment in AD, but NFTs also occur in a variety of degenerative, traumatic, and toxic neuro-logical conditions. AD neuropathological changes evolve slowly over a very long time period and have a specific pattern of distribution in the brain that is nearly symmetrical in the two cerebral hemispheres (Braak & Braak, 1998).

Neuroanatomical distribution of NFTs and NPs in the Alzheimer brain

A striking feature of the neuropathology of AD is the highly selective, hierarchical distribution of NFTs (Arnold, 2000). Based on the distribution of NFTs, Braak and Braak (1991b) described the gradual evolution of NFTs and dendritic NTs in AD and proposed six neuropathological stages of AD ranging from a few NFTs in the medial temporal lobe to marked NFT changes throughout the cortex.

Stages I and II are referred to as the transentorhinal stages, III and IV as the limbic stages, and V and VI as the neocortical stages. Slender NTs appear in the twisted, dilated distil dendritic segments of neurons that are in the process of developing NFTs in the cell body (Braak & Braak, 1998). Although neurons with NFTs may survive for a considerable period of time (estimates range from 4 to 20 years), it is likely that the functional capabilities of entangled neurons are increasingly dysfunctional long before cell death (Braak & Braak, 1998). NFTs first appear in the structures of the medial temporal lobe, then somewhat later occur in the temporal, parietal, and frontal neocortical association areas, and in the final stage involve the primary motor and sensory neocortex (Arnold, Hyman, Flory, Damasio, & Van Hoesen, 1991; Braak & Braak, 1991b; Hyman, 1998).

A reasonable correlation exists between Braak stages and severity of cognitive impairment (Geddes et al., 1997; Hyman, 1998). For example, a strong association was found between Braak stage of neurofibrillary pathology and the percentage of sisters from the Nun Study who displayed impaired delayed word recall on a word-list learning test at the last examination before death (Riley, Snowdon, & Markesbery, 2002). None of the sisters in Braak stage 0 (sparse NFTs) displayed memory impairment on delayed recall, whereas 42% had impaired delayed recall in stages I and II, 68% in stages III and IV, and 93% in stages V and VI (Riley et al., 2002; Snowdon, 2003).

In clinicopathologic correlation studies, the severity of antemortem dementia correlated more highly with density of NFTs than with density of senile plaques (Arnold, 2000; Braak, Tredici, & Braak, 2003) or β-amyloid deposition (Hyman, 1998; Kay & Roth, 2002; Neuropathology Group, 2001; Riley et al., 2002). Virtually all elderly have some NFTs in the entorhinal cortex (EC) and hippocampus, and some individuals without dementia have a relatively high load of NFTs in the hippocampal formation (Arnold, 2000). Dementia is almost always displayed when NFTs are present in the neocortical association areas. Neuritic plaques, but not diffuse plaques, correlate with dementia, but the association is not as strong as that between NFTs and dementia (Arnold, 2000). One study reported that the density of neocortical synapses in the midfrontal regions, but not plaques or tangles, correlated very highly with the global scores on each of three widely used mental status tests (Terry et al., 1991). Based on a longitudinal clinicopathologic cohort study of patients with clinically diagnosed AD and individuals without dementia from the Religious Orders Study, Bennett, Schneider,

Wilson, Bienias, and Arnold (2004) concluded that NFTs appear to mediate the effect of amyloid deposition on clinically diagnosed AD and on level of global cognitive function proximate to death.

Arnold et al. (1991) examined the distributions of both NFTs and NPs in a group of patients who met both clinical and neuropathologic criteria for AD. The distribution of neuropathology in AD was found to affect specific cortical areas and specific laminae within those cortical areas. Furthermore, NFTs and NPs had different patterns of distribution in the Alzheimer brain. The brain areas that were found to be most severely and consistently affected with NFTs were in the ventromedial temporal lobe, followed by the neocortical areas of the lateral temporal lobe. The limbic and temporal lobes had significantly more NFTs than the frontal, parietal, and occipital lobes. The nonprimary and primary sensory association areas had less NFTs than the ventromedial and lateral temporal lobe areas, and the motor and primary sensory cortices had the lowest densities of NFTs. NFT density in the nucleus basalis of Meynert was highly variable among patients.

In general, NPs were more evenly distributed throughout the cortex (Arnold et al., 1991). However, the EC (area 28), hippocampus (subiculum/CA1 zone and CA2) and nucleus basalis of Meynert consistently had the *lowest* density of NPs compared to other cortical regions, whereas, as previously mentioned, the EC and subiculum/CA1 zone consistently had the *highest* density of NFTs of any brain area. The limbic lobe had significantly *fewer* NPs than temporal, parietal, or occipital lobes. The frontal lobe had significantly *fewer* NPs than temporal and occipital lobes, and the parietal lobes were intermediate in NP density.

Functional brain imaging (cerebral blood flow, PET, functional MRI) studies indicate that dysfunction predominates in the temporoparieto-occipital areas of AD patients. Damage to these regions in the left hemisphere likely causes the following impairments in AD: fluent aphasia, ideomotor apraxia, ideational apraxia, and constructional dyspraxia characterized by omission errors when copying geometrical figures. Damage to these brain areas in the posterior right hemisphere in AD likely results in fragmentation and poor spatial relations on figure copying tests. For additional information on this topic see Chapter 7 in this volume. A discussion of the neuroanatomy and neuropathology of Alzheimer amnesia is given below in the subsection titled Neuroanatomy of the Anterograde Amnesia in AD.

Neuropathologic criteria for the diagnosis of AD

Alzheimer's description of the neuropathological changes in AD remains the basis of a succession of neuropathologic criteria that have been proposed over the past 30 years (Arnold, 2000). Khachaturian criteria, which were proposed in 1984, required that minimum densities of senile plaques per microscopic field be exhibited in the neocortex as a function of age and as a function of whether clinically diagnosed dementia was present or absent (Khachaturian,

1985). The Consortium to Establish a Registry for AD (CERAD) neuro-pathologic criteria were later proposed to address methodological problems with the Khachaturian criteria (Mirra et al., 1991). The CERAD criteria specified semiquantitative counts of neuritic plaques, and de-emphasized diffuse plaques, in three neocortical regions (i.e., superior temporal gyrus, lateral prefrontal cortex, and inferior parietal lobule) in conjunction with Bielchowsky silver staining or thioflavin S fluorescent staining (Arnold, 2000). These CERAD criteria provided neuropathologic definitions for the normal brain and for different levels of diagnostic certainty of AD, i.e., definite, probable, and possible (Mirra et al., 1991).

Both the Khachaturian and CERAD sets of neuropathologic criteria for AD were criticized for having conceptual problems (Arnold, 2000). Because numerous senile plaques can be found in elderly individuals without dementia, older people were required to have more pathology to meet neuropathologic criteria. In addition, both sets of criteria adjusted for whether or not there had been a clinical dementia, which interfered with determining the sensitivity and specificity of the neuropathologic criteria in the prediction of clinical status.

More recently, the National Institute on Aging—Reagan Institute (NIA-RI) neuropathologic criteria for AD were proposed (National Institute on Aging, and Reagan Institute Working Group, 1997). In these criteria, the probability of a diagnosis of AD is based on semiquantitative ratings of both senile plaques *and* NFTs (Arnold, 2000). These criteria specify that the protocols for histologic staining and region sampling described in the CERAD criteria be employed. Furthermore, these new criteria recognize that AD is a heterogeneous disorder and that other types of neuropathologic lesions (e.g., cerebrovascular lesions and Lewy bodies) could contribute to whether and how severe a dementia is expressed. An estimate of the probability that AD neuropathology is causing the dementia is selected from several categories. The neuropathologic criteria do not, however, adjust the minimum amount of neuropathology that needs to be present as a function of age nor do the criteria require a clinical diagnosis of dementia to assess the probability of neuropathologic AD. A "high" likelihood of AD is assigned when there is a high density of both NFTs and neuritic plaques in the neocortex. An "intermediate" likelihood is assigned when there are moderate densities of neocortical neuritic plaques and NFTs confined to limbic regions. A "low" likelihood is assigned when there are few neuritic plaques and few NFTs confined to the limbic regions (Arnold, 2000). Inclusion of NFTs in the NIA-RI neuropathologic criteria may improve both the sensitivity and specificity in diagnosing AD (Schmitt et al., 2000).

The use of neuropsychological assessment in the diagnosis of Alzheimer's disease

The diagnosis of clinically probable AD based on established criteria is highly associated with autopsy-confirmed definite AD based on established neuropathologic criteria (Galasko et al., 1994). Clinical criteria for AD are set forth by both the *Diagnostic and Statistical Manual IV* (DSM-IV) and by the National Institute for Neurological and Communicative Disorders and Stroke—Alzheimer's Disease and Related Disorders (NINCDS-ADRDA) (American Psychiatric Association, 1994; McKhann et al., 1984). These criteria identify AD when a clear dementia is present. In order to meet standardized criteria for dementia and/or AD (DSM-III–R, American Psychiatric Association, 1987, or DSM-IV for dementia and NINCDS-ADRDA for AD), the patient must display clear impairment in general cognitive functioning, activities of daily living (ADLs), and in memory and at least one other nonmemory cognitive domain.

NINCDS-ADRDA criteria for the clinical diagnosis of probable AD requires that the dementia be confirmed by neuropsychological tests in addition to being established by clinical examination and documented by the Mini-Mental State Examination (MMSE) or some similar examination (McKhann et al., 1984). There must be a deficit in memory and at least one other area of cognition, e.g., attention, language, visuospatial functioning, problem solving, or executive functioning. In addition, a progressive decline in memory and overall cognitive functioning must be documented.

The NINCDS-ADRDA task force operationally defined impairment in a domain of cognitive functioning as a score at or below the fifth percentile compared to appropriate normative data controlling for age, gender, and education. Adequate demographic normative data for cognitive test measures employed are needed in order to accurately judge whether a score is abnormal or not for a given patient. See Ivnik et al. (2001) for an in-depth discussion of statistics not typically reported in neuropsychological studies (e.g., sensitivity, specificity, hit rates, positive and negative predictive values, odds ratios, and likelihood ratios) that describe a cognitive test's ability to classify individuals as either "impaired" or "normal."

A clinical neuropsychological evaluation can measure the severity, pattern, and progression of the cognitive strengths and weaknesses, which provides information that is useful in the early detection and differential diagnosis of AD and other dementias. The confirmation of dementia with a neuropsychological evaluation is especially important when the dementia is mild, whereas cases of more severe dementia may be obvious without formal cognitive testing. However, even when a patient has obvious cognitive/functional impairment, a neuropsychological assessment can still provide a profile of the patient's cognitive strengths and weakness, i.e., areas of relatively preserved versus impaired abilities.

A cognitive profile should be interpreted in the context of a thorough history. In a dementia evaluation, a history should be taken by separately interviewing the patient and a reliable informant, and also by reviewing the patient's medical records. The history should include information regarding the nature, severity and course of any cognitive changes, and information regarding the patient's medical, psychosocial, and psychiatric background.

The objective cognitive test results and history information will help form an impression of the degree of cognitive decline and its possible causes. This information should be helpful in the diagnosis and management of the patient. If the patient reports little or no cognitive/functional decline, whereas a reliable informant reports clinically significant decline in the patient, then this discrepancy may be an indication that the patient lacks awareness of his or her cognitive decline (see Awareness of Deficit section later in this chapter). The reader is referred to Chapter 1 of this volume for thorough coverage of the neuropsychological interview.

The differential diagnosis of early dementia versus aging can be challenging because AD begins insidiously and normal aging is associated with some declines in memory and other cognitive abilities. In the past, a lack of elderly normative data, especially for age 75 and above, compromised the ability to detect early (i.e., mild) Alzheimer dementia. However, considerably improved normative data has become available in recent years, including normative data for minorities. See Chapter 6 in this volume for a discussion of the effects of race, ethnicity, and cultural background on neuropsychological performance and the issue and availability of separate norms for African-Americans and other racial/ethnic groups.

Early detection of Alzheimer dementia

A typical pattern of neuropsychological test results in mild to moderate AD is anterograde amnesia, intellectual impairment, a lower Performance IQ than Verbal IQ, constructional problems, reduced verbal fluency, and variable language deficits including impaired confrontation naming (Salmon & Hodges, 2001; Zec, 1993). In early AD not all of these impairments may be present. Motor disorders are rare in AD patients until the advanced stages, and sensory functions generally remain intact (Mendez & Cummings, 2003). A screening cognitive evaluation for dementia taking an hour or less can provide an assessment of major cognitive functions. A longer assessment (2 hours or more) can provide a more comprehensive evaluation, which is useful in cases of mild dementia.

Anterograde memory impairment is an almost universal initial presenting feature in AD, which is typically followed by impairment in abstract reasoning and complex attention, and then in language and visuospatial abilities (Grady et al., 1988). New declarative learning and memory (e.g., episodic memory) is almost always impaired in early AD, and continues to decline over the course of the disorder (Zec, 1993). Multiple trial word-list learning and retention tests are especially useful and should include immediate and delayed recall, and delayed recognition. AD patients display rapid forgetting of new information, which is evident when memory on a delayed retention measure is compared to immediate memory performance on the last learning trial (Moss, Albert, Butters, & Payne, 1986). There is some evidence, however, that the rate of forgetting is not abnormal when short-delay and long-delay recall are compared.

These findings indicate that it is the failure to consolidate new information during learning that accounts for the rapid forgetting (Salmon & Hodges, 2001).

There are published cases of AD confirmed by biopsy or autopsy that initially presented atypically with either a progressive right parietal lobe syndrome (Crystal, Horoupian, Katzman, & Jotkowitz, 1982) or a progressive aphasia (Kirshner, Webb, Kelly, & Wells, 1984). Furthermore, AD patients with impairments in memory and intellectual functioning may display additional impairment only in semantic knowledge (e.g., word-finding ability) or only in visuospatial abilities during a phase of their illness (Martin, 1987). AD patients with predominant word-finding deficits were found to have significantly greater hypometabolism in the left temporal lobe compared to other cortical regions, whereas patients with predominant constructional impairment displayed significantly greater hypometabolism in the right temporal and parietal areas (Martin, 1987).

The sensitivity of a given test measure to the progressive cognitive decline in AD is in part a function of the patient's initial level of performance on that test (Mohs, Kim, Johns, Dunn, & Davis, 1986). Test measures on which the patient displays an intermediate level of impairment are more likely to be sensitive to further decline. Test measures that are too difficult will have "floor" effects and will not be able to detect further decline. Tests that are too easy will have "ceiling" effects and may be useful later in the course of the disorder but are not likely to detect further decline in the near term (e.g., next year or two). For example, Mohs et al. (1986) reported that recall was more impaired than recognition memory on a baseline assessment, but recognition memory was a better measure of the progressive decline over the next 12 months. Neither a *difficult* task like learning low-frequency paired associates or an *easy* task like naming common objects were sensitive to change over 12 months, whereas tests of *intermediate* difficulty (e.g., sentence reading and paired-associate learning) were sensitive to decline over that period.

Brief mental status tests and neuropsychological batteries for evaluation of dementia

The clinical diagnosis of probable AD using NINCDS-ADRDA Work Group criteria requires that the dementia be "established by clinical examination and documented by the Mini-Mental Status, Blessed Dementia Scale, or some similar examination, and confirmed by neuropsychological tests" (McKhann et al., 1984). Brief mental status tests are reliable and valid measures of moderate to severe dementia (Kaszniak, 1986). Among the commonly used brief mental status tests taking 5–10 minutes to administer are the Mini-Mental State Examination (MMSE; Folstein, Folstein, & McHugh, 1975), the Information Memory Concentration test (IMC; Blessed, Tomlinson, & Roth, 1968), and the short Blessed IMC test (Katzman et al., 1983). The MMSE and Blessed IMC decline at an average rate of 2.8 and 3.2 points per year, respectively, in patients with probable AD (Salmon, Thal,

Butters, & Heindel, 1990). One of these mental status tests should be part of a dementia workup in order to provide a widely accepted quantitative index of dementia severity. The brief mental status tests have a very high false-negative rate for patients with mild dementia (Pfeffer et al., 1981; Wilson & Kaszniak, 1986). They are not adequate for the detection and description of mild dementia or in providing a cognitive profile, and should be only one part of a comprehensive neuropsychological evaluation for dementia (Bondi, Salmon, Galasko, Thomas, & Thal, 1999; Mathuranath, Nestor, Berrios, Rakowicz, & Hodges, 2000; Tombaugh & McIntyre, 1992). For additional information on this topic see Chapter 2 in this volume.

A cognitive evaluation for dementia needs to assess a wide range of memory and nonmemory cognitive abilities. A comprehensive assessment can provide a good description of the patient's cognitive profile and also can determine whether a patient exhibits the two or more areas of cognitive impairment required to meet DSM-IV criteria for dementia and NINCDS-ADRDA neuropsychological criteria for AD.

By providing a description of the patient's pattern of cognitive strengths and weaknesses across different cognitive domains, a neuropsychological assessment can aid in the early detection and differential diagnosis of dementing disorders (including mild cognitive impairment) and provide a baseline against which to measure change over time and response to treatment. These test results need to be interpreted in the context of the patient's history. The cognitive tests used should be standardized psychometric measures with established test–retest reliability and discriminative validity for which there is adequate demographic normative data for the patient being evaluated. There should also be data available describing the typical cognitive profile displayed by patients with different dementing disorders.

There are many alternative test measures that can be used to evaluate the multiple cognitive areas that become impaired in patients with AD (Salmon & Butters, 1992; Salmon & Hodges, 2001). There is a variety of neuropsychological test batteries for the evaluation of dementia, but typically each battery includes measures of mental status, intellect, memory, language, and visuospatial functioning. In general, the more comprehensive the cognitive test battery, the more information that is provided regarding the patient's cognitive strengths and weaknesses across and within cognitive domains. Neuropsychological batteries are discussed in Chapter 3 of this volume and thus this topic will only be briefly discussed here. In a later section of this chapter, the cognitive profiles characteristic of various dementing disorders are discussed along with the test measures that are useful in differential diagnosis.

At Southern Illinois University (SIU) Center for Alzheimer Disease and Related Disorders, dementia referrals receive an initial short cognitive assessment using an extended version of the Alzheimer's Disease Assessment Scale (ADAS), which takes approximately 1 hour to administer (Zec, 1993; Zec et al., 1994; Zec, Landreth, Vicari, Belman et al., 1992; Zec, Landreth, Vicari, Feldman et al., 1992). If the results on the ADAS are equivocal or atypical (e.g., memory is not disproportionately impaired), we often bring the patient back for a more comprehensive dementia assessment using the SIU Comprehensive Cognitive Battery for Dementia (CCBD), which takes approximately 2.5 hours to administer (for a description of this battery see Zec, 1993). For a list of tests comprising another comprehensive neuropsychological test battery used in dementia assessments see Salmon and Butters (1992).

There are several short cognitive assessment instruments used in dementia evaluations that each take approximately 30 minutes to administer. These include the Mattis Dementia Rating Scale (MDRS; Mattis, 1976; Salmon et al., 1990), the Repeatable Battery for the Assessment of Neuropsychological Status (RBANS; Randolph, Tierney, Mohr, & Chase, 1998), the Cambridge Cognitive Examination (CAMCOG; Huppert, Brayne, Gill, Paykel, & Beardsall, 1995), the Alzheimer Disease Assessment Scale (ADAS-Cog; Grundman et al., 2004; Rosen, Mohs & Davis, 1984; Zec, Landreth, Vicari, Belman et al., 1992; Zec, Landreth, Vicari, Feldman et al., 1992), and the Consortium to Establish a Registry for Alzheimer's Disease (CERAD) neuropsychological battery (Welsh, Butters, Hughes, Mohs, & Heyman, 1991, 1992).

Attention

Based on both cross-sectional and longitudinal data, episodic memory is typically the first presenting cognitive impairment in AD followed by attentional impairment (e.g., Trail Making Test B and Stroop test), and then visuospatial and language dysfunction (Grady et al., 1988). Perry, Watson, and Hodges (2000) reported that a mildly demented AD group (MMSE = 18–23) was impaired on all measures in a battery of attentional tests assessing sustained, divided, and selective attention. A minimally demented AD group (MMSE ≥ 24) was intact on sustained attention and divided attention based on a dual-task paradigm, but was impaired on response inhibition and speed of attentional switching. Overall, attentional impairment was more common than semantic memory impairment, and least common were deficits in visuospatial functions. Episodic memory was impaired in all patients including the 40% of AD patients who displayed no impairments in attention or any other cognitive domain, indicating that anterograde amnesia is often the only cognitive deficit in the very early stages of AD (Perry et al., 2000). In another recent study, tasks emphasizing three different aspects of selective attention, i.e., inhibition, visuospatial selective attention, and decision making, were compared in mild AD patients and healthy elderly controls (Levinoff, Li, Murtha, & Chertkow, 2004). Inhibition was found to be the most impaired aspect of selective attention in the early AD patients.

Higher levels of selective and divided attention were also found to be clearly and disproportionately impaired in AD, whereas psychomotor speed and lower levels of attention (i.e., sensorimotor) were disproportionately impaired in subcortical dementias like multi-infarct dementia even though matched with the

AD group in terms of overall dementia severity (Gainotti, Marra, & Villa, 2001). AD patients are particularly affected on visual search tasks (ability to detect a target among a set of distractors) in which the target is defined by a conjunction of features (e.g., orientation and lightness) and where performance depends on shifting of attention (Tales et al., 2002). The poor performance of AD patients on visual search tasks is probably the result of both a deficit in the ability to shift attention from item to item and inefficient processing of each item within the search set (Tales, Muir, Jones, Bayer, & Snowden, 2004).

Early AD patients are typically impaired on tests that place strong demands on working memory (Sahakian, Jones, Levy, Gray, & Warburton, 1989). For example, patients with AD are impaired on dual task perform- ance, i.e., the capacity to combine performance on two simultaneous tasks (Baddeley, Della Sala, & Spinnler, 1991; Baddeley, Baddeley, Bucks, & Wilcock, 2001). These findings support the hypothesis that there is impair- ment in the central executive component of working memory that controls and directs attentional resources.

General cognitive slowing in aging and AD

Aging is associated with a general mental slowing, but there is greater general slowing of cognitive processing in AD (Nebes & Brady, 1992). The difference in reaction time (RT) in AD versus normal aging increases linearly but pro- portionately with increasing task complexity across a wide variety of cogni- tive tasks, i.e., the difference between AD patients and normal controls becomes larger the more complex the task. Because a significant group by condition interaction may be due to general cognitive slowing, evidence for a specific cognitive deficit in AD is more convincing if the AD group is *disproportionately* slow on a specific task. The magnitude of this general slowing increases with severity of dementia.

Executive functioning and problem solving

Executive functioning and problem solving in AD has not received as much research attention as memory, language, or visuospatial functioning, but it is believed to be impaired relatively early in the clinical course of the disorder. Although abstract problem-solving ability declines in aging, there is addi- tional decline in early AD, along with a decline in episodic memory. However, it should be kept in mind that tests of abstraction are often quite sensitive to the effects of age and education and can be sensitive to psychi- atric disorders such as depression and other neurological disorders like Pick's disease (Raskin, Friedman, & DiMascio, 1982). Considerable intrasubject variability in performance on abstraction measures can be seen in many depressed patients as a function of mood state (LaRue, Spar, & Hill, 1986).

Executive functions involving the concurrent manipulation of information including set shifting, self-monitoring, and sequencing (as measured by FAS word fluency test, Trails B, and the Self-Ordering Test) and the ability to perceive and synthesize visual patterns of relationships in increasingly complex visual stimuli (Hukok Test) were reported to be impaired in early AD (Lafleche & Albert, 1995). On the other hand, executive functions involved in cue-directed attention (Cued Reaction Time Test) and verbal concept formation (Similarities and Proverb Interpretation) were found to be relatively spared. AD patients with mild to moderate dementia, however, have been reported to be impaired relative to age-matched elderly controls on the WAIS–R Similarities and Comprehension subtests, which measure verbal abstraction and judgment (Moss & Albert, 1988).

Abstraction deficits in dementia patients have been reported on tests of proverb interpretation, card sorting, picture absurdities, Raven's Colored Progressive Matrices, and Piaget's abstract problem-solving tasks. Compared to a group of age- and education-matched controls, AD patients had difficulty verbally interpreting proverbs, although they could choose the correct answers on a recognition test (Andree, Hittmair, & Benke, 1992). Patients with mild AD generally do well on the easy visual abstractions on the MDRS but performance declines as the dementia progresses (Mattis, 1976). Impairment of basic arithmetic skills can appear early in AD (Cummings, 1990), which may be due to impaired problem-solving skills or to impairments in other cognitive functions like attention and semantic memory.

Drawing to command (i.e., spontaneous drawing or drawing from memory) is more sensitive than copying (i.e., reproduction drawings) early in the course of AD (Strub & Black, 1988). On a clock to command test, the patient is asked to draw a clock with all the numbers on it and draw the hands to indicate a specific time, e.g., "10 after 11" (Salmon & Butters, 1992). Impairment on clock to command is often found as AD advances as manifested by misplacement of the hands and/or incorrectly numbering the clock. If the patient can correctly copy the clock face from a model, then impairment on clock to command is likely due to difficulty in conceptualizing time on a clock rather than due to visuoconstructional deficits. Performance on a clock-drawing test requires semantic memory, visuospatial ability, and executive skills (Ueda et al., 2002). In a SPECT study with a group of AD patients, it was found that the clock-drawing test correlated significantly with MMSE score and with metabolism in the left posterior temporal area (Ueda et al., 2002).

Awareness of deficit

Anosognosia for one's own dementia is most common in "cortical" dementias like AD or Pick's disease. Some loss of insight or awareness of one's own cognitive/functional deficits has been reported in mild AD with decreasing awareness as the severity of dementia increases (Frederiks, 1985). Considerable variability in insight among dementia patients has been reported (Neary et al., 1986). The loss of insight can vary in terms of the degree of unawareness and across different cognitive/functional domains, and can fluctuate over time. AD patients' self-ratings significantly underestimate impairments on objective memory measures and on ratings of everyday memory and cognitive functioning, and activities of daily living compared with ratings by relatives (McGlynn & Kaszniak, 1991a, 1991b; Ott et al., 1996). Measures of awareness of deficits have been found to correlate with performance on tests of executive and visuospatial functioning. It is possible that the severe impairment in episodic memory and the resultant lack of an enduring record for personal events in AD patients is a contributing factor to their lack of insight. Poor self-predictions of AD patients have also been attributed to impairment in metacognitive processes or executive functions, including self-monitoring, which may be due to disruption of frontal-sub-cortical circuits. Behavioral problems in everyday life displayed by AD patients that may be expressions of their unawareness of deficit include delu-sions, risky behavior, and failure to use compensatory techniques (Kaszniak, 1992). It should also be said that unawareness of deficit may have the beneficial effect of emotionally protecting the AD patient from the painful awareness of their cognitive loss.

Memory impairment in AD

All stages of memory *eventually* decline in AD, including sensory, primary (i.e., short-term memory), secondary (i.e., long-term memory), and tertiary (remote) memory, whereas only secondary memory declines in normal aging (Kaszniak, Poon, & Riege, 1986). In this section, the following topics are dis-cussed: forgetfulness in daily life, anterograde memory impairment, multiple memory systems in AD, neuroanatomy of the anterograde amnesia in AD, and assessment of memory in AD. In this chapter, the terms anterograde memory, recent memory, new declarative learning and memory, secondary memory, and episodic memory are used interchangeably.

Forgetfulness in daily life

Forgetfulness increases with progression of AD. Patients with AD may repeatedly ask the same question and repeat the same story. Patients with AD forget people's names, telephone numbers, conversations, and events. They forget appointments and to take their medications. They may leave tasks unfinished because of forgetting to resume an activity after being interrupted, e.g., may forget to turn off the stove or leave the faucet running. Patients with AD frequently misplace objects and forget why they entered a room. AD patients typically become progressively disoriented to time, place, and then person (Ashford, Kolm, Colliver, Bekian, & Hsu, 1989).

In the early stages, AD patients may increasingly write many reminder notes and often need to be reminded by family members to compensate for their for-getfulness. AD patients, especially in the earlier stages, often appear to recall events from the very distant past better than those from the recent past. More recent memory is impaired because of an anterograde memory impairment, whereas remote memories are less affected in the early stages of the disorder.

Forgetfulness can also increase with normal aging. When memory lapses become frequent and reminder cues become less helpful in jogging one's memory, then abnormal forgetting is likely being exhibited and should be a source of concern. Conversely, if memory lapses are not frequent and reminder cues successfully jog a person's memory, then this milder forgetfulness is more likely due to normal aging.

Anterograde memory impairment

The central cognitive deficit in AD is a progressive anterograde memory impairment, which begins insidiously, progresses gradually, and is usually the first presenting symptom. This memory impairment will progress to the point of floor effects on most standardized tests of memory recall relatively early in the clinical course of the disorder. Anterograde memory impairment remains a prominent and often disproportionate cognitive deficit in patients with AD throughout its clinical course. A small minority of AD patients exhibit language or visuospatial deficits as the initial presenting symptom and only later become amnesic.

Virtually all aspects and types of new declarative learning and memory (including both learning and delayed retention, recall and recognition memory, verbal and visual memory) are typically severely impaired by the middle stages of AD. This impairment can be demonstrated in AD patients on a variety of memory measures, including word-list learning, story memory, and paired-associate learning, although word-list learning tests appear to be especially useful.

Anterograde amnesia in AD is characterized by a dramatic loss of information over a short delay (e.g., 2–10 minutes) compared to immediate memory on the last learning trial (Hart, Kwentus, Harkins, & Taylor, 1988; Moss et al., 1986). This rapid forgetting including on retention measures with low retrieval demands (cued recall and recognition memory) suggests that the anterograde memory impairment in AD is due to a failure to store information in long-term memory (LTM), rather than being only a retrieval problem.

Multiple memory systems in AD

Multiple memory systems in the brain have been identified (Squire, 1992), including declarative and nondeclarative memory. Declarative or explicit memory is memory for facts and events (i.e., semantic and episodic memory, respectively) in which the information can be consciously declared or described verbally or visually. New declarative learning and memory is dependent upon the integrity of the medial temporal lobe memory system (MTLMS) (i.e., hippocampus and related structures, including entorhinal, perirhinal, and parahippocampal cortices) (Squire & Zola-Morgan, 1991). The MTLMS establishes new long-term declarative memories for facts and events via its extensive and reciprocal connections with widespread neocortical association areas (Squire & Zola-Morgan, 1991).

Nondeclarative or implicit memory includes a variety of different learning and memory abilities in which there is activation of a memory trace and a change in performance as a result of experience that does not depend on conscious awareness of what is being learned or the context of the learning. There are different types of implicit memory, including lexical priming as can be measured by stem-completion, perceptual priming as measured by identification of fragmented line drawings of objects, motor skill learning as can be measured by a motor pursuit task, and weight-biasing skill. Priming can be perceptual or semantic. Nondeclarative memory is not mediated by the MTLMS.

Both types of declarative memory (i.e., semantic and episodic memory) and *some* types of nondeclarative memory (i.e., lexical and semantic priming) are impaired in AD (Salmon, Shimamura, Butters, & Smith, 1988). On the other hand, perceptual priming and procedural (i.e., skill) learning are types of nondeclarative memory that remain preserved in AD. Impaired priming in AD patients was attributed to damage to association neocortex, whereas the basal ganglia are generally not damaged in AD, which presumably accounts for their intact procedural (i.e., skill) learning (Butters, Heindel, & Salmon, 1990).

Episodic memory is new declarative learning and memory for information or events that requires temporal and spatial contextual cues for retrieval (Tulving, 1983). AD patients display gradually progressive anterograde memory impairment for the acquisition and retention of new episodic memories. This deficit in episodic memory can also be conceptualized as a difficulty in transferring information from primary memory (i.e., short-term memory) to secondary memory (long-term memory). Episodic memory impairment can be measured using any of a wide variety of standardized tests. These include the Rey Auditory Verbal Learning Test, the California Verbal Learning Test–II, the Buschke Selective Reminding Test, the Wechsler Memory Scale–III, the Memory Assessment Scale, the Fuld Object-Memory Evaluation, the Hopkins Verbal Learning Test, and the Delayed Recognition Span Test (see Zec, 1993).

In addition to an anterograde amnesia, AD patients exhibit a temporally graded retrograde amnesia (RA) that eventually progresses to a temporally extended, severe RA (Albert, 1981). RA is difficulty remembering previously learned information including both public and autobiographical facts and events. Earlier in the clinical course of AD, more remote memories from childhood and adolescence are initially better preserved than more recent memories. However, this temporally graded aspect is gradually lost and the RA becomes flat as AD progresses into the moderate dementia stage. In AD, the medial temporal lobe is the brain region first to be damaged, but eventually both the medial and lateral temporal lobes become severely damaged, which is known to be sufficient to cause a very extensive RA in human amnesic patients (Reed & Squire, 1998). The findings of Reed and Squire suggest that RA can be quite limited or very extensive, depending on whether the damage is restricted to the hippocampal formation or also involves additional temporal cortex. In AD, there is progressive damage to all the structures in the MTLMS, including the hippocampal formation and surrounding medial temporal lobe structures. As the disease progresses, damage in the medial temporal lobe spreads to the neighboring lateral temporal cortical areas, which likely cause a more severe and temporally extensive RA. Damage to neocortical association areas in general eventually impairs semantic memory and thereby also contributes to the RA.

Semantic memory is well-learned information that is part of one's fund of knowledge (i.e., crystallized knowledge) and no longer dependent upon temporal and spatial contextual cues for retrieval. Information in semantic memory for most people includes common historical facts, facts about geography, number facts, and vocabulary. The WAIS–III Information and Vocabulary subtests are tests of semantic memory. AD patients in the very early stages primarily display impairment in episodic memory (i.e., an anterograde amnesia) with relatively preserved semantic memory, but both episodic and semantic memory will be impaired as the dementia becomes more severe (Butters, Granholm, Salmon, Grant, & Wolfe, 1987).

Neuroanatomy of the anterograde amnesia in AD

Converging evidence from both animal and human studies has established that a group of interconnected structures in the medial temporal lobe (MTL) are critical to new declarative learning and memory (Squire & Zola-Morgan, 1991). The medial temporal lobe memory system (MTLMS) includes the hippocampal formation (especially the CA1 field and subiculum), the entorhinal cortex (Brodmann area 28), perirhinal cortex (Brodmann areas 35 and 36), and the parahippocampal cortex (Squire & Zola-Morgan, 1991). Sufficient bilateral damage to the structures in the MTLMS can cause an anterograde amnesia (Squire & Zola-Morgan, 1991). In general, the greater the degree of damage to these structures, the more severe the anterograde memory impairment (Squire & Zola-Morgan, 1991). In addition to AD, the MTLMS can be damaged by viral encephalitis, posterior cerebral artery occlusions, anoxia, carbon monoxide poisoning, and anterior temporal lobectomy in cases of intractable epilepsy.

In AD, all the major components of the MTLMS undergo progressive damage due to the slow accumulation of pathological changes (especially neurofibrillary tangles and neuronal loss). The MTLMS is the brain region in which neuropathological changes characteristic of AD first appear and first reach a clinically significant threshold of damage. All the major components of the MTLMS are major sites in the regional cortical distribution of neurofibrillary tangles (NFTs) in AD. NFTs and neuronal loss progressively destroy the following major medial temporal lobe structures: the perirhinal and posterior parahippocampal areas, the entorhinal cortex, and the CA1 region of the hippocampus and subiculum (Van Hoesen, 2002; Van Hoesen, Augustinack, Dierking, Redman, & Thangavel, 2000).

Progressive degeneration of the MTLMS and a disconnection of the flow of information through this system at multiple critical points is likely the primary cause of the progressive anterograde memory impairment in AD patients. Early and progressive damage to perirhinal cortex and somewhat later to the parahippocampal cortex increasingly interrupts communication between the association neocortex and the entorhinal cortex (EC). Early and progressive damage to layers II and IV of the EC, and to the EC as a whole, increasingly interrupts communication between the hippocampal formation and the perirhinal and parahippocampal cortices. Early and progressive damage to the CA1/subiculum increasingly interrupts the unidirectional flow of information through the trisynapic circuit of the hippocampus and the output from the hippocampus to the EC. In the later stages of AD, there is complete or near complete destruction and disconnection of all the major critical components of the MTLMS that culminates in a very profound anterograde amnesia in which there is little or no residual capacity for new declarative learning and memory.

The damage to brain areas outside of the MTLMS may also contribute to the anterograde memory impairment by decreasing an individual's functional reserve capacity for new learning and memory. As AD progresses, there is damage to structures in the midline diencephalon (Braak & Braak, 1991a) and basal forebrain (Arendt, Bigl, Arendt, & Tennstedt, 1983) that can also cause anterograde memory impairment and thus may further contribute to the anterograde amnesia in AD. In the midline diencephalon, there are numerous NFTs and neuropil threads in several thalamic nuclei in AD, including the anterior nuclear complex, and numerous amyloid deposits were found in almost all thalamic nuclei (Braak & Braak, 1991a). Although damage in brain areas outside the medial temporal lobe may contribute to Alzheimer amnesia, the progressive damage to the MTLMS is sufficient to cause progressive anterograde memory impairment in AD from mild forgetfulness to very profound or end-stage anterograde amnesia.

Assessment of memory in AD

A memory evaluation of a patient referred for possible dementia should include both a cognitive history and an objective memory assessment using appropriate standardized test measures. The patient and a reliable informant should be separately interviewed regarding the following aspects of the patient's memory decline: premorbid level of functioning, nature and time of onset, course, rate of progression, current status, examples of everyday memory difficulty and its impact on daily functioning, and possible causes or contributing factors. Verbal memory measures, especially word-list learning tests, are the most useful cognitive tests for the early detection of clinical AD and amnestic MCI. In order to adequately test anterograde memory in AD using a word-list paradigm, one should administer a supraspan list of words (i.e., the list should at minimum include 10 words) over multiple learning trials (i.e., at least 3) followed by measures of short-delay recall and recognition memory. The word list should exceed the 7 ± 2 items of information that can typically be temporarily stored in short-term (i.e., primary) memory. A minimum of three learning trials are needed to generate a learning curve and to provide the subject with an adequate opportunity to acquire and store new information. The three learning trials will also increase the likelihood that the subject has paid adequate attention to the words on the list, and thus poor delayed recall would more likely be due to impaired memory rather than to concentration difficulty.

In general, on multiple trial word-list learning and retention tasks, elderly controls display a clear learning curve, good recall, and good recognition memory with minimal false positive errors, whereas AD patients with mild dementia display little learning over trials, poor recall, and poor recognition memory with many false positive errors if a demanding recognition paradigm is used. The memory impairment increases with progression of AD, but floor effects on delayed recall measures are often reached early in the course of the disorder. Delayed recall has been reported to be the most sensitive measure to early AD (Welsh et al., 1991, 1992). Other measures of verbal memory include story recall (such as the Logical Memory portion of the WMS–III) or verbal paired-associate learning (e.g., from the WMS–III; Wechsler, 1997). Tests of visual memory include the WMS–III Visual Immediate and Delayed indexes and its subtests, the Benton Visual Retention Test, immediate and delay recall of the Rey-Osterreith Complex Figure Test, and the Warrington Visual Memory Test.

Language

Aphasia

Aphasia is common as AD progresses (Appell, Kertesz, & Fisman, 1982; Cummings, Benson, Hill, & Read, 1985). To classify the type of aphasic syndrome, the following three language characteristics need to be assessed: auditory comprehension, repetition, and fluency of speech (i.e., phrase length) (Helm-Estabrooks & Albert, 1991). A commonly used aphasia classification system identifies eight aphasia syndromes, including anomic, transcortical sensory, Wernicke's, global, conduction, Broca's, transcortical motor, and mixed aphasia. Lexical retrieval problems, i.e., word-finding difficulties, are found in all aphasic syndromes (Helm-Estabrooks & Albert, 1991). Anomic aphasia in the context of relatively intact articulation, repetition, speech fluency, and auditory comprehension, is usually displayed in early AD (Appell et al., 1982; Cummings et al., 1985; Kertesz, 1979). In terms of a differential diagnosis, it should be kept in mind that an anomic aphasia is also common after head injury and in metabolic or toxic disorders, and a slowly progressive anomic aphasia can result from a brain tumor in either cerebral hemisphere (Mesulam, 2000). Alzheimer aphasia increasingly resembles a transcortical sensory aphasia as the dementia progresses and comprehension deficits become more severe (Cummings et al., 1985). These patients exhibit fluent paraphasic output but relatively preserved repetition. In the late stages of the disease, repetition declines and the language disorder resembles a Wernicke's aphasia (Cummings et al., 1985). A global aphasia may be displayed in end-stage AD (Appell et al., 1982). The four types of fluent aphasia associated with AD (i.e., anomic, transcortical sensory, Wernicke's, and global) can all be caused by focal left temporal damage depending on the location and extent of the lesion (Benson, 1979). It can be inferred that left posterior frontal cortex is not significantly damaged in AD because AD patients do not display either Broca's aphasia or transcortical motor aphasia.

Confrontation naming

Word finding difficulty, semantic paraphasias and circumlocutions are evident relatively early in AD (Appell et al., 1982). Although naming difficulties are found in aphasic syndromes of different etiologies (Kertesz, 1979), the types of naming errors may have value in differential diagnosis. AD patients exhibit frequent circumlocutions (e.g., "horse with a horn" for unicorn) and semantic paraphasias (e.g., "plane" for helicopter), but do not display phonemic paraphasias (e.g., "harmotica" for harmonica) or transpositions until the late stages (Appell et al., 1982).

Impairment in confrontation naming as measured by the Boston Naming Test (BNT) becomes more common as AD progresses. Initial BNT impairment is associated with increased risk of a subsequent diagnosis of AD, but it is not as useful a predictor as impairment in delayed recall (Testa et al., 2004). Hodges, Salmon, and Butters (1991) reported that on the BNT, AD patients made a disproportionate number of semantic-superordinate and semantic-associative errors. Semantic-superordinate errors are responses that indicate the general semantic category to which the object belongs (e.g., "vegetable" for asparagus). In semantic-associative errors, there is a clear semantic association with the target object (e.g., "painting" for easel; "ice" for igloo; "ocean" for octopus, or "Vesuvius" for volcano). Over a 3-year follow-up period, confrontation naming scores declined and there was a significant increase in the percentage of semantic associative errors and visual errors. The findings were interpreted as indicating that there is a progressive breakdown in semantic processing in AD and that visuoperceptual impairment will increasingly contribute to the naming difficulty. Phonemic processes are relatively preserved in AD.

Generative naming

Generative naming (i.e., word fluency) tasks are another important part of a cognitive assessment of dementia (Bayles, Kaszniak, & Tomoeda, 1987). Along with tests of episodic memory, generative naming tests (which measure language and semantic memory) are useful in differentiating mild AD patients and normal elderly (Storandt, Botwinick, Danziger, Berg, & Hughes, 1984). On tests of generative naming, subjects are asked to generate exemplars from a particular semantic category (i.e., semantic word fluency; SWF) or words that begin with a certain letter of the alphabet (i.e., phonemic word fluency; PWF) within a specific time limit (e.g., 60 seconds). AD patients, even in the early clinical stages, tend to generate fewer correct words than normal elderly. Generative naming declines with increasing severity of dementia (Bayles et al., 1987) and has been reported in several studies to be more sensitive than confrontation naming in early dementia (Appell et al., 1982; Bayles et al., 1987; Zec, 1993).

The majority of studies have found that SWF is superior to PWF in discriminating patients with AD (including mild AD) from elderly controls (Monsch et al., 1992; Salmon, Heindel, & Lange, 1999; also see Zec, 1993). The greater impairment of AD patients on SWF versus PWF tasks may be due to a breakdown in the hierarchical structure of semantic knowledge (Martin, 1987) that interferes with the ability to generate exemplars of an abstract concept. Using sensitivity and specificity to calculate predictive values, both category fluency and letter fluency were useful in differentially diagnosing AD versus nondemented elderly, but category fluency was superior in correctly categorizing subjects in these two groups (Cerhan et al., 2002). It has been suggested that AD patients are relatively less impaired on PWF tasks because they can rhyme their way through the list rather than having to use semantic processes (Butters et al., 1987). Generative naming in AD may be reduced both by aphasia and increased sensitivity to interference (Butters et al., 1987).

Visuospatial functioning

Visuospatial deficits in both perceptual and constructional abilities are exhibited in dementias of different etiologies and are commonly displayed by the middle stages of AD. Impaired visuospatial functioning is likely due to the disproportionate neuropathological changes and brain dysfunction which are found in posterior cortical areas (e.g., parietal lobes) as AD progresses. Sometimes, albeit rarely, an impairment in visuospatial functioning is the first presenting cognitive impairment in AD (Martin, 1987). Everyday expression of impaired visuospatial functioning in AD patients includes getting lost in familiar and unfamiliar surroundings, getting lost when driving, and difficulty recognizing familiar faces (Cummings & Benson, 1992). Visuospatial functioning can be measured in AD patients using the following types of tests: constructional, drawing and copying, judgment of line orientation, visuointegration, facial discrimination, mental rotation, map reading, and mazes.

Visuoperceptual deficits

Visuoperceptual deficits in AD are not typically the first presenting cognitive deficit but do increase with dementia severity (Bayles et al., 1987). However, Ska, Poissant, and Joanette (1990) reported impaired performance on the Benton Line Orientation test in a group of early AD patients compared to controls. Eslinger and Benton (1983) reported that a group of patients with dementia due to a variety of etiologies scored significantly worse than a matched normal group (with a large effect size) on two visuoperceptual tests, i.e., the Benton Facial Recognition Test (Benton & van Allen, 1968) and the Benton Line Orientation Test (Benton, Varney, & deS. Hamsher, 1978). Both tests are sensitive to right posterior damage (Benton, deS. Hamsher, Varney, & Spreen, 1983). Dissociations in performance on these two visuoperceptual tests are common in dementia patients suggesting that the two tests are measuring different aspects of visuoperceptual decline.

Object form discrimination correlated significantly ($r = .60$) with performance in visually based instrumental activities of daily living (IADL) (e.g., judging distances, driving, and recognizing familiar people) in a group of dementia patients (most diagnosed with probable AD) (Glosser et al., 2002). Other visuoperceptual functions did not correlate with IADL, and object form recognition only correlated with visually based IADL. The authors inferred that bilateral inferotemporal visuoperceptual systems are important for the performance of IADL in elderly patients with neurodegenerative dementia.

Impairment in *visuoconstructional* ability, i.e., block construction and drawing and copying geometrical figures, is commonly found in AD and increases with progression of dementia. The Wechsler block design subtest, a measure of visuoconstructional problem solving, is impaired in mildly demented AD patients, although this is likely due to a decline in both visuospatial functioning and problem-solving ability (Storandt et al., 1984). Drawing tests that have been used to evaluate AD patients include the Clock Drawing Test, Clock Setting Test, and Copy-a-Cube Test (Salmon & Butters, 1992). AD patients, including those with mild dementia, often have difficulty copying two- and three-dimensional figures (Storandt et al., 1984; Zec, 1993). AD patients sometimes exhibit the "closing-in" phenomenon when copying geometrical figures, i.e., inappropriately tracing over the lines of the model or tracing lines from the model to the surrounding space when drawing a freestanding figure is the required task.

Spatial disorientation

Spatial disorientation (i.e., geographical or topographical disorientation), a form of visual agnosia, can occur as AD progresses and have a profound adverse effect on daily functioning (Strub & Black, 1988). A variety of functional impairments are considered manifestations of spatial disorientation, including wandering and getting lost, difficulty locating a public building or even one's room at home, or describing how to get to a specific place using verbal descriptions or indicating on a map (Mesulam, 2000). Spatial orientation is a complex process involving attentional, perceptual, and memory components (Maguire, 1999). The functional impairments associated with spatial disorientation can be caused by agnosia, hemispatial neglect, or global amnesia (Mesulam, 2000). Brain areas that if damaged can result in topographical disorientation include the posterior parietal lobe, the occipital lobe, the hippocampal formation, and parahippocampal gyrus (Maguire, 1999). A variety of structures in both inferior and superior visual association cortices, especially the right occipitoparietal region, are likely involved in spatial orientation (Mesulam, 2000).

Mild cognitive impairment

Research has indicated that in individuals destined to develop an Alzheimer dementia, normal cognitive aging is followed by a prodromal or transition period of cognitive impairment before the full development of dementia (Petersen, 2000, 2003). This transitional or intermediate stage has been labeled with several different terms, including incipient dementia, prodromal AD, isolated memory impairment, and most recently mild cognitive impairment (MCI). A theoretical continuum or course of progression has been proposed in persons who are destined to develop AD from normal aging to MCI to probable AD and definite AD (Petersen, 1995). There is an overlap in cognitive functioning between normal aging and MCI, and between MCI and AD. The most common presenting complaint of patients with MCI who eventually progress to meet diagnostic criteria for AD is impairment in new learning and memory. Early diagnosis of MCI in the incipient or prodromal stages of AD will become critical when effective treatments for the early stages of dementia become available.

The clinical criteria for MCI (amnestic type) include the following: (1) memory complaint, preferably corroborated by an informant, (2) objective memory impairment given the patient's age and education, (3) largely intact general cognitive functioning, (4) essentially preserved activities of daily living (ADLs), and (5) no dementia (Petersen et al., 1999). Petersen (2003) has emphasized that the criteria for MCI are clinical rather than actuarial. Thus, while neuropsychological testing is important, it is the clinical interpretation of the test results in the context of relevant information from the patient's history that is the basis for assigning this diagnosis. Amnestic MCI can be considered a prodromal, at-risk condition for AD because the vast majority of amnestic MCI subjects eventually develop clinically probable AD, although it is also important to emphasize that a small minority of these patients appear not to progress to dementia (Petersen & Morris, 2003).

At the Mayo Clinic, the diagnosis of dementia (e.g., AD) and MCI are made by consensus in a meeting of behavioral neurologists, neuropsychologists, a geriatrician, and nurses who have examined the patient. The determination of memory impairment is a clinical judgment based on the patient's history, the clinician's examination, and the objective neuropsychological test results. For a diagnosis of amnestic MCI, impairment in new learning and memory that is disproportionate to other cognitive test results is the key finding. Although no rigid cutoff scores have been proposed to establish objective memory impairment, Petersen et al. (1999) have reported that the delayed recall scores of subjects meeting clinical criteria for MCI tend to fall 1.5 *SD* or greater below age- and education-matched subjects, but they add that there is a range of scores around this mean. New learning and memory has typically been evaluated by learning or delayed recall on a multiple-trial free-recall task such as the Rey Auditory Verbal Learning Test and sometimes by delayed story recall (i.e., Logical Memory II) or delayed recall for geometrical figures (i.e., Visual Reproduction II) on the Wechsler Memory Scale–Revised or III.

In general, nonmemory cognitive domains, including attention, language, visuospatial function, and problem solving, should have little or no impairment (e.g., z-score of 0.5 or less compared to normative values), i.e., insufficient to meet criteria for dementia. Judgment about the ADLs is based on the history obtained from the subject and informant, and can be documented using questionnaires or rating scales. By definition, a patient who meets criteria for dementia cannot be diagnosed with MCI.

Neuroimaging data (e.g., hippocampal and EC volumes on structural MRI) may be helpful in predicting which MCI individuals will progress to dementia (Jack et al., 1999, 2000; Xu et al., 2000). Depressed perfusion on single photon emission computed tomography (SPECT) was found in the hippocampal-amygdaloid complex, posterior cingulate, anterior thalamus, and caudal portion of the anterior cingulate at baseline in subjects with questionable AD who would later progress to AD within a 3-year follow-up period (Johnson et al., 1998). Positron emission tomography (PET) abnormalities in metabolism have been found in presymptomatic family members of AD patients who are APOE-4 carriers (Reiman et al., 1996; Small et al., 1995). Tabert et al. (2002) found that patients with a lack of self-awareness of functional deficits, which were reported by an informant, strongly predicted progression to probable AD in MCI patients. It may be that a combination of clinical, genetic, and neuroimaging markers will provide the best predictions of which MCI subjects will progress to AD (Petersen & Morris, 2003).

Differential diagnosis of AD and other dementing disorders

In addition to early detection of a dementia and providing a detailed description of the cognitive profile, a neuropsychological evaluation can aid in differential diagnosis. In a fundamental sense, dementing disorders are neuropsychological disorders because the neuropsychological deficits (cognitive, personality, and behavioral) define the core features of the dementia. However, the differential diagnosis of the cause of the cognitive impairment also depends on an examination by a neurologist, psychiatrist, or other physician, e.g., to detect neurological signs and symptoms, and to interpret appropriate laboratory tests. Thus, ideally the differential diagnosis is an interdisciplinary process.

There are more than 50 causes of dementia in the elderly, but AD accounts for 55–70% of all cases. A diagnosis of AD depends on excluding other possible causes of the cognitive decline including neurological, medical, or psychiatric causes, or side effects of medications. Causes of dementia or chronic cognitive impairment include neurodegenerative disorders, cerebrovascular disease, endocrine disorders, vitamin deficiencies, systemic diseases, brain infection, traumatic brain injury, and other neurological disorders.

A comprehensive neuropsychological evaluation to detect and differentially diagnose a dementia consists of a relevant history and cognitive assessment. The best guideline for diagnosing AD versus other conditions is to keep in mind the natural evolution of cognitive impairment in the typical AD patient. In AD, memory impairment is usually the first presenting symptom, which begins insidiously and progresses gradually to an anterograde amnesia (i.e., amnestic MCI) before criteria for dementia are clearly met by having clear impairment in other cognitive domains. If personality, behavioral, or emotional changes are the first presenting symptoms or a nonmemory cognitive impairment is disproportionate to the memory impairment, then a diagnosis other than AD should be seriously considered. However, AD can sometimes present atypically, thus an atypical pattern does not in itself rule out this diagnosis. Other signs and symptoms that are atypical for AD and thus raise the likelihood of another dementing disorder include the following: duration of illness is less than 6 months, sudden onset of symptoms, a stepwise or lack of progression, early dramatic changes in personality, early visual hallucinations or other psychotic behavior, early severe disturbance in language in the context of preserved memory, seizures early in the course of the dementia, early gait disturbance, early urinary incontinence, or other abnormal motor or sensory signs, including parkinsonism (rigidity and bradykinesia with or without pill-rolling rest tremor), chorea, weakness on one side of the body, dysarthria, primary sensory loss, and visual field cut.

Petersen (2003) proposed three subtypes of MCI defined by different cognitive patterns, which are associated with dementing disorders of different etiologies. These three subtypes are amnestic MCI, multiple-domain MCI, and single nonmemory domain MCI. These MCI subtypes provide a useful conceptual framework for thinking about the differential diagnosis of dementing disorders. The most common presentation is amnestic MCI and it typically represents a degenerative disorder, which usually is AD. However, it needs to be emphasized that each of the three basic subtypes of MCI can progress to AD and each can be caused by degenerative, vascular, traumatic, or metabolic disorders. For example, amnestic MCI may also be caused by hippocampal sclerosis, head trauma, ischemia, depression, argyrophilic grain disease, and alcohol or other substance abuse, which may progress (e.g., ischemia may progress to vascular dementia) or remain static. Any of these different forms of MCI might progress to a vascular dementia because infarcts can affect different brain regions and thus different cognitive functions (Chui, 2000).

In *amnestic MCI* there is prominent impairment in episodic memory and these subjects progress to AD at a rate of 10–15% per year (Petersen, 2003). In *multiple-domain MCI*, there is mild impairment in more than one cognitive domain but not severe enough to meet criteria for dementia. It is thought that this type of MCI could be prodromal to AD or vascular dementia, or could be normal aging. In *single nonmemory domain MCI*, individuals have impairment in a single nonmemory cognitive domain in the context of otherwise intact cognitive functioning. For example, executive dysfunction may progress to frontotemporal dementia (Rosen, Lengenfelder, & Miller, 2000), visuospatial deficits may progress to Lewy body dementia (Ferman et al., 1999), and a prominent anomia may progress to primary progressive aphasia (Mesulam, 2001).

AD needs to be differentially diagnosed from other conditions that can cause cognitive impairment, including other irreversible progressive dementing disorders, and conditions that are fully or at least partially treatable. Other irreversible dementias include vascular dementia, Parkinson's disease, Lewy body dementia, frontotemporal dementia (e.g., Pick's disease), Huntington's disease, progressive supranuclear palsy, and Jakob-Creutzfeldt disease. Approximately 13% of dementia cases have potentially reversible causes of their dementia, but most show a partial response with only 1% displaying a complete reversal with treatment. The most common causes of reversible or partially reversible dementia are drugs, depression, metabolic causes (thyroid disease, vitamin B12 deficiency, calcium disturbance, liver disease), normal pressure hydrocephalus, subdural hematoma, and tumor (Eastley & Wilcock, 2002). Other treatable conditions that need to be considered are neurosyphilis, chronic meningitis, sleep apnea, and systemic disorders like renal failure.

The differential diagnosis of AD versus these other conditions usually depends on information beyond that provided by a cognitive assessment, i.e., on neurological signs or symptoms and the results of various medical laboratory tests. In AD, there typically is a normal neurological exam in the early stages. Parkinson's disease is characterized by rigidity, bradykinesia, and rest tremor. In Jakob-Creutzfeldt disease, there is rapid progression, myoclonus, ataxia, cortical blindness, and an abnormal EEG. In normal pressure hydrocephalus, there is a symptom triad that includes dementia, gait disturbance, urinary incontinence, and enlargement of the frontal horn of the lateral ventricle. In vascular dementia, there are focal motor and sensory signs in patients with a history of one or more strokes that has affected memory and cognition. In progressive supranuclear palsy, there is a mixture of parkinsonism, ataxia, and impairment in voluntary eye movement, especially in the downward direction.

Two of the most common causes of a misdiagnosis of dementia are delirium and depression, which may occur as comorbid conditions and may each coexist with dementia (Eastley & Wilcock, 2002). Any acute illness has the potential to cause delirium in the elderly, but urinary tract or respiratory system infections are common causes. Unlike dementia, delirium is characterized by rapid onset over hours or days associated with a medical condition, a fluctuation in consciousness and severity of symptoms (but this is also true of dementia with Lewy bodies) and confusion tends to be worse at night. In depression, there is impairment in attention and concentration that can affect memory functioning. Depression and dementia frequently co-occur. Depression pseudodementia, which improves with treatment of the depression, often over time progresses to dementia.

Studies indicate that 55–70% of dementia cases have significant AD neuropathological changes; although the percentage of "pure AD" is lower because a significant proportion of cases with AD neuropathology also have coexisting cerebrovascular disease or cortical Lewy bodies (Mendez & Cummings, 2003). Three dementing disorders, i.e., AD, vascular dementia (VaD), and dementia with Lewy bodies (DLB), account for 70–80% of cases of dementia (Mendez & Cummings, 2003). Mixed causes of dementia are common, e.g., approximately one-third of AD patients (clinically diagnosed and neuropathologically confirmed) have Lewy body pathology and another third have cerebrovascular lesions (Mendez & Cummings, 2003). The relative percentages of different dementing diseases based on both clinical and neuropathological studies are as follows: pure AD 35%, mixed vascular AD 15%, DLB 15%, pure VaD 10%, frontotemporal lobar degeneration 5%, normal pressure hydrocephalus 2.5%, other movement disorders 6%, toxic-metabolic 4%, psychiatric 4%, infectious 3%, and miscellaneous <1% (Mendez & Cummings, 2003).

In the remainder of this section, the three most common progressive dementing disorders after AD, i.e., dementia with Lewy bodies, frontotemporal lobar degeneration, and vascular dementia, will be discussed in greater detail and compared to AD. Included under frontotemporal lobar degeneration are frontotemporal dementia, progressive nonfluent aphasia, semantic dementia, and hippocampal sclerosis dementia. For additional information on neurological and psychiatric disorders that can cause cognitive impairment or dementia, see Chapters 9–12 in this volume.

Dementia with Lewy bodies

DLB is the most common degenerative dementia after AD representing 15–20% of all elderly dementia cases who go to autopsy (McKeith et al., 2003). DLB is a neurodegenerative dementia sharing clinical and pathological characteristics with both PD and AD (McKeith et al., 2003). In DLB, there is mild to moderate bradykinesia and rigidity, typically without rest tremor, and visual hallucinations. DLB often presents early prominent and disproportionate impairments in attention, problem solving, and visuospatial functioning (McKeith et al., 1996). DLB is more associated than AD with fluctuations in cognitive functioning. A relative preservation of medial temporal lobe volume is found on structural MRI. Cognitive impairment in DLB is most strongly associated with cortical LB and Lewy neurites (LNs) rather than Alzheimer type pathology. In addition, persistent well-formed visual hallucinations and parkinsonism motor symptoms are core features of DLB and help differentiate DLB from AD and other dementias (McKeith et al., 1996).

For patients with MMSE scores greater than 12 (i.e., mild to moderate dementia), greater impairment in copying overlapping pentagons has been reported in neuropathologically confirmed DLB versus AD (Ala, Hughes, Kyrouac, Ghobrial, & Elble, 2001, 2002). Furthermore, the attention and construction subtest scores of the DLB group were significantly worse than those of the AD group, whereas there was a trend for the memory subscores to be worse in the AD group (Ala et al., 2002).

Walker, Allen, Shergill, and Katona (1997) reported that the DLB group was better on recall but worse on praxis than the AD group even though the groups displayed a similar overall degree of cognitive impairment. Ballard et al. (1999) reported similar findings in which the DLB group had significantly better performance on recent memory than the AD or VaD groups, but were more impaired on visuospatial praxis than the AD group. Using optimal cutoff points for the recent memory/praxis ratio, good discrimination was attained between DLB and the other two dementias.

Patients with diffuse Lewy body disease (DLBD) *without* concomitant AD pathology were reported to display visuoconstructive and psychomotor impairments that were significantly worse than those of AD patients at the same level of dementia, whereas the memory performance of the AD patients was worse than that of the DLBD patients (Salmon et al., 1996). In addition to severe impairment in visuospatial and visuoconstructive functioning, the DLBD without AD group also displayed a global dementia that included deficits in attention, memory, language, psychomotor performance, and executive functions (Salmon et al., 1996).

Patients with the Lewy body variant of AD (LBV), i.e., AD with concomitant Lewy body pathology, were also reported to have relatively greater impairment on visuospatial and executive tests than patients with pure AD (Galasko, Katzman, Salmon, & Hansen, 1996). In another study, patients with LBV performed worse than patients with pure AD on the Construction and Initiation/Perseveration subscales of the MDRS, but better on the Memory subscale (Connor et al., 1998). The two groups did not differ on the total MDRS score, and this differential pattern of impairment between the groups was also found when subgroups with mild to moderate and moderate to severe dementia were separately analyzed (Connor et al., 1998).

Frontotemporal lobar degeneration

Frontotemporal lobar degeneration (FTLD) may be the most common primary degenerative dementia occurring *before* the age of 65 years. The three clinical syndromes associated with FTLD are frontotemporal dementia (FTD or dementia of the frontal type), progressive nonfluent aphasia (or frontal variant FTD), and semantic dementia (or temporal variant FTD), each associated with a different predominant site of pathology (Neary et al., 1998). FTLD can be caused by a variety of different non-AD neuropathological changes, and only a small percentage of cases have classic Pick bodies. The clinical syndrome correlates with site, not the type, of neuropathology. More than one-third of FTLD cases have a positive family history. Hippocampal Sclerosis Dementia has also been proposed to be a FTD.

Frontotemporal dementia

In FTD or dementia of the frontal type, there are major changes in personality and social behavior due to orbitobasal involvement, including stereotypical behavior, reduced motivation, poor concentration, reduced speech output, changes in eating habits, disinhibition, blunted affect, and loss of empathy in the context of relatively preserved memory. Both functional and structural brain imaging may be initially normal in patients with FTD even when the patient clearly exhibits abnormal behavior; orbitobasal changes on functional brain imaging appear before atrophy on structural imaging. FTD is a cause of atypical parkinsonism, and thus may be confused with Parkinson's disease and LBD (Goedert, Ghetti, & Spillantini, 2000).

Some patients with FTD, i.e., those with dorsolateral prefrontal cortex damage, display impairments on "frontal executive" tasks, including the Wisconsin Card Sorting Test and phonemic word fluency (Hodges & Miller, 2001). However, traditional tests of executive functioning are not sensitive to orbitobasal pathology. Unlike in the typical AD patient, memory (i.e., recall of recent events), orientation, visuospatial functions, and language comprehension are relatively well preserved in early FTD. However, patients with FTD generally display poor recall on tests of episodic memory, but intact recognition memory in the early stages. With disease progression, a severe anterograde amnesia often emerges along with impairment in remote memory. Although spontaneous conversation often decreases, performance on semantic tasks typically remains intact. Patients with FTD generally display intact visuospatial ability, although they may display impulsivity and poor strategizing on the Rey Complex Figure Test.

Patients with FTD almost always lack insight and usually are brought in by family or friends because of the patient's gradual onset of personality and behavioral changes. The disinhibition and inappropriate social behavior due to orbitobasal involvement are often presenting symptoms and occur in 50% of FTD patients. For example, common behaviors include stealing, hit-and-run accidents, and public exposure. It has been suggested that patients with asymmetric right-sided frontal lobe involvement are more likely to display socially inappropriate behavior.

In one study, stereotypic behavior, changes in eating behavior/preference, disinhibition, and poor social awareness reliably separated FTD and AD groups (Bozeat, Gregory, Ralph, & Hodges, 2000). For example, FTD patients often ate the same food at the same time each day. Also, the patients often displayed a change in food preference toward wanting to eat sweet things and frequently used "catch phrases." The patients with frontal variant FTD and temporal variant FTD (i.e., semantic dementia) displayed similar behavioral profiles, which the authors attributed to common involvement of the ventral frontal lobe, temporal pole, and amygdala. Apathy and dysexecutive symptoms (e.g., deficits in planning and organization) were common, but were not found to discriminate FTD from AD (Bozeat et al., 2000). Symptoms of dysexecutive functioning, poor self-care, and restlessness increased with disease severity in both FTD and AD, which the authors speculated may be due to involvement of dorsolateral prefrontal cortex in the later stages of both disorders. Mental rigidity and depression were more common in the semantic dementia group compared with those with frontal variant FTD, whereas the latter group showed greater disinhibition. The patients frequently displayed a lack of empathy and concern for others. The Neuropsychiatric Inventory (Cummings et al., 1994), which is based on an interview with the caregiver, appears to be useful in differentiating patients with FTD and AD (Levy, Miller, Cummings, Fairbanks, & Craig, 1996).

Progressive nonfluent aphasia

In progressive nonfluent aphasia, there is clear impairment in the phonological and syntactic aspects of language associated with left perisylvian brain atrophy (Hodges & Miller, 2001). These patients display markedly reduced speech output, word-finding difficulties, and distorted speech with frequent phonological substitutions and grammatical errors that make communication difficult (in the late stages, the patients may be mute and in effect "word deaf"). On the other hand, the semantic aspects of language, e.g., language comprehension, are relatively well preserved in the early stages, except on tests requiring speech.

In progressive nonfluent aphasia, conversational speech is severely impaired, but picture naming is usually only mildly impaired due to some phonological mispronunciations. Phoneme discrimination also becomes impaired, which patients attribute to poor hearing. Semantic category fluency is less affected than phonemic word fluency. Performance is poor on tests of phonological competence, including repetition of multisyllabic words, blending word segments, and rhyming. These patients usually exhibit reduced digit span. Syntactic comprehension, e.g., matching pictures to sentences of increasing complexity, is clearly impaired (Hodges & Patterson, 1996). However, as with other FTD variants, visuospatial and perceptual functioning is generally intact. Memory for recent events and other cognitive functions are typically intact or only mildly impaired until the late stages of the disease when a more global dementia appears. Structural brain imaging reveals widening of the Sylvian fissure and atrophy of the insula, and inferior frontal and superior temporal lobes.

Semantic dementia

Semantic dementia is the mirror opposite of progressive nonfluent aphasia in terms of symptoms. In semantic dementia, patients display a fluent aphasia in which speech remains fluent with normal syntax and phonology but there is a progressive breakdown in semantic memory, including severe impairment in naming and language comprehension. Patients display clear impairment on tests of semantic memory, especially when a verbal response is required, including category fluency, picture naming, and giving verbal definitions to words and pictures. These patients are also impaired on "odd-man out" synonym tasks (e.g., pond, lake, *river*). In addition, semantic dementia patients are impaired on tests requiring matching words with pictures and matching one picture with another. Nonverbal semantic knowledge is also impaired, e.g., as measured by the Pyramids and Palm Trees Test in which the subject must make judgments regarding the semantic relatedness of pictures. The patients have difficulty reading and spelling irregular words like on the National Adult Reading Test in which the word is not spelled the way it sounds.

Conversely, episodic nonverbal memory, working memory (as measured by digit span), nonverbal problem solving (e.g., Raven's Colored Progressive Matrices), visuospatial functioning, and activities of daily living remain relatively preserved until the late stages (Hodges & Miller, 2001). Patients with semantic dementia are typically well oriented and exhibit good recall of recent events (Hodges & Miller, 2001). However, their severe semantic deficit and anomia interferes with performance on tests of episodic verbal memory, including story memory and word-list learning tests, whereas they will be intact on nonverbal memory measures like reproductive memory on the Complex Figure Test.

In semantic dementia, structural brain imaging reveals severe atrophy in the anterolateral temporal lobe that is typically greater in the left hemisphere (Hodges & Miller, 2001). An average volume loss of 50% has been reported in the temporal pole, fusiform, and inferolateral gyri that is greater in the left than the right temporal lobe, and a 20% volume loss in the hippocampal region. In AD, the hippocampal and parahippocampal regions have a greater volume loss than the temporal polar and inferolateral structures. A less common type of semantic dementia, associated with selective *right* temporal atrophy, presents with an inability to recognize faces (i.e., prosopagnosia) and a progressive loss of knowledge about people.

Hippocampal sclerosis dementia

It has been recommended that hippocampal sclerosis dementia (HSD) be added to the list of possible diagnoses causing memory loss (Lippa & Dickson, 2004). Among dementia patients, the prevalence of autopsy-proven HSD is 0.4–2%. Although mesial temporal sclerosis is often found in children and nonelderly adults with epilepsy, it is almost always associated with dementia in the elderly and rarely with a seizure disorder (Hatanpaa et al., 2004). Elderly with dementia due to a variety of causes also often are found to have hippocampal sclerosis. HSD is considered "pure" if there are no other neuropathologic findings sufficient to explain the dementia.

The clinical symptoms and course of HSD are more similar to that of FTD than AD, and it has been recommended that HSD be considered a FTD (Blass et al., 2004; Hatanpaa et al., 2004). Blass et al. (2004) reported that the majority of patients with "pure" HSD met diagnostic criteria for FTD. Abnormal behaviors such as poor grooming, socially inappropriate behavior, mutism, and stereotyped behavior were more common in HSD and FTD than AD. Inappropriate behavior, decreased interest and hyperorality were found to have an earlier onset in HSD and FTD than AD. On the other hand, certain cognitive symptoms (i.e., disorientation, dyscalculia, apraxia, and agnosia) and psychiatric symptoms (i.e., hallucinations, delusions, and aggression) were more common in AD. Previous studies with HSD patients who *also* met criteria for other neurologic disorders emphasized the similarities in the cognitive presentations of AD and HSD, including memory decline in the context of general cognitive decline (Leverenz et al., 2002). However, compared to AD, visuomotor problem solving has been found to be less impaired in HSD and cognitive decline may be slower (Kuslansky et al., 2004).

In HSD, there is severe neuronal loss and gliosis in the hippocampal CA1 region and subiculum. Patients with AD, FTD, and HSD all display hippocampal atrophy. Blass et al. (2004) speculated that because the CA1 subregion of the hippocampus projects to the medial orbitofrontal cortex (OFC), CA1 damage in HSD may cause OFC dysfunction, which in turn may be responsible for the abnormal changes in personality, social behavior, and basic drives such as eating. The etiology of HSD is unknown, but it likely has a variety of causes (Lippa & Dickson, 2004). The hippocampus is known to be vulnerable to neurotoxicity from excitatory amino acids like glutamate, and thus glutamate neurotoxicity is one possible cause.

Vascular dementia

A typical pattern of cognitive impairments in VaD consists of mild impairment in episodic memory, more severely impaired executive functioning, and psychiatric symptoms (Hodges & Graham, 2001). In VaD versus AD, there is generally greater impairment in executive and motor functioning, and perhaps attention, but less impairment in episodic memory (Hodges & Graham, 2001). The general pattern of cognitive impairments in VaD is similar to that found when there is frontal or subcortical involvement. However, distinguishing the pattern of cognitive deficits in VaD and AD can often be difficult.

It appears that performance on measures of executive functioning, e.g., the WCST and Porteus mazes, is worse in VaD (Hodges & Graham, 2001).

There is also some evidence of greater impairment in attention in VaD than AD, as measured by tests like the Digit Symbol Modalities Test and Trail Making. Overall, episodic memory impairment is less severe in VaD than in AD, but some patients with VaD display severe anterograde amnesia similar to patients with AD. It has been reported that both VaD and AD groups display an equal severity of impairment on tests of semantic memory. However, it has been speculated that loss of knowledge underlies the semantic memory deficit in AD, whereas impaired retrieval underlies the semantic deficit in VaD. Patients with VaD tend to display greater changes in personality and affect than AD patients, including anxiety, agitation, irritability, and emotional lability. The severity of apathy and depression is greater in VaD.

The pattern of language deficits is similar in VaD and AD, except that phonemic word fluency is more impaired in VaD. Category fluency is equally impaired in these two dementias. There is some evidence that reading and writing are more impaired in VaD than AD. VaD patients are found to be more impaired at writing single dictated letters and in copying sentences on the writing subtest from the Western Aphasia Battery. Compared to AD patients, VaD patients have been found to make more spelling errors, produce grammatically simpler sentences, and have more difficulty writing in straight lines. In terms of spontaneous speech in patients with moderate dementia, the mechanics of speech tends to be more impaired in VaD patients, while the linguistic aspects of speech are more affected in AD patients. VaD patients tend to have reduced phrase length, reduced grammatical complexity, and abnormal prosody and articulation, but their speech tends to be more informative than AD patients.

No consistent differences have been reported in studies comparing VaD and AD groups on tests of visuospatial functioning, including block design, copying the Rey complex figure, or clock drawing (Hodges & Graham, 2001). Patients with VaD are more impaired on tests of motor functioning than AD patients, including timed finger tapping and fist clenching. Increasing evidence indicates that vascular risk factors increase the risk for both VaD and AD and actual cerebrovascular damage increases the probability that clinical AD will be expressed.

VaD can be classified into three clinical syndromes: multi-infarct dementia, subcortical ischemic infarction, and strategic infarctions of critical brain areas (e.g., medial thalamic nuclei and basal forebrain) (Hodges & Graham, 2001). *Multi-infarct dementia* (MID), in which there are repeated clinically evident large vessel and lacunar strokes, accounts for one-third of VaD cases. *Subcortical ischemic dementia* (including lacunar states and Binswanger's encephalopathy) due to small vessel disease (i.e., diffuse white matter pathology) represents the majority of VaD cases (Hodges & Graham, 2001). A *strategic infarction* can result in dementia if a lesion affects a critical brain region (Hodges & Graham, 2001). A large left hemisphere stroke can result in a severe aphasia with alexia and/or agraphia, and some degree of memory and/or attentional impairment. However, small strategic infarcts can also produce severe cognitive impairment in the absence of focal neurological signs like hemiplegia. A posterior cerebral artery infarction can damage the hippocampal formation and result in impaired verbal or visual memory or severe amnesia if the damage is bilateral. After a basal forebrain infarction, an anterograde amnesia and apathy often results.

The language disorders typically associated with AD versus stroke often can be distinguished, but the left angular gyrus syndrome (AGS) is commonly misdiagnosed as AD (Benson, Cummings, & Tsai, 1982). This syndrome can be caused by infarction of the posterior branch of the medial cerebral artery in which Wernicke's area in the posterior portion of the superior temporal gyrus is not affected. The symptoms of AD overlap with the symptoms of AGS, which include posterior aphasia, alexia with agraphia, and Gerstmann's syndrome (i.e., finger agnosia, right–left confusion, agraphia, and acalculia) (Benson, et al., 1982). Thus, both AGS patients and AD patients display fluent aphasias, empty paraphasic output, and impaired language comprehension. Focal neurological deficits (especially right-sided abnormalities, including motor symptoms) may be evident in AGS, whereas no neurological symptoms are found in AD. Unlike AD, AGS has an abrupt onset, usually does not progress, and memory is intact except on verbal memory tests. AD patients are typically unaware of their language problems, whereas AGS patients have insight into their deficit.

Treatment and case management

Although no cure for AD is presently available, good planning and medical and social management may ease the burdens on the patient and family. The focus of this section is the various pharmacological and behavioral treatments for the cognitive, emotional, and behavioral symptoms of Alzheimer's disease.

Medications: Cholinesterase inhibitors and memantine

There is currently no medical treatment to cure, prevent or stop the progression of AD. However, there are five drugs that have been approved by the FDA for treatment of the symptoms of AD. These drugs may temporarily improve symptoms related to the disease to a modest extent, but they do not reverse the disease. Four of the approved drugs are cholinesterase inhibitors, i.e., inhibit the enzyme that breaks down the neurotransmitter acetylcholine thereby making more acetylcholine available at the synapse. The brand names (and associated generic names) of the four cholinesterase inhibitors are Cognex (tacrine) approved in 1993, Aricept (donepezil) approved in 1996, Exelon (rivastigmine) approved in 2000, and Reminyl (galantamine) approved in 2001.

There is a cholinergic deficit in AD that is due to atrophy of the nucleus basalis of Meynert and associated loss of the enzyme choline acetyltransferase and reduced synthesis of the neurotransmitter acetylcholine leading to limbic and neocortical cholinergic deficits (Cummings, 2003b). In an evidenced-based review on the efficacy of cholinesterase inhibitors (ChE-Is) (i.e., donepezil, rivastigmine, and galantamine) in the treatment of AD, Cummings (2003b) concluded that double-blind, placebo-controlled trials demonstrate that ChE-Is exert *modest* reproducible effects on global and cognitive measures and on measures of activities of daily living and behavior in patients with mild-to-moderate AD. Cummings also concludes that there are some indications from clinical trials that early initiation of a ChE-I is associated with greater long-term benefits and that withdrawal and reinitiation of treatment may result in loss of benefit. Open-label extensions of clinical trials suggest that benefits for patients treated with a ChE-I continue for several years. There are few studies directly comparing the major ChE-Is, but existing data suggests no major differences in efficacy. The most common side effects of ChE-Is are nausea, vomiting, diarrhea, and anorexia, which occur more frequently during dose escalation than maintenance therapy. Cummings points out that the efficacy data from clinical trials is based on carefully selected patient groups and thus the findings should be generalized with caution to the unselected populations of AD patients in clinical practice.

In 2003, the FDA approved memantine (brand name Namenda) as the first treatment for moderate to severe Alzheimer's dementia. Memantine blocks excess amounts of the neurotransmitter glutamate that can damage or kill nerve cells. As with the ChE-Is, the average effect is modest in magnitude, i.e., helps to maintain basic activities of daily living for a few months longer. Whereas the ChE-Is have only been tested on AD patients in the milder dementia stages, memantine has only been tested on patients in the later stages, but there are ongoing studies designed to address whether memantine might be effective in the earlier stages of AD. The findings of one study demonstrated a significantly greater beneficial effect when both Aricept and Namenda were used together.

Neuropsychiatric behavioral disturbances

Neuropsychiatric behavioral disturbances, including agitation, assault/aggression, screaming, wandering, and depression/apathy/withdrawal, are common in AD and cause distress to the patient and caregiver (Mega, Cummings, Fiorello, & Gornbein, 1996; Teri et al., 1992). Often there are multiple problem behaviors simultaneously present and each type of abnormal behavior is associated with specific neurobiologic changes (Mega et al., 1996). Teri, Larson, and Reifler (1988) reported that the total number of behavioral problems in AD patients increased significantly with increased cognitive impairment and that some types of problems (e.g., wandering, agitation, incontinence, and poor personal hygiene) varied as a function of cognitive severity. Thus, behavioral problems become more common with disease progression. It has been reported that dementia-related problem behaviors in poor, frail, demented elderly shorten the time of nursing home placement by approximately 2 years, thus demonstrating the importance of developing and implementing effective intervention strategies for these behaviors (Phillips & Diwan, 2003). Controlled research trials have shown that caregivers can acquire specific behavioral techniques through caregiver training programs that decrease problematic behaviors and delay institutionalization in dementia patients (Teri & Logsdon, 2000; Teri, Logsdon, & McCurry, 2002).

The treatment of AD generally involves one of the cholinesterase inhibitor drugs, environmental interventions, and, if necessary, pharmacologic treatment of residual behavioral disturbances. With respect to nonpharmacologic behavioral interventions, the 3 Rs and the ABCs are good general approaches to basic behavioral management. The 3 Rs refer to repeat, reassure, and redirect as a way of addressing problem behaviors. The ABCs behavioral analysis (i.e., antecedents, behavior, and consequences) involves identifying the antecedent stimulus conditions and the consequences that are controlling a disruptive behavior so that the environment can be modified to improve behavior (Weiner & Teri, 2003). The cholinesterase inhibitors have been shown to have some beneficial effects in treating behavioral disturbances (Cummings, 2003a; Cummings, Schneider, Tariot, Kershaw, & Yuan, 2004), and psychotropic agents (e.g., antidepressants, antipsychotic and antiagitation agents) can provide additional treatment if needed (De Deyn et al., 2004; Street et al., 2000; Teri et al., 2000).

Mega et al. (1996) investigated the frequency and severity of different behavioral disturbances occurring in the month prior to an interview using the Neuropsychiatric Inventory (NPI) in AD. The most common behavioral disturbance was apathy, which was displayed by 72% of patients, followed by agitation (60%), anxiety (48%), irritability (42%), dysphoria and aberrant motor behavior (both 38%), disinhibition (36%), delusions (22%), and hallucinations (10%). Levy, Cummings et al. (1996) studied neuropsychiatric symptoms in patients with probable AD over 1 year and reported that the recurrence rates were 95% for psychosis, 93% for agitation, and 85% for depression.

Teri (1994) proposed that the behavioral theory of depression, i.e., that decreased positive person–environment interactions initiate and maintain a cycle of depression, can be applied to demented adults, and can thus help guide treatment. Behavioral therapy for depression focuses on changing the aversive events and interactions that maintain depression and on increasing pleasant events and interactions. It also teaches caregivers techniques for behavior change and problem solving. Behavioral treatment has been shown to decrease depression in both AD patients and their caregivers in controlled clinical trials (Teri, 1994; Teri, Logsdon, Uomoto, & McCurry, 1997). In another randomized controlled trial, exercise training combined with teaching caregivers behavioral management techniques was found to improve physical health and depression in patients with AD (Teri et al., 2003).

Both cognitive therapy and behavioral interventions have been used successfully in treating depression in AD patients (Teri & Gallagher-Thompson,

1991). In mildly demented AD patients, cognitive therapy has been success-ful in challenging the patient's negative thought patterns, reducing cognitive distortions, and increasing more adaptive perspectives on specific events. In moderately or severely demented AD patients, behavioral intervention strate-gies increased the level of positive activities and decreased negative activities. Depressive symptoms in dementia patients have been treated with selective serotonin reuptake inhibitors, tricyclic agents, and combined serotonergic and noradrenergic reuptake inhibitors (Lyketsos et al., 2003; Reifler et al., 1989; Teri et al., 1991).

The most common sleep problem in AD is diurnal rhythm disturbance, which can result in an overall decrease in sleep time and increased daytime napping and thus decrease the patient's energy, alertness, and level of cogni-tive functioning. Other sleep disorders found in patients with AD include REM behavior disorders, myoclonus, periodic leg movements, fragmented sleep, early morning awakening, and delayed sleep onset. Current treatments for sleep problems in AD include pharmacological treatments, cognitive-behavioral or psychoeducational strategies, and biological/circadian therapies (McCurry, Reynolds, Ancoli-Israel, Teri, & Vitiello, 2000). Sleep problems in AD are multifactorial in that they are affected by a variety of demographic, physical, psychiatric, and situational factors, and thus the treatment interven-tion needs to target underlying causes in the context of the sleep problem (McCurry et al., 2000). McCurry, Gibbons, Logsdon, Vitiello, and Teri (2003) reported that caregivers can successfully implement sleep hygiene interven-tions with AD patients, but they need active assistance implementing a sleep hygiene program because education alone is usually not sufficient (McCurry et al., 2003).

General principles of behavioral management

The general principles of psychological and behavioral management, which take into account the AD patient's impairment in learning ability, include correcting sensory impairment, acceptance, nonconfrontation, optimal autonomy, simplification, structuring, multiple cueing, repetition, guiding and demonstration, reinforcement, reducing choices, optimal stimulation, determining and using overlearned skills, avoiding new learning, minimizing anxiety, and using redirection (Weiner & Teri, 2003).

The first principle in managing an AD patient is correctly recognizing and accepting the patient's present level of functioning, including valuing what is still preserved, and not being preoccupied by what has been lost. It is impor-tant to use a nonconfrontational approach when interacting with an AD patient who is unaware of his/her deficits, which will help decrease patient agitation. Where possible, minimize danger through environmental change, e.g., disconnect the gas or electric supply to a stove, remove weapons from the house, and remove poisons from locations where they might be confused with foods. Optimize autonomy to the level of the patient's needs and ability (Weiner & Teri, 2003).

Use simplification where appropriate by reducing the number and complexity of environmental demands and by providing instructions one step at a time. Caregivers need to help structure daily activities and the environment for patients with AD, especially when there is more severe cognitive impairment. A structured environment including a daily routine can help provide environmental constancy or predictability. Individual patient preferences for activities should be taken into account. Multiple external cueing, including nonverbal cues, can be used to initiate and maintain an activity, e.g., handing items of clothing to the person one at a time when getting dressed. Repetition will often be needed because of attention/concentration problems and slow information processing speed. Guiding and demonstrating verbal commands reinforces communication and acts as a reminder of how to do something (Weiner & Teri, 2003).

Use immediate, positively reinforcing feedback, e.g., praise, to encourage positive behaviors. Reduce the number of choices confronting the AD patient in order to lessen confusion. Optimal stimulation level should be determined for each person for different times of the day and will vary depending on many factors, including level of cognitive functioning, alertness, and emotional status. It is recommended that overlearned skills be identified and utilized, e.g., musicians may be able to continue to play their instruments. Overlearned activities are more likely to be failure-free activities that will be enjoyable and provide stimulation to the patient without feelings of frustration or failure. Avoid activities that require new learning because these will be frustrating to the AD patients due to their severe impairment in new learning and memory (Weiner & Teri, 2003).

Anxiety can be triggered in the AD patient when unable to comprehend their environment and anxiety can increase suspiciousness and delusions. Minimize anxiety by keeping the environment simple, providing a structured routine, reducing choices, avoiding new learning, reducing anticipatory anxiety, and keeping the patient focused on the current day. Redirection or distraction is an effective technique for managing anxiety, anger, or depression in AD patients by interrupting self-perpetuating emotional cycles and thus helping the patient calm down (Weiner & Teri, 2003).

Activity-focused care (AFC), in which the patient is given the opportunity and encouraged to engage in activities that are suitable for his/her cognitive level and interests, is a helpful way to approach caring for a person with a progressive dementia like Alzheimer disease. AFC is appropriate because many AD patients exhibit apathy and impaired executive functioning along with impairments in memory and other cognitive abilities, which prevent the patient from being able to initiate and maintain enjoyable activities without the structure and planning provided by others. If the patients can't make their own activity, they may substitute problem behaviors like pacing. A good reference book on this subject is *Alzheimer's Disease: Activity-Focused Care* by C. R. Hellen (1998).

Cognitive changes in AD that can adversely affect driving competence include impaired memory, disorientation regarding time and place, difficulty performing familiar tasks, poor judgment, poor concentration/inattention, slower reaction time, and impaired problem-solving abilities. These impairments can lead to unsafe driving, including driving in the wrong lane, ignoring traffic lights and other road signs, not responding appropriately in emergency situations, misjudging directions, and getting lost (van Zomeren, Brouwer, & Minderhoud, 1987). A consensus statement on the issue of driving and dementia was reached by a group of researchers in conjunction with the Swedish National Road Administration stating that a diagnosis of moderate-to-severe dementia precludes driving and that some individuals with mild dementia need to have an evaluation of their driving competence (Lundberg et al., 1997). Alternative transportation should be identified, including having others do the driving (e.g., friends and relatives), using public transportation or taxis, and reducing the need to drive.

Caregiving

Caregivers are a critical part of the treatment for AD patients. They provide the most patient care and administer the most treatments. They are also reported to suffer high rates of illness and stress. Caregiving can be an overwhelming task. In order to improve caregiving while reducing the burden and stress on the caregiver, the following coping strategies may be helpful: develop a daily schedule for the patient, set aside personal time, coordinate caregiving with others, make time for some relaxing activity every day, attend a support group, obtain individual counseling, hire professional help, and consider adult day service programs or long-term care placement if appropriate. Because caregivers of AD patients have significant responsibilities and challenges, they need to be aware of available resources. The Alzheimer's Association is an important resource for caregivers of AD patients. The Alzheimer's Association has more than 200 chapters, which provide programs and services within local communities to assist AD patients, their families, and caregivers.

Conclusions

A neuropsychological assessment of a patient suspected of having AD or another dementing disorder is necessary to quantitatively measure the severity, extent, and pattern of deficits in memory and other cognitive abilities. The clinical presentation of AD typically begins with an insidious onset of impairment in new declarative learning and memory that progresses gradually over time to severe memory impairment (i.e., anterograde amnesia) before impairment in other cognitive domains clearly emerge. Although memory impairment is a nearly universal first presenting symptom of Alzheimer disease, there is considerable variability in what cognitive impairment is next to emerge. A common neuropsychological profile for an AD patient with mild to moderate dementia includes impairments in new declarative learning and memory (i.e., recent memory), general intellectual functioning, visuoconstructional skills, word generation (especially semantic word fluency), and confrontation naming. Basic sensory and motor functions are typically preserved until the advanced stages of AD.

A thorough description of the patient's cognitive functioning is essential to the early detection of a dementing disorder, including in the prodromal phase (i.e., mild cognitive impairment). A neuropsychological evaluation is also helpful in the differential diagnosis of the type of dementia (e.g., Alzheimer disease, Lewy body disease, frontotemporal dementia, vascular dementia) and provides useful information for treatment planning. Adequate demographic normative data for the cognitive test measures used are necessary in order to make an accurate determination of whether a test score is abnormal or not for a given patient. Serial cognitive testing can quantitatively chart the course of the disorder, help confirm the diagnosis (e.g., of a progressive dementia), and aid in evaluating the efficacy of treatment interventions. This chapter also addressed treatment (both pharmacological and behavioral) for the symptoms of AD and provided recommendations for caregivers.

References

Ala, T. A., Hughes, L. F., Kyrouac, G. A., Ghobrial, M. W., & Elble R. J. (2001). Pentagon copying is more impaired in dementia with Lewy bodies than in Alzheimer's disease. *Journal of Neurology, Neurosurgery, and Psychiatry*, *70*(4), 483–488.

Ala, T. A., Hughes, L. F., Kyrouac, G. A., Ghobrial, M. W., & Elble, R. J. (2002). The Mini-Mental State exam may help in the differentiation of dementia with Lewy bodies and Alzheimer's disease. *International Journal of Geriatric Psychiatry*, *17*(6), 503–509.

Albert, M. S. (1981). Geriatric neuropsychology. *Journal of Consulting and Clinical Psychology*, *49*(6), 835–850.

Albert, M. S., & Drachman, D. A. (2000). Alzheimer's disease: What is it, how many people have it, and why do we need to know? *Neurology*, *55*(2), 166–168.

Alzheimer, A. (1907). Uber eine eignartige Erkrankung der Hirnrinde. *Allgemeine Zeitschrift für Psychiatrie und psychisch-gerichtliche Medizin*, *64*, 146–148.

Alzheimer, A. (1977). A unique illness involving the cerebral cortex. In D. A. Rottenbert & F. H. Hochberg (Eds: C. N. Hochberg & F. H. Hochberg, Trans.), *Neurological classics in modern translation* (pp. 41–43). New York: Haffner Press.

American Psychiatric Association. (1987). *Diagnostic and statistical manual of mental disorders* (3rd ed., rev.). Washington, DC: Author.

American Psychiatric Association. (1994). *Diagnostic and statistical manual of mental disorders* (4th ed.). Washington, DC: Author.

Andree, B., Hittmair, M., & Benke, T. H. (1992). Recognition and explanation of proverbs in Alzheimer's disease. *Journal of Clinical and Experimental Neuropsychology*, *14*(3), 372.

Appell, J., Kertesz, A., & Fisman, M. (1982). A study of language functioning in Alzheimer's patients. *Brain and Language, 17*(1), 73–91.

Arendt, T., Bigl, V., Arendt, A., & Tennstedt, A. (1983). Loss of neurons in the nucleus basalis of Meynert in Alzheimer's disease. *Acta Neuropathologica, 61,* 101–108.

Arnold, S. E. (2000). Part III. Neuropathology of Alzheimer's disease. *Disease Monitor, 46*(10), 687–705.

Arnold, S. E., Hyman, B. T., Flory, J., Damasio, A. R., &. Van Hoesen, G. W. (1991). The topographical and neuroanatomical distribution of neurofibrillary tangles and neuritic plaques in the cerebral cortex of patients with Alzheimer's disease. *Cerebral Cortex, 1*(1), 103–116.

Ashford, J. W., Kolm, P., Colliver, J. A., Bekian, C., & Hsu, L. H. (1989). Alzheimer patient evaluation and the Mini-Mental State: Item characteristic curve analysis. *Journal of Gerontology, 44*(5), 139–146.

Baddeley, A., Della Sala, S., & Spinnler, H. (1991). The two-component hypothesis of memory deficit in Alzheimer's disease. *Journal of Clinical and Experimental Neuropsychology, 13*(2), 372–380.

Baddeley, A. D., Baddeley, H. A., Bucks, R. S., & Wilcock, G. K. (2001). Attentional control in Alzheimer's disease. *Brain, 124*(8), 1492–1508.

Ballard, C. G., Ayre, G., O'Brien, J., Sahgal, A., McKeith, I. G., Ince, P. G., et al. (1999). Simple standardized neuropsychological assessments aid in the differential diagnosis of dementia with Lewy bodies from Alzheimer's disease and vascular dementia. *Dementia and Geriatric Cognitive Disorders, 10*(2), 104–108.

Bayles, K. A., Kaszniak, A. W., & Tomoeda, C. K. (1987). *Communication and cognition in normal aging and dementia.* Boston: College Hill Little, Brown & Company.

Bennett, D. A., Schneider, J. A., Wilson, R. S., Bienias, J. L., & Arnold, S. E. (2004). Neurofibrillary tangles mediate the association of amyloid load with clinical Alzheimer disease and level of cognitive function. *Archives of Neurology, 61*(3), 378–384.

Benson, D. F. (1979). *Aphasia, alexia, and agraphia.* New York: Churchill Livingstone.

Benson, D. F., Cummings, J. L., & Tsai, S. Y. (1982). Angular gyrus syndrome simulating Alzheimer disease. *Archives of Neurology, 39*(10), 616–620.

Benton, A. L., deS. Hamsher, K., Varney, N. R., & Spreen, O. (1983). *Contributions to neuropsychological assessment: A clinical manual.* New York: Oxford University Press.

Benton, A. L., & van Allen, M. W. (1968). Impairment in facial recognition in patients with cerebral disease. *Transactions of the American Neurological Association, 93,* 38–42.

Benton, A. L., Varney, N. R., & deS. Hamsher, K. (1978). Visuospatial judgment. *Archives of Neurology, 35*(6), 364–367.

Blass, D. M., Hatanpaa, K. J., Brandt, J., Rao, V., Steinberg, M., Troncoso, J.C., et al. (2004). Dementia in hippocampal sclerosis resembles frontotemporal dementia more than Alzheimer disease. *Neurology, 63*(3), 492–497.

Blessed, G., Tomlinson, B. E., & Roth, M. (1968). The association between quantitative measures of dementia and senile change in the cerebral gray matter of elderly subjects. *International Journal of Geriatric Psychiatry, 11*(12), 1036–1038.

Bondi, M. W., Salmon, D. P., Galasko, D., Thomas, R. G., & Thal, L. J. (1999). Neuropsychological function and apolipoprotein E genotype in the preclinical detection of Alzheimer's disease. *Psychology and Aging, 14*(2), 295–303.

Bozeat, S., Gregory, C. A, Ralph, M. A., & Hodges, J. R. (2000). Which neuropsychiatric and behavioural features distinguish frontal and temporal variants of frontotemporal dementia from Alzheimer's disease? *Journal of Neurology, Neurosurgery, and Psychiatry, 69*(2), 178–186.

Braak, H., & Braak, E. (1991a). Alzheimer's disease affects limbic nuclei of the thalamus. *Acta Neuropathologica, 81*(3), 261–268.

Braak, H., & Braak, F. (1991b). Neuropathological staging of Alzheimer-related changes. *Acta Neuropathologica, 82*(4), 239–259.

Braak, H., & Braak, E. (1993). Entorhinal–hippocampal interaction in amnestic disorders. *Hippocampus, 3*, 239–246.

Braak, H., & Braak, E. (1994). Morphological criteria for the recognition of Alzheimer's disease and the distribution pattern of cortical changes related to this disorder. *Neurobiology of Aging, 15*(3), 355–356.

Braak, H., & Braak, E. (1998). Evolution of neuronal changes in the course of Alzheimer's disease. *Journal of Neural Transmission, 53*(Suppl.), 127–140.

Braak, H., Tredici, K. D., & Braak, E. (2003). Spectrum of pathology. In R. Petersen (Ed.), *Mild cognitive impairment: Aging to Alzheimer's disease* (pp. 149–189). New York: Oxford University Press.

Brookmeyer, R., Gray, S., & Kawas, C. (1998). Projections of Alzheimer's disease in the United States and the public health impact of delaying disease onset. *American Journal of Public Health, 88*(9), 1337–1342.

Butters, N., Granholm, E., Salmon, D. P., Grant, I., & Wolfe, J. (1987). Episodic and semantic memory: A comparison of amnestic and dementia patients. *Journal of Clinical and Experimental Neuropsychology, 9*(5), 479–497.

Butters, N., Heindel, W. C., & Salmon, D. P. (1990). Dissociation of implicit memory in dementia: Neurological implications. *Bulletin of the Psychonomic Society, 28*(4), 359–366.

Cerhan, J. H., Ivnik, R. J., Smith, G. E., Tangalos, E. C., Petersen, R. C., & Boeve, B. F. (2002). Diagnostic utility of letter fluency, category fluency, and fluency difference scores in Alzheimer's disease. *The Clinical Neuropsychologist, 16*(1), 35–42.

Chui, H. (2000). Vascular dementia, a new beginning: Shifting focus from clinical phenotype to ischemic brain injury. *Neurologic Clinics, 18*(4), 951–978.

Connor, D. J., Salmon, D. P., Sandy, T. J., Galasko, D., Hansen, L. A., & Thal, L. J. (1998). Cognitive profiles of autopsy-confirmed Lewy body variant vs. pure Alzheimer disease [erratum in *Archives of Neurology*, 1998, *55*(10), 1352]. *Archives of Neurology, 55*, 994–1000.

Crystal, H. A., Horoupian, D. S., Katzman, R., & Jotkowitz, S. (1982). Biopsy-proven Alzheimer disease presenting as a right parietal lobe syndrome. *Annals of Neurology, 12*, 186–188.

Cummings, J. L. (1990). Clinical diagnosis of Alzheimer's disease. In J. L. Cummings & B. L. Miller (Eds.), *Alzheimer's disease: Treatment and long-term management* (pp. 3–22). New York: Marcel Dekker.

Cummings, J. L. (2003a). The impact of depressive symptoms on patients with Alzheimer's disease. *Alzheimer Disease and Associated Disorders, 7*(2), 61–62.

Cummings, J. L. (2003b). Use of cholinesterase inhibitors in clinical practice: Evidence-based recommendations. *American Journal of Geriatric Psychiatry, 11*(2), 131–145.

Cummings, J. L., & Benson, D. F. (1992). *Dementia: A clinical approach*. Boston: Butterworth-Heinemann.

Cummings, J. L., Benson, D. F., Hill, M., & Read, S. (1985). Aphasia in dementia of the Alzheimer type. *Neurology, 35*(3), 394–397.

Cummings, J. L., Mega, M., Gray, K., Rosenberg-Thompson, S., Carusi, D. A., & Gornbein, J. (1994). The Neuropsychiatric Inventory: Comprehensive assessment of psychopathology in dementia. *Neurology, 44*(12), 2308–2314.

Cummings, J. L., Schneider, L., Tariot, P. N., Kershaw, P. R., & Yuan, W. (2004). Reduction of behavioral disturbances and caregiver distress by galantamine in patients with Alzheimer's disease. *American Journal of Psychiatry, 161*(3), 532–538.

Davies, C. A., & Mann, D. M. (1993). Is the "preamyloid" of diffuse plaques in Alzheimer's disease really nonfibrillar? *American Journal of Pathology, 143*(6), 1594–1605.

De Deyn, P. P., Carrasco, M. M., Deberdt, W., Jeandel, C., Hay, D. P., Feldman, P. D., et al. (2004). Olanzapine versus placebo in the treatment of psychosis with or without associated behavioral disturbances in patients with Alzheimer's disease. *International Journal of Geriatric Psychiatry, 19*(2), 115–126.

Eastley, R., & Wilcock, G. (2002). Assessment and differential diagnosis of dementia. In J. Obrien, D. Ames, & A. Burns (Eds.), *Dementia* (2nd ed., pp. 41–47). New York: Oxford University Press.

Eslinger, P. J., & Benton, A. L. (1983). Visuoperceptual performances in aging and dementia: Clinical and theoretical implications. *Journal of Clinical Neuropsychology, 5*, 213–220.

Evans, D. A., Bennett, D. A., Wilson, R. S., Bienias, J. L., Morris, M. C., Scherr, P. A., et al. (2003). Incidence of Alzheimer disease in a biracial urban community: Relation to apolipoprotein E allele status. *Archives of Neurology, 60*(2), 185–189.

Ferman, T. J., Boeve, B. F., Smith, G. E., Silber, M. H., Kokmen, E., Petersen, R. C., et al. (1999). REM sleep behavior disorder and dementia: Cognitive differences when compared with AD. *Neurology, 52*(5), 951–957.

Folstein, M. F., Folstein, S. E., & McHugh, P. R. (1975). "Mini-mental state": A practical method for grading the mental state of patients for clinicians. *Journal of Psychiatric Research, 12*(3), 189–198.

Frederiks, J. A. M. (1985). The neurology of aging and dementia. In J. A. M. Frederiks (Ed.), *Handbook of clinical neurology* (pp. 199–219). Amsterdam: Elsevier.

Gainotti, G., Marra, C., & Villa, G. (2001). A double dissociation between accuracy and time of execution on attentional tasks in Alzheimer's disease and multi-infarct dementia. *Brain, 124*(4), 731–738.

Galasko, D., Hansen, L. A., Katzman, R., Wiederholt, W., Masliah, E., Terry, R., et al. (1994). Clinical-neuropathological correlations in Alzheimer's disease and related dementias. *Archives of Neurology, 51*(9), 888–895.

Galasko, D., Katzman, R., Salmon, D. P., & Hansen, L. (1996). Clinical and neuropathological findings in Lewy body dementias. *Brain and Cognition, 31*(2), 166–175.

Geddes, J. W., Tekirian, T. L., Soultanian, N. S., Ashford, J. W., Davis, D. G., & Markesbery, W. R. (1997). Comparison of neuropathologic criteria for the diagnosis of Alzheimer's disease. *Neurobiology of Aging, 18*(4), S99–S105.

Glosser, G., Gallo, J., Duda, N., de Vries, J. J., Clark, C. M., & Grossman, M. (2002). Visual perceptual functions predict instrumental activities of daily living in patients with dementia. *Neuropsychiatry, Neuropsychology, and Behavioral Neurology, 15*(3), 198–206.

Goedert, M., Ghetti, B., & Spillantini, M. G. (2000). Tau gene mutations in frontotemporal dementia and parkinsonism linked to chromosome 17 (FTDP-17): Their relevance for understanding the neurogenerative process. *Annals of the New York Academy of Sciences, 920,* 74–83.

Grady, C. L., Haxby, J. V., Horwitz, B., Sundaram, M., Berg, G., Schapiro, M., et al. (1988). Longitudinal study of the early neuropsychological and cerebral metabolic changes in dementia of the Alzheimer type. *Journal of Clinical and Experimental Neuropsychology, 10*(5), 576–596.

Graeber, M. B., Kosel, S., Grasbon-Frodl, E., Moller, H. J., & Mehraein, P. (1998). Histopathology and APOE genotype of the first Alzheimer disease patient, Auguste D. *Neurogenetics, 1*(3), 223–228.

Grundman, M., Petersen, R. C., Ferris, S. H., Thomas, R. G., Aisen, P. S., Bennett, D. A., et al. (2004). Alzheimer's Disease Cooperative Study: Mild cognitive impairment can be distinguished from Alzheimer disease and normal aging for clinical trials. *Archives of Neurology, 61*(1), 59–66.

Hansen, L. A., & Terry, R. D. (1997). Position paper on diagnostic criteria for Alzeimer disease. *Neurobiology of Aging, 18*(4 Suppl.), S71–S73.

Hart, R. P., Kwentus, J. A., Harkins, S. W., & Taylor, J. R. (1988). Rate of forgetting in mild Alzheimer's-type dementia. *Brain and Cognition, 7*(1), 31–38.

Hatanpaa, K. J., Blass, D. M., Pletnikova, O., Crain, B. J., Bigio, E. H., Hedreen, J. C., et al. (2004). Most cases of dementia with hippocampal sclerosis may represent frontotemporal dementia. *Neurology, 63*(3), 538–542.

Hebert, L. E., Beckett, L. A., Scherr, P. A. & Evans, D. A. (2001). Annual incidence of Alzheimer disease in the United States projected to the years 2000 through 2050. *Alzheimer Disease and Associated Disorders, 15*(4), 169–173.

Hebert, L. E., Scherr, P. A., Bienias, J. L., Bennett, D. A., & Evans, D. A. (2003). Alzheimer disease in the US population: Prevalence estimates using the 2000 census. *Archives of Neurology, 60*(8), 1119–1122.

Hellen, C. R. (1998). *Alzheimer's disease: Activity-focused care* (2nd ed.). Boston: Butterworth Heinemann.

Helm-Estabrooks, N., & Albert, M. L. (1991). *Manual of aphasia therapy.* Austin, TX: Pro-Ed.

Hodges, J. R., & Graham, N. L. (2001). Vascular dementias. In J. Hodges (Ed.), *Early-onset dementia: A multi-disciplinary approach* (pp. 319–337). New York: Oxford University Press.

Hodges, J. R., & Miller, B. (2001). Frontotemporal dementia (Pick's disease). In J. Hodges (Ed.), *Early-onset dementia: A multi-disciplinary approach* (pp. 284–303). New York: Oxford University Press.

Hodges, J. R., & Patterson, K. (1996). Nonfluent progressive aphasia and semantic dementia: A comparative neuropsychological study. *Journal of the International Neuropsychological Society, 2,* 511–24.

Hodges, J. R., Salmon, D. P., & Butters, N. (1991). The nature of the naming deficit in Alzheimer's and Huntington's disease. *Brain, 114*(4), 1547–1558.

Huppert, F. A., Brayne, C., Gill, C., Paykel, E. S., & Beardsall, L. (1995). CAM-COG—a concise neuropsychological test to assist dementia diagnosis: Socio-demographic determinants in an elderly population sample. *British Journal of Clinical Psychology, 34*(4), 529–541.

Hy, L. X., & Keller, D. M. (2000). Prevalence of AD among whites: A summary by levels of severity. *Neurology, 55*(2), 198–204.

Hyman, B. T. (1998). New neuropathological criteria for Alzheimer disease. *Archives of Neurology, 55*(9), 1174–1176.

Ivnik, R. J., Smith, G. E., Cerhan, J. H., Boeve, B. F., Tangalos, E. G., & Petersen, R. C. (2001). Understanding the diagnostic capabilities of cognitive tests. *The Clinical Neuropychologist, 15*(1), 114–124.

Jack, C. R., Jr., Petersen, R. C., Xu, Y. C., O'Brien, P. C., Smith, G. E., Ivnik, R. J., et al. (1999). Prediction of AD with MRI-based hippocampal volume in mild cognitive impairment. *Neurology, 52*(7), 1397–1403.

Jack, C. R., Jr., Petersen, R. C., Xu, Y., O'Brien, P. C., Smith, G. E., Ivnik, R. J., et al. (2000). Rates of hippocampal atrophy correlate with change in clinical status in aging and AD. *Neurology, 55*(4), 484–489.

Johnson, K. A., Jones, K., Holman, B. L., Becker, J. A., Spiers, P. A., Satlin, A., et al. (1998). Preclinical prediction of Alzheimer's disease using SPECT. *Neurology, 50*(6), 1563–1571.

Kaszniak, A. W. (1986). The neuropsychology of dementia. In I. Grant & K. M. Adams (Eds.), *Neuropsychological assessment of neuropsychiatric disorders* (pp. 172–220). New York: Oxford University Press.

Kaszniak, A. W. (1992). *Awareness of cognitive and behavioral deficit in Alzheimer's dementia.* Paper presented at the meeting of American Psychological Association, Washington, DC.

Kaszniak, A. W., Poon, L. W., & Riege, W. (1986). Assessing memory deficits: An information-processing approach. In L. W. Poon (Ed.), *Handbook for clinical memory assessment of older adults* (pp. 277–284). Washington, DC: American Psychological Association.

Katzman, R. (1976). Editorial: The prevalence and malignancy of Alzheimer disease: A major killer. *Archives of Neurology, 33*, 217–218.

Katzman, R., Brown, T., Fuld, P., Peck, A., Schecter, R., & Schimmel, H. (1983). Validation of a short orientation-memory-concentration test of cognitive impairment. *American Journal of Psychiatry, 140*(6), 734–739.

Kay, D. W., & Roth, M. (2002). Pathological correlates of dementia. *Lancet, 359*(9306), 624–625.

Kertesz, A. (1979). *Aphasia and associated disorders.* New York: Grune & Stratton.

Khachaturian, Z. S. (1985). Diagnosis of Alzheimer's disease. *Archives of Neurology, 42*(11), 1097–1105.

Kirshner, H. S., Webb, W. G., Kelly, M. P., & Wells, C. E. (1984). Language disturbance: An initial symptom of cortical degenerations and dementia. *Archives of Neurology, 41*(5), 491–496.

Kuslansky, G., Verghese, J., Dickson, D., Katz, M., Busche, H., & Lipton, R. (2004). Hippocampal sclerosis: Cognitive consequences and contributions to dementia. *Neurology, 62*(7), 128–129.

Lafleche, G., & Albert, M. (1995). Executive function deficits in mild Alzheimer's disease. *Neuropsychology, 9*(3), 313–320.

LaRue, A., Spar, J., & Hill, C. D. (1986). Cognitive impairment in late-life depression: Clinical correlates and treatment implications. *Journal of Affective Disorders, 11*(3), 179–184.

Leverenz, J. B., Agustin, C. M., Tsuang, D., Peskind, E. R., Edland, S. D., Nochlin, D., et al. (2002). Clinical and neuropathological characteristics of hippocampal sclerosis: A community-based study. *Archives of Neurology, 59*(7), 1099–1106.

Levinoff, E. J., Li, K. Z., Murtha, S., & Chertkow, H. (2004). Selective attention impairments in Alzheimer's disease: Evidence for dissociable components. *Neuropsychology, 18*(3), 580–588.

Levy, M. L., Cummings, J. L., Fairbanks, L. A., Bravi, D., Calvani, M., & Carta, A. (1996). Longitudinal assessment of symptoms of depression, agitation, and psychosis in 181 patients with Alzheimer's disease. *American Journal of Psychiatry, 153*(11), 1438–1443.

Levy, M. L., Miller, B. L., Cummings, J. L., Fairbanks, L. A., & Craig, A. (1996) Alzheimer disease and frontotemporal dementias: Behavioral distinctions. *Archives of Neurology, 53*(7), 681–690.

Lippa, C. F., & Dickson, D. W. (2004). Hippocampal sclerosis dementia: Expanding the phenotypes of frontotemporal dementias? *Neurology, 63*(3), 414–415.

Lundberg, C., Johansson, K., Ball, K., Bjerre, B., Blomqvist, C., Braekhus, A., et al. (1997). Dementia and driving: An attempt at consensus. *Alzheimer Disease and Associated Disorders, 11*(1), 28–37.

Lyketsos, C. G., DelCampo, L., Steinberg, M., Miles, Q., Steele, C. D., Munro, C., et al. (2003). Treating depression in Alzheimer disease: efficacy and safety of sertraline therapy, and the benefits of depression reduction: The DIADS. *Archives of General Psychiatry, 60*(7), 737–746.

Maguire, E. A. (1999). Hippocampal and parietal involvement in human topographical memory: Evidence from functional neuroimaging. In N. Nurgess, K. J. Jeffery, & J. O'Keefe (Eds.), *The hippocampal and parietal foundations of spatial cognition* (pp. 404–415). New York: Oxford University Press.

Martin, A. (1987). Representation of semantic and spatial knowledge in Alzheimer's patients: Implications for models of persevered learning in amnesia. *Journal of Clinical and Experimental Neuropsychology, 9*(2), 191–224.

Mathuranath, P. S., Nestor, P., Berrios, G. E., Rakowicz, W., & Hodges, J. R. (2000). A brief cognitive test battery to differentiate Alzheimer's disease and frontotemporal dementia. *Neurology, 55*(11), 1613–1620.

Mattis, S. (1976). Mental status examination for organic mental syndrome in the elderly patient. In L. Bellack & T. E. Karasu (Eds.), *Geriatric psychiatry: A handbook for psychiatrists and primary care physicians* (pp. 77–121). New York: Grune & Stratton.

McCurry, S. M., Gibbons, L. E., Logsdon, R. G., Vitiello, M., & Teri, L. (2003). Training caregivers to change the sleep hygiene practices of patients with dementia: The NITE-AD project. *Journal of the American Geriatrics Society, 51*(10), 1455–1460.

McCurry, S. M., Reynolds, C. F., Ancoli-Israel, S., Teri, L., & Vitiello, M. V. (2000). Treatment of sleep disturbance in Alzheimer's disease. *Sleep Medicine Reviews, 4*(6), 603–628.

McGlynn, S. M., & Kaszniak, A. W. (1991a). Unawareness of deficits in dementia and schizophrenia. In G. P. Prigatano & D. L. Schacter (Eds.), *Awareness of deficit after brain injury: Clinical and theoretical issues* (pp. 84–110). New York: Oxford University Press.

McGlynn, S. M., & Kaszniak, A. W. (1991b). When metacognition fails: Impaired awareness of deficit in Alzheimer disease. *Journal of Cognitive Neuroscience, 3*(2), 183–189.

McKeith, I. G., Burn, D. J., Ballard, C. G., Collerton, D., Jaros, E., Morris, C. M., et al. (2003). Dementia with Lewy bodies. *Seminars in Clinical Neuropsychiatry, 8*(1), 46–57.

McKeith, I. G., Galasko, D., Kosaka, K., Perry, E. K., Dickson, D. W., Hansen, L. A., et al. (1996). Consensus guidelines for the clinical and pathologic diagnosis of dementia with Lewy bodies (DLB): Report of the consortium on DLB international workshop. *Neurology, 47*(5), 1113–1124.

McKhann, G., Drachman, D., Folstein, M., Katzman, R., Price, D., & Stadlin, E. M. (1984). Clinical diagnosis of Alzheimer's disease: Report of the NINCDS-ADRDA work group under the auspices of the Department of Health and Human Services Task Force on Alzheimer's Disease. *Neurology, 34*(7), 939–944.

Mega, M. S., Cummings, J. L., Fiorello, T., & Gornbein, J. (1996). The spectrum of behavioral changes in Alzheimer's disease. *Neurology, 46*(1), 130–135.

Mendez, M. F., & Cummings, J. L. (2003). *Dementia: A clinical approach* (3rd ed.). Philadelphia: Butterworth-Heinemann.

Mesulam, M. M. (2000). *Principles of behavioral and cognitive neurology* (2nd ed.). New York: Oxford University Press.

Mesulam, M. M. (2001). Primary progressive aphasia. *Annals of Neurology, 49*(4), 425–432.

Mirra, S. S., Heyman, A., McKeel, D., Sumi, S. M., Crain, B. J., Brownlee, L. M., et al. (1991). The Consortium to Establish a Registry for Alzheimer's Disease (CERAD). Part II. Standardization of the neuropathologic assessment of Alzheimer's disease. *Neurology, 41*(4), 479–486.

Mohs, R. C., Kim, Y., Johns, C. A., Dunn, D. D., & Davis, K. L. (1986). Assessing changes in Alzheimer's disease: Memory and language. In L. W. Poon (Ed.), *Handbook for clinical memory assessment of older adults* (pp. 149–155). Washington, DC: American Psychological Association.

Monsch, A. U., Bondi, M. W., Butters, N., Salmon, D. P., Katzman, R., & Thal, L. J. (1992). Comparisons of verbal fluency tasks in the detection of dementia of the Alzheimer type. *Archives of Neurology, 49*(12), 1253–1258.

Moss, M., & Albert, M. (1988). Alzheimer's disease and other dementing *disorders*. In M. S. Albert & M. B. Moss (Eds.), *Geriatric neuropsychology* (pp. 145–178). New York: Guilford Press.

Moss, V. B., Albert, M. S., Butters, N., & Payne, M. (1986). Differential patterns of memory loss among patients with Alzheimer disease, Huntington's disease, and Alcoholic Korsakoff's syndrome. *Archives of Neurology, 43*(3), 239–246.

National Institute on Aging, and Reagan Institute Working Group on Diagnostic Criteria for the Neuropathological Assessment of Alzheimer's Disease. (1997). Consensus recommendations for the postmortem diagnosis of Alzheimer's disease. *Neurobiology of Aging, 18*(4), S1–2.

Neary, D., Snowden, J. S., Bowen, D. M., Sims, N. R., Mann, D. M. A., Benton, J. S., et al. (1986). Neuropsychological syndromes in presenile dementia due to cerebral atrophy. *Journal of Neurology, Neurosurgery, and Psychiatry, 49*(2), 163–174.

Neary, D., Snowden, J. S., Gustafson, L., Passant, U., Stuss, D., Black, S., et al. (1998). Frontotemporal lobar degeneration: A consensus on clinical diagnostic criteria. *Neurology, 51*(6), 1546–1554.

Nebes, R. D., & Brady, C. B. (1992). Generalized cognitive slowing and severity of dementia in Alzheimer's disease: Implications for the interpretation of response-time data. *Journal of Clinical and Experimental Neuropsychology, 14*(2), 317–326.

Neuropathology Group of the Medical Research Council Cognitive Functioning and Aging Study (MRC CFAS). (2001). Pathological correlates of late-onset dementia in a multi-center community-based population study in England and Wales. *Lancet, 357*(9251), 169–175.

Ott, B. R., Lafleche, G., Whelihan, W. M., Buongiorno, G. W., Albert, M. S., & Fogel, B. S. (1996). Impaired awareness of deficits in Alzheimer disease. *Alzheimer Disease and Associated Disorders, 10*(2), 68–76.

Perry, R. J., Watson, P., & Hodges, J. R. (2000). The nature and staging of attention dysfunction in early (minimal and mild) Alzheimer's disease: Relationship to episodic and semantic memory impairment. *Neuropsychologia, 38*(3), 252–271

Petersen, R. C. (1995). Normal aging, mild cognitive impairment, and early Alzheimer's disease. *Neurologist, 1*(6), 326–344.

Petersen, R. C. (2000). Mild cognitive impairment: Transition between aging and Alzheimer's disease. *Neurologia, 15*(3), 93–101.

Petersen, R. C. (2003). Conceptual overview. In R. C. Petersen (Ed.), *Mild cognitive impairment: Aging to Alzheimer's disease* (pp. 1–14). New York: Oxford University Press.

Petersen, R. C., & Morris, J. C. (2003). Clinical features. In R. C. Petersen (Ed.), *Mild cognitive impairment: Aging to Alzheimer's disease* (pp. 15–39). New York: Oxford University Press.

Petersen, R. C., Smith, G. E., Waring, S. C., Ivnik, R .J., Tangalos, E. G., & Kokmen, E. (1999). Mild cognitive impairment: Clinical characterization and outcome [erratum in *Archives of Neurology, 56*(6), 760]. *Archives of Neurology, 56*(3), 303–308.

Pfeffer, R. I., Kurosaki, T. T., Harrah, C. H., Chance, J. M., Bates, D., Detels, R., et al. (1981). A survey diagnostic tool for senile dementia. *American Journal of Epidemiology, 114*(4), 515–527.

Phillips, V. L., & Diwan, S. (2003). The incremental effect of dementia-related problem behaviors on the time to nursing home placement in poor, frail, demented older people. *Journal of the American Geriatrics Society, 51*(2), 188–193.

Price, J. L., & Morris, J. C. (1999). Tangles and plaques in nondemented aging and "preclinical" Alzheimer's disease. *Annals of Neurology, 45*(3), 358–368.

Randolph, C., Tierney, M. C., Mohr, E., & Chase, T. N. (1998). The Repeatable Battery for the Assessment of Neuropsychological Status (RBANS): Preliminary clinical validity. *Journal of Clinical and Experimental Neuropsychology, 20*(3), 310–319.

Raskin, A., Friedman, A. S., & DiMascio, A. (1982). Cognitive and performance deficits in depression. *Psychopharmacology Bulletin, 18*(4), 196–202.

Reed, J. M., & Squire, L. R. (1998). Retrograde amnesia for facts and events: Findings from our new cases. *Journal of Neuroscience, 18*(10), 3943–3954.

Reifler, B. V., Teri, L., Raskind, M., Veith, R., Barnes, R., White, E., et al. (1989). Double-blind trial of imipramine in Alzheimer's disease patients with and without depression. *American Journal of Psychiatry, 146*(1), 45–49.

Reiman, E. M., Caselli, R. J., Yun, L. S., Chen, K., Bandy, D., Minoshima, S., et al. (1996). Preclinical evidence of Alzheimer's disease in persons homozygous for the E4 allele for apolipoprotein E. *New England Journal of Medicine, 334*(12), 752–758.

Riley, K. P., Snowdon, D. A., & Markesbery, W. R. (2002). Alzheimer's neurofibrillary pathology and the spectrum of cognitive function: Findings from the Nun Study. *Annals of Neurology, 51*(5), 567–577.

Rosen, H. J., Lengenfelder, J., & Miller, B. (2000). Frontotemporal dementia. *Neurologic Clinics, 18*(4), 972–992.

Rosen, W. G., Mohs, R. C., & Davis, K. L. (1984). A new rating scale for Alzheimer disease. *American Journal of Psychiatry, 141*(11), 1356–1364.

Sahakian, B. J., Jones, G., Levy, R., Gray, J., & Warburton, D. (1989). The effects of nicotine on attention, information processing, and short-term memory in patients with dementia of the Alzheimer type. *British Journal of Psychiatry, 154,* 797–800.

Salmon, D. P., & Butters, N. M. (1992). Neuropsychology assessment of dementia in the elderly. In R. Katzman & J. W. Rowe (Eds.), *Principles of geriatric neurology* (pp. 144–163). Philadelphia: F. A. Davis Company.

Salmon, D. P., Galasko, D., Hansen, L. A., Masliah, E., Butters, N., Thal, L. J., et al. (1996). Neuropsychological deficits associated with diffuse Lewy body disease. *Brain and Cognition, 31*(2), 148–165.

Salmon, D. P., Heindel, W. C., & Lange, K. L. (1999). Differential decline in word generation from phonemic and semantic categories during the course of Alzheimer's disease: Implications for the integrity of semantic memory. *Journal of the International Neuropsychological Society, 5*(7), 692–703.

Salmon, D. P., & Hodges, J. R. (2001). Neuropsychological assessment of early onset dementia. In J. Hodges (Ed.), *Early-onset dementia: A multi-disciplinary approach* (pp. 47–73). New York: Oxford University Press.

Salmon, D. P., Shimamura, A. P., Butters, N., & Smith, S. (1988). Lexical and semantic priming deficits in patients with Alzheimer disease. *Journal of Clinical and Experimental Neuropsychology, 10*(4), 477–494.

Salmon, D. P., Thal, L. J., Butters, N., & Heindel, W. C. (1990). Longitudinal evaluation of dementia of the Alzheimer type: A comparison of three standardized mental state examinations. *Neurology, 40*(8), 1225–1230.

Schmitt, F. A., Davis, D. G., Wekstein, D. R., Smith, C. D., Ashford, J. W., & Markesbery, W. R. (2000). "Preclinical" AD revisited: Neuropathology of cognitively normal older adults. *Neurology, 55*(3), 370–376.

Ska, B., Poissant, A., & Joanette, Y. (1990). Line orientation judgment in normal elderly and subjects with dementia of Alzheimer's type. *Journal of Clinical and Experimental Neuropsychology, 12*(5), 695–702.

Small, G. W., Mazziotta, J. C., Collins, M. T., Baxter, L. R., Phelps, M. E., Mandelkern, M. A., et al. (1995). Apolipoprotein E type 4 allele and cerebral glucose metabolism in relatives at risk for familial Alzheimer disease. *Journal of the American Medical Association, 273*(12), 942–947.

Snowdon, D. A. (2003). Healthy aging and dementia: Findings from the Nun Study. *Annals of Internal Medicine, 139,* 450–454.

Squire, L. R. (1992). Memory and the hippocampus: A synthesis from findings with rats, monkeys, and humans [erratum in *Psychological Review, 99*(3), 582]. *Psychological Review, 99*(2), 195–231.

Squire, L. R., & Zola-Morgan, S. (1991). The medial temporal lobe memory system. *Science, 253*(5026), 1380–1385.

Storandt, M., Botwinick, J., Danziger, W. L., Berg, L., & Hughes, C. P. (1984). Psychometric differentiation of mild senile dementia of the Alzheimer's type. *Archives of Neurology, 41*(5), 497–499.

Street, J. S., Clark, W. S., Gannon, K. S., Cummings, J. L., Bymaster, F. P., Tamura, R. N., et al. (2000). Olanzapine treatment of psychotic and behavioral symptoms in patients with Alzheimer disease in nursing care facilities: A double-blind, randomized, placebo-controlled trial. The HGEU Study Group. *Archives of General Psychiatry, 57*(10), 968–976.

Strub, R. L., & Black, F. W. (1988). *Neurobehavioral disorders: A clinical approach.* Philadelphia: F. A. Davis Company.

Tabert, M. H., Albert, S. M., Borukhova-Milov, L., Camacho, Y., Pelton, G., Liu, X., et al. (2002). Functional deficits in patients with mild cognitive impairment: Prediction of AD. *Neurology, 58*(5), 758–764.

Tales, A., Butler, S. R., Fossey, J., Gilchrist, I. D., Jones, R. W., & Troscianko, T. (2002). Visual search in Alzheimer's disease: A deficiency in processing conjunctions of features. *Neuropsychologia, 40*(12), 1849–1857.

Tales, A., Muir, J., Jones, R., Bayer, A., & Snowden, R. J. (2004). The effects of saliency and task difficulty on visual search performance in ageing and Alzheimer's disease. *Neuropsychologia, 42*(3), 335–345.

Teri, L. (1994). Behavioral treatment of depression in patients with dementia. *Alzheimer Disease and Associated Disorders, 8*(Suppl. 3), 66–74.

Teri, L., & Gallagher-Thompson, D. (1991). Cognitive-behavioral interventions for treatment of depression in Alzheimer's patients. *The Gerontologist, 31*(3), 413–416.

Teri, L., Gibbons, L. E., McCurry, S. M., Logsdon, R. G., Buchner, D. M., Barlow, W. E., et al. (2003). Exercise plus behavioral management in patients with Alzheimer disease: A randomized controlled trial. *Journal of the American Medical Association, 290*(15), 2015–2022.

Teri, L., Larson, E. B., & Reifler, B. V. (1988). Behavioral disturbance in dementia of the Alzheimer's type. *Journal of the American Geriatrics Society, 36*(1), 1–6.

Teri, L., & Logsdon, R. G. (2000). Assessment and management of behavioral disturbances in Alzheimer disease. *Comprehensive Therapy, 26*(3), 169–175.

Teri, L., Logsdon, R. G., & McCurry, S. M. (2002). Nonpharmacologic treatment of behavioral disturbance in dementia. *Medical Clinics of North America, 86*(3), 641–656.

Teri, L., Logsdon, R. G., Peskind, E., Raskind, M., Weiner, M. F., Tractenberg, R. E., et al. (2000). Alzheimer's Disease Cooperative Study. Treatment of agitation in AD: A randomized, placebo-controlled clinical trial. *Neurology, 55*(9), 1271–1278.

Teri, L., Logsdon, R. G., Uomoto, J., & McCurry, S. M. (1997). Behavioral treatment of depression in dementia patients: A controlled clinical trial. *Journals of Gerontology, Series B: Psychological Sciences and Social Sciences, 52*(4), 159–166.

Teri, L., Rabins, P., Whitehouse, P., Berg, L., Reisberg, B., Sunderland, T., et al. (1992). Management of behavior disturbance in Alzheimer disease: Current knowledge and future directions. *Alzheimer Disease and Associated Disorders, 6*(2), 77–88.

Teri, L., Reifler, B. V., Veith, R. C., Barnes, R., White, E., McLean, P., et al. (1991). Imipramine in the treatment of depressed Alzheimer's patients: Impact on cognition. *Journal of Gerontology, 46*(6), 372–377.

Terry, R. D., Masliah, E., Salmon, D. P., Butters, N., DeTeresa, R., Hill, R., et al. (1991). Physical basis of cognitive alterations in Alzheimer's disease: Synapse loss is the major correlate of cognitive impairment. *Annals of Neurology, 30*(4), 572–580.

Testa, J. A., Ivnik, R. J., Boeve, B., Petersen, R. C., Pankratz, V. S., Knopman, D., et al. (2004). Confrontation naming does not add incremental diagnostic utility in MCI and Alzheimer's disease. *Journal of the International Neuropsychological Society, 10*(4), 504–512.

Tombaugh, T. N., & McIntyre, N. J. (1992). The mini-mental state examination: A comprehensive review. *Journal of the American Geriatrics Society, 40*(9), 922–935.

Tulving, E. (1983). *Elements of episodic memory*. New York: Oxford University Press.

Ueda, H., Kitabayashi, Y., Narumoto, J., Nakamura, K., Kita, H., Kishikawa, Y., et al. (2002). Relationship between clock drawing test performance and regional cerebral blood flow in Alzheimer's disease: A single photon emission computed tomography study. *Psychiatry and Clinical Neurosciences, 56*(1), 25–29.

Van Hoesen, G. W. (2002). The human parahippocampal region in Alzheimer's disease, dementia, and ageing. In M. Witter & F. Wouterlood (Eds.), *The parahippocampal region: Organization and role in cognitive function* (pp. 271–295). New York: Oxford University Press.

Van Hoesen, G. W., Augustinack, J. C., Dierking, J., Redman, S. J., & Thangavel, R. (2000). The parahippocampal gyrus in Alzheimer's disease: Clinical and preclinical neuroanatomical correlates. *Annals of the New York Academy of Sciences, 911*, 254–274.

Van Zomeren, A. H., Brouwer, W. H., & Minderhoud, J. M. (1987). Acquired brain damage and driving: A review. *Archives of Physical Medicine and Rehabilitation, 68*(10), 697–705.

Walker, Z., Allen, R. L., Shergill, S., & Katona, C. L. (1997). Neuropsychological performance in Lewy body dementia and Alzheimer's disease. *British Journal of Psychiatry, 170*, 156–158.

Wechsler, D. (1997). *WAIS–III and WMS–III technical manual*. San Antonio, TX: Psychological Corporation.

Weiner, M. F., & Teri, L. (2003). Psychological and behavioral management. In M. F. Weiner & A. M. Lipton (Eds.), *The dementias: Diagnosis, treatment, and research* (3rd ed., pp. 181–218). Washington, DC: American Psychiatric Publishing, Inc.

Welsh, K., Butters, N., Hughes, J., Mohs, R., & Heyman, A. (1991). Detection of abnormal memory decline in mild cases of Alzheimer's disease using CERAD neuropsychological measures. *Archives of Neurology, 48*(3), 278–281.

Welsh, K. A., Butters, N., Hughes, J. P., Mohs, R. C., & Heyman, A. (1992). Detection and staging of dementia in Alzheimer's disease: Use of the neuropsychological measures developed for the Consortium to Establish a Registry for Alzheimer's Disease. *Archives of Neurology, 49*(5), 448–452.

Wilson, R. S., & Kaszniak, A. W. (1986). Longitudinal changes: Progressive idiopathic dementia. In L. W. Poon, B. J. Gurland, C. Eisdorfer, T. Crook, L. W. Thomas, A. W. Kaszniak, & K. Davis (Eds.), *The handbook of clinical memory assessment of older adults* (pp. 285–293). Washington, DC: American Psychological Association.

Xu, Y., Jack, C. R., Jr., O'Brien, P. C., Kokmen, E., Smith, G. E., Ivnik, R. J., et al. (2000). Usefulness of MRI measures of entorhinal cortex versus hippocampus in AD. *Neurology, 54*(9), 1760–1767.

Zec, R. F. (1993). Neuropsychological functioning in Alzheimer's disease. In R. W. Parks, R. F. Zec, & R. S. Wilson (Eds.), *Neuropsychology of Alzheimer's disease and other dementias* (pp. 1–80). New York: Oxford University Press.

Zec, R. F., Landreth, E. S., Bird, E., Harris, R. B., Robbs, R., Markwell, S. J., et al. (1994). Psychometric strengths and weaknesses of the Alzheimer Disease Assessment Scale in clinical testing: Recommendations for improvements. In E. Giacobini & R. Becker (Eds.), *Advances in Alzheimer disease therapy* (pp. 444–449). Boston: Birkhauser.

Zec, R. F., Landreth, E. S., Vicari, S. K., Belman, J., Feldman, E., Andrise, A., et al. (1992). Alzheimer Disease Assessment Scale: A subtest analysis. *Alzheimer Disease and Related Disorders—An International Journal, 6*(3), 164–181.

Zec, R. F., Landreth, E. S., Vicari, S. K., Feldman, E., Belman, J., Andrise, A., et al. (1992). Alzheimer Disease Assessment Scale: Useful for both early detection and staging of dementia of the Alzheimer type. *Alzheimer Disease and Related Disorders An International Journal, 6*(2), 89–102.

9 Cerebrovascular disorders: Neurocognitive and neurobehavioral features

Stephen N. Macciocchi, Amy L. Alderson, and Sara L. Schara

Cerebrovascular disorders (CVDs) are common in the elderly. Some cerebrovascular abnormalities are caused by specific disease processes such as infections and hematologic disorders, which appear generally unrelated to the aging process, while other CVDs (e.g., stroke) commonly occurring in the elderly are associated with risk factors such as age, hypertension, diabetes, atrial fibrillation, hyperlipidemia and smoking (Victor & Ropper, 2001). The etiology of stroke is to some extent age dependent, with the elderly having greater rates of thombotic and embolic occlusive disease (Brown, Whisnant, & Sicks, 1996). Stroke in the elderly has been shown to result in considerable neurocognitive, neurobehavioral, and functional morbidity, depending on a person's age, prior medical history, and lesion volume-location (Macciocchi, Diamond, Alves, & Mertz, 1998). Because the base rate of stroke is high in the elderly, neuropsychologists working in geriatric settings are frequently involved in the assessment and treatment of persons with stroke, particularly in acute care hospitals and neurorehabilitation programs. Consequently, becoming familiar with common stroke syndromes, methods of neurocognitive and neurobehavioral assessment, and interventions for the disabling consequences of stroke are important for any neuropsychologist or clinical psychologist working with the elderly.

In this chapter, we review the most common clinical syndromes following stroke. While stroke can produce untold variability in clinical presentation, we attempt to focus on clinical presentations most commonly encountered by neuropsychological practitioners. Our discussion is organized around a core of basic parameters for each syndrome including neurocognitive and neurobehavioral features, recommended assessment strategies, potential interventions, and general issues relevant for clinical decision making in medical settings. Before we discuss neurovascular syndromes, a brief review of the epidemiology and pathophysiology of stroke is provided for heuristic purposes.

Epidemiology and risk

A stroke or cerebrovascular accident (CVA) is a sudden interruption in blood supply to the brain. CVAs represent the fifth most common neurological disease and the third leading cause of death in the United States (Elkind, 2003; Williams, Jiang, Matacher, & Samsa, 1999). Epidemiologic studies indicate that in the United States alone, there are more than 4.7 million CVA survivors, and at least 500,000 persons will experience their first CVA each year. On average, someone in the United States suffers a stroke every 45 seconds, and stroke-related deaths occur every 3.1 minutes (Williams et al., 1999). In the year 2000, stroke accounted for approximately 1 in 14 deaths in the United States. Worldwide, there were 20.5 million strokes in 2001, with 5.5 million of those resulting in fatalities. Approximately 25% of individuals who suffer a CVA die within 1 year of their stroke, and 14% of persons who have a CVA experience a second stroke within the first year (American Heart Association [AHA], 2003). Fang and Alderman (2001) suggest that the national incidence of stroke may be increasing, since age-adjusted stroke hospitalization rates have increased 18.6% from 1988 to 1997. Despite increased incidence and hospitalization, mortality rates appear to have declined (Fang & Alderman, 2001; Muntner, Garrett, Klag, & Coresh, 2002).

Various studies have estimated demographic and clinical characteristics of stroke survivors. Among demographic characteristics, age seems to be the most important determinant of stroke (Elkind, 2003). Brown et al. (1996) and Wolf, DiAgostino, and O'Neal (1992) found that for every successive 10 years beyond the age of 55 the rate of stroke for both men and women more than doubles. Olindo et al. (2003) concur, finding the incidence rate of stroke increases with age, even beyond 85 years of age. Total stroke incidence rates exponentially increased with age for both men and women (Williams et al., 1999). More specifically, individuals aged 65–74, 75–84, and 85+ had incident total stroke rates that were 1.5, 2, and 3 times higher than first ever stroke incidence rates, suggesting older persons were more likely to sustain recurrent strokes (Williams et al., 1999).

Men are known to have a higher stroke incidence rate than women (Elkind, 2003; Hollander et al., 2003; Olindo et al., 2003; Williams et al., 1999), although in the very elderly, the incidence is higher among women, presumably because women live longer. Further examination of clinical characteristics of stroke patients by Williams et al. (1999) revealed the distribution of stroke subtypes among hospitalized patients to include 3.4% subarachnoid hemorrhages, 10.5% intracerebral hemorrhages, and 86.1% ischemic strokes. Fang and Alderman's (2001) analysis of stroke trends over a 10-year period also supported the higher incidence of ischemic stroke. Likewise, Abbott et al. (2003) conducted a study on the 6-year incidence rate of strokes, finding the overall occurrence of thromboembolic strokes at 15.3/1000, as compared to 5.3/1000 for hemorrhagic strokes.

There are a number of potentially modifiable or controllable risk factors for stroke. Cigarette smoking is the most preventable risk factor for stroke. Smoking not only reduces the amount of blood oxygen available to the brain, but also damages blood vessel walls. Smoking is particularly dangerous for individuals also taking estrogen-containing birth control pills, although such combination is rare in the elderly. Hypertension ($\geq$ 140/90 mm Hg) is also a significant risk factor for stroke. Diabetes mellitus, particularly in combination with hypertension, significantly increases the risk of CVA. Heart disease, prior myocardial infarction, atrial fibrillation, and other blood vessel diseases are all potentially modifiable risk factors, as are hyperlipidemia and obesity (AHA, 2003). One of the most important "warning signs" or risk factors for stroke is transient ischemic attacks (TIA) or "ministrokes" that produce stroke-like symptoms but no overt, persisting change in function. Nonetheless, TIAs have ominous implications and signal the need for medical assessment and intervention. Heredity and racial factors also appear to pose risk factors for stroke, with African-Americans at greater risk for CVAs and stroke-related fatalities than Caucasians (AHA, 2003).

Pathophysiology

CVAs are commonly classified according to the underlying pathological processes. There are two main categories of CVAs, ischemic and hemorrhagic. In an ischemic stroke, the most common type of stroke, there is an abrupt blockage of cerebral arteries or their distributions resulting in a reduction in blood flow to sections of the brain served by vascular areas downstream from the blockage. In contrast, hemorrhagic strokes result when cerebral blood vessels burst, causing bleeding into surrounding brain tissue (Blumenfeld, 2002). As mentioned previously, ischemic CVAs account for approximately 85% of all strokes, and there are two basic subtypes. Ischemic-thrombotic CVAs are caused by the formation of blood clots within a given cerebrovascular region. Thrombi are most likely to form in vessels already narrowed by atherosclerosis. Thrombotic strokes most often occur at night or early in the morning, when blood pressure is low. They are sometimes preceded by TIAs. In contrast, ischemic-embolic strokes result when particles formed at sites distant from the brain are transported via vessels and eventually block normal cerebral blood flow. Most emboli are believed to form in the heart, particularly during atrial fibrillation, when inadequately pumped blood pools and clots before being pumped back into the bloodstream (Victor & Ropper, 2001).

In both thrombotic and embolic CVAs, the vessel blockage diminishes blood flow and transport of oxygen and other nutrients to neurons. The risk of necrosis and neuronal death secondary to ischemia from either thrombotic or embolic stroke increases when cerebral vessels remain blocked for more than a few minutes. Because there is redundancy in cerebral blood flow, the effects of a single site of occlusion may be modulated by the location of the occlusion and the availability of collateral blood supply from unblocked cerebral vessels. Nonetheless, the specific neurologic and neurocognitive deficits observed following CVA are typically artery specific and relate to the location and size of the infarction (AHA, 2003).

In contrast to ischemic CVAs, when someone suffers a hemorrhagic CVA, blood vessels within the brain or along the surface of the brain rupture and bleed into the surrounding cerebral space. Hemorrhagic strokes typically have a much greater fatality rate than ischemic strokes (Victor & Ropper, 2001). When the hemorrhage occurs between the brain and skull, it is referred to as a subarachnoid hemorrhage (SAH). In this case, the vessels do not bleed directly into the brain, but in the subarachnoid space. SAH is often caused by aneurysms, regional areas of vascular weakness, resulting in balloon-shaped deformities in the vessel wall. The chances of aneurysmal rupture are significantly increased by hypertension. In contrast, intracerebral hemorrhages result when vessels within the cerebrum proper rupture, releasing blood into the surrounding brain matter.

When cerebral hemorrhage occurs, neuronal dysfunction occurs from at least two separate processes. First, there is a loss of a constant blood supply downstream from the rupture, and second, the blood is released in the region surrounding the hemorrhage. The amount of pressure placed on surrounding brain tissue by the hemorrhage interferes with normal neuronal functioning and can lead to brain herniation, and death, if not medically or surgically relieved. The treatment of cerebral hemorrhage may involve evacuation of accumulated blood and/or removal of portions of the skull (craniotomy) to reduce pressure effects. Unlike ischemic strokes, the clinical picture in hemorrhagic strokes is often more complex because it involves more than one arterial distribution and causes a number of secondary features as a result of pressure effects and deep extension (Victor & Ropper, 2001).

Neurocognitive–neurobehavioral networks and stroke

Neuroanatomical structure and organization obviously are important factors in understanding the consequences of stroke. In fact, some of the most interesting and robust neuropsychological syndromes occur secondary to focal cerebral infarction and hemorrhage. Apraxia, aphasia, amnesia, and neglect are well-described neuropsychological consequences of ischemic and hemorrhagic CVAs (Victor & Ropper, 2001). In most cases, the neuropsychological consequences of stroke are related to damage inflicted on cerebral structures known to underlie neurocognitive and neurobehavioral systems. Mesulam (2000) has identified various types of cerebral cortex, which work in concert to form the substrate for various neurocognitive and neurobehavioral networks. The implications of Mesulam's work are for reaching, but several aspects of his theoretical model are important for understanding the consequences of CVAs. First, Mesulam describes various types of cortical types including idiotypic cortex, unimodal association cortex, heteromodal cortex, and paralimbic cortex (2000). Idiotypic cortex is highly programmed, modality specific cortex typified by primary sensory (visual) and motor cortex.

CVA involving primary or idiotypic cortex would result in modality specific impairment. As an example, stroke affecting primary visual cortex would significantly impair visual processing, but leave language and motor skills relatively unaffected. In contrast, CVA involving more integrative, heteromodal cortical structures such as the prefrontal or posterior parietal cortex may result in multimodality deficits. As an example, stroke in the area of the angular gyrus can produce apraxia, aphasia, acalculia, astereognosis, and other deficits associated with angular gyrus syndrome. In other words, not all cortical structures contribute equally to neurocognitive and neurobehavioral functioning, although the overall integrity of neurocognitive networks is dependent on the interaction of primary, secondary and tertiary cortical systems (Mesulam, 2000). When considering disorders such as stroke, the implications of Mesulam's model are straightforward. Simply put, CVAs may disrupt neurocognitive and neurobehavioral functioning in variable, but generally predictable ways depending upon the location of the stroke and the cortical-subcortical structures involved.

Executive, language, attention, visuospatial and memory networks have been well described by many neuroscientists (Alexander, 1997, 2003; Cummings, 1993; Mesulam, 2000; Zola, 1997). In most cases, the concept of a neurocognitive and neurobehavioral network also is helpful in understanding the consequences of focal cerebral lesions such as those observed following CVAs. For instance, the language network has been described and debated for decades and continues to be the focus of discussion (Alexander, 2003). Despite debate about interaction of various components of the language network, clinical studies have shown that lesions in certain areas (Broca's and Wernicke's areas) severely disrupt communication (Damasio & Damasio, 2000).

More recently, Cummings (1993) proposed a cortical-subcortical model of executive functioning. In brief, Cummings describes three neurocognitive–neurobehavioral circuits composed of various cortical and subcortical structures. Cortical structures included medial, orbital, and dorsolateral neocortex, and subcortical structures included the thalamus, putamen, and globus pallidus. Cummings used lesion studies to show that damage to components of this executive system can result in similar clinical disorders despite differences in lesion location. For instance, a relatively circumscribed globus pallidus CVA can produce a dysexecutive disorder virtually indistinguishable from what might be expected following a significantly larger orbitofrontal stroke. Consequently, knowledge of cortical types, cortical organization, and neurocognitive networks can help neuropsychologists to better understand the consequences of stroke. Although an extended discussion of the anatomical components of specific neurocognitive networks is beyond the scope of this chapter, the interested reader may find neurocognitive networks discussed in detail in Feinberg and Farah (2003) and Mesulam (2000). In order to completely grasp the neuropsychological consequences of stroke, a basic understanding of cerebrovascular anatomy and underlying neocortical organization and neurocognitive networks is required.

Neurovascular organization

The cerebrovascular system provides blood supply to the entire brain (for visual depictions, see Blumenfeld, 2002; Netter, 1972; Victor & Ropper, 2001). The major arterial blood supply to the brain arises from an anterior and posterior system. Anterior cerebral circulation is provided by bilateral internal carotid arteries, which arise from the common carotid branches of the aorta. The primary posterior circulation is provided by the vertebral-basilar system. The vertebral arteries arise from the subclavian arteries and then join to form a single basilar artery. The anterior and posterior systems meet along the base of the brain at a junction called the Circle of Willis (CW). The CW has multiple components and connections, including the right and left anterior cerebral arteries (ACA), the right and left middle cerebral arteries (MCA), and the right and left posterior cerebral arteries (PCA). There also are two arteries that complete the circle. The anterior communicating artery (ACoA) joins the right and left ACA, and the posterior communicating arteries (PCoA) joins the anterior and posterior circulatory systems. In effect, the anterior and posterior circulation is connected by the CW, which allows for one vessel of the circulatory system to compensate for ischemia in another vessel depending on the location of the ischemic event. In other words, the vascular system is interconnected despite having numerous arteries dedicated to specific aspects of cerebral circulation.

The largest divisions of the ICA are the ACA and the MCA. The MCA supplies the largest part of the cerebral circulation and is divided into superior and inferior branches. Taken as a whole, the MCA territory encompasses most of the dorsolateral cortical convexity. The MCA superior division provides the blood supply to the inferior lateral frontal lobe, parietal lobe, and angular and supramarginal gyri. The inferior division supplies the cortex below the Sylvian fissure, most notably superior portions of the temporal lobe and the insula. Deep branches of the MCA form the lenticulostriate arteries, which supply the putamen, portions of the caudate, the lateral globus pallidus, the corona radiata, and the posterior limb of the internal capsule (Blumenfeld, 2002).

The ACA provides blood supply for approximately 75% of the medial surface of the cerebral hemispheres as well as 80% of the anterior corpus callosum, the medial-orbital frontal lobes, the medial sensorimotor cortex, and a strip of the lateral surface of the cerebral hemisphere along the superior border. Deep branches of the ACA supply the anterior internal capsule, and anterior portions of the caudate and globus pallidus. The ACA also gives rise to the anterior choroidal artery, which provides circulation to various subcortical structures, including the internal globus pallidus, posterior internal capsule, and various components of the optic tract. The territory between the ACA and MCA circulation distributions is often called the watershed zone and is a frequent site of ischemic stroke.

As mentioned previously, the vertebral arteries join to form a single basilar artery. The basilar artery then bifurcates again into bilateral PCAs. The cortical branches of the PCA supply the occipital cortex and inferomedial portions of the temporal lobe, including large portions of the hippocampus. More proximal branches of the PCA, near the bifurcation of the basilar artery, supply important parts of the brainstem circulation. More distally, the PCA also gives rise to the thalamoperforate artery, which supplies inferior, medial and anterior aspects of the thalamus (Blumenfeld, 2002).

Neurovascular syndromes: Neurobehavioral and neurocognitive features

Dominant middle cerebral artery CVA

The MCA is one of the most common sites for ischemia and associated infarction of cortical and subcortical structures. As mentioned previously, the vascular territory of the MCA includes a large portion of the lateral surface of the cerebral cortex and underlying white matter. A lesion involving the superior and inferior divisions of the dominant (most commonly left) MCA (DMCA) typically produces deficits in speech, language, praxis, attention, and emotional regulation. In some cases, learning and memory are affected, but typically memory is spared relative to other neurocognitive functions (see Table 9.1 for an overview of neurobehavioral and neurocognitive features of strokes involving ACA, MCA, and PCA distributions).

Persons with occlusions below the bifurcation of the MCA experience similar deficits, but may also evidence significant incontinence and visual defects (hemianopsia-quadrantanopsia). Prominent anosognosia is somewhat rare in most DMCA stroke survivors, especially following resolution of the acute confusional period, but right neglect can occur following DMCA stroke, although it is much less common, and in most cases less pervasive than neglect observed following nondominant (right) MCA strokes.

DMCA stroke may affect speech, language or both, and it is important to distinguish between speech and language dysfunction. Impairment in speech refers to limitations in word production as seen in dysarthria or aphemia in the absence of a more systemic impairment in semantics and syntax. In contrast, a true language disorder may include a disturbance in reading, writing, naming and comprehension (Alexander, 2003). Sometimes DMCA strokes produce symptoms of both speech and language impairment. As an example, speech may be severely dysarthric secondary to poor motor control, while verbal expression is also impaired secondary to damage to cortical structures dedicated to the cognitive components of language functioning (Alexander, 2003). Language disorders associated with DMCA stroke vary depending on the volume and location of the lesion, but common disorders include Broca's aphasia (BA), global aphasia (GA) and transcortical motor aphasia (TMA). All of these disorders typically have an associated hemiplegia, which complicates many aspects of functioning (Alexander, 2003; Damasio & Damasio, 2000). In some cases, inferior MCA stroke can produce a disturbance in

Table 9.1 Neurobehavioral and neurocognitive features of stroke

	Left hemisphere lesion	Bilateral lesion	Right hemisphere lesion
ACA		Impaired initiation Motor impersistence Utilization behavior Perseveration Confabulation Aphemia Apraxia Anosmia Impaired proprioception Astereognosis Agraphesthesia Anosognosia Alien hand syndrome Apathy/akinesis	
MCA	Impaired auditory discrimination Impaired auditory attention Receptive aphasia Expressive aphasia Impaired speech production Anomia Alexia Agraphia Acalculia Asymbolia Right–left discrimination Gerstman's syndrome Astereognosis Agraphesthesia Hemiparesis Visual imperception Agnosia Apraxia	Impaired proprioception Kluver-Bucy syndrome	Visuospatial deficit Neglect Allesthesia Prosopagnosia Anosoagnosia Astereognosis Agraphesthesia Hemiparesis Visual imperception Agnosia Apraxia Aprosodia Impaired arousal Misidentification
PCA	Visual impairment Ataxia Hemianesthesia Paresthesias Hemiballismus Alexia Agraphia Memory deficits Prosopagnosia Achromatopsia	Optic ataxia Hyperpathia (thalamic pain syndrome) Weber syndrome Benedikt syndrome Anton's syndrome Balint syndrome Amnestic (Korsakoff's) syndrome Apathetic akinetic mutism Alexia without agraphia	Visual impairment Ataxia Hemianesthesia Paresthesias Hemiballismus Memory deficits Prosopagnosia Achromatopsia

language comprehension (Wernicke's aphasia), although Wernicke's aphasia is less commonly observed than nonfluent language disorders.

There are a number of variants of Broca's aphasia, but persons with any form of BA, GA, or TCMA almost always evidence moderate to severe problems in communication (Alexander, 2003). Typically speech is nonfluent, and written communication is similarly impaired. Oral reading is also compromised. In BA and TCMA, comprehension is relatively spared in comparison to expression, but complex comprehension is typically quite impaired. Global aphasia is the most severe form of DMCA communication disturbance and is typically associated with large lesions involving cortical and subcortical structures. In GA, comprehension is severely impaired, at a level equal to, or greater than, expression.

An inability to communicate effectively has obvious functional limitations, and persons with BA, GA, and TCMA often need to communicate via gestures, pictures, communication boards, and other augmentative communication aids. In general, persons with nonfluent aphasias appear aware of their language disorders and seem willing to use adaptive communication skills. In contrast, persons with Wernicke's aphasia typically appear grossly unaware of language deficits and have considerable difficulty. Language disorders can affect performance of most activities of daily living and in many cases diminish the capacity necessary for decision making, which often raises legal and ethical issues, depending upon the clinical context. Persons with aphasia are sometimes unable to understand or communicate complex medical or financial decisions, which produces a need for surrogate decision makers, typically family members, but in some cases, legally appointed guardians. The more profound the comprehension deficit, the greater the need for surrogate decision makers.

Emotional changes are common following DMCA stroke. Apathy and depression have both been found to be related to DMCA stroke. The incidence of secondary depression has been debated, but appears to range from 25% to 35% depending on the study referenced. Lesion location is believed to play a role in the development of poststroke depression, and lesions in the dorsolateral frontal lobe and basal ganglia are believed to be most strongly associated with poststroke depression (Mayberg, 2001). Because of language deficits, persons with DMCA stroke often have problems articulating their mood and thoughts, as well as their particular frustrations related to impairment and changes in functioning. Thus, in most cases, clinicians use affect as the primary index of an emotional disorder. Unfortunately, using affect as a diagnostic sign can be problematic. In general, CVAs are known to cause both apathy and depression as well as pathological affect. Apathy differs from depression in several respects although the disorders have overlapping symptoms. In general, apathy is characterized by decreased arousal, impaired intention—motivation, and indifference (anosodiaphoria). Depression on the other hand may present with dysphoria, melancholia, and other cognitive features of depression, such as hopelessness and helplessness. While dysphoria and apathy are commonly observed, in some cases, pathological affect is observed. Pathological affect is a disturbance in the regulation of affect characterized by the rapid onset of tearfulness or, in some cases, profound weeping or crying that is sometimes referred to as pseudobulbar affect or "emotional incontinence" (Absher & Toole, 1996).

Although the relationship between the cognitive and emotional components of pathologic affect is generally consistent, the degree of affective change is rapid, disproportionate, and troublesome for many stroke survivors. Persons who are used to controlling their emotions suddenly find themselves embarrassed by their uncontrolled emotionality. In most cases, simple distraction or redirection can serve as a valuable tool in terminating unwanted tearfulness or lability. Discriminating between apathy, depression and pathologic affect is an important diagnostic role for most neuropsychologists, since many healthcare and rehabilitation professionals have trouble using self-reported symptoms or outward appearances to reach an accurate diagnosis.

Because of potential deficits in motor functions, language skills, attention, cognition, and functional skills, persons with dominant MCA infarction usually require extended neurorehabilitation in an inpatient setting, subacute nursing home, and/or outpatient setting, depending upon the severity of the initial neurologic deficit. Neuropsychologists may encounter DMCA patients during the acute medical-neurologic stage, during rehabilitation, or subsequently in outpatient settings where return to independent functioning, placement, capacity, and other disability questions predominate. In reality, during the acute stage following stroke, extended assessment and treatment are very rarely needed or possible. During rehabilitation and postacute stages, more in-depth assessment and, in some cases treatment, may be beneficial. In many cases, elderly persons with stroke have a number of other medical comorbidities, as well as neurologic morbidities, such as prior strokes and/or vascular or other dementias. In some cases, persons with serious medical problems require long-term institutional placement simply due to extensive care needs. In other cases, well-educated and determined family members manage stroke survivors in a home setting, but the complexity and severity of functional and neurocognitive disorders is a significant factor in determining who needs placement.

Assessment and intervention

In most cases of DMCA stroke, assessment is significantly complicated by motor, and especially language, deficits. Overt right hemiplegia is almost always accompanied by some form of communication deficit. Consequently, the first order of assessment is to determine the level of communication ability. Language may be assessed using a variety of standardized language measures or aphasia batteries. While many neuropsychologists are not formally trained in assessing language using comprehensive aphasia batteries, clinicians who work with persons who have suffered CVAs must become familiar with language assessment or rely on speech therapists to provide an index of communication skills. In the long run, neuropsychologists would be well served by acquiring skills in formal language assessment. In any case, at a minimum, assessment of naming, fluency, repetition, reading, and auditory comprehension at various levels of complexity must be undertaken. There are various ways to assess fluency, but an interview is usually sufficient for obtaining a global index. In many ways, comprehension is more important than fluency, although impaired fluency is troublesome for most stroke survivors. Both oral and reading comprehension should be assessed. Single word as well as basic and complex sentence comprehension should be assessed in both written and oral modalities. Such information is very relevant for determining what other measures can be administered as well as for planning functional and educational interventions. Nondominant apraxia, which is common with DMCA, may also complicate assessment above and beyond language deficits, particularly if a complex motor response is required as part of visuospatial cognitive tasks (Alexander, Baker, & Naeser, 1992).

In general, assessment of comprehension often helps to determine what nonverbal tests may be administered to aphasic persons. Following stroke, most persons must learn to perform many activities of daily living in a novel manner, including dressing, bathing, ambulating, and making transfers. The extent to which persons with DMCA stroke can learn and retain visual information is critical, so utilization of visuoperceptual and visuospatial learning and memory measures can be very helpful in indexing learning capacity, even in the absence of functional verbal communication. In many cases, adaptive language strategies are practiced in speech therapy, and patient responses to these interventions provides critical, but nonpsychometric, data for assessing learning.

Assessment questions with DMCA syndrome are usually pragmatic, as opposed to esoteric. The extent and level of decision-making capacity is important. Medical decision making is typically important in the acute phase of recovery and becomes even more important if there are disagreements between family members on the plan of care. Concern about a person's capacity to participate in their care and follow medical instructions regarding medications and therapy instructions are also common. Safety, broadly defined, is a significant concern. As such, neuropsychologists may be asked to assess a person's poststroke capacity to make decisions and function independently and to provide input into whether a surrogate power of attorney or guardianship is required. Sometimes constraints on autonomy are necessary (Macciocchi & Stringer, 2002). As an example, following DMCA stroke, persons may not be able to fully care for themselves, but they may also resist having a guardian or refuse placement in a nursing home. In such cases, there is no standard test battery or approach that has been empirically determined to be optimal. For such determinations, clinicians must use common sense and consider the affected neocortical networks. At a minimum, an attempt should be made to index orientation, attention, language, memory, and executive functions. We have argued that constraints on autonomy based on beneficence must be supported by strong clinical evidence as opposed to conjecture. In other words, if health care professionals feel the need to act paternally, neuropsychological evidence of incapacity should be clear and convincing (Macciocchi & Stringer, 2002).

In addition to neurocognitive functioning, all persons with DMCA syndrome should have a neurobehavioral assessment to insure that there are no signs of apathy, anosognosia, disinhibition, emotional liability, or aggressive behavior. Much of this assessment must be observational and is not readily available via psychometric techniques. As discussed previously, depression is common following DMCA stroke and may become more prevalent as recovery proceeds past the acute stage. Documenting adjustment to deficits and disability is an important aspect of the neuropsychological assessment, particularly for health care providers or physicians who are managing the elderly poststroke request referrals. Observational data can also be helpful in documenting the effectiveness of medical interventions, especially psychopharmacologic treatment for apathy, depression, and pathological affect. Assessing safety (risk and harm) is a complicated endeavor performed by many health care professionals on a daily basis. Fortunately, neuropsychologists are uniquely trained in many areas relevant to these assessments.

As far as treatment is concerned, most traditional applications of counseling, cognitive therapy, education, and psychopharmacology are applicable with DMCA syndrome. All interventions may be complicated by language problems, and persons with aphasias very often do not fare well in counseling or psychotherapy, either because they cannot readily comprehend the nature of the session or because they are easily frustrated by their expressive limitations. When counseling is not effective for persons with stroke, pharmacologic interventions for depression may be beneficial (Absher & Toole, 1996), although many of the emotional problems following stroke appear existential. Patient and family education can be helpful, and these interventions can sometimes mitigate distress secondary to unrealistic expectations for recovery and/or functional disability following stroke. In reality, most elderly persons with stroke are remarkably well adjusted considering the significant deficits and limitations typically apparent post stroke.

Nondominant middle cerebral artery CVA

In contrast to persons with DMCA-related lesions, persons with nondominant MCA (NDMCA) lesions evidence a similar, but different set of symptoms. As with persons who experience DMCA stroke, persons with NDMCA stroke initially may be incontinent. Deficits in motor function also are typically apparent, and mobility is usually affected secondary to hemiplegia. In contrast to DMCA stroke, dysarthria may be present, but true cognitive-linguistic deficits (semantics and syntax) are rarely observed, unless cerebral dominance is atypical (Alexander, 2003). Crossed aphasia is observed in a small percentage of NDMCA strokes. When present, about two-thirds of right cerebral hemisphere aphasias mirror DMCA language disorders, while about one-third are atypical language disorders (Alexander, 2003). Deficits in formulation of narrative and discourse are typically apparent following NDMCA stroke, and these deficits affect communication in a variety of ways (Alexander, 2003).

Disturbances in affective expression are also observed following NDMCA stroke, and these disorders (dyprosodias) appear to affect communication pragmatics (Ross, 2000). Visuospatial deficits are common, and attentional (neglect) disorders are frequently observed, depending on lesion volume (Heilman, Watson, & Valenstein, 2003). Persons with NDMCA strokes are often apathetic and amotivated. In some cases, anosodiaphoria (indifference) predominates; in other cases anosognosia is observed. Clinically speaking, the presence of a right gaze preference is pathognomonic for multimodality neglect and anosognosia and, in some cases, somatoparaphrenia or delusional denial of the affected limb or side of the body (Mesulam, 2000). In some cases, NDMCA stroke produces misidentification disorders. While the type of misidentification disorder varies, reduplicative paramensia (place) appears more common than health care professionals seem to report.

Communication problems in NDMCA syndrome are typically one of pragmatics, as opposed to semantics and syntax. Mutism may be apparent early following stroke, but during rehabilitation, speech typically becomes more fluent, although possibly dysarthic. Language comprehension is rarely affected, but apathy may reduce verbal responses. While basic communication is typically functional, NDMCA persons often communicate in a digressive manner and have considerable problems with nonpropositional aspects of communication. Sarcasm, wit, and humor are affected, although many persons with NDMCA syndrome appear to be capable of considerable caustic sarcasm. Speech may be fluent but characterized by dyprosdy, resulting in a monotone presentation reminiscent of someone who is depressed or sedated. When neurocognitive functioning is not severely affected, persons with NDMCA syndrome can communicate sufficiently to complete most neuropsychological tests, including verbal learning and memory measures.

Neglect is well described in the scientific and clinical literature (Heilman et al., 2003). When neglect is present, a myriad of other neuropsychological and neurobehavioral symptoms may also present. Symptoms of neglect typically include a right gaze preference and nondominant extinction of simultaneous stimuli in multiple sensory modalities. Persons with neglect usually have decreased motivation or intention, particularly in the affected (nondominant) hemispace. Decreased attention to and persistence on tests and functional tasks is common. Bradyphrenia is apparent and may affect performance on any learning task or test. Visual field defects and/or deficits in visuoperceptual and/or visuospatial processing may be present secondary to damage to cortical-subcortical systems in the right parietal lobe. In some cases, rather unique and interesting modality-specific knowledge deficits such as prosopagnosia are observed, but these disorders in pure form are rare (Damasio, Tranel, & Rizzo, 2000).

While modality-specific knowledge deficits are somewhat uncommon, dyprosodias are quite common following NDMCA stroke. According to Ross (2000), "damage to the right hemisphere selectively impairs the production, comprehension, and repetition of affective prosody without disrupting the prepositional elements of language" (p. 319). Disorders in prosody are believed to generally mirror language disorders, so that disturbances may be expressive (motor, transcortical motor, or global) or receptive (sensory or transcortical sensory) in nature. The practical implications of theoretical models of dysprosdy are that persons with NDMCA stroke typically have difficulty perceiving the emotional content of communication provided by health care professionals or family members. Since emotional components of language are critical for effective communication, NDMCA persons frequently lose crucial information necessary for understanding the directives, wishes and emotional states of those around them. As a result, persons with NDMCA stroke may not be able to discern when others are angry or frustrated with them or simply providing subtle or overt cues intended to motivate a change in behavior. On the expressive side, NDMCA persons' limited affective prosody often makes them appear depressed and apathetic, which in some cases are coexisting disorders. Nonetheless, in many cases, the absence of affect, melody, and tone in speech is not diagnostic of depression. When questioned about mood and depressogenic cognition, many persons with NDMCA syndrome deny being dysphoric and/or having melancholic thoughts.

Visuoperceptual and visuospatial deficits may be observed following NDMCA stroke depending on lesion volume. Deficits in visual information processing may affect functional skills such as spatial orientation and route finding. In some cases, visuoperceptual-spatial deficits are complicated by neglect/hemispatial inattention and/or a visual field defect, which makes performance of functional tasks even more difficult. In addition, symptoms of apathy and impaired intention may decrease visual processing even more. In general, persons with NDMCA stroke may appear to be confused for longer periods of time, have more difficulty learning new environments, struggle to benefit from therapies, and have poorer functional outcomes when compared to their DMCA peers (Macciocchi et al., 1998).

From a neurobehavioral perspective, persons with NDMCA stroke often appear apathetic and are frequently disinhibited. Judgment may be significantly impaired, especially when lesions are large and involve both the frontal and the parietal lobes, as well as subcortical structures. In such cases, anosognosia may be present; that is, awareness of deficits in motor, visual, and cognitive functions may be limited (McGlynn & Schacter, 1989). In general, the relationship between lesion volume, cognitive deficits, and neurobehavioral disturbance is variable, but as the severity of cognitive impairment increases so do behavioral problems. As an example, when hemispatial inattention is mild, it is rare to observe prominent anosognosia. In contrast, when a person with NDMCA stroke has a strong right gaze preference, prominent multimodality neglect, significant apathy, and anosognosia are common and may involve unawareness of motor, cognitive, and neurobehavioral deficits. In some cases, awareness of hemiplegia is intact, but awareness of neglect and cognitive and behavioral problems is impaired. Not surprisingly, in such cases, impairment in judgment regarding the impact of stroke on functional skills and independence is also quite common.

Assessment and intervention

In the acute stage following NDMCA stroke, extensive neurocognitive testing is not necessary or particularly useful. In most cases, a thorough neurobehavioral mental status examination can address typical referral questions. As persons become oriented, a brief assessment can be undertaken that focuses on attention, visuospatial perceptual skills, learning-memory, and executive functions. Since neglect is common following NDMCA stroke, various measures of visual attention can be administered. Cancellation tasks are helpful, although subtle signs of resolving visual neglect can be documented on many perceptual and spatial tasks. Parenthetically, rehabilitation therapists often use cancellation and other visual perceptual tests in therapy, so performance on such tests may be influenced by practice. When neglect is severe, practice effects are limited, but some persons with mild neglect may have benefited from practice on tests, so behavioral observation of functional skills can be important. Tests for perceptual problems may be very helpful in documenting deficits that may have functional implications. Tests of memory functioning, as well as executive skills, may also be helpful, particularly if questions of competency and decision making arise. There are many attention, visuoperceptual and executive tests available, and no specific set of tests has proven superior to another set. Clinicians must address referral questions using instruments that are reliable, sensitive, and valid for elderly persons who have significant neurocognitive problems. Extensive testing is often taxing and may not provide critical information above and beyond shorter batteries that are focused on functional cognition and ecological application.

In many cases, neurobehavioral assessment is more important than neurocognitive testing. Persons with NDMCA stroke often have problems with self-regulation and may be impulsive and or dangerous to themselves. They may be at risk for falls secondary to motor impairment and/or or aspiration secondary to hyperphagia. Unawareness complicates rehabilitation interventions, and developing behavior plans for persons with anosognosia can be challenging (Schacter & Prigatano, 1991). Assessment of affect and mood is important, and distinguishing between depression and apathy is often important for families and health care providers alike. As an example, apathetic persons typically are not at risk for self-injurious (suicidal) behavior, and educating families can mitigate concerns about such behavior. In terms of treatment, pharmacologic interventions designed to enhance arousal (dopamine agonists) and reduce apathy can improve therapy compliance and functional capacity. Treatment with various antidepressants can also be beneficial depending on the particular pattern of neurobehavioral dysfunction.

Anterior cerebral artery stroke

ACA syndromes do occur in the elderly, but neuropsychologists are more likely to see MCA syndromes in geriatric clinical practice. In general, ACA syndromes are related to anurysmal rupture, which most often occurs in middle, rather than late, age (Victor & Ropper, 2001). Ruptures of the anterior communicating artery or proximal branch (A1) of the anterior cerebral artery are common causes of ACA syndrome. When ACA stroke or anurysmal rupture do occur in the elderly, the neurocognitive and neurobehavioral deficits typically observed are strongly related to medial frontal and/or orbital frontal cerebral dysfunction. Cummings (1993) has articulated specific marker behaviors for medial and orbital syndromes. To summarize, orbitofrontal lesions have been found to produce disinhibition in the absence of significant neurocognitive dysfunction, while medial lesions result in apathy, which may initially present as mutism and akinesis, particularly following bilateral lesions. In general, depending on lesion volume and location, persons with dominant or nondominant ACA syndrome may have a number of deficits including motor weakness in the contralateral lower extremity, communication abnormalities, behavioral changes, and neurocognitive dysfunction. Behavioral changes vary and may include apathy, anergia, depression, and/or disinhibition. In persons with apathy or an intentional deficit, disinhibition may be quiescent until recovery proceeds. Often, persons with ACA syndromes retain some capacity for mobility and may not evidence severe deficits in language or cognitive functioning other than memory skills.

In some cases, right-sided ACA lesions will produce a neglect syndrome, but in many cases the disturbance in attention is more related to general inattentiveness than to the vector dysfunction observed in true neglect. Persons with ACA lesions are often distractible and have difficulty regulating their attention even when in highly structured environments. When persons with ACA lesions have significant memory disorders, disorientation and confabulation are commonly observed (DeLuca, 1992). Confabualtion may be provoked or spontaneous, although in many cases, provocation is necessary to produce confabualtion, particularly if apathy is also present. Nonetheless, spontaneous and fantastic confabulation is sometimes observed, particularly if significant deficits in neurocognitive regulation and anosognosia are also present. Memory disorders can be significant, and in some cases ACA strokes may produce extended periods of confusion.

When persons with ACA stroke are not hemiplegic and do not have significant lower extremity weakness, they are able to ambulate and pose a safety risk to themselves, and sometimes to others, depending on their level of disinhibition and aggressiveness. When disinhibition is accompanied by amnesia, behavior management concerns become significant. ACA lesions are known to cause significant memory problems, particularly with declarative memory (DeLuca, Bryant, & Myers, 2003), which limit patients' ability to benefit from therapy. In many cases, procedural learning may be possible and facilitate route finding, and environmental awareness can be facilitated by orientation and repetition. In other cases, dense anterograde amnesia is present and presents a considerable challenge for staff and family.

Assessment and intervention

In general, assessment following ACA stroke should focus on cognitive and behavioral functioning. In most cases, delirium will be present in the initial stages of recovery and complex cognitive assessment will not be possible. If attention recovers to the point that testing is possible, language skills, memory functions, and executive capacity should be assessed. Assessment of language should include examination of fluency, repetition and comprehension, as well as formulation of narrative and discourse. If language is functional and attention is not severely impaired, memory skills can be assessed. List learning, narrative learning, and visuospatial learning may all be appropriate targets for assessment. If persons with ACA stroke are amnestic, there is usually enough information from behavioral observations to support the diagnosis, but testing will rapidly confirm clinical observations since anything ranging from moderate memory dysfunction to dense anterograde amnesia can be observed.

Since cognition is most often preserved, neurobehavioral assessment may take precedence. Testing for behavioral dysfunction is typically observational in nature, although awareness of cognitive and behavioral problems can be indexed in a variety of ways. Luria (1966) offered a number of methods for examining awareness, and more recent methods have also been developed (Prigatano & Schacter, 1991). In many cases, clinicians can simply build in a self-evaluation scale after each test and have the patient rate their skills relative to their prior functioning. In most cases, basic interview data can establish that awareness for current functioning is impaired, particularly in persons who are disoriented and/or truly amnestic. Prolonged periods of confusion and amnesia are common, and disturbances in attention and memory are especially problematic when mobility is functional. In such cases, close supervision is required, even when persons are in a secure environment. For the most part, environmental control and monitoring are most important, but mass repetition and situational orientation may help to facilitate adjustment, especially if persons with ACA are not aggressive. If aggressive behavior is prominent, medical interventions (medication) may be necessary to insure the safety of the patient, family, and staff, particularly if anosognosia is severe.

Posterior cerebral artery syndrome

As in the case of ACA syndrome, pure PCA syndrome appears to be less common than MCA syndrome in the elderly, although base rates of the disorder seem to vary based on the clinical setting. As an example, PCA may be more commonly observed in an acute neurological setting as opposed to a rehabilitation setting, where prominent motor deficits are necessary for admission. Nonetheless, PCA stroke can produce a number of neurocognitive and neurobehavioral deficits. A PCA stroke can involve many structures including the visual cortex, thalamus, internal capsule, hippocampus, and corpus callosum. PCA stroke is known to be associated with classic neuropsychological disorders such as alexia without agraphia. Sensory integration impairments are common in individuals with PCA strokes. Such individuals often have difficulty incorporating their sensory experiences into a cognitive schema despite apparently intact orientation. Visual field defects are common and may complicate assessment and treatment. In some cases, unawareness of visual deficits is observed (Anton's syndrome), although this disorder is somewhat uncommon in general clinical practice.

Assessment and intervention

Clinical examinations in PCA stroke should address visual perceptual, memory, and language functioning. If cerebellar involvement is present, motor functions may be impaired and require assessment. Deficits in memory function may be apparent, and systematic assessment of learning and recall in multiple modalities is prudent. Many cases of amnesia documented in the literature involve ischemic damage to the hippocampal region secondary to hypoxic ischemic effects of cardiac arrest. Persons with PCA ischemia may evidence similar impairments in memory. In many ways, interventions are similar to those following other CVAs. Assessment data should be used to educate the patient and family. Cognitive therapy should be used to increase functional skills, when possible. Finally, pharmacologic interventions for arousal, depression, and apathy should be considered.

Functional outcome

The prevalence of stroke, increased rate of survival, and expense of rehabilitation have resulted in pressure to identify valid, reliable predictors of outcome. Many predictors of outcome have been studied, sometimes with conflicting results. Some authors have shown that increasing age is associated with poorer outcome after stroke (Alexander, 1994; Kotila, 1986), whereas other researchers maintain that age is not an independent predictor of functional outcome (Samuelsson, Soderfeldt, & Olsson, 1996). Alexander (1994) found initial severity of stroke and age to be the most powerful predictors of functional recovery. Similarly, Kotila, Waltimo, Niemi, Laaksonen, and Lempinen (1984) showed that age greater than 65 years had a significant negative impact on discharge from the hospital, adequate performance of activities of daily living (ADL), and return to work. Moreover, other researchers have found survival to be decreased in each successive age group (Chen & Ling, 1985). Differences in association between age and outcome across studies might be due to the correlation of age with comorbidities such as medical, psychosocial, and psychiatric disorders, which obscure predictors of outcome. For instance, history of prior stroke, as well as, as history of hypertension, diabetes, or cardiac disease, have been associated with poorer outcome after stroke, and the impact of these comorbid disorders may be greater in older persons (Cifu & Lorish, 1994).

In addition to age and medical comorbidities, initial stroke severity appears strongly related to functional outcomes (Alexander, 1994). Stroke severity and side of lesion have also been shown to interact. In some studies, persons with severe functional impairment on admission following right hemisphere lesions appeared to demonstrate less improvement than those with left hemisphere lesions (Alexander, 1994). Although these findings are not unique, some researchers have not found a difference in outcome related to lesion location, and literature reviews suggest that hemisphere of stroke does not predict outcome (Cifu & Lorish, 1994; Kotila, 1986). Consequently, additional outcome data is needed in order to address outcome following stroke, particularly with respect to various parameters such as age, lesion location-volume, and the effects of medical comorbidities.

Despite the need for valid outcome data, differences in methodology complicate the interpretation of results across studies. Problems frequently identified in stroke studies include heterogeneity of the stroke samples, including variability in diagnosis (cerebral hemorrhage vs. ischemia), mixing of single and recurrent stroke, failure to control for prior stroke, and combining levels of acuity of strokes and treatment settings (Anderson, 1990; Jongbloed, 1990). In addition to these concerns, studying only the most severely affected stroke patients is problematic when improved scores on functional measures could be attributed to statistical regression to the mean rather than to genuine functional improvement. Moreover, the instruments used to measure outcomes are not necessarily quantitatively or qualitatively interchangeable, thereby making study comparisons difficult. Finally, many stroke studies are retrospective, quasiexperimental designs, which enhance potential threats to internal validity (selection bias, for example). Retrospective studies that do not take into account patient selection and attrition due to mortality run the risk of biased results and misrepresentation of the larger stroke population.

Because findings on the effects of age and lesion location on outcome were being debated, Macciocchi et al. (1998) decided to prospectively identify predictors of stroke outcome. Based on past research, age, gender, lesion location (right vs. left; cortical vs. subcortical), initial neurologic deficit, history of previous stroke, and comorbid medical disorders were all examined in a prospective study of outcome following stroke in a large cohort ($N = 328$).

Standardized protocols were used to study participants from stroke onset to 3 months post stroke. Participant's neurologic status and functional skills were documented using clinical scales, and lesions were quantified using neuroimaging studies (Macciocchi et al., 1998). In this study, multiple sites were used to recruit stroke patients, which reduced the bias introduced by a single center or enrollment site. Standardized inclusion/exclusion criteria provided a homogeneous stroke population with general equivalent frequencies of dominant and nondominant ischemic lesions of generally comparable size. The frequency of right and left hemisphere lesions was essentially equivalent and lesion location was equally distributed in both cerebral hemispheres. Most importantly, patients were followed prospectively from onset of stroke to 3 months after their initial hospitalization, a period of time when much, but not all, restitution in function is observed.

The results of the study by Macciocchi et al. (1998) supported several previous findings. First, age did have a significant effect on functional outcome. Moreover, this effect appeared generally linear. As age increases, functional outcome following ischemic stroke worsens. Somewhat surprisingly, comorbid medical disorders did not appear to significantly contribute to functional status post stroke. This finding is encouraging and suggests that patients with medical comorbidities are likely to demonstrate functional recovery despite their medical disorders. Previous research on side of lesion has yielded contradictory results. Despite reviews that found no differences in outcome between dominant and nondominant cerebral lesions, our study supports findings obtained by other researchers who found poorer functional outcomes in patients with nondominant (right) hemisphere strokes. The difference in functional outcome related to lesion side did not appear to be due to differences in lesion volume and location, since lesion distribution was statistically equivalent across groups. As mentioned previously, persons with nondominant (right) hemisphere strokes are known to evidence neurobehavioral problems, such as apathy, neglect, and anosognosia, which may play a role in determining functional skill acquisition post stroke. Finally, persons with cortical strokes appeared to fare better, whether they experienced a right or a left CVA. In contrast, not surprisingly, a history of prior stroke was strongly related to higher risk of impaired functional skills at 3 months after a second stroke.

While the study by Macciocchi et al. (1998) did not directly address neurocognitive and neurobehavioral functioning, functional capacity was clearly affected by age, severity of initial neurologic deficit, a history prior stroke, and lesion location and volume. While more research replicating these findings is necessary, the implications of the study for neuropsychologists are relatively straightforward. Older persons will likely have greater functional deficits post stroke, which will have implications for stroke survivors as well as family members. The degree of initial neurologic deficit is a reasonable marker for expectations for recovery, particularly in functional skills. Clinicians should pay close attention to persons with right hemisphere lesions, particularly lesions involving subcortical as well as cortical structures. These persons probably will have poorer outcomes and require more attention during hospitalization and post discharge.

Summary and conclusions

Strokes produce both fascinating and severely debilitating neuropsychological deficits. Aphasia, apraxia, agnosia, anosognosia, and amnesia are commonly observed following stroke. In some cases, clinicians will not have the opportunity to observe these disorders in pure form unless they work in a setting where persons with stroke are diagnosed and treated. Alternatively, many elderly persons experience severe neuropsychological and functional deficits following stroke, which significantly affect their independence and lifestyle. Clinicians working in geriatric settings will certainly encounter many persons who have suffered a stroke of one type or another. In general, neuropsychological practitioners must be able to perform brief, but reliable and valid, assessments of neurocognitive and neurobehavioral functioning. Elderly persons are often not able to tolerate more traditional, extended test batteries. Moreover, many of the questions raised by referral sources relate to self-care, independence, and decision making as opposed to return to school or work. Other more formal issues such as testamentary capacity, disability determination, and dispositional placement may also be encountered. Clinicians must also be able to use neuropsychological knowledge to educate and intervene with the common clinical problems that arise post stroke.

We have provided an overview of cognitive and behavioral problems associated with stroke. In no way does our review mitigate clinicians' need to become familiar with the literature on cortical organization, neurocognitive networks, and research on neuropsychological deficits associated with stroke or outcome following stroke. Many texts providing information relevant for clinical practice in the area of stroke have been cited and could be incorporated into training and educational programs. In many ways, clinicians in training should have an opportunity to work in a geriatric setting dedicated to stroke survivors. Clinicians will not only learn a tremendous amount about classic neuropsychological disorders, but elderly persons with stroke are typically some of the most interesting, motivated, cooperative, and gracious persons clinicians will encounter.

References

Abbott, R., Curb, J., Rodriguez, B., Masaki, K., Popper, J., Ross, G., & Petrovitich, H. (2003). Age-related changes in risk factor effects on the incidence of thromboembolic and hemorrhagic stroke. *Journal of Clinical Epidemiology, 56*, 479–486.

Absher, J., & Toole, J. (1996). Neurobehavioral features of cerebrovascular disease. In B. S. Fogel & R. B. Schiffer (Eds.), *Neuropsychiatry* (pp. 895–912). Baltimore: Williams & Wilkins.

Alexander, M. P. (1994). Stroke rehabilitation outcome: A potential use of predictive variables to establish levels of care. *Stroke, 25,* 128–134.

Alexander, M. P. (1997). Aphasia: Clinical and anatomic aspects. In T. E. Feinberg & M. J. Farah (Eds.), *Behavioral neurology and neuropsychology* (pp. 133–150). New York: McGraw-Hill.

Alexander, M. P. (2003). Aphasia: Clinical and anatomic issues. In T. E. Feinberg & M. J. Farah (Eds.), *Behavioral neurology and neuropsychology* (2nd ed., pp. 147–164). New York: McGraw-Hill.

Alexander, M. P., Baker, E., & Naeser, M. A. (1992). Neuropsychological and neuroanatomical dimensions of ideomotor apraxia. *Brain, 118,* 87–107.

American Heart Association. (2003). *Heart disease and stroke facts.* Retrieved June 1, 2005, from http://www.americanheart.org/downloadable/heart/1056719919740 HSFacts2003text.pdf

Anderson, T. P. (1990). Studies up to 1980 on stroke rehabilitation outcomes. *Stroke, 21*(Suppl. 2), 43–45.

Blumenfeld, H. (2002). *Neuroanatomy through clinical cases.* Sunderland, MA: Sinauer Associates.

Brown, R., Whisnant, J., & Sicks, R. (1996). Stroke incidence, prevalence and survival: Secular trends in Rochester, Minnesota, through 1989. *Stroke, 27,* 373–380.

Chen, Q., & Ling, R. (1985). A 1–4 year follow-up study of 306 cases of stroke. *Stroke, 16,* 323–327.

Cifu, D. X., & Lorish, T. R. (1994). Stroke rehabilitation outcome. *Archives of Physical Medicine and Rehabilitation, 75*(Suppl.), 56–60.

Cummings, J. (1993). Frontal-subcortical circuits and human behavior. *Archives of Neurology, 50,* 873–880.

Damasio, A. R., & Damasio, H. (2000). Aphasia and the neural basis of language. In M. M. Mesulam (Ed.), *Principles of behavioral and cognitive neurology* (2nd ed., pp. 294–315). New York: Oxford University Press.

Damasio, A. R., Tranel, D., & Rizzo, M. (2000). Disorders of complex visual processing. In M. M. Mesulam (Ed.), *Principles of behavioral and cognitive neurology* (2nd ed., pp. 332–372). New York: Oxford University Press.

DeLuca, J. (1992). Cognitive dysfunction after aneurysm of the anterior communicating artery. *Journal of Clinical and Experimental Neuropsychology, 14*(6), 924–934.

DeLuca, J., Bryant, D., & Myers, C. E. (2003). Memory impairment following anterior communicating artery aneurysm. In T. E. Feinberg & M. J. Farah (Eds.), *Behavioral neurology and neuropsychology* (2nd ed., pp. 477–486). New York: McGraw-Hill.

Elkind, M. (2003). Stroke in the elderly. *Mount Sinai Journal of Medicine, 70*(1), 27–37.

Fang, J., & Alderman, M. (2001). Trend of stroke hospitalization, United States, 1988–1997. *Stroke, 32,* 2221–2226.

Feinberg, T. E., & Farah, M. J. (2003). *Behavioral neurology and neuropsychology* (2nd ed.). New York: McGraw-Hill.

Heilman, K. M., Watson, R. T., & Valenstein, E. (2003). Neglect and related disorders. In K. M. Heilman & E. Valenstein (Eds.), *Clinical neuropsychology* (4th ed., pp. 296–346). New York: Oxford University Press.

Hollander, M., Koudstaal, P., Bots, M., Grobbee, D., Hofman, A., & Breteler, M. (2003). Incidence, risk and case fatality of first ever stroke in the elderly population:

The Rotterdam study. *Journal of Neurology and Neurosurgical Psychiatry, 74,* 317–321.

Jongbloed, L. (1990). Problems of methodological heterogeneity in studies predicting disability after stroke. *Stroke, 21*(Suppl. 2), 32–34.

Kotila, M. (1986). Four year prognosis of patients under the age of 65 surviving their first ischemic brain infarction. *Annals of Clinical Research, 18,* 76–79.

Kotila, M., Waltimo, O., Niemi, M. J., Laaksonen, R., & Lempinen, M. (1984). The profile of recovery from stroke and factors influencing outcome. *Stroke, 15,* 1039–1044.

Luria, A. R. (1966). *Higher cortical functions in man.* New York: Basic Books.

Macciocchi, S. N., Diamond, P. D., Alves, W. A., & Mertz, T. (1998). Ischemic stroke: Relation of age, lesion location, and initial neurologic deficit to functional outcome. *Archives of Physical Medicine and Rehabilitation, 79,* 1255–1257.

Macciocchi, S. N., & Stringer, A. Y. (2002). Assessing risk and harm: The convergence of ethical and empirical considerations. *Archives of Physical Medicine and Rehabilitation, 82*(Suppl. 2), S15–S19.

Mayberg, H. (2001). Depression and frontal-subcortical circuits: Focus on prefrontal-limbic interactions. In D. G. Lichter & J. L. Cummings (Eds.), *Frontal-subcortical circuits in psychiatric and neurological disorders* (pp. 177–206). New York: Guilford Press.

McGlynn, S. M., & Schacter, D. I. (1989). Unawareness of deficits in neuropsychological syndromes. *Journal of Clinical and Experimental Neuropsychology, 11,* 143–205.

Mesulam, M. (2000). Behavioral neuroanatomy: Large-scale networks, association cortex, frontal syndromes, the limbic system, and hemispheric specialization. In M. M. Mesulam (Ed.), *Principles of behavioral and cognitive neurology* (2nd ed., pp. 1–120). New York: Oxford University Press.

Muntner, P., Garrett, E., Klag, M., & Coresh, J. (2002). Trends in stroke prevalence between 1973 and 1991 in the US population 25 to 74 years of age. *Stroke, 33,* 1209–1213.

Netter, F. H. (1972). *The CIBA collection of medical illustrations: Vol. I. Nervous system.* New York: Colorpress.

Olindo, S., Cabre, P., Deschamps, R., Chatot-Henry, C., Rene-Corail, P., Fournerie, P., et al. (2003). Acute stroke in the very elderly: Epidemiological features, stroke subtypes, management and outcome in Martinique, French West Indies. *Stroke, 34,* 1593–1597.

Prigatano, G. P., & Schacter, D. L. (1991). *Awareness of deficit after brain injury: Clinical and theoretical issues.* New York: Oxford University Press.

Ross, E. D. (2000). Affective prosody and the aprosodias. In M. M. Mesulam (Ed.), *Principles of behavioral and cognitive neurology* (2nd ed., pp. 316–331). New York: Oxford University Press.

Samuelsson, M., Soderfeldt, B., & Olsson, G. B. (1996). Functional outcome in patients with lacunar infarction. *Stroke, 27,* 842–846.

Schacter, D. L., & Prigatano, G. P. (1991). Forms of unawareness. In G. P. Prigatano & D. L. Schacter (Eds.), *Awareness of deficit after brain injury: Clinical and theoretical issues* (pp. 258–262). New York: Oxford University Press.

Victor, M., & Ropper, A. (2001). *Adam's and Victor's principles of neurology* (7th ed.). New York: McGraw-Hill.

Williams, G., Jiang, J., Matachar, D., & Samsa, G. (1999). Incidence and occurrence of total (first-ever and recurrent) stroke. *Stroke, 30*, 2523–2528.

Wolf, P., D'Agostino, R., & O'Neal, M. (1992). Secular trends in stroke incidence and mortality: The Framingham Study. *Stroke, 23*, 1551–1555.

Zola, S. (1997). Amnesia: Neuroanatomic and clinical aspects. In T. F. Feinberg & M. J. Farah (Eds.), *Behavioral neurology and neuropsychology* (pp. 447–462). New York: McGraw-Hill.

10 Neuropsychology of Parkinson's disease and its dementias

Alexander I. Tröster and Steven Paul Woods

Historical perspectives

The illness bearing his name was first described by James Parkinson in 1817. In that description of six patients (of whom Parkinson had personally examined three), it was categorically asserted that intellect and senses were preserved, but the author's recognition of depression in these patients is suggested by his use of terms such as melancholia (Parkinson 1817; see also Darvesh & Freedman 1996). Though the assertion that Parkinson's disease (PD) leaves cognition unscathed was challenged by Charcot and Vulpian (1861, 1862) and by isolated reports in the late nineteenth and early twentieth centuries, many outside France remained unconvinced of cognitive compromise in PD probably until the middle of the twentieth century (Goetz, 1992). Naville (1922) introduced the term "bradyphrenia" to capture the phenomena of slowed information processing and diminished attention in postencephalitic parkinsonians without dementia. Dementia was rarely a topic of early medical manuscripts concerned with paralysis agitans (PD). Interestingly, Fritz Lewy, whose name the eosinophilic, neuronal inclusion bodies have borne since 1918 (Schiller, 2000), did not distinguish depression and dementia when he described the neuropathology and mental alterations of PD (Lewy, 1912, 1923). Furthermore, Lewy apparently did not appreciate the significance of the inclusion bodies he had identified, and the entity of dementia with Lewy bodies (DLB) was not recognized until the last 30 years of the twentieth century (Holdorff, 2002).

Neuropsychological investigations using standardized, psychometric tests were rarely carried out in early studies of PD, but the likely first published use of such tests can be traced to Shaskin, Yarnell, and Alper's (1942) administration of the Wechsler Bellevue Scale, an intelligence scale, to postencephalitic parkinsonians. A further catalyst for neuropsychological evaluation (using projective tests and tests of cognition and intelligence) in PD was the advent of the neurosurgical treatment of parkinsonism (idiopathic, postencephalitic, and vascular) in the 1950s (Diller, Riklan, & Cooper, 1956). Though the number of surgical interventions for PD declined dramatically after the introduction of levodopa in the late 1960s (Siegfried & Blond, 1997), numerous psychometric studies of the neuropsychological effects of thalamotomy and pallidotomy were carried out both in North America (Jurko & Andy 1964; Riklan & Levita, 1969; Shapiro, Sadowsky, Henderson, & van Buren, 1973) and on the other side of the Atlantic (Almgren, Andersson, & Kullberg, 1969; Asso, Crown, Russell, & Logue, 1969; Christensen, Juul-Jensen, Malmros, & Harmsen, 1970; Fünfgeld, 1967; McFie, 1960; Vilkki & Laitinen, 1974; Welman, 1971).

The clinical focus of early neuropsychological studies of PD was maintained by investigators examining the cognitive effects of levodopa in the 1960s and 1970s (Beardsley & Puletti, 1971). By the 1980s, clinically oriented studies concerned themselves with the neuropsychological characterization of dementia in PD and its discriminability from other dementias (Huber, Shuttleworth, Paulson, Bellchambers, & Clapp, 1986; Pillon, Dubois, Lhermitte, & Agid, 1986; Pirozzolo, Hansch, Mortimer, Webster, & Kuskowski, 1982). In parallel, studies increasingly informed by cognitive psychological theory began to provide more detailed and sophisticated descriptions of neuropsychological deficits in PD (Boller, Mizutani, Roessmann, & Gambetti, 1980; Brown & Marsden, 1988; Cooper, Sagar, Jordan, Harvey, & Sullivan, 1991; Lees & Smith, 1983; Levin, Llabre, & Weiner, 1989; Taylor, Saint-Cyr, & Lang, 1986). Advances in understanding the neural substrates and cognitive mechanisms underlying neuropsychological deficits in PD continue as functional neuroimaging technology matures and becomes more readily available (Cools, Stefanova, Barker, Robbins, & Owen, 2002; Dagher, Owen, Boecker, & Brooks, 1999; Feigin et al., 2003; Owen, Doyon, Dagher, Sadikot, & Evans, 1998). The 1990s saw a renaissance of neurobehavioral studies of surgical treatments of PD, including deep brain stimulation, which holds promise of allowing researchers a window on the neurobehavioral functions of the basal ganglia (Fields & Tröster, 2000; Tröster & Fields, 2003b). Studies are now beginning to address possible neuropsychological differences between Parkinson's disease with dementia and dementia with Lewy bodies (DLB), but it remains unknown whether these clinical diagnostic entities are in fact neuropathologically and phenomenologically distinct or two sides of one coin (McKeith et al., 2003).

Epidemiology and genetics

Zhang and Roman (1993) reported worldwide prevalence rates of PD ranging from 18 to 418 per 100,000. Prevalence rates in Western countries, once differences in study methodology and the age of study populations are taken into consideration, vary less widely, namely from 102 to 190 per 100,000. Because prevalence is impacted by survival and survival-related factors that vary geographically and temporally (with long survival associated with larger prevalence than a disease with comparable incidence but short survival), incidence might be a more accurate index of the frequency with which PD occurs. Few incidence estimates exist, but Bower, Maraganore, McDonnell, &

Rocca (1999) reported an annual incidence of 26 per 100,000 of parkinsonism, and a Parkinson's disease incidence of 11 per 100,000 in Minnesota. In that study, PD incidence increased from 0 per 100,000 among those aged 0–29 years, to 93 per 100,000 among those aged 70–79 years.

Parkinson's disease rarely occurs before age 50 years, and age-specific prevalence increases until the ninth decade (Tanner, Hubble, & Chan, 1997). Gender and race differences in PD prevalence remain controversial. However, in studies that do report gender differences, a higher prevalence is consistently found among males than females (Baldereschi et al., 2000). Because the lower prevalence of PD among blacks than whites and Hispanics found in one study was accompanied by a higher death rate among incident black cases (Mayeux et al., 1995), the lower prevalence among blacks reported by some studies may be an artifact of apparently diminished survival.

In addition to age and possibly gender, several environmental factors, a common denominator of which is exposure to potential neurotoxins, have been identified that heighten the risk of developing PD. These include exposure to 1-methyl-4-phenyl-1,2,3,6-tetrahydropiridine (MPTP) (which also produces neuropsychological impairments resembling those of PD) (Stern & Langston, 1985), herbicides, pesticides, and metals such as manganese and iron, and drinking of well water (Hubble, Cao, Hassanein, Neuberger, & Koller, 1993; Kuopio, Marttila, Helenius, & Rinne, 1999b; Seidler et al., 1996). Other environmental factors include residence in industrialized or rural areas, and employment in farming, wood pulp, chemical and steel manufacturing industries (Gorell, Johnson, Rybicki, Peterson, & Richardson, 1998; Tanner, 1989; Tanner et al., 1987).

Genetic factors do not play a dominant role in the causation of PD. There is accumulating evidence, however, that a minority of cases is etiologically linked to genetic factors, and that in other cases genetics may confer susceptibility to PD, perhaps via a synergistic interaction with exposure to toxins. Genetic polymorphisms have only been inconsistently and inconclusively associated with PD (Tanner, Goldman, & Ross, 2002). Many of the studies have focused on genes that code for metabolic enzymes, free-radical detoxifying enzymes, and proteins involved in dopaminergic transmission, and on dopamine transporter and receptor genes. Were genetic factors to play a major role in the etiology of PD, then concordance rates for PD ought to be higher among monozygotic (identical) than dizygotic (fraternal) twins. This appears not to be the case, except perhaps in some early onset cases, meaning in persons who develop the disease before age 50 years (Tanner et al., 1999).

Over the past few years several genetic mutations and loci have been identified and linked to parkinsonism (often of early onset) in a small number of families (Dekker, Bonifati, & van Duijn, 2003). The term parkinsonism is used because the constellation of clinical features (and underlying neuropathology), despite commonalities, varies between genetic mutations and loci and often differs from idiopathic PD. Though the relevance of these findings to sporadic cases of PD and parkinsonism remains unknown, it is hoped that the findings will help identify molecular pathways of therapeutic relevance (Hardy, Cookson, & Singleton, 2003). To date, linkage studies have identified six genetic loci that cosegregate with parkinsonism in families with autosomal dominant inheritance patterns of parkinsonism. Four loci have been linked to autosomal recessive forms of parkinsonism. Only one locus has been linked to sporadic, late-onset, nonmendelian Parkinson's disease. Although the various loci have all been mapped to chromosomes 1, 2, 4, 6, or 12, mutations of only five genes have been identified. From a neuropsychological standpoint, of particular interest are the Iowa kindred with early dementia (PARK 4, with a locus on chromosome 4p) (Farrer et al., 1999), and the Contursi kindred (PARK 1) (Golbe et al., 1996), in which atypical clinical features include fluent aphasia and palilalia.

Potential genetic contributions to the variability of neuropsychological profiles in PD have not received sufficient empirical attention. Dujardin, Defebvre, Grunberg, Becquet, and Destee (2001) compared small groups of patients with sporadic and familial PD and found that while both groups demonstrated executive dysfunction, only the sporadic PD group had memory impairments. Although intriguing, the basis and significance of this finding remains to be determined. While the apoliopoprotein E ε4 genotype has been linked to an increased risk of Alzheimer's disease and poorer memory test performance among healthy elderly, this genotype has not consistently been linked to dementia in PD (Koller et al., 1995) and thus probably does not account for possible differences in memory in PD subgroups. Indeed, Tröster and Fields (2003a), despite replicating the finding of slightly lower (but not abnormal) verbal memory test scores among healthy elderly with at least one ε4 allele as compared to those without such an allele, did not find similar memory differences between PD groups with and without ε4 alleles. Whether ε4 relates to nonmemory cognitive differences among dementias in PD remains to be studied.

Neuropathology and pathophysiology

Parkinson's disease involves the loss of pigmented cells from the substantia nigra (especially the ventrolateral part), which is the main source of the brain's dopamine. Though all the dopaminergic systems are eventually compromised in PD, the most pronounced core deficit is in the nigrostriatal system, and it is estimated that 70–80% of this system's neurons have been lost when PD symptoms first emerge (Bernheimer, Birkmayer, Hornykiewicz, Jellinger, & Seitelberger, 1973). Braak et al. (2003) attempted to define the sequence of neuropathological changes in PD by developing a staging system analogous to their system for staging Alzheimer's disease pathology. These stages, and their core features, are presented in Table 10.1.

Dopamine depletion in the striatum is more profound in the putamen than the caudate. Cognitive and affective changes accompanying PD, when attributable to dopaminergic system pathology, are probably linked to mesocortical and mesolimbic, rather than nigrostriatal system abnormalities. It has

Table 10.1 Braak staging of neuropathology in Parkinson's disease

Stage	Primary brain region affected	Loci of pathology
1	Medulla	Dorsal IX/X motor nucleus and/or immediate reticular zone
2	Medulla and pontine tegmentum	Stage 1 + caudal raphe nuclei, gigantocellular reticular nucleus and caeruleus-subcaeruleus complex
3	Midbrain	Stage 2 + midbrain (esp. pars compacta of substantia nigra)
4	Basal prosencephalon and mesocortex	Stage 3 + prosencephalon (confined to transentorhinal region and CA2-plexus)
5	Neocortex	Stage 4 + high order sensory association areas of the neocortex and prefrontal cortex
6	Neocortex	Stage 5 + first order sensory association neocortical areas and premotor areas; may be some mild changes in primary sensory areas and primary motor field

been argued too that neurobehavioral changes in PD may reflect non-dopaminergic system dysfunction (Pillon, Boller, Levy, & Dubois, 2001), because cognitive deficits tend to correlate with the motor symptoms that are least, if at all, responsive to levodopa (e.g., gait abnormality, dysarthria), but not with motor symptoms responsive to levodopa (Pillon et al., 1989). While it is probably the case that many neurobehavioral abnormalities in PD result from nondopaminergic system dysfunction, the lack of correlation between cognitive deficits and levodopa-responsive motor systems (and the relatively limited impact levodopa has on cognition) does not exclude a dopaminergic system role in neurobehavioral deficits. First, levodopa's principal effect is on the nigrostriatal system, leaving the possibility that neurobehavioral changes are related, at least partly, to mesocortical (Mattay et al., 2002) and mesolimbic system dysfunction. Second, the dopaminergic system's role in neurobehavioral alterations may differ as a function of disease stage, as suggested by the findings of Owen et al. (1995). Third, traditional neuropsychological tests may not be adequately sensitive to dopamine-related cognitive deficits in PD. These deficits may be subtle and highly specific. Several studies have shown that levodopa may affect only selected aspects of executive function, and even affect different facets of executive function in apparently opposite manner (Fournet, Moreaud, Roulin, Naegele, & Pellat, 2000; Lange et al., 1992; Owen et al., 1995). Fourth, functional neuroimaging advances continue to facilitate the elucidation of the role of different neural systems, including the dopaminergic systems, in the various neurobehavioral changes of PD (Cools et al., 2002; Feigin et al., 2003; Mattay et al., 2002; Mentis et al., 2002).

Certainly some cognitive and behavioral changes are likely to be dopamine related given the fluctuation of nonmotor symptoms in PD.

Nondopaminergic system changes in PD include cell loss in the locus caeruleus (noradrenergic), the dorsal raphe nuclei (serotonergic), the nucleus basalis of Meynert (cholinergic), and the dorsal vagal nucleus. Dysfunction of these various neurotransmitter systems has also been linked to cognitive (especially executive) and affective changes in PD (Dubois et al., 1987; Dubois, Pillon, Lhermitte, & Agid, 1990; Mayeux, Stern, Cote, & Williams, 1984; Stern, Mayeux, & Cote, 1984). Indeed, such neurobehavioral fluctuations may be more troubling to the patient than the analogous fluctuations in motor function (Witjas et al., 2002).

An important additional feature of the neuropathology of PD is the presence of Lewy bodies. The presence of these spherical, eosinophilic, intracytoplasmic neuronal inclusions in pigmented brainstem nuclei, especially the substantia nigra, together with neuronal loss and gliosis in this region, are a hallmark of PD. While brainstem Lewy bodies have a filamentous and granular core, cortical Lewy bodies lack this "core and halo" appearance. Kosaka, Matsushita, Oyanagi, and Mehraein (1980) proposed a pathological classification of Lewy body disease encompassing three topographical categories: brainstem, transitional, and cortical. The brainstem category corresponds to PD, in which Lewy bodies are confined to the pigmented brainstem nuclei. The transitional category (also called the limbic category) describes the additional distribution of Lewy bodies in the limbic cortices, most prominently in the insula, cingulate, and parahippocampal gyrus. In the cortical type, Lewy bodies are abundant in the isocortex.

Considerable debate continues about the role of Lewy bodies in the dementia of Parkinson's disease, and whether the clinical entities of dementia with Lewy bodies (DLB) and Parkinson's disease with dementia (PDD) are neuropathologically and neuropsychologically distinct. While dementia and overall severity of cognitive impairment have been associated with cortical Lewy body density, especially in frontal and temporal cortices (Gomez-Tortosa et al., 1999; Hurtig et al., 2000), there are cases of PD with dementia that lack cortical pathology (Perry et al., 1985; Xuereb et al., 1990). Furthermore, a subset of patients with a clinical diagnosis of PD, but meeting neuropathological criteria for DLB at necropsy, may lack a history of significant cognitive impairment (Colosimo, Hughes, Kilford, & Lees, 2003). To complicate matters further, in a series of patients with PD and dementia but no neuropathologic changes of Alzheimer's disease (AD) (e.g., plaques and tangles), the severity of dementia was related to density of Lewy neurites in the hippocampal CA2 cell field (Churchyard & Lees, 1997).

Changes in cognition and emotion accompanying PD (and many of its motor signs) can also be understood by considering the pathophysiology of basal ganglionic-thalamo-cortical circuits. Although the traditional model of five frontal-basal ganglionic-thalamic-frontal circuits (Alexander, DeLong, & Strick, 1986; Mega & Cummings, 1994) needs updating in light of recent anatomical findings (Middleton & Strick, 2000; Saint-Cyr, 2003), it is still a simple heuristic for understanding in broad brushstrokes some of the cognitive and behavioral changes in PD. According to this model, the frontal cortex and basal ganglia are linked by five loops (circuits) that, although anatomically and functionally segregated, retain their relative position and proximity to each other in shared anatomic structures, and utilize the same neurotransmitters at each point. The circuits, while closed, have open elements that allow communication with other cortical regions implicated in functions similar to those of a given circuit (Joel, 2001). The five circuits are named for their origin: the dorsolateral, orbitofrontal, anterior cingulate, motor, and oculomotor circuits. The first three circuits are particularly important in the regulation of cognition, affect, and motivation, respectively. The five circuits (actually better conceptualized as categories of loops) have both direct and indirect pathways linking the striatum with the substantia nigra and internal globus pallidus, with the indirect pathway involving the external globus pallidus and subthalamic nucleus (see Figure 10.1).

In PD, in the indirect pathway, the subthalamic nucleus is overactive and thus excessively activates the internal globus pallidus. The internal globus pallidus' overactivity is amplified by the direct pathway's diminished inhibition of the internal globus pallidus. A consequence of the overactivity of the internal globus pallidus is an excessive braking of the thalamus, and the subsequent dampening of the thalamus' excitatory influence on the frontal cortical

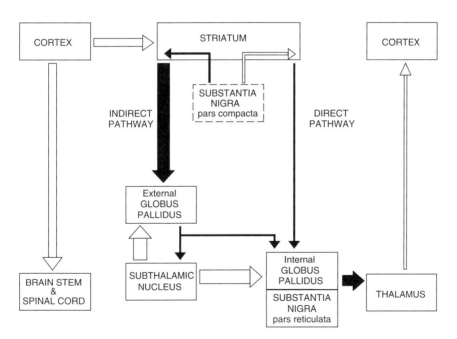

Figure 10.1   Frontostriatal circuit dysfunction in Parkinson's disease. Solid arrows: inhibitory influence; open arrows: excitatory influence; narrow arrows: underactive relative to normal; medium arrows: relatively unaffected in PD; broad arrows: overactive relative to normal.

regions. It is not possible to map a specific neurobehavioral change in PD to dysfunction in a single circuit. Instead, changes in these and other neural circuits probably interact to produce complex behavioral syndromes.

Neurobehavioral features of Parkinson's disease

Idiopathic PD is not synonymous with parkinsonism. The former is a specific disease, while the latter is a syndrome with four cardinal motor signs: tremor, rigidity, bradykinesia, and postural abnormalities. Parkinsonism is not only seen in PD, but can be produced by a host of infectious, toxic, metabolic, neurodegenerative, neurovascular, pharmacologic, psychogenic, and hereditary conditions (Tröster, Fields, & Koller, 2000). Because PD is thought to have a lengthy prodromal phase (Koller & Montgomery, 1997), early diagnosis can be challenging. Consequently, frequent use is made of various probabilistic diagnostic schemes (Gelb, Oliver, & Gilman, 1999). Autopsy reveals the accuracy of the clinical diagnosis of idiopathic PD to be about 76%. Although use of stricter clinical diagnostic criteria (including, for example, asymmetric symptom onset, and absence of other parkinsonism-producing conditions) increases true positives, there is an accompanying sizable increase in false negatives (Hughes, Ben-Shlomo, Daniel, & Lees, 2001). Table 10.2 provides probabilistic criteria for the diagnosis of Parkinson's disease.

Parkinson's disease is no longer considered exclusively a movement disorder. Lieberman's (1998) review revealed that about 19% (17–53% across various studies) of treated and untreated PD patients without dementia demonstrate cognitive dysfunction. Neurobehavioral changes in PD, when present early in the disease course, can be thought of as reflecting a pre/frontal-subcortical syndrome characterized by slowness of thought, inefficient learning and recall, diminished working memory, mild executive dysfunction, and mood disturbance (Bondi & Tröster, 1997; Pillon et al., 2001). Careful neuropsychological testing, often using experimental paradigms, reveals other subtle cognitive alterations that, while of academic interest, may lack clinical significance. In addition, whether such other subtle changes (for example, visuospatial dysfunction and reduced syntactic comprehension) are primary or secondary to executive dysfunction remains a matter of debate. Though deficits are most apparent on tasks requiring spontaneous development and deployment of efficient information processing strategies (Taylor & Saint-Cyr, 1995), and such difficulty can account for many early test performance decrements (Bondi, Kaszniak, Bayles, & Vance, 1993), executive deficits cannot account for the full range of cognitive deficits described in PD (Tröster & Fields, 1995). Hallmarks of cortical dysfunction (e.g., apraxia, amnesia, aphasia, and agnosia) are absent, and if present prior to or within the first year of onset of motor (extrapyramidal) signs, raise the index of suspicion of another condition (e.g., AD, DLB, vascular dementia, or major depression).

Dementia prevalence rates vary widely (8–93%), depending upon diagnostic criteria, sampling, and case ascertainment methods used. The most

Table 10.2 Probabilistic criteria for the diagnosis of Parkinson's disease

Clinically possible
1. Presence of two of the following, of which at least one is tremor or bradykinesia:
   resting tremor
   rigidity
   bradykinesia
   asymmetric onset

2. Absence of the following in the first 3 years (or absence to date if symptoms present less than 3 years):
   freezing
   postural instability
   hallucinations not related to medications

3. Dementia cannot precede onset of motor symptoms or occur within 1 year of motor symptom onset.

4. Absence of:
   supranuclear gaze palsy
   severe dysautonomia unrelated to medications
   another condition known to produce parkinsonism

5. Notable, sustained response to levodopa or dopamine agonist, or inadequate trial of such.

Clinically probable
1. At least three of the following:
   resting tremor
   rigidity
   bradykinesia
   asymmetric onset

2. Absence of the following in the first 3 years (thus, symptoms must have been present at least 3 years):
   freezing
   postural instability
   hallucinations not related to medications

3. Dementia cannot precede onset of motor symptoms or occur within 1 year of motor symptom onset.

4. Absence of:
   supranuclear gaze palsy
   severe dysautonomia unrelated to medications
   another condition known to produce parkinsonism

5. Notable, sustained response to levodopa or dopamine agonist.

Clinically definite
All criteria for "possible" Parkinson's disease are met
AND
Histopathologic confirmation of Parkinson's disease at autopsy by all of the following: substantial cell loss and gliosis in the substantia nigra; presence of at least one Lewy body in the substantia nigra or locus caeruleus; no pathologic evidence of another parkinsonism-producing condition.

commonly accepted prevalence rates are 20–40% (Mohr, Mendis, & Grimes, 1995). Because dementia increases risk of mortality, incidence may be a more accurate gauge of dementia frequency in PD. Unfortunately few studies have been published, but it is estimated that dementia incidence is about 3% for persons with PD younger than 60 years and 15% or less for persons with PD older than 80 years (Biggins et al,. 1992; Marder, Tang, Cote, Stern, & Mayeux, 1995; Mayeux et al., 1990). The dementia in PD is probably more accurately referred to as "the dementias" of PD, because the underlying neuropathology (and neuropsychological profile) is heterogeneous. Nonetheless, omnibus between-group comparisons reveal an average profile resembling that of a "subcortical" dementia.

Attention

Performance on simple attention tasks, such as digit span (which requires repetition of increasingly long number strings in forward or backward order) and spatial span (requiring the tapping in given order of increasingly long series of blocks in different spatial arrangements), is preserved in PD (Huber, Shuttleworth, Paulson, Bellchambers et al., 1986; Pillon et al., 1986; Sullivan & Sagar, 1989). As similar tasks increase demands on the manipulation of information within working memory, performance becomes impaired. For example, even newly diagnosed patients with PD are impaired on the Digit Ordering Task during which examinees are read a randomly ordered string of seven digits and then are asked to repeat the digits in ascending order (Stebbins, Gabrieli, Masciari, Monti, & Goetz, 1999). Similarly, on tasks requiring divided or selective attention (or the self-allocation of attention), patients with PD are likely to demonstrate difficulty, though impairments may be task dependent (cf. Gauntlett-Gilbert, Roberts, & Brown, 1999; Lee, Wild, Hollnagel, & Grafman, 1999). Both limited attentional resources and/or attentional set shifting may contribute to parkinsonians' poor performance on Stroop-like tasks that require naming of the color of the ink in which a word (the name of an incongruent color) is printed, thus necessitating selective attention and inhibition of the prepotent verbal response (Dujardin, Degreef, Rogelet, Defebvre, & Destee, 1999; Woodward, Bub, & Hunter, 2002). As the disease progresses, patients may demonstrate impairments even on attention tasks that provide external cues (Yamada, Izyuuinn, Schulzer, & Hirayama, 1990).

Executive functions

Executive functions comprise a variety of cognitive operations (including planning, abstraction, conceptualization, flexibility of thought, insight, judgment, self-monitoring, and regulation) that are critical to the realization of goals. Though the term has likely become too broad to be conceptually meaningful, it probably remains a useful phrase that captures the "managerial" or "higher order" essence of the processes (*vis-à-vis* more basic functions such as arousal and attention) subsumed by the term. The assessment of these functions in PD is of particular importance given (1) the relationship between executive function and the capacity to consent to medical treatment (Dymek, Atchison, Harrell, & Marson, 2001), (2) the ability to engage in instrumental activities of daily living (IADL), meaning those activities allowing independence within the community (Cahn, Sullivan, Shear, Pfefferbaum et al., 1998), and (3) their role in efficiently and correctly completing domestic tasks such as preparing a meal (Bedard, Paquet, Chouinard, & Blanchet, 2001). Furthermore, poor performance on various tests of executive (or "frontal lobe") function may be an early indicator of subsequent dementia in PD (Jacobs et al., 1995; Mahieux et al., 1998; Piccirilli, D'Alessandro, Finali, Piccinin, & Agostini, 1989; Woods & Tröster, 2003). An issue of particular importance to neuropsychological evaluation is whether potential diminution of awareness of deficits is likely to compromise the validity of information obtained on interview and self-report measures. While advancing disease and cognitive impairment in PD might bring with it metacognitive compromise (meaning reduced awareness of deficits and functioning) (Seltzer, Vasterling, Mathias, & Brennan, 2001; Starkstein et al., 1996), research indicates that in patients with PD, when considered as a group, there is no significant compromise in metacognition (Seltzer et al., 2001). Furthermore, the work of Brown, MacCarthy, Jahanshahi, and Marsden (1989) shows that persons with PD and mild cognitive impairment, even when depressed, are able to adequately and accurately complete self-report measures of various disabilities.

Planning is frequently assessed using the Tower of London task or one of its variants (e.g., Tower of Toronto, Tower of Hanoi). Although some studies reveal PD patients to show normal accuracy (number of moves) but a slowness in solving the Tower problems (Morris et al., 1988), other studies reveal also diminished accuracy in planning (Owen et al., 1995; Saint-Cyr, Taylor, & Lang, 1988) and greater stimulus-bound responses, especially among demented patients with PD (Culbertson, Moberg, Duda, Stern, & Weintraub, 2004).

Card sorting tests such as the Wisconsin Card Sorting Test (WCST; Grant & Berg, 1948; Heaton, Chelune, Talley, Kay, & Curtiss, 1993) or the California Card Sorting Test, which is now a part of the Delis-Kaplan Executive Function System (D-KEFS; Delis, Kaplan, & Kramer, 2001) are used to evaluate, among other functions, the ability to conceptualize or form, maintain, and switch set. The D-KEFS Sorting test is similar, but differs from the well-known WCST in that the examinee is not provided feedback about the correctness of the sort, and the examinee has to sort six cards into two decks of three, so that the two decks of cards differ according to an unambiguous semantic or visuoperceptual characteristic. Studies using card sorting tasks, with few exceptions, have shown patients with PD to have difficulty with one or more of set formation, set maintenance, and set shifting. The California Card Sorting task may be more sensitive to deficits in PD than the

WCST (Beatty & Monson, 1990b), but deficits may be apparent in only those PD patients with declining mental status (Beatty & Monson, 1990b; Dimitrov, Grafman, Soares, & Clark, 1999). The number of categories or sorts completed on the WCST, a measure of concept formation, is often reduced even in early PD when overall level of cognitive function is preserved (Bondi et al., 1993; Pillon, Dubois, Ploska, & Agid, 1991). Patients with PD may also: (a) be slow to conceptualize, as evidenced by an increased number of sorting trials required to complete the first series of 10 consecutive correct sorts (Bowen, Kamienny, Burns, & Yahr, 1975; Taylor et al., 1986); (b) have difficulty shifting set, as witnessed by an elevated number of perseverative errors (continuing to sort to the same incorrect principle despite feedback) (Cooper et al., 1991; Levin et al., 1989); and (c) lose attention or set, especially later in the disease, as indicated by an elevated number of nonperseverative errors or failures to maintain set (Bowen et al., 1975, Taylor et al., 1986).

Because impairment in cognitive set shifting may be a critical determinant of whether patients with PD demonstrate difficulty on various executive function tasks (Cronin-Golomb, Corkin, & Growdon, 1994), the nature of the attentional and cognitive set shifting difficulties in PD has been investigated in more detail by several authors. This research suggests that an interesting disassociation may exist between extradimensional and intradimensional set shifting (Robbins, Owen, & Sahakian, 1998). Extradimensional shifting requires the patient to respond to a new, previously irrelevant stimulus dimension (e.g., to switch from responding to the color of a stimulus to responding to its shape). In contrast, an intradimensional set shift occurs when the patient switches from responding to one characteristic of a stimulus dimension to another characteristic of the same dimension (e.g., when continuing to respond to the dimension "color," but switching from responding to "blue" stimuli to responding to "yellow" stimuli). Studies have generally found that patients with PD have difficulty with extradimensional set shifting in the presence of spared intradimensional set shifting, even in early disease stages and before pharmacotherapy has been initiated (Downes et al., 1989; Owen et al., 1992). It has been speculated that failure to make extradimensional shifts in PD is less related to a perseverative tendency (continued responding to the previously correct dimension) than to the phenomenon of enhanced learned irrelevance (i.e., slow conditioning to a stimulus dimension that was previously incorrect, irrelevant, or unrewarded). While this explanation has been supported by some research (Owen et al., 1993), it has not been supported by other studies (Gauntlett-Gilbert et al., 1999; van Spaendonck, Berger, Horstink, Borm, & Cools, 1995).

An experimental task that has been used to investigate decision making, judgment, and impulsivity is the gambling task developed by Bechara, Damasio, Damasio, and Anderson (1994). In general, the concept underlying the task is straightforward. Patients are instructed to maximize their gambling winnings by choosing cards (indicating winnings and/or losses) from different card decks. The card decks have either a high payoff (but involve high risk), or low payoff at low risk (much like the stock market). In the long run, the low payoff, low risk decks are advantageous, resulting in net winnings, while the high payoff, high risk decks are designed to yield net losses. Patients with ventromedial frontal lobe damage (Bechara et al., 1994) accumulate heavy losses on the task, while healthy persons typically learn over time which decks (i.e., strategies) are advantageous and preferentially draw cards from those decks. Stout, Rodawalt, and Siemers (2001) examined performance on the gambling task in groups with either Huntington's disease (HD) or PD. While the group with HD was impaired relative to its younger control group, the PD group performed comparably to its elderly control group. In contrast, Czernecki et al. (2002) found that patients' performance on the gambling task did not improve across trials, and this deficit was apparent regardless of medication state. However, another recent study suggests that the observation of deficits on the gambling task may depend on medication state, with deficits perhaps observable in the "on," but not the "off" state (Cools, Barker, Sahakian, & Robbins, 2003). Such a finding would not be particularly surprising given the phenomenon of pathological gambling that has been associated with dopaminergic therapy in PD (Gschwandtner, Aston, Renaud, & Fuhr, 2001; Molina et al., 2000) and the possible alleviation of this aberrant behavior with dopaminergic antagonists such as risperidone (Seedat, Kesler, Niehaus, & Stein, 2000). These conflicting preliminary findings remain to be reconciled and substantial research might be involved in decomposing the motivational, affective, cognitive, and response processes underlying potential deficits on this complex task.

Theory-of-mind is a term that to some extent relates to the social psychological process of attribution. More specifically, it refers to the ability to recognize and understand the mental state of others and to utilize this inference or attribution to predict their actions. Several studies have shown persons with frontal lobe damage to be impaired on theory-of-mind tasks (Rowe, Bullock, Polkey, & Morris, 2001; Stuss, Gallup, & Alexander, 2001). While one study has found HD, a frontal-basal ganglionic dementia, to leave theory-of-mind task performance uncompromised (Snowden et al., 2003), one study with a very small number of subjects provides tentative indication that patients with PD, even in the absence of dementia, may show impairments on some theory-of-mind tasks (Saltzman, Strauss, Hunter, & Archibald, 2000). Another feature of possibly impaired social cognition in PD is a diminution in the generation of counterfactuals and impaired ability to make inferences based on counterfactuals, that is, mental representations of possible alternatives to events as they have actually unfolded. Thus, patients with PD are less likely to consider "what if I had done X instead of Y when Z occurred," and are likely to differ from normal controls in identifying which of several actors in a given scenario would be more likely to engage in counterfactual thinking (McNamara, Durso, Brown, & Lynch, 2003).

Their consistency notwithstanding, findings of various executive function deficits in PD still need elaboration in terms of underlying cognitive and biological mechanisms. Observations of executive dysfunction in PD are, however, increasingly being accompanied by functional neuroimaging data that permit a clearer understanding of these deficits' neural correlates. Functional neuroimaging (positron emission tomography or PET) studies have shown reduced blood flow in the globus pallidus (Owen et al., 1998) and the caudate and dorsolateral frontal cortex of PD patients compared to controls in response to activation with the Tower of London planning task (Dagher, Owen, Boecker, & Brooks, 2001). There is a possibility that patients with PD compensate for poor working memory while carrying out the Tower of London task by relying to a greater extent on declarative memory, given enhanced hippocampal activation (Dagher et al., 2001), though the latter finding might also be interpreted as indicative of neural rather than cognitive plasticity. That is, the hippocampus may be recruited to a greater extent in PD than in normal elderly when engaging in similar working memory (rather than different declarative memory) processes. Of much interest is the recent report that performance on the Tower of London task is improved by levodopa administration in PD, and that this improvement is accompanied by normalization of dorsolateral frontal cortex blood flow relative to healthy elderly. Furthermore, levodopa-induced decreases in dorsolateral frontal cortex activation occurred during the planning task, suggesting that levodopa might ameliorate certain executive deficits by inducing dorsolateral prefrontal blood flow changes in response to tasks (Cools et al., 2002). While these neuroimaging findings are intriguing and consonant with known brain–behavior relationships, their reliability remains to be evaluated given that they are based on studies with very few subjects. It must also be conceded that there is variability in regional activations and deactivations reported in different studies (sometimes by the same research groups despite using similar activation and control tasks), and these apparent inconsistencies remain to be explicitly reconciled.

Language

Motor speech abnormalities such as dysarthria and hypophonia are frequently observed in advanced PD (Cummings, Darkins, Mendez, Hill, & Benson, 1988), and these may underlie rarely reported sentence repetition impairments (Matison, Mayeux, Rosen, & Fahn, 1982). Though certain aspects of language are compromised in parkinsonians with dementia, these patients rarely have a frank aphasia (Levin & Katzen, 1995). Whether these language changes are a consequence of pathology related to PD, DLB, or coexisting AD pathology is unknown. Careful investigation also reveals subtle alterations in performance on language tasks in parkinsonians without dementia, but these changes are often attributed to diminished attention, working memory, or inefficient information processing strategy development and deployment.

One language task on which patients with PD may have difficulty is verbal fluency using letter or category constraints. These tasks require the patient to orally generate within a time limit as many words as possible that either begin with a given letter of the alphabet, or belong to a semantic category. Not surprisingly, patients with dementia perform more poorly on these tasks than do parkinsonians without dementia (Azuma et al., 1997; Cummings et al., 1988; Tröster et al., 1998; Troyer, Moscovitch, Winocur, Leach, & Freedman, 1998), and indeed patients without dementia may demonstrate intact performance (Cohen, Bouchard, Scherzer, & Whitaker, 1994; Lewis, Lapointe, & Murdoch, 1998). Interestingly, in PD without dementia, there is a tendency for poorer performance on letter than category fluency (Azuma et al., 1997; Bayles, Trosset, Tomoeda, Montgomery, & Wilson, 1993; Hanley, Dewick, Davies, Playfer, & Turnbull, 1990). While a similar discrepancy has been observed in PD with dementia, it is unclear whether this difference between letter and category fluency performance is specific to PD (Suhr & Jones, 1998). It is also unclear whether the difference reflects the specific lexical or semantic categories chosen for the task (Azuma et al., 1997) or the greater demand placed by letter than category fluency tasks on systematic word search and retrieval strategies (Auriacombe et al., 1993; Nelson & McEvoy, 1979). Research suggests that diminished verbal fluency is related to retrieval deficits in PD (Randolph, Braun, Goldberg, & Chase, 1993).

Two verbal fluency tasks that may be especially sensitive to cognitive alterations in PD are alternating word fluency and verb fluency tasks. Alternating fluency requires persons to retrieve consecutive words from alternate semantic or letter categories. On such tasks, which make greater demands on attentional and executive resources, patients with PD are fairly consistently impaired, and sometimes more so than on nonalternating tasks (Gotham, Brown, & Marsden, 1988; Zec et al., 1999). Although verbal fluency tasks are mediated by multiple brain regions, the retrieval of verbs may depend more on frontal than temporal lobe integrity, while the retrieval of nouns may depend more critically on the temporal than the frontal lobes (Damasio & Tranel, 1993). Using this reasoning, Piatt, Fields, Paolo, and Tröster (1999) hypothesized that a fluency task demanding retrieval of verbs (in this case actions) would be more sensitive to PD than would letter or category fluency. Consistent with this hypothesis, these authors found that while patients with PD without significant cognitive impairment were not impaired on letter, semantic category, or verb fluency tasks, patients with PD and dementia were disproportionately impaired on the verb fluency task.

Visual confrontation naming tasks, requiring naming of pictured or actual objects, typically reveal no impairment in PD without dementia (Freedman, Rivoira, Butters, Sax, & Feldman, 1984; Levin et al., 1989; Lewis et al., 1998), though some studies have found subtle naming impairments even in early PD (Globus, Mildworf, & Melamed, 1985; Matison et al., 1982). Patients with PD with more notable cognitive impairment, on the other hand, do show impairments in naming (Beatty & Monson, 1989b; Lewis et al., 1998), though the naming impairment is less severe in PD than in AD when overall severity of dementia is comparable (Cummings et al., 1988; Frank, McDade, & Scott, 1996; Tröster, Fields, Paolo, Pahwa, & Koller, 1996) and may emerge later in PD dementia than AD (Stern et al., 1998).

A growing body of literature points to relatively subtle impairments in syntactic comprehension and production in PD. Illes (1989) and Lieberman, Friedman, & Feldman (1990) found the spontaneous speech output of mild PD patients to be syntactically simplified, and Murray (2000) observed that patients with PD produced a smaller proportion of grammatical sentences. A sizable subgroup of patients with PD without dementia (45–65%) (Grossman et al., 2002) demonstrated difficulty comprehending the noncanonical, object-centered clause-containing sentences. The cognitive mechanisms underlying sentence comprehension deficits in PD remain controversial. Some have attributed this to grammatical processing deficits (Cohen et al., 1994; Ullman et al., 1997); others to slowed information processing speed (Grossman et al., 2002), diminished attention (Lee, Grossman, Morris, Stern, & Hurtig, 2003), or compromised working memory (Grossman, Carvell, Stern, Gollomp, & Hurtig, 1992); though others have not confirmed a relationship between working memory and sentence comprehension deficits (Skeel et al., 2001). Grossman et al. (2003) have published preliminary functional neuroimaging data that implicates attentional and information processing resource limitations in PD sentence comprehension deficits. Specifically, left anteromedial prefrontal, striatal, and right posterior-lateral temporal cortical activations were reduced during sentence processing in patients with PD compared to healthy persons. Striatal and anteromedial activations have previously been associated with information processing speed and attention, respectively. Though the study generally failed to find convincing differences in fMRI activation in PD as a function of sentence complexity, it was observed that patients with good comprehension, in comparison to those with poorer comprehension, appeared to have compensatory upregulation of activation in left posterior-lateral temporal cortex and inferior frontal cortex bilaterally. While the temporal cortical activation is putatively linked to linguistic processing, the inferior frontal activation may reflect compensatory working memory network recruitment.

A few studies suggest that there may be mild phonetic impairment in early PD. Grossman et al. (1992) and Lee et al. (2003) observed that patients had difficulty detecting phonetic errors in words, regardless of the clausal structure of sentences. Two PD patients' errors in the temporal organization and coordination of American Sign Language have also been interpreted as reflecting a phonetic deficit (Brentari, Poizner, & Kegl, 1995).

Pragmatics (or the study of discourse within social context) has rarely been studied in PD. One recent study (McNamara & Durso, 2003) reported that patients with PD, in comparison to healthy elderly, were rated as having impairments in conversational appropriateness, turn taking, prosody, and proxemics (i.e., perception and use of personal space). Though the pragmatics rating score was related to performance on tests of "frontal lobe function" such as the Stroop and Tower of London tasks, it remains to be determined to what extent motor impairments, speech impairments, and motivational and emotional factors such as apathy and depression might contribute to diminished pragmatic communication skills. Whether patients with PD generally develop pragmatic compensatory strategies, as have been observed among three patients with PD (who cannot hear or speak) using sign language (Kegl & Poizner, 1998), also remains to be investigated.

Visuoperceptual and spatial functions

The existence and nature of visuoperceptual and spatial deficits in PD remains debated. Although some have argued that visuospatial deficits are among the earliest and most readily observable neurobehavioral deficits in PD (Passafiume, Boller, & Keefe, 1986), others suggest that such deficits are not primary visuoperceptual deficits, but rather, might be secondary to increased saccadic eye movements (Bodis-Wollner, 2003), motor impairments, or limitations in information processing resources and their strategic allocation (Brown & Marsden, 1986). Thus, the observation that patients with PD might perform poorly in following a route, assembling blocks to match a pattern, and drawing, tracing, or copying complex figures (Bowen, Hoehn, & Yahr, 1972; Pirozzolo et al., 1982; Stern, Mayeux, & Rosen, 1984) may relate to motor demands of the tasks. However, impairments on visuoperceptual and spatial tasks are also observed when motor demands of tasks are minimized (Boller et al., 1984; Lee, Harris, & Calvert, 1998; Levin et al., 1991). Still other investigators have failed to find visuoperceptual or spatial impairments in their samples of patients with PD (Brown & Marsden, 1986; Taylor, Saint-Cyr, & Lang, 1987), or have observed impairments on one set of tasks but not another (Ransmayr et al., 1987).

One task that minimizes motor demands and on which patients with PD may demonstrate particular difficulty is a facial matching task (Levin et al., 1989). Facial identification relies on perceptual processing of both individual features and feature configurations. Cousins, Hanley, Davies, Turnbull, and Playfer (2000) administered a facial recognition (memory) task to non-demented persons with PD, along with tests of configural (a variant of Mooney's Faces Closure Test) and componential (the 15-objects test) visuoperceptual processing (and there is no reason to expect that one process is more demanding of information processing resources than the other). Patients with PD were impaired in facial recognition, configural processing, but not componential processing. Importantly, the facial recognition impairment was significantly associated with deficient configural processing, even after controlling for intelligence, age, and depressive symptoms, and the impairment was evident even in some recently diagnosed patients. Thus, impairments in basic visuoperceptual processes occur at least in a subset of patients, and these impairments are observable independent of motor impairments or limitations in information processing resources. Parkinsonians are also impaired in the perception and production of emotional expressions (Blonder, Gur, & Gur, 1989; Borod et al., 1990; Scott, Caird, & Williams, 1984). Most recently, a reduction in recognition of "angry" faces, but not other emotions, was observed during bilateral deep brain stimulation of the subthalamic nucleus in 10 patients with PD (Schroeder et al., 2004). Although such impairments are not limited to facial expressions of emotion, more basic visuoperceptual impairments in analyzing facial features probably contribute significantly to parkinsonians' difficulty in identifying facial emotional expressions (Beatty, Goodkin et al., 1989).

Memory and learning

Numerous taxonomies of memory exist, but one of the most common distinguishes between declarative and nondeclarative memory. Declarative memory refers to facts and data acquired via learning processes that are accessible to conscious recollection. Nondeclarative memory, in contrast, refers to "knowing how" and is expressed only via the performance of task operations. Thus, the content of nondeclarative memory is not available to conscious recollection.

Declarative memory impairments are circumscribed in PD without dementia. Although this is not an invariant finding, the learning of new information may be slowed in PD (Faglioni, Saetti, & Botti, 2000), and while free recall is impaired, recognition is relatively preserved (Beatty, Staton, Weir, Monson, & Whitaker, 1989). The mild recall impairment in PD without dementia is evident on a variety of tasks: word lists (Buytenhuijs et al., 1994; Sommer, Grafman, Clark, & Hallett, 1999; Taylor et al., 1986), prose passages (Taylor et al., 1986; Tröster, Stalp, Paolo, Fields, & Koller, 1995), paired associates (Huber, Shuttleworth, & Paulson, 1986), complex figure reproduction (Bowen, Burns, & Yahr, 1976; Stefanova, Kostic, Ziropadja, Ocic, & Markovic, 2001), spatial locations on maps (Beatty, Staton et al., 1989), and abstract designs (Sullivan & Sagar, 1989). As patients develop more global cognitive impairments or dementia, both recall and recognition are compromised (Beatty, Staton et al., 1989), and impairments particularly in delayed recall become evident with longer disease duration (Zakzanis & Freedman, 1999). Memory impairment in PD is also significantly exacerbated by depression (Fields, Norman, Straits-Tröster, & Tröster, 1998; Kuzis, Sabe, Tiberti, Leiguarda, & Starkstein, 1997; Norma, Tröster, Fields, & Brooks, 2002; Tröster, Paolo et al., 1995; Tröster, Stalp et al., 1995), though depression may have to reach a certain severity threshold before it compromises memory (Boller, Marcie, Starkstein, & Traykov, 1998).

Several studies have been carried out to elucidate the mechanisms underlying the verbal memory impairment in PD. Although the mechanisms may be quite heterogeneous across patients (Filoteo, Rilling et al., 1997), the relative preservation of recognition *vis-à-vis* free recall has often been interpreted to mean that patients with PD have retrieval deficits. Recognition impairments, though typically mild, can, however, be observed in PD without dementia (Whittington, Podd, & Kan, 2000), and it is clear that even patients without dementia may also have encoding difficulties. Not only is semantic clustering reduced in PD (Buytenhuijs et al., 1994), but the rate with which this strategy evolves across the five learning trials is slow in comparison to healthy elderly (Berger et al., 1999; Buytenhuijs et al., 1994). In contrast, serial encoding, indexed by the extent to which a patient recalls the words in the same order in which they were presented, appears to be preserved (Berger et al., 1999; Buytenhuijs et al., 1994). Similarly, serial position effects, that is, the tendency to recall more words from the beginning (primacy) and the end (recency) than from the middle of a list, are comparable in early PD and healthy elderly (Stefanova et al., 2001). One explanation for these findings is that serial encoding reflects the use of an externally imposed strategy, whereas semantic encoding relies to a greater extent on the spontaneous self-initiated deployment of an efficient learning strategy, something patients with PD find difficult (Taylor & Saint-Cyr, 1995). It is likely that as more widespread and severe cognitive impairment develops, a multiplicity of memory mechanisms becomes affected. For example, in patients with PD and more severe cognitive impairment, rates of forgetting are accelerated (Beatty, Staton et al., 1989), suggesting that storage mechanisms also become disrupted.

Deficits in prospective memory may also be evident in PD. First described by Loftus (1971), prospective memory refers to one's memory for future intentions or, in other words, "remembering to remember." A form of episodic (i.e., declarative) memory, prospective memory describes the complex process of forming, monitoring, and executing a future intention *vis-à-vis* ongoing distractions; for example, remembering to take one's medications at a particular time during the day. Prospective memory is singly (but not doubly) dissociable from retrospective memory whereby a deficit in the latter function will result in failures in the former (Burgess & Shallice, 1997). A growing convergence of evidence from the cognitive neuropsychology and neuroimaging literatures indicates that prospective memory is intimately linked to the integrity of prefrontal-striatal circuits (Burgess, Quayle, & Frith, 2001) and is thereby of relevance to the neuropsychology of PD. The prospective memory impairment in PD has been found not to be attributable to forgetting task instructions, but rather to difficulty retrieving and executing the intention in response to a cue (Katai, Maruyama, Hashimoto, & Ikeda, 2003). Moreover, research in brain injured populations indicates that consideration of prospective memory may enhance the prediction of—and interventions related to enhancing—IADLs (van den Broek, Downes, Johnson, Dayus, & Hilton, 2000). In contrast to the mild difficulty that patients without dementia have recalling new information and future intentions, their recollection of information from the past is typically preserved (Fama et al., 2000; Freedman et al., 1984; Huber, Shuttleworth, & Paulson, 1986; Leplow et al., 1997).

Two studies have found impairments in remote memory. Whereas Sagar, Cohen, Sullivan, Corkin, and Growdon (1988) found a mixed sample of patients with and without dementia to have difficulty dating events but to have difficulty recognizing famous scenes only from the most recent past (past decade), Venneri et al. (1997) found patients without dementia to be impaired in recalling and dating public events (but not in recognizing these events). There is consistent evidence that patients with PD and dementia have impairments in remote memory (Freedman et al., 1984; Huber, Shuttleworth, & Paulson, 1986; Leplow et al., 1997). However, unlike in AD, in which the impairment is often characterized by a temporal gradient (revealing of more dramatic impairment of recent than remote information), the impairment in PD is equally severe for information across past decades. Although spatial (geographical) remote memory (assessed by patients' ability to locate cities on maps of the USA and various states) was also found to be impaired, it remains to be investigated whether the loss of spatial information follows a temporal gradient (i.e., might be more pronounced for the regions in which the person has lived more recently than during adolescence and early adulthood) (Beatty & Monson, 1989a).

Another aspect of memory that is consistently revealed to be impaired in PD is working memory. Working memory is a limited-capacity, multicomponent system that permits temporary, online manipulation and storage of information to guide and control action. In PD, impairments in working memory have been related to both reduced capacity of the system (Gabrieli, Singh, Stebbins, & Goetz, 1996) and difficulty inhibiting responses (Kensinger, Shearer, Locascio, & Growdon, 2003; Rieger, Gauggel, & Burmeister, 2003). Whether deficits in updating the content of working memory might be due to increased susceptibility to the entry of irrelevant information or resistance of existing information to deletion remains to be resolved. Regardless of the underlying difficulty, deficits in working memory can significantly impact performance on other declarative memory tasks (Higginson et al., 2003).

Several other memory tasks that are sensitive to frontal dysfunction have also been found to reveal impairments in PD, though most of these tasks are experimental and not standardized, clinical tests. Thus, patients with PD may have difficulty on tasks of conditional associative learning (Pillon et al., 1998; Postle, Locascio, Corkin, & Growdon, 1997; Taylor, Saint-Cyr, & Lang, 1990), aspects of source memory (Hsieh & Lee, 1999; Taylor et al., 1990), metamemory (Ivory, Knight, Longmore, & Caradoc-Davies, 1999), recency discrimination (Fischer, Kendler, & Goldenberg, 1990; Sullivan & Sagar, 1989), temporal ordering (Cooper, Sagar, & Sullivan, 1993; Vriezen & Moscovitch, 1990), and subject-ordered pointing (Gabrieli et al., 1996; West, Ergis, Winocur, & Saint-Cyr, 1998).

Findings with respect to nondeclarative memory in PD are inconsistent and this form of memory is rarely assessed in clinical contexts. One type of nondeclarative memory task involves priming. In these tasks a person is exposed to verbal or visuoperceptual stimuli but is not told that their memory for this material will be assessed. Instead, the examinee is later presented with a series of partial or degraded stimuli, some of which are unrelated to the stimuli the person was exposed to earlier, while others are related to the initially presented stimuli. Several studies have reported that priming is preserved in PD without dementia (Appollonio et al., 1994; Bondi & Kaszniak, 1991; Filoteo et al., 2003; Heindel, Salmon, Shults, Walicke, & Butters, 1989; Huberman, Moscovitch, & Freedman, 1994; Ivory et al., 1999; Spicer, Brown, & Gorell, 1994) and even in PD with dementia (Kuzis et al., 1999), but conflicting results are reported in the case of PD with dementia (Beatty, 1992; Heindel et al., 1989).

Procedural memory tasks are another heterogeneous class of nondeclarative memory tasks. These tasks require the acquisition of perceptual, motor, or cognitive skills through exposure to an activity that is constrained by certain rules. Tasks that fall into this category include mirror reading, a serial reaction time task, learning of an artificial grammar, and the pursuit rotor task. Classical conditioning is another form of procedural memory, and one that appears to be preserved in PD (Sommer et al., 1999). Patients with PD also perform comparably to healthy control groups in learning artificial grammar (Reber & Squire, 1999; Witt, Nuhsman, & Deuschl, 2002b), and reading of mirror-reversed words (Bondi & Kaszniak, 1991; Harrington, Haaland, Yeo, & Marder, 1990; but see Yamadori, Yoshida, Mori, & Yamashita, 1996, who found an impairment; and Koenig, Thomas-Antérion, & Laurent, 1999, and Roncacci, Troisi, Carlesimo, Nocentini, & Caltagirone, 1996, who observed that improvement occurs for repeated, but not nonrepeated words). In contrast, patients with PD are likely to show impairments on probabilistic classification tasks (Knowlton, Mangels, & Squire, 1996; Witt, Nuhsman, & Deuschl, 2002a), pursuit rotor learning (Harrington et al., 1990, but see Heindel et al., 1989), and in learning how to solve the Tower of Toronto (Saint-Cyr et al., 1988). Impairments on the serial reaction time task (Ferraro, Balota, & Connor, 1993) may be observed only among patients with executive dysfunction (Jackson, Jackson, Harrison, Henderson, & Kennard, 1995), if longer sequences are used (Pascual-Leone et al., 1993), if longer skill retention delays are imposed (Doyon et al., 1997), or only when shifts occur between predictive and nonpredictive sequences (Kaszniak, Trosset, Bondi, & Bayles, 1992). One possible interpretation of these findings is that the striatum is critical to those procedural memory tasks not involving highly predictive information or involving shifts between predictive and less predictive information. It has also been suggested that the inconsistency in findings pertaining to procedural memory may relate to the types of patients being assessed, and that impairments on some tasks may be evident in patients with the akinetic-rigid form of PD, but not in tremor-predominant patients (Vakil & Herishanu-Naaman, 1998).

Purposes of clinical neuropsychological assessment

As outlined by Tröster and Woods (2003), neuropsychological evaluation contributes to the management of the patient with PD by providing information about and assistance with: (1) the determination of a likely etiology of recent onset cognitive deterioration; (2) assessment of competence to consent to medical treatment; (3) the facilitation of financial, legal, and living situation decision making; (4) the planning and requesting of adaptive changes in the home or at work to minimize handicap; and (5) the development of strategies that minimize the impact of cognitive changes on day-to-day functioning. More recently, it has become clear that neuropsychological evaluation can be a useful adjunct in identifying the appropriateness of certain medical and surgical interventions for patients with PD (Saint-Cyr & Trépanier, 2000; Tröster & Fields, 2003b). Neuropsychological evaluation can also assist in identifying persons with psychogenic movement disorders (Koller, Marjama, & Tröster, 2002).

It bears emphasizing that although group comparisons of cognitive profiles in various dementias and movement disorders (e.g., AD, DLB, PDD, progressive supranuclear palsy) show that these conditions are associated with different (though sometimes overlapping) cognitive deficits, these studies do not typically report the diagnostic sensitivity and specificity of cognitive profiles. Consequently, it is advisable to use neuropsychological test results to formulate etiologic hypotheses and to comment on the consistency or inconsistency of a given test result profile with the various conditions (Tröster, 1998).

Various test batteries have been proposed for evaluating patients with PD. While these efforts are meritorious and well-intentioned, there is probably greater agreement about the neurobehavioral domains one should assess than about the specific tests that should be employed. The selection of tests in the clinical setting should rest on the referral question(s), patient and caregiver questions, the clinician's familiarity with the tests, the normative and psychometric properties of the tests, the patient's ability to tolerate and cooperate with the tests, and a thorough awareness of how manifestations of PD can impact evaluation (e.g., motor "on–off" fluctuations, wearing off, sleep disturbance, and fatigability, and choreiform and dystonic dyskinesias). Thus, a careful interview with the patient that inquires about his or her symptoms, their time course, and medication schedule is indispensable in planning a successful psychometric evaluation (Tröster, 1998).

Process-oriented assessment of the patient with Parkinson's disease

Cognitive screening examinations

Cognitive screening examinations can be helpful and cost effective in deciding whether a patient might benefit from a full neuropsychological evaluation and for providing a rough estimate of rate of cognitive change. Unfortunately, the shortcomings of screening instruments are probably as widely appreciated as is their efficiency. In particular, many screening instruments employ cutoff scores, and these cutoff scores often are not corrected (or are inadequately corrected) for demographic factors or base rates. With these provisos in mind, it is helpful to look at score patterns and errors on two commonly used screening instruments, the Mini Mental State Exam (MMSE; Folstein, Folstein, & McHugh, 1975) and the Dementia Rating Scale (DRS and DRS–2; Mattis, 1988, 2001).

Though the MMSE was designed for use with patients with AD, it appears to be employed with a wide range of clinical populations that may experience cognitive compromise. Because the MMSE deemphasizes assessment of working memory and executive functions, one might expect it to lack sensitivity to the early cognitive changes associated with PD. Some empirical evidence confirms this suspicion. In a study comparing MMSE in PD patients with and without mild cognitive impairment (defined by a separate neuropsychological test battery), the average score of the mildly impaired group was only 1.5 points lower than that of the cognitively intact group, and in the normal range (mean 28.0, standard deviation 2.1) (Janvin, Aarsland, Larsen, & Hugdahl, 2003). However, the MMSE probably has adequate sensitivity and specificity in detecting cognitive impairment among unequivocally demented patients with PD. Using the DSM-IV criteria for dementia as the "gold standard," one study of 126 patients with PD reported the MMSE cutoff of 23/24 to have a sensitivity of 98% and a specificity of 77%, although the mean MMSE scores of the PD groups with and without dementia per DSM-IV did not differ significantly (Hobson & Meara, 1999).

A recent study compared the qualitative MMSE performance patterns of a small group of patients with PD and dementia to those of groups of patients with AD or ischemic vascular dementia (IVD) whose total MMSE scores were comparable (Jefferson et al., 2002). Although diagnostic sensitivity and specificity were not addressed by the study, it found that a greater proportion of patients with PD than IVD failed to correctly draw the intersecting pentagons, a finding consonant with the observation that patients with DLB have greater difficulty with this task than do patients with AD (Ala, Hughes, Kyrouac, Ghobrial, & Elble, 2001). In comparison to patients with AD, a greater proportion of patients with PD failed to correctly spell "world" backwards (an item the authors designate as evaluating working memory) and to draw the pentagons. On the other hand, patients with PD were more likely than patients with AD to correctly identify the day of the week.

Paolo, Tröster, Glatt, Hubble, and Koller (1995) compared DRS performance in AD and PD groups matched for overall severity of dementia (total DRS score). Whereas the AD group earned lower Memory subtest scores than the PD group, the PD group attained lower Construction subtest scores. Discriminant function analyses using Memory, Initiation/Perseveration, and Construction subtest scores correctly classified the diagnoses of about 75% of the sample. Brown et al. (1999) also have shown that the Construction and Initiation/Perseveration subtest scores are the most helpful in distinguishing PD patients from healthy controls. Though PDD and DLB may differ minimally in their DRS profiles (with perhaps lower conceptualization scores in

DLB early on), Aarsland et al. (2003) again found Memory, Construction, and Initiation/Perseveration scores to best distinguish between PDD/DLB and AD. Studies determining sensitivity and specificity of the DRS–2 in detecting dementia in PD remain to be carried out.

Given concerns about the possible lack of sensitivity of the MMSE in detecting cognitive impairment in PD (McFadden, Sampson, & Mohr, 1994), several researchers have developed brief screening tests that put greater emphasis on '"frontal" function assessment. Although the Mini-Mental Parkinson (MMP; Mahieux et al., 1995), Frontal/Subcortical Assessment Battery (FSAB; Rothlind & Brandt, 1993), and the Frontal Assessment Battery (FAB; Dubois, Slachevsky, Litvan, & Pillon, 2000) show promise as brief, valid screening instruments of cognitive function in PD, they remain to be validated in independent studies.

Intelligence tests

The only published research describing the performance of persons with PD on the WAIS–III is detailed in the *WAIS–III/WMS–III Technical Manual* (Psychological Corporation, 1997). These data should be considered highly preliminary given the small sample ($n = 10$). In that sample, the Verbal IQ was about 12 points higher than the Performance IQ, an observation consonant with the general finding that when differences between persons with PD and healthy control groups do emerge on WAIS–III predecessors, persons with PD perform more poorly on Performance but not Verbal subtests (Bondi et al., 1993; Brown & Marsden, 1988; Mohr et al., 1990; Ross et al., 1996).

Two studies have used the WAIS–R NI (Kaplan, Fein, Morris, & Delis, 1991) in an attempt to apply process analyses to WAIS–R test performance in PD. Tröster, Fields, Paolo, and Koller (1996) compared free recall and recognition performance, and examined intrasubtest scatter, on the Vocabulary and Information subtests in persons with PD without dementia and in healthy elderly. The elderly and PD groups attained similar raw and scaled scores on the WAIS–R Information and Vocabulary subtests and derived similar benefit from the provision of the WAIS–R NI recognition format *vis-à-vis* recall. A similar, negligible proportion of the PD and elderly groups had abnormal intrasubtest scatter as defined by the WAIS–R NI normative standards. It was concluded that among patients with average or above test scores, the WAIS–R NI did not reveal the retrieval deficits (evident from disproportionately better recognition than recall) ascribed to PD, a finding consistent with the test authors' proposal that standard and multiple choice test scores rarely differ in individuals with above average subtest scores. It might be noted that these findings were replicated by another study of PD patients of above average intelligence (Peavy et al., 2001), though in that study patients with PD did benefit more than a control group from the multiple choice than the standard format on the Comprehension subtest evaluating knowledge of social conventions.

Peavy et al. (2001) found that patients, relative to a normal control group, earned significantly lower scores on only the Digit Symbol subtest of the WAIS–R. Trends toward lower scores were observed for Picture Arrangement and Object Assembly. However, qualitative analyses via the WAIS–R NI indicated that patients earned lower scores on the Symbol Copy task (suggesting that reduced visuomotor speed contributes significantly to patient's poorer Digit Symbol test performance), and had extended response latencies on the Picture Arrangement, Sentence Arrangement, and Object Assembly tests. Although motor slowing may contribute to poor WAIS Performance scale subtest performance (Knight, Godfrey, & Shelton, 1988), it is unlikely to be the sole determinant. Because patients had lower spatial spans than the control group in the study by Peavy et al., it is possible that visual attention deficits contribute to poor performance on Picture Arrangement and Object Assembly. It has also been suggested that more general sequencing deficits may underlie poor Picture Arrangement performance in PD (Beatty & Monson, 1990a; Sullivan, Sagar, Gabrieli, Corkin, & Growdon, 1989). Another interesting finding of the study by Peavy et al. is that patients performed more poorly than the control group when asked to recount the story told by the Picture Arrangement sequences and, specifically, they identified fewer main point and key elements. Patients' weaker performance on the Sentence Arrangement task probably did not reflect only sequencing problems, because they tended to make more "capture errors"; linking two highly related words though such a construction would preclude a meaningful sentence (e.g., "the *hair brush* long clogged" vs. "long hair clogged the brush"). It is possible that such errors reveal the grammatical and syntactic difficulties ascribed to PD by Grossman et al. (2003).

Executive function tests

The two executive function tests probably most commonly administered to patients with PD are the Wisconsin Card Sorting Test (WCST) and one of a variety of "Tower" tests. The patterns of errors on these tests, and the cognitive mechanisms implicated, were described earlier on. It is worth noting that the Delis-Kaplan Executive Function System (D-KEFS; Delis et al., 2001) holds promise for use with PD, although validity studies remain to be carried out and published. Potential advantages of the D-KEFS over other available clinical tests of executive function are the availability of norms for a wide age range (8–89 years), a common normative base across multiple tests (enhancing direct comparability of standard scores), and, most important for a process approach to assessment, the tests include subtests that allow fractionation of component skills and elucidation of the nature of the deficit. Thus, the D-KEFS includes modified versions of clinically well-established tests such as verbal fluency, design fluency, Trailmaking, the Stroop task, and card sorting, as well as standardized versions of experimental tasks such as the Tower test, proverb interpretation, 20 questions, and a word context test.

Language

Several studies have examined the cognitive mechanisms that might underlie verbal fluency decrements in PD. One theoretical framework (Gruenewald & Lockhead, 1980) suggests that optimal performance on semantic fluency tasks relies on searching for semantic subcategories and producing semantically related groups of words from these subcategories. Extending this framework to score the qualitative aspects of lexical and semantic verbal fluency performance, Troyer, Moscovitch, and Winocur (1997) devised two indexes: switching and clustering. Switching refers to disengaging from one subcategory of words (related semantically or phonemically; that is, in meaning or sound) and moving onto another category. Clustering, in contrast, refers to the production of consecutive items from the same semantic or phonemic subcategory. Presumably, the most efficient strategy involves retrieval of highly related words within a subcategory followed by highly related items from another subcategory rather than an attempt to search for and retrieve tenuously related words from the same category. Studies generally demonstrate that switching impairments are more readily observed among patients with PD and dementia than in AD, while deficits in clustering are more pronounced in AD than PD dementia (Tröster et al., 1998; Troyer et al., 1998). Even when verbal fluency output is diminished in PD patients without dementia, clustering appears to be preserved (Heiss, Kalbe, & Kessler, 2001). These findings might be interpreted as consistent with the view that switching is heavily reliant on intact executive or frontal-subcortical functions and the observation that fluency decrements after pallidal surgery in PD are related to further declines in switching (Tröster, Woods, Fields, Hanisch, & Beatty, 2002).

Few studies have attempted to identify the error types committed by patients with PD on visual confrontation naming tests, perhaps because PD does not involve a marked compromise unless dementia is also present. Tröster, Fields, Paolo, Pahwa et al. (1996) utilized the error categorization system for the Boston Naming Test described by Hodges, Salmon, and Butters (1991) and compared the performances of a normal control (NC) group to those of AD and PDD groups equated for overall severity of cognitive impairment. Both AD and PDD groups named fewer items than the control group, but the impairment of the AD group was more severe than that of PDD. The error types also differentiated the two dementia groups. The AD group made more phonemic errors (responses that were mispronunciations or distortions of the target but shared at least one syllable with it) and "don't know" responses than the control and PDD groups, which did not differ in the number of these errors. Although both PDD and AD made more semantic errors than the control group, the PDD group's proportion of semantic errors that were predominantly of the associative type exceeded that of either the AD or NC groups. That is, the PD group had a proclivity to produce responses that had a clear association with the target, such as describing an associated action or function, a physical attribute, a contextual associate, or a subordinate or proper noun example of the target. These findings were interpreted to indicate that in PDD category knowledge is available but insufficient to generate item names, whereas in AD category knowledge is often unavailable, consistent with the notion that AD involves a degradation of the semantic networks.

Fields, Paolo, and Trösters (1996), comparing PD and PDD groups' errors on the Boston Naming Test, found that when semantic errors were made, those of the normal control group were largely within category errors. Such within-category errors are responses from the same semantic category as the target but are visually dissimilar (e.g., "spinach" for "asparagus"). In contrast, the PDD group's semantic errors were largely associative errors. The PD group did not differ significantly from either the control or the PDD groups in the proportion of semantic errors that were associative in nature. This again suggests retrieval difficulties in PDD, rather than a degradation of semantic networks *per se*.

Visuoperceptual and spatial functions

Few "process" analyses have been undertaken of parkinsonians' performance on clinical tests of visuospatial perception and construction. Patients with PD tend to demonstrate impairments on tests such as the Benton Judgment of Line Orientation, Facial Recognition tests, the Hooper Visual Organization Test, embedded figures tests, mental object rotation, tests of visual attention, and constructional tasks such as Block Design and drawing of complex figures (Levin et al., 1991), though impairments may be a function of disease duration, disease severity, sex (Crucian et al., 2003), and presence of dementia (Alegret, Pere, Junqué, Valldeoriola, & Tolosa, 2001; Levin et al., 1991). Both Alegret et al. (2001) and Finton, Lucas, Graff-Radford, and Uitti (1998) found that a group with PD made more egregious errors on the Judgment of Line Orientation (JLO) test (which requires the examinee to match pairs of lines of similar orientation) than a control group. Specifically, PD patients made more errors that involve the confusion of an oblique line with one from the same quadrant that was displaced by two or three 18° segments from the target line. In contrast, when controls made errors, they tended to involve no more than a single 18° displacement. In the study by Alegret et al., patients with PD also made more errors than controls involving mismatching of a horizontal line.

Freeman et al. (2000) recently described the errors made by patients with PD and dementia on the Rey-Osterrieth Complex Figure test. Compared to controls and AD patients, the PD patients made more placement errors, configural errors, errors of omission, perseverations, and produced more fragmented drawings that lacked more of the clusters of elements within the figure. However, recognition of the figure after a delay was much better in the PD than the AD group. The PD group differed from the IVD group only in that the IVD group accurately reproduced more of the clusters of features and made fewer perseverative errors.

In an attempt to isolate and identify the nature of visual attention deficits underlying PD patients' difficulty with a clinical visual search and cancellation task, Filoteo, Williams, Rilling, and Roberts (1997) slightly modified the administration of the Visual Search and Attention Test (VSAT; Trennerry, Crosson, deBoe, & Leber, 1990). This task usually requires examinees to scan each of four pages containing monochromatic or colored stimuli that are either letters of the alphabet or symbols (targets and distractors), and to cross out as many targets in the stimulus array as quickly as possible within a time limit. In this study, the task was modified to allow persons to complete the task without a time limit. The study's authors suggested that the tasks requiring cancellation of monochromatic targets tap selective attention because the person needs to focus on one target feature (shape). In contrast, the last two parts of the test that require cancellation of a target of a specific color require divided attention because the person has to divide their attention between stimuli's color and shape. The PD patients were slower than healthy controls only when the search involved single feature stimuli, and the numbers of omission and commission errors were comparable across the groups. Interestingly, right-hand performance on the Grooved Pegboard was not related to completion time, suggesting that motor speed is unlikely to account for the finding. Instead, losses of set on the WCST correlated significantly with completion time and commission errors. The findings in tandem suggest that PD patients may have particular difficulty on tasks demanding of selective attention and perhaps vigilance.

Memory

As noted earlier, declarative memory deficits in PD have typically been ascribed to retrieval deficits given impoverished recall but relatively, if not entirely, normal recognition. Examination of performance patterns by patients with PD on the CVLT suggest that encoding difficulties may contribute to poor free recall. Massman, Delis, Butters, Levin, and Salmon (1990) observed among 19 patients, 10 of whom were in the more advanced stages of PD, that immediate and delayed recall and recognition were impaired compared to a normal control group. In addition, patients made more intrusion errors during delayed recall, showed reduced semantic encoding (but intact serial encoding), and had poorer recall consistency. However, retention over time was normal, and the intrusion errors (production of nonlist words during recall) were mostly semantically related to the words on the list and, thus, qualitatively similar to those of the control group, a finding similar to that reported by Rouleau, Imbault, Laframboise, and Bedard (2001) for the Rey Auditory Verbal Learning Test. The learning slope, serial position effects, and number of perseverations (repeated words) were comparable in the PD and control groups.

Filoteo, Williams et al. (1997) observed that, among a group of 39 patients with PD (some with dementia and some taking anticholinergic medications that may affect memory), the CVLT profile was qualitatively and quantitatively heterogeneous. Using a discriminant function algorithm, Filoteo, Williams et al. classified 20 of the 39 patients with PD as having normal CVLT profiles, while 10 patients had a profile resembling that of HD, and 9 had AD-like CVLT profiles. Because the patients with the AD-like verbal memory test score patterns did not differ from the other groups in score on a cognitive screening examination and several other tests known to be compromised by AD, the authors concluded that it was unlikely that the AD-like pattern observed in some patients was due to coexisting early AD. Difference in memory impairment patterns may also relate to predominant motor symptoms and their severity. For example, Berger et al. (1999) noted that those persons with more severe bradykinesia tended to have encoding difficulty and rely on less efficient, externally guided, serial encoding. Given diminished encoding, it is not surprising that PD patients may benefit more from the external retrieval guidance afforded by cuing (Knoke, Taylor, & Saint-Cyr, 1998) or recognition formats (van Oostrom et al., 2003). Indeed, among patients with dementia, PD patients earn better recognition scores than do AD patients (Tierney et al., 1994).

Mood and affect

Depression occurs in about half of all patients with PD, with 50% of those having minor mood disturbance or dysthymia, and 50% have major depression (Tröster & Letsch, 2004). Assessment of depression in PD can be complicated because several symptoms of depression overlap those of PD, such as psychomotor retardation, anergia, stooped posture, amimia, sleep disturbance, dry mouth, and sexual dysfunction. It has been recommended that early morning awakening, anergia, and psychomotor slowing be excluded from consideration when diagnosing depression in PD (Starkstein, Bolduc, Mayberg, Preziosi, & Robinson, 1990). Because depression and PD symptoms overlap, there is concern that self-report and rating instruments might overdiagnose depression in PD. Several scales have been evaluated for use in PD, and scales such as the Beck Depression Inventory, Montgomery-Åsberg Depression Rating Scale, Geriatric Depression Scale, Hamilton Rating Scale for Depression, Zung Depression Rating Scale, Hospital Anxiety and Depression Scale, and the Neuropsychiatric Inventory have successfully been used in PD. Indeed, for several scales specific cutoff scores have been proposed to screen for and diagnose depression in PD (see Table 10.3).

Similar symptom overlap considerations apply to the assessment of anxiety in PD, though rating instruments' validity and reliability have not been widely studied. Higginson, Fields, Koller, and Tröster (2001) observed that the Beck Anxiety Inventory and Profile of Mood States both yielded scores associated with clinical levels of anxiety in PD more frequently than did interview. However, elimination of items loading on autonomic and neurophysiologic factors of anxiety was not advised as it was believed that this adjustment would lead to serious underestimation of anxiety in PD. Other symptom inventories

Table 10.3 Self-report and rating scales with empirically modified cutoff scores to detect depression in Parkinson's disease

Scale (reference)	Number of items; maximum score; traditional cutoff (*)	PD cutoffs recommended by:	Recommended cutoff to distinguish depressed PD vs. non-depressed PD (sensitivity/specificity)	Recommended screening cutoff for PD (sensitivity/specificity)	Recommended diagnostic cutoff for PD (sensitivity/specificity)
Beck Depression Inventory (Beck, Ward, Mendelson, Mock, & Erbaugh, 1961)	21 items; maximum = 63; 10 = mild; 12 = moderate; 30 = severe	Leentjens, Verhey, Luijckx, & Troost (2000)	13/14 (0.67/0.88)	8/9 (0.92/0.59)	16/17 (0.42/0.98)
Hamilton Rating Scale for Depression (17-item) (Hamilton, 1960)	17 items; maximum = 50; 8 = mild; 14 = moderate; 19 = severe; 23 = very severe	Leentjens, Verhey, Lousberg, Spitsbergen, & Wilmink (2000) Naarding, Leentjens, van Kooten, & Verhey (2002)	13/14 (0.88/0.89) 12/13 (0.80/0.92)	11/12 (0.94/0.75) 9/10 (0.95/0.98)	16/17 (0.75/0.98) 15/16 (0.99/0.93)
Montgomery-Åsberg Depression Rating Scale (Montgomery & Åsberg, 1979)	10 items; maximum = 60; 15 = mild; 25 = moderate; 31 = severe; 44 = very severe	Leentjens, Verhey, Lousberg et al. (2000)	14/15 (0.88/0.89)	14/15 (0.88/0.89)	17/18 (0.63/0.94)

Traditional cutoffs from test manuals or per task force for the *Handbook of Psychiatric Measures* (American Psychiatric Association, 2000).

that have been used to assess various aspects of anxiety in PD include the State–Trait Anxiety Inventory and the Yale-Brown Obsessive Compulsive Scale.

Comments on differentiating Lewy body, Parkinson's, and Alzheimer's dementias

Few studies have dealt with the neuropsychological differentiation of DLB, PDD, and AD. Perhaps because the majority of DLB cases involve pathological changes of AD (most often plaques) (McKeith et al., 2003) rather than pure cases (also called diffuse Lewy body disease), the emphasis has been on comparing neuropsychological performance in AD and DLB. In general, these studies indicate that AD is characterized by more prominent memory impairment, whereas DLB is associated with more pronounced visuoperceptual, attentional, and verbal fluency impairments (Aarsland et al., 2003; Connor et al., 1998; Galasko, Katzman, Salmon, & Hansen, 1996; Gnanalingham, Byrne, Thornton, Sambrook, & Bannister, 1997; Sahgal et al., 1992; Salmon & Galasko, 1996; Salmon et al., 1996; Shimomura et al., 1998; Walker, Allen, Shergill, & Katona, 1997).

Only three studies have compared the performances of PDD and DLB on rather circumscribed neuropsychological test batteries (excluding cognitive screening measures). Gnanalingham et al.'s (1997) finding of greater attentional and frontal function impairments in DLB than PD is difficult to interpret since the overall severity of cognitive impairment was greater in the DLB than PD group. In groups matched for age, education, estimated premorbid IQ, and overall severity of cognitive impairment (MMSE score), Downes et al. (1998) found DLB to demonstrate more severe impairments than PDD on tasks involving attention and working memory (WAIS–R Arithmetic; Stroop), and verbal fluency (letter, category, and alternating fluency tasks). The finding of greater impairment of attention in DLB is especially intriguing because fluctuating cognition, a putative hallmark of DLB, has been linked to attention impairment (Walker et al., 2000). Unfortunately, using computerized simple and choice reaction time and vigilance tasks, Ballard et al. (2002) were unable to demonstrate differences in attention between DLB and PDD. While group differences on neuropsychological test batteries promise to inform differential diagnosis and neuroanatomical bases of cognitive deficits in DLB, PDD, and AD, large prospective studies evaluating the predictive power, sensitivity, and specificity of such differences remain to be carried out.

Impact of pharmacological and surgical treatments on cognition

Tables 10.4 and 10.5 summarize the neurobehavioral impact of medical and surgical therapies for PD. Empirical findings concerning the impact of levodopa and dopamimetics on cognitive functions are inconsistent, revealing improvements, decrements, and an absence of significant cognitive changes

Table 10.4 Possible neurobehavioral effects of mediations commonly used in the treatment of Parkinson's disease

Drug category	Generic name(s)	Trade name(s)	Possible neurobehavioral adverse effects in PD	Possible neurobehavioral therapeutic effects in PD
Dopamine replacement	Levodopa + carbidopa	Sinemet Atamet	Hallucinations; delusions; euphoria; confusion; depression; anxiety; agitation; nightmares; hedonistic homeostatic dysregulation syndrome (Giovannoni et al., 2000); cognitive ("frontal") effects vary by disease stage	May improve working memory early in disease (Costa et al., 2003); may improve dysphoria
Combined dopamine replacement and COMT-inhibitors Dopamine agonists	Levodpa + carbidopa + entacapone	Stalevo	Depression; psychosis; generally unstudied due to novelty of drug	
Ergot alkaloids	bromocriptine	Parlodel	As for levodopa, possibly more severe; minimal effect on cognition (Cooper et al., 1993; Piccirilli et al., 1986; Weddell & Weiser, 1995)	
	pergolide	Permax	As for levodopa, possibly more severe somnolence; minimal cognitive effect (Stern et al., 1984)	
Nonergot alkaloids	pramipexole	Mirapex	Similar to levodopa; fatigue, somnolence	
	ropinirole	Requip	Similar to levodopa; fatigue, somnolence	

COMT-inhibitors	entacapone tolcapone	Comtan Tasmar	Hallucinations	Possible attention and memory improvement when used as adjunct to levodopa (Gasparini et al., 1997)
MAO-inhibitors	selegiline	Eldepryl Deprenyl	Rare confusion or hallucinations	Small, uncontrolled studies suggest possible cognitive benefits (Finali et al., 1994; Hietanen, 1991) but not confirmed in large prospective study
Anticholinergics	trihexyphenidyl biperiden benztropine	Artane Akineton Cogentin	Sedation; delirium; memory impairment; executive dysfunction (Bedard et al., 1999; Koller, 1984; Meco et al., 1984; Reid et al., 1992)	
Antiglutamatergics	amantadine	Symmetrel		

Source: Tröster & Arnett (in press).

Table 10.5 Possible neurobehavioral effects of modern surgical interventions for Parkinson's disease

Procedure type	Target	Possible adverse effects in PD	Possible beneficial effects in PD
Ablation	Globus pallidus interna (GPi)	Confusion; depression; hypomania; cognitive impairment (especially after bilateral procedure)	Reduction in obsessive-compulsive symptoms
	Ventralintermediate nucleus of thalamus (Vim)	Confusion; rare cognitive impairment	Reduction in depressive and obsessive symptoms
	Subthalamic nucleus (modern target)	Not reported	Not reported
Deep brain stimulation	GPi	Rare cognitive dysfunction, hypomania, depression	Mildly improved performance on some memory tests (probably not a true memory improvement); reduced anxiety and depressive symptoms
	Vim		Reduction in depressive symptoms; mild naming improvement
	STN	Apathy; depression (including suicidality); (hypo)mania; psychosis; euphoria/mirth; hypersexuality; dopamine; dysregulation syndrome; cognitive impairment	Reduction in depressive and anxiety symptoms
Transplantation	Putamen and/or caudate	Psychosis; depression; cognitive dysfunction	Transient memory improvement

Source: Burn & Tröster (2004).

associated with levodopa therapy or its withdrawal (Kulisevsky et al., 2000). Levodopa probably has at least short-term effects on selected aspects of memory and executive functions, though effects may reveal themselves only in some disease stages. Kulisevsky et al. reported short-term improvements in learning and memory, visuoperception, and certain executive functions with dopamine replacement, but these improvements were not maintained over time. Owen et al. (1995) also found that some executive functions (i.e., planning accuracy) were improved by levodopa therapy early in the disease, but other aspects (response latency) were unaffected by therapy. That levodopa affects only certain functions is consistent with the findings of Fournet et al. (2000) and Lange et al. (1992) who reported poorer performance only on a small number of tasks (e.g., working memory) after levodopa withdrawal. Levodopa's rather selective cognitive effects may be related to its mediation of dorsolateral frontal cortical blood flow changes in response to executive task activation (Cools et al., 2002).

Anticholinergic medications used to treat motor symptoms (e.g., benztropine and trihexyphenidyl) can adversely affect memory, executive functions, and overall cognitive state (Bedard et al., 1999). Memory decrements related to anticholinergic therapy are especially likely to be induced in patients with preexisting cognitive impairment (Saint-Cyr, Taylor, & Lang, 1993). Anticholinergics should be avoided in elderly patients who are susceptible to developing confusional states (Pondal, Del Ser, & Bermejo, 1996).

Cholinesterase inhibitors used in the treatment of AD were initially used only cautiously in PDD and DLB due to possible worsening of motor symptoms by these agents. However, cholinesterase inhibitors, such as rivastigmine, are well tolerated by patients with PD and may improve cognitive and neuropsychiatric symptoms in DLB and PDD (Bullock & Cameron, 2002; Kaufer, 2002; McKeith et al., 2000; Reading, Luce, & McKeith, 2001).

Modern ablative surgical interventions for PD that involve the stereotactic lesioning of the globus pallidus, thalamus, or subthalamic nucleus, at least when carried out unilaterally, appear relatively safe from a cognitive perspective. The most common postoperative decline after pallidotomy occurs in verbal fluency (observed in about 75% of studies that included a measure of verbal fluency) (Alegret et al., 2001; Cahn, Sullivan, Shear, Heit et al., 1998; de Bie et al., 2001; Green et al., 2002; Tröster, Woods, & Fields, 2003). Attention, memory, and executive function decrements (usually mild and transient) have been reported more occasionally, and significant cognitive complications even more rarely (de Bie et al., 2002). Preexisting cognitive impairment, advanced age, and dominant hemisphere surgery are putative risk factors for postoperative cognitive deficits. Bilateral pallidotomy may entail limited cognitive decline (Scott et al., 1998, 2002), gains in memory (Iacono et al., 1997), or marked morbidity (Ghika et al., 1999; Trépanier, Kumar, Lozano, Lang, & Saint-Cyr, 2000). Modern thalamotomy is associated with minimal cognitive morbidity (Fukuda, Kameyama, Yoshino, Tanaka, & Narabayashi, 2000; Hugdahl & Wester, 2000; Lund-Johansen et al., 1996). Initial reports of the apparent cognitive safety of unilateral subthalamotomy (Alvarez et al., 2001; McCarter, Walton, Rowan, Gill, & Palomo, 2000) remain to be replicated.

Deep brain stimulation (DBS), a nonablative therapy, involves unilateral or bilateral implantation of electrodes into thalamus (ventralis intermedius), globus pallidus (internus), or subthalamic nucleus and the application of high frequency electrical stimulation from an implanted pulse generator to these structures. Unilateral pallidal (GPi) DBS is relatively safe from a neurobehavioral standpoint (Fields & Tröster, 2000; Kalteis, Tröster, & Alesch, 2002; Tröster & Fields, 2003b), although a few studies have demonstrated postoperative declines in verbal fluency (Merello et al., 1999; Tröster, Fields, Wilkinson, Pahwa et al., 1997), likely related to diminished switching between semantic categories, rather than a diminution of the semantic memory networks *per se* (Tröster et al., 2002). Even bilateral GPi stimulation is cognitively well tolerated (Ardouin et al., 1999; Fields, Tröster, Wilkinson, Pahwa, & Koller, 1999; Pillon et al., 2000), but in isolated cases, cognitive declines can occur (Dujardin, Krystkowiak, Defebvre, Blond, & Destee, 2000; Trépanier et al., 2000). Similarly, unilateral thalamic DBS appears to be well tolerated (Caparros-Lefebvre, Blond, Pécheux, Pasquier, & Petit, 1992; Tröster, Fields, Wilkinson, Busenbark et al., 1997; Woods et al., 2001).

Most DBS procedures now target the subthalamic nucleus (STN). Findings regarding possible postoperative declines and/or improvements in global cognitive abilities, memory, attention, and executive functions are inconsistent, though, as with other stereotactic procedures in PD, verbal fluency decrements and improvement in self-reported symptoms of depression are commonly reported (Tröster & Fields, 2003b; Woods, Fields, & Tröster, 2002). Preliminary evidence indicates that elderly patients (older than 69 years), and patients displaying presurgical cognitive deficits, might be at greater risk for neurobehavioral morbidity after STN DBS. In general, however, it appears that for most patients with PD, the risk of mild, transient neurocognitive deficits does not outweigh the notable improvements in motor symptoms of the disease after STN DBS.

Acknowledgement

The authors thank Julie A. Fields for assistance with manuscript and figure preparation.

References

Aarsland, D., Litvan, I., Salmon, D., Galasko, D., Wentzel-Larsen, T., & Larsen, J. P. (2003). Performance on the Dementia Rating Scale in Parkinson's disease with dementia and dementia with Lewy bodies: Comparison with progressive supranuclear palsy and Alzheimer's disease. *Journal of Neurology, Neurosurgery, and Psychiatry, 74*, 1215–1220.

Ala, T. A., Hughes, L. F., Kyrouac, G. A., Ghobrial, M. W., & Elble, R. J. (2001). Pentagon copying is more impaired in dementia with Lewy bodies than in Alzheimer's disease. *Journal of Neurology, Neurosurgery, and Psychiatry, 70*, 483–488.

Alegret, M., Pere, V., Junqué, C., Valldeoriola, F., & Tolosa, E. (2001). Visuospatial deficits in Parkinson's disease assessed by Judgment of Line Orientation Test: Error analyses and practice effects. *Journal of Clinical and Experimental Neuropsychology, 23*, 592–598.

Alexander, G. E., DeLong, M. R., & Strick, P. L. (1986). Parallel organization of functionally segregated circuits linking basal ganglia and cortex. *Annual Review of Neuroscience, 9,* 357–381.

Almgren, P. E., Andersson, A. L., & Kullberg, G. (1969). Differences in verbally expressed cognition following left and right ventrolateral thalamotomy. *Scandinavian Journal of Psychology, 10,* 243–249.

Alvarez, L., Macias, R., Guridi, J., Lopez, G., Alvarez, E., Maragoto, C., et al. (2001). Dorsal subthalamotomy for Parkinson's disease. *Movement Disorders, 16,* 72–78.

American Psychiatric Association. (2000). *Handbook of psychiatric measures.* Washington, DC: Author.

Appollonio, I., Grafman, J., Clark, K., Nichelli, P., Zeffiro, T., & Hallett, M. (1994). Implicit and explicit memory in patients with Parkinson's disease with and without dementia. *Archives of Neurology, 51,* 359–367.

Ardouin, C., Pillon, B., Peiffer, E., Bejjani, P., Limousin, P., Damier, P., et al. (1999). Bilateral subthalamic or pallidal stimulation for Parkinson's disease affects neither memory nor executive functions: A consecutive series of 62 patients. *Annals of Neurology, 46,* 217–223.

Asso, D., Crown, S., Russell, J. A., & Logue, V. (1969). Psychological aspects of the stereotactic treatment of parkinsonism. *British Journal of Psychiatry, 115,* 541–553.

Auriacombe, S., Grossman, M., Carvell, S., Gollomp, S., Stern, M. B., & Hurtig, H. I. (1993). Verbal fluency deficits in Parkinson's disease. *Neuropsychology, 7,* 182–192.

Azuma, T., Bayles, K. A., Cruz, R. F., Tomoeda, C. K., Wood, J. A., McGeagh, A., & Montgomery, E. B., Jr. (1997). Comparing the difficulty of letter, semantic, and name fluency tasks for normal elderly and patients with Parkinson's disease. *Neuropsychology, 11,* 488–497.

Baldereschi, M., Di Carlo, A., Rocca, W. A., Vanni, P., Maggi, S., Perissinotto, E., et al. (2000). Parkinson's disease and parkinsonism in a longitudinal study: Two-fold higher incidence in men. Italian Longitudinal Study on Aging. *Neurology, 55,* 1358–1363.

Ballard, C. G., Aarsland, D., McKeith, I., O'Brien, J., Gray, A., Cormack, F., et al. (2002). Fluctuations in attention: PD dementia vs DLB with parkinsonism. *Neurology, 59,* 1714–1720.

Bayles, K. A., Trosset, M. W., Tomoeda, C. K., Montgomery, E. B., Jr., & Wilson, J. (1993). Generative naming in Parkinson disease patients. *Journal of Clinical and Experimental Neuropsychology, 15,* 547–562.

Beardsley, J., & Puletti, F. (1971). Personality (MMPI) and cognitive (WAIS) changes after L-DOPA treatment. *Archives of Neurology, 25,* 145–150.

Beatty, W. W. (1992). Memory dysfunction in the subcortical dementias. In L. Bäckman (Ed.), *Memory functioning in dementia* (pp. 153–173). Amsterdam: Elsevier.

Beatty, W. W., Goodkin, D. E., Weir, W. S., Staton, R. D., Monson, N., & Beatty, P. A. (1989). Affective judgments by patients with Parkinson's disease or chronic progressive multiple sclerosis. *Bulletin of the Psychonomic Society, 27,* 361–364.

Beatty, W. W., & Monson, N. (1989a). Geographical knowledge in patients with Parkinson's disease. *Bulletin of the Psychonomic Society, 27,* 473–475.

Beatty, W. W., & Monson, N. (1989b). Lexical processing in Parkinson's disease and multiple sclerosis. *Journal of Geriatric Psychiatry and Neurology, 2,* 145–152.

Beatty, W. W., & Monson, N. (1990a). Picture and motor sequencing in Parkinson's disease. *Journal of Geriatric Psychiatry and Neurology, 3,* 192–197.

Beatty, W. W., & Monson, N. (1990b). Problem solving in Parkinson's disease: Comparison of performance on the Wisconsin and California Card Sorting Tests. *Journal of Geriatric Psychiatry and Neurology*, *3*, 163–171.

Beatty, W. W., Staton, R. D., Weir, W. S., Monson, N., & Whitaker, H. A. (1989). Cognitive disturbances in Parkinson's disease. *Journal of Geriatric Psychiatry and Neurology*, *2*, 22–33.

Bechara, A., Damasio, A. R., Damasio, H., & Anderson, S. W. (1994). Insensitivity to future consequences following damage to human prefrontal cortex. *Cognition*, *50*, 7–15.

Beck, A. T., Ward, C. H., Mendelson, M., Mock, J., & Erbaugh, J. (1961). An inventory for measuring depression. *Archives of General Psychiatry*, *4*, 53–63.

Bedard, M.-A., Paquet, F., Chouinard, S., & Blanchet, P. (2001). Impact of the frontal behavioral disturbances in Parkinson's disease during a daily activity [Abstract]. *Neurology*, *56*(Suppl. 3), A50.

Bedard, M. A., Pillon, B., Dubois, B., Duchesne, N., Masson, H., & Agid, Y. (1999). Acute and long-term administration of anticholinergics in Parkinson's disease: Specific effects on the subcortico-frontal syndrome. *Brain and Cognition*, *40*, 289–313.

Berger, H. J., van Es, N. J., van Spaendonck, K. P., Teunisse, J. P., Horstink, M. W., van 't Hof, M. A., & Cools, A. R. (1999). Relationship between memory strategies and motor symptoms in Parkinson's disease. *Journal of Clinical and Experimental Neuropsychology*, *21*, 677–684.

Bernheimer, H., Birkmayer, W., Hornykiewicz, O., Jellinger, K., & Seitelberger, F. (1973). Brain dopamine and the syndromes of Parkinson and Huntington. *Journal of the Neurological Sciences*, *20*, 415–455.

Biggins, C. A., Boyd, J. L., Harrop, F. M., Madeley, P., Mindham, R. H., Randall, J. I., & Spokes, E. G. (1992). A controlled, longitudinal study of dementia in Parkinson's disease. *Journal of Neurology, Neurosurgery, and Psychiatry*, *55*, 566–571.

Blonder, L. X., Gur, R. E., & Gur, R. C. (1989). The effects of right and left hemiparkinsonism on prosody. *Brain and Language*, *36*, 193–207.

Bodis-Wollner, I. (2003). Neuropsychological and perceptual defects in Parkinson's disease. *Parkinsonism and Related Disorders*, *9*, S83–S89.

Boller, F., Marcie, P., Starkstein, S., & Traykov, L. (1998). Memory and depression in Parkinson's disease. *European Journal of Neurology*, *5*, 291–295.

Boller, F., Mizutani, T., Roessmann, U., & Gambetti, P. (1980). Parkinson disease, dementia, and Alzheimer disease: Clinicopathological correlations. *Annals of Neurology*, *7*, 329–335.

Boller, F., Passafiume, D., Keefe, N. C., Rogers, K., Morrow, L., & Kim, Y. (1984). Visuospatial impairment in Parkinson's disease: Role of perceptual and motor factors. *Archives of Neurology*, *41*, 485–490.

Bondi, M. W., & Kaszniak, A. W. (1991). Implicit and explicit memory in Alzheimer's disease and Parkinson's disease. *Journal of Clinical and Experimental Neuropsychology*, *13*, 339–358.

Bondi, M. W., Kaszniak, A. W., Bayles, K. A., & Vance, K. T. (1993). Contributions of frontal system dysfunction to memory and perceptual abilities in Parkinson's disease. *Neuropsychology*, *7*, 89–102.

Bondi, M. W., & Tröster, A. I. (1997). Parkinson's disease: Neurobehavioral consequences of basal ganglia dysfunction. In P. D. Nussbaum (Ed.), *Handbook of neuropsychology and aging* (pp. 216–245). New York: Plenum.

Borod, J. C., Welkowitz, J., Alpert, M., Brozgold, A. Z., Martin, C., Peselow, E., & Diller, L. (1990). Parameters of emotional processing in neuropsychiatric disorders: Conceptual issues and a battery of tests. *Journal of Communication Disorders*, *23*, 247–271.

Bowen, F. P., Burns, M., & Yahr, M. D. (1976). Alterations in memory processes subsequent to short- and long-term treatment with L-Dopa. In W. Birkmayer & O. Hornykiewicz (Eds.), *Advances in parkinsonism* (pp. 488–491). Geneva, Switzerland: Roche.

Bowen, F. P., Hoehn, M. M., & Yahr, M. D. (1972). Parkinsonism: Alterations in spatial orientation as determined by a route-walking test. *Neuropsychologia*, *10*, 355–361.

Bowen, F. P., Kamienny, R. S., Burns, M. M., & Yahr, M. (1975). Parkinsonism: Effects of levodopa treatment on concept formation. *Neurology*, *25*, 701–704.

Bower, J. H., Maraganore, D. M., McDonnell, S. K., & Rocca, W. A. (1999). Incidence and distribution of parkinsonism in Olmsted County, Minnesota, 1976–1990. *Neurology*, *52*, 1214–1220.

Braak, H., Tredici, K. D., Rüb, U., de Vos, R. A., Jansen Steur, E. N., & Braak, E. (2003). Staging of brain pathology related to sporadic Parkinson's disease. *Neurobiology of Aging*, *24*, 197–211.

Brentari, D., Poizner, H., & Kegl, J. (1995). Aphasic and parkinsonian signing: Differences in phonological disruption. *Brain and Language*, *48*, 69–105.

Brown, G. G., Rahill, A. A., Gorell, J. M., McDonald, C., Brown, S. J., Sillanpaa, M., & Shults, C. (1999). Validity of the Dementia Rating Scale in assessing cognitive function in Parkinson's disease. *Journal of Geriatric Psychiatry and Neurology*, *12*, 180–188.

Brown, R. G., MacCarthy, B., Jahanshahi, M., & Marsden, C. D. (1989). Accuracy of self-reported disability in patients with parkinsonism. *Archives of Neurology*, *46*, 955–959.

Brown, R. G., & Marsden, C. D. (1986). Visuospatial function in Parkinson's disease. *Brain*, *109*, 987–1002.

Brown, R. G., & Marsden, C. D. (1988). Internal versus external cues and the control of attention in Parkinson's disease. *Brain*, *111*, 323–345.

Bullock, R., & Cameron, A. (2002). Rivastigmine for the treatment of dementia and visual hallucinations associated with Parkinson's disease: A case series. *Current Medical Research and Opinion*, *18*, 258–264.

Burgess, P. W., Quayle, A., & Frith, C. D. (2001). Brain regions involved in prospective memory as determined by positron emission tomography. *Neuropsychologia*, *39*, 545–555.

Burgess, P. W., & Shallice, T. (1997). The relationship between prospective and retrospective memory: Neuropsychological evidence. In M. A. Conway (Ed.), *Cognitive models of memory* (pp. 247–272). Cambridge, MA: MIT Press.

Burn, D. J., & Tröster, A. I. (2004). Neuropsychiatric complications of medical and surgical therapies for Parkinson's disease. *Journal of Geriatric Psychiatry and Neurology*, *17*(3), 172–180.

Buytenhuijs, E. L., Berger, H. J., van Spaendonck, K. P., Horstink, M. W., Borm, G. F., & Cools, A. R. (1994). Memory and learning strategies in patients with Parkinson's disease. *Neuropsychologia*, *32*, 335–342.

Cahn, D. A., Sullivan, E. V., Shear, P. K., Heit, G., Lim, K. O., Marsh, L., et al. (1998). Neuropsychological and motor functioning after unilateral anatomically guided posterior ventral pallidotomy: Preoperative performance and three-month follow-up. *Neuropsychiatry, Neuropsychology, and Behavioral Neurology*, *11*, 136–145.

Cahn, D. A., Sullivan, E. V., Shear, P. K., Pfefferbaum, A., Heit, G., & Silverberg, G. (1998). Differential contributions of cognitive and motor component processes to physical and instrumental activities of daily living in Parkinson's disease. *Archives of Clinical Neuropsychology*, *13*, 575–583.

Caparros-Lefebvre, D., Blond, S., Pécheux, N., Pasquier, F., & Petit, H. (1992). Evaluation neuropsychologique avant et après stimulation thalamique chez 9 parkinsoniens. *Revue Neurologique*, *148*, 117–122.

Charcot, J. M., & Vulpian, A. (1861). De la paralysie agitante. *Gazette Hebdomadaire de Médecine et Chirurgie*, *8*, 765–767.

Charcot, J. M., & Vulpian, A. (1862). De la paralysie agitante. *Gazette Hebdomadaire de Médecine et Chirurgie*, *9*, 54–59.

Christensen, A. L., Juul-Jensen, P., Malmros, R., & Harmsen, A. (1970). Psychological evaluation of intelligence and personality in parkinsonism before and after stereotaxic surgery. *Acta Neurologica Scandanavica*, *46*, 527–537.

Churchyard, A., & Lees, A. J. (1997). The relationship between dementia and direct involvement of the hippocampus and amygdala in Parkinson's disease. *Neurology*, *49*, 1570–1576.

Cohen, H., Bouchard, S., Scherzer, P., & Whitaker, H. (1994). Language and verbal reasoning in Parkinson's disease. *Neuropsychiatry, Neuropsychology, and Behavioral Neurology*, *7*, 166–175.

Colosimo, C., Hughes, A. J., Kilford, L., & Lees, A. J. (2003). Lewy body cortical involvement may not always predict dementia in Parkinson's disease. *Journal of Neurology, Neurosurgery, and Psychiatry*, *74*, 852–856.

Connor, D. J., Salmon, D. P., Sandy, T. J., Galasko, D., Hansen, L. A., & Thal, L. J. (1998). Cognitive profiles of autopsy-confirmed Lewy body variant vs pure Alzheimer disease. *Archives of Neurology*, *55*, 994–1000.

Cools, R., Barker, R. A., Sahakian, B. J., & Robbins, T. W. (2003). L-Dopa medication remediates cognitive inflexibility, but increases impulsivity in patients with Parkinson's disease. *Neuropsychologia*, *41*, 1431–1441.

Cools, R., Stefanova, E., Barker, R. A., Robbins, T. W., & Owen, A. M. (2002). Dopaminergic modulation of high-level cognition in Parkinson's disease: The role of the prefrontal cortex revealed by PET. *Brain*, *125*, 584–594.

Cooper, J. A., Sagar, H. J., Jordan, N., Harvey, N. S., & Sullivan, E. V. (1991). Cognitive impairment in early, untreated Parkinson's disease and its relationship to motor disability. *Brain*, *114*, 2095–2122.

Cooper, J. A., Sagar, H. J., & Sullivan, E. V. (1993). Short-term memory and temporal ordering in early Parkinson's disease: Effects of disease chronicity and medication. *Neuropsychologia*, *31*, 933–949.

Cousins, R., Hanley, J. R., Davies, A. D., Turnbull, C. J., & Playfer, J. R. (2000). Understanding memory for faces in Parkinson's disease: The role of configural processing. *Neuropsychologia*, *38*, 837–847.

Cronin-Golomb, A., Corkin, S., & Growdon, J. H. (1994). Impaired problem solving in Parkinson's disease: Impact of a set-shifting deficit. *Neuropsychologia*, *32*, 579–593.

Crucian, G. P., Barrett, A. M., Burks, D. W., Riestra, A. R., Roth, H. L., Schwartz, R. L., et al. (2003). Mental object rotation in Parkinson's disease. *Journal of the International Neuropsychological Society*, *9*, 1078–1087.

Culbertson, W. C., Moberg, P. J., Duda, J. E., Stern, M. B., & Weintraub, D. (2004). Assessing the executive function deficits of patients with Parkinson's disease: Utility of the Tower of London-Drexel. *Assessment, 11*, 27–39.

Cummings, J. L., Darkins, A., Mendez, M., Hill, M. A., & Benson, D. F. (1988). Alzheimer's disease and Parkinson's disease: Comparison of speech and language alterations. *Neurology, 38*, 680–684.

Czernecki, V., Pillon, B., Houeto, J. L., Pochon, J. B., Levy, R., & Dubois, B. (2002). Motivation, reward, and Parkinson's disease: Influence of dopatherapy. *Neuropsychologia, 40*, 2257–2267.

Dagher, A., Owen, A. M., Boecker, H., & Brooks, D. J. (1999). Mapping the network for planning: A correlational PET activation study with the Tower of London task. *Brain, 122*, 1973–1987.

Dagher, A., Owen, A. M., Boecker, H., & Brooks, D. J. (2001). The role of the striatum and hippocampus in planning: A PET activation study in Parkinson's disease. *Brain, 124*, 1020–1032.

Damasio, A. R., & Tranel, D. (1993). Nouns and verbs are retrieved with differently distributed neural systems. *Proceedings of the National Academy of Sciences, USA, 90*, 4957–4960.

Darvesh, S., & Freedman, M. (1996). Subcortical dementia: A neurobehavioral approach. *Brain and Cognition, 31*, 230–249.

De Bie, R. M., de Haan, R. J., Schuurman, P. R., Esselink, R. A., Bosch, D. A., & Speelman, J. D. (2002). Morbidity and mortality following pallidotomy in Parkinson's disease: A systematic review. *Neurology, 58*, 1008–1012.

De Bie, R. M., Schuurman, P. R., Bosch, D. A., de Haan, R. J., Schmand, B., & Speelman, J. D. (2001). Outcome of unilateral pallidotomy in advanced Parkinson's disease: Cohort study of 32 patients. *Journal of Neurology, Neurosurgery, and Psychiatry, 71*, 375–382.

Dekker, M. C. J., Bonifati, V., & van Duijn, C. M. (2003). Parkinson's disease: Piecing together a genetic jigsaw. *Brain, 126*, 1722–1733.

Delis, D. C., Kaplan, E., & Kramer, J. H. (2001). *Delis-Kaplan Executive Function System (D-KEFS)*. San Antonio, TX: Psychological Corporation.

Diller, L., Riklan, M., & Cooper, I. S. (1956). Preoperative response to stress as a criterion of the response to neurosurgery in Parkinson's disease. *Journal of the American Geriatrics Society, 4*, 1301–1308.

Dimitrov, M., Grafman, J., Soares, A. H., & Clark, K. (1999). Concept formation and concept shifting in frontal lesion and Parkinson's disease patients assessed with the California Card Sorting Test. *Neuropsychology, 13*, 135–143.

Downes, J. J., Priestley, N. M., Doran, M., Ferran, J., Ghadiali, E., & Cooper, P. (1998). Intellectual, mnemonic, and frontal functions in dementia with Lewy bodies: A comparison with early and advanced Parkinson's disease. *Behavioural Neurology, 11*, 173–183.

Downes, J. J., Roberts, A. C., Sahakian, B. J., Evenden, J. L., Morris, R. G., & Robbins, T. W. (1989). Impaired extra-dimensional shift performance in medicated and unmedicated Parkinson's disease: Evidence for a specific attentional dysfunction. *Neuropsychologia, 27*, 1329–1343.

Doyon, J., Gaudreau, D., Laforce, R., Jr., Castonguay, M., Bedard, P. J., Bedard, F., & Bouchard, J. P. (1997). Role of the striatum, cerebellum, and frontal lobes in the learning of a visuomotor sequence. *Brain and Cognition, 34*, 218–245.

Dubois, B., Danze, F., Pillon, B., Cusimano, G., Lhermitte, F., & Agid, Y. (1987). Cholinergic-dependent cognitive deficits in Parkinson's disease. *Annals of Neurology*, *22*, 26–30.

Dubois, B., Pillon, B., Lhermitte, F., & Agid, Y. (1990). Cholinergic deficiency and frontal dysfunction in Parkinson's disease. *Annals of Neurology*, *28*, 117–121.

Dubois, B., Slachevsky, A., Litvan, I., & Pillon, B. (2000). The FAB: A Frontal Assessment Battery at bedside. *Neurology*, *55*, 1621–1626.

Dujardin, K., Defebvre, L., Grunberg, C., Becquet, E., & Destee, A. (2001). Memory and executive function in sporadic and familial Parkinson's disease. *Brain*, *124*, 389–398.

Dujardin, K., Degreef, J. F., Rogelet, P., Defebvre, L., & Destee, A. (1999). Impairment of the supervisory attentional system in early untreated patients with Parkinson's disease. *Journal of Neurology*, *246*, 783–788.

Dujardin, K., Krystkowiak, P., Defebvre, L., Blond, S., & Destee, A. (2000). A case of severe dysexecutive syndrome consecutive to chronic bilateral pallidal stimulation. *Neuropsychologia*, *38*, 1305–1315.

Dymek, M. P., Atchison, P., Harrell, L., & Marson, D. C. (2001). Competency to consent to medical treatment in cognitively impaired patients with Parkinson's disease. *Neurology*, *56*, 17–24.

Faglioni, P., Saetti, M. C., & Botti, C. (2000). Verbal learning strategies in Parkinson's disease. *Neuropsychology*, *14*, 456–470.

Fama, R., Sullivan, E. V., Shear, P. K., Stein, M., Yesavage, J. A., Tinklenberg, J. R., & Pfefferbaum, A. (2000). Extent, pattern, and correlates of remote memory impairment in Alzheimer's disease and Parkinson's disease. *Neuropsychology*, *14*, 265–276.

Farrer, M., Gwinn-Hardy, K., Muenter, M., DeVrieze, F. W., Crook, R., Perez-Tur, J., et al. (1999). A chromosome 4p haplotype segregating with Parkinson's disease and postural tremor. *Human Molecular Genetics*, *8*, 81–85.

Feigin, A., Ghilardi, M. F., Carbon, M., Edwards, C., Fukuda, M., Dhawan, V., et al. (2003). Effects of levodopa on motor sequence learning in Parkinson's disease. *Neurology*, *60*, 1744–1749.

Ferraro, F. R., Balota, D. A., & Connor, L. T. (1993). Implicit memory and the formation of new associations in nondemented Parkinson's disease individuals and individuals with senile dementia of the Alzheimer type: A serial reaction time (SRT) investigation. *Brain and Cognition*, *21*, 163–180.

Fields, J. A., Norman, S., Straits-Tröster, K. A., & Tröster, A. I. (1998). The impact of depression on memory in neurodegenerative disease. In A. I. Tröster (Ed.), *Memory in neurodegenerative disease: Biological, cognitive, and clinical perspectives* (pp. 314–337). New York: Cambridge University Press.

Fields, J. A., Paolo, A. M., & Tröster, A. I. (1996). Visual confrontation naming in Parkinson's disease with and without dementia [Abstract]. *The Clinical Neuropsychologist*, *10*, 321–322.

Fields, J. A., & Tröster, A. I. (2000). Cognitive outcomes after deep brain stimulation for Parkinson's disease: A review of initial studies and recommendations for future research. *Brain and Cognition*, *42*, 268–293.

Fields, J. A., Tröster, A. I., Wilkinson, S. B., Pahwa, R., & Koller, W. C. (1999). Cognitive outcome following staged bilateral pallidal stimulation for the treatment of Parkinson's disease. *Clinical Neurology and Neurosurgery*, *101*, 182–188.

Filoteo, J. V., Friedrich, F. J., Rilling, L. M., Davis, J. D., Stricker, J. L., & Prenovitz, M. (2003). Semantic and cross-case identity priming in patients with Parkinson's disease. *Journal of Clinical and Experimental Neuropsychology*, *25*, 441–456.

Filoteo, J. V., Rilling, L. M., Cole, B., Williams, B. J., Davis, J. D., & Roberts, J. W. (1997). Variable memory profiles in Parkinson's disease. *Journal of Clinical and Experimental Neuropsychology*, *19*, 878–888.

Filoteo, J. V., Williams, B. J., Rilling, L. M., & Roberts, J. W. (1997). Performance of Parkinson's disease patients on the Visual Search and Attention Test: Impairment in single-feature but not dual-feature visual search. *Archives of Clinical Neuropsychology*, *12*, 621–634.

Finton, M. J., Lucas, J. A., Graff-Radford, N. R., & Uitti, R. J. (1998). Analysis of visuospatial errors in patients with Alzheimer's disease or Parkinson's disease. *Journal of Clinical and Experimental Neuropsychology*, *20*, 186–193.

Fischer, P., Kendler, P., & Goldenberg, G. (1990). Recency-primacy recognition in Parkinson's disease. *Journal of Neural Transmission*, *2*, 71–77.

Folstein, M. F., Folstein, S. E., & McHugh, P. R. (1975). "Mini-mental state": A practical method for grading the cognitive state of patients for the clinician. *Journal of Psychiatric Research*, *12*, 189–198.

Fournet, N., Moreaud, O., Roulin, J. L., Naegele, B., & Pellat, J. (2000). Working memory functioning in medicated Parkinson's disease patients and the effect of withdrawal of dopaminergic medication. *Neuropsychology*, *14*, 247–253.

Frank, E. M., McDade, H. L., & Scott, W. K. (1996). Naming in dementia secondary to Parkinson's, Hungtington's, and Alzheimer's diseases. *Journal of Communication Disorders*, *29*, 183–197.

Freedman, M., Rivoira, P., Butters, N., Sax, D. S., & Feldman, R. G. (1984). Retrograde amnesia in Parkinson's disease. *Canadian Journal of Neurological Sciences*, *11*, 297–301.

Freeman, R. Q., Giovannetti, T., Lamar, M., Cloud, B. S., Stern, R. A., Kaplan, E., & Libon, D. J. (2000). Visuoconstructional problems in dementia: Contribution of executive systems functions. *Neuropsychology*, *14*, 415–426.

Fukuda, M., Kameyama, S., Yoshino, M., Tanaka, R., & Narabayashi, H. (2000). Neuropsychological outcome following pallidotomy and thalamotomy for Parkinson's disease. *Stereotactic and Functional Neurosurgery*, *74*, 11–20.

Fünfgeld, E. W. (1967). *Psychopathologie und Klinik des Parkinsonismus vor und nach stereotaktischen Operationen*. Berlin: Springer-Verlag.

Gabrieli, J. D. E., Singh, J., Stebbins, G., & Goetz, C. G. (1996). Reduced working memory span in Parkinson's disease: Evidence for the role of a frontostriatal system in working and strategic memory. *Neuropsychology*, *10*, 322–332.

Galasko, D., Katzman, R., Salmon, D. P., & Hansen, L. (1996). Clinical and neuropathological findings in Lewy body dementias. *Brain and Cognition*, *31*, 166–175.

Gauntlett-Gilbert, J., Roberts, R. C., & Brown, V. J. (1999). Mechanisms underlying attentional set-shifting in Parkinson's disease. *Neuropsychologia*, *37*, 605–616.

Gelb, D. J., Oliver, E., & Gilman, S. (1999). Diagnostic criteria for Parkinson disease. *Archives of Neurology*, *56*, 33–39.

Ghika, J., Ghika-Schmid, F., Fankhauser, H., Assal, G., Vingerhoets, F., Albanese, A., et al. (1999). Bilateral contemporaneous posteroventral pallidotomy for the treatment of Parkinson's disease: Neuropsychological and neurological side effects.

Report of four cases and review of the literature. *Journal of Neurosurgery, 91,* 313–321.

Globus, M., Mildworf, B., & Melamed, E. (1985). Cerebral blood flow and cognitive impairment in Parkinson's disease. *Neurology, 35,* 1135–1139.

Gnanalingham, K. K., Byrne, E. J., Thornton, A., Sambrook, M. A., & Bannister, P. (1997). Motor and cognitive function in Lewy body dementia: Comparison with Alzheimer's and Parkinson's diseases. *Journal of Neurology, Neurosurgery, and Psychiatry, 62,* 243–252.

Goetz, C. G. (1992). The historical background of behavioral studies in Parkinson's disease. In S. J. Huber & J. L. Cummings (Eds.), *Parkinson's disease: Neurobehavioral aspects* (pp. 3–9). New York: Oxford University Press.

Golbe, L. I., Di Iorio, G., Sanges, G., Lazzarini, A. M., La Sala, S., Bonavita, V., & Duvoisin, R. C. (1996). Clinical genetic analysis of Parkinson's disease in the Contursi kindred. *Annals of Neurology, 40,* 767–775.

Gomez-Tortosa, E., Newell, K., Irizarry, M. C., Albert, M., Growdon, J. H., & Hyman, B. T. (1999). Clinical and quantitative pathologic correlates of dementia with Lewy bodies. *Neurology, 53,* 1284–1291.

Gorell, J. M., Johnson, C. C., Rybicki, B. A., Peterson, E. L., & Richardson, R. J. (1998). The risk of Parkinson's disease with exposure to pesticides, farming, well water, and rural living. *Neurology, 50,* 1346–1350.

Gotham, A. M., Brown, R. G., & Marsden, C. D. (1988). "Frontal" cognitive function in patients with Parkinson's disease "on" and "off" levodopa. *Brain, 111,* 299–321.

Grant, D. A., & Berg, E. A. (1948). A behavior analysis of damage of reinforcement and ease of shifting to new responses in a Weigl-type card sorting problem. *Journal of Experimental Psychology, 38,* 404–411.

Green, J., McDonald, W. M., Vitek, J. L., Haber, M., Barnhart, H., Bakay, R. A., et al. (2002). Neuropsychological and psychiatric sequelae of pallidotomy for PD: Clinical trial findings. *Neurology, 58,* 858–865.

Grossman, M., Carvell, S., Stern, M. B., Gollomp, S., & Hurtig, H. I. (1992). Sentence comprehension in Parkinson's disease: The role of attention and memory. *Brain and Language, 42,* 347–384.

Grossman, M., Cooke, A., DeVita, C., Lee, C., Alsop, D., Detre, J., et al. (2003). Grammatical and resource components of sentence processing in Parkinson's disease: An fMRI study. *Neurology, 60,* 775–781.

Grossman, M., Zurif, E., Lee, C., Prather, P., Kalmanson, J., Stern, M. B., & Hurtig, H. I. (2002). Information processing speed and sentence comprehension in Parkinson's disease. *Neuropsychology, 16,* 174–181.

Gruenewald, P. J., & Lockhead, G. R. (1980). The free recall of category examples. *Journal of Experimental Psychology: Human Learning and Memory, 6,* 225–240.

Gschwandtner, U., Aston, J., Renaud, S., & Fuhr, P. (2001). Pathologic gambling in patients with Parkinson's disease. *Clinical Neuropharmacology, 24,* 170–172.

Hamilton, M. (1960). A rating scale for depression. *Journal of Neurology, Neurosurgery, and Psychiatry, 23,* 56–62.

Hanley, J. R., Dewick, H. C., Davies, A. D., Playfer, J., & Turnbull, C. (1990). Verbal fluency in Parkinson's disease. *Neuropsychologia, 28,* 737–741.

Hardy, J., Cookson, M. R., & Singleton, A. (2003). Genes and parkinsonism. *Lancet Neurology, 2,* 221–228.

Harrington, D. L., Haaland, K. Y., Yeo, R. A., & Marder, E. (1990). Procedural memory in Parkinson's disease: Impaired motor but not visuoperceptual learning. *Journal of Clinical and Experimental Neuropsychology, 12,* 323–339.

Heaton, R. K., Chelune, G. J., Talley, J. L., Kay, G. G., & Curtiss, G. (1993). *Wisconsin Card Sorting Test manual.* Odessa, FL: Psychological Assessment Resources.

Heindel, W. C., Salmon, D. P., Shults, C. W., Walicke, P. A., & Butters, N. (1989). Neuropsychological evidence for multiple implicit memory systems: A comparison of Alzheimer's, Huntington's, and Parkinson's disease patients. *Journal of Neuroscience, 9,* 582–587.

Heiss, C., Kalbe, E., & Kessler, J. (2001). Quantitative und qualitative Analysen von verbalen Flüssigkeitsaufgaben bei Parkinsonpatienten. *Zeitschrift für Neuropsychologie, 12,* 188–199.

Higginson, C. I., Fields, J. A., Koller, W. C., & Tröster, A. I. (2001). Questionnaire assessment potentially overestimates anxiety in Parkinson's disease. *Journal of Clinical Psychology in Medical Settings, 8,* 95–99.

Higginson, C. I., King, D. S., Levine, D., Wheelock, V. L., Khamphay, N. O., & Sigvardt, K. A. (2003). The relationship between executive function and verbal memory in Parkinson's disease. *Brain and Cognition, 52,* 343–352.

Hobson, P., & Meara, J. (1999). The detection of dementia and cognitive impairment in a community population of elderly people with Parkinson's disease by use of the CAMCOG neuropsychological test. *Age and Ageing, 28,* 39–43.

Hodges, J. R., Salmon, D. P., & Butters, N. (1991). The nature of the naming deficit in Alzheimer's and Huntington's disease. *Brain, 114,* 1547–1558.

Holdorff, B. (2002). Friedrich Heinrich Lewy (1885–1950) and his work. *Journal of the History of the Neurosciences, 11,* 19–28.

Hsieh, S., & Lee, C.-Y. (1999). Source memory in Parkinson's disease. *Perceptual and Motor Skills, 89,* 355–367.

Hubble, J. P., Cao, T., Hassanein, R. E., Neuberger, J. S., & Koller, W. C. (1993). Risk factors for Parkinson's disease. *Neurology, 43,* 1693–1697.

Huber, S. J., Shuttleworth, E. C., & Paulson, G. W. (1986). Dementia in Parkinson's disease. *Archives of Neurology, 43,* 987–990.

Huber, S. J., Shuttleworth, E. C., Paulson, G. W., Bellchambers, M. J., & Clapp, L. E. (1986). Cortical vs subcortical dementia: Neuropsychological differences. *Archives of Neurology, 43,* 392–394.

Huberman, M., Moscovitch, M., & Freedman, M. (1994). Comparison of patients with Alzheimer's and Parkinson's disease on different explicit and implicit tests of memory. *Neuropsychiatry, Neuropsychology, and Behavioral Neurology, 7,* 185–193.

Hugdahl, K., & Wester, K. (2000). Neurocognitive correlates of stereotactic thalamotomy and thalamic stimulation in Parkinsonian patients. *Brain and Cognition, 42,* 231–252.

Hughes, A. J., Ben-Shlomo, Y., Daniel, S. E., & Lees, A. J. (2001). What features improve the accuracy of clinical diagnosis in Parkinson's disease: A clinicopathologic study 1992? *Neurology, 57,* S34–S38.

Hurtig, H. I., Trojanowski, J. Q., Galvin, J., Ewbank, D., Schmidt, M. L., Lee, V. M., et al. (2000). Alpha-synuclein cortical Lewy bodies correlate with dementia in Parkinson's disease. *Neurology, 54,* 1916–1921.

Iacono, R. P., Carlson, J. D., Kuniyoshi, S., Mohamed, A., Meltzer, C., & Yamada, S. (1997). Contemporaneous bilateral pallidotomy [Electronic version]. *Neurosurgical Focus, 2,* Manuscript 5.

Illes, J. (1989). Neurolinguistic features of spontaneous language production dissociate three forms of neurodegenerative disease: Alzheimer's, Huntington's, and Parkinson's. *Brain and Language, 37*, 628–642.

Ivory, S.-J., Knight, R. G., Longmore, B. E., & Caradoc-Davies, T. (1999). Verbal memory in non-demented patients with idiopathic Parkinson's disease. *Neuropsychologia, 37*, 817–828.

Jackson, G. M., Jackson, S. R., Harrison, J., Henderson, L., & Kennard, C. (1995). Serial reaction time learning and Parkinson's disease: Evidence for a procedural learning deficit. *Neuropsychologia, 33*, 577–593.

Jacobs, D. M., Marder, K., Cote, L. J., Sano, M., Stern, Y., & Mayeux, R. (1995). Neuropsychological characteristics of preclinical dementia in Parkinson's disease. *Neurology, 45*, 1691–1696.

Janvin, C., Aarsland, D., Larsen, J. P., & Hugdahl, K. (2003). Neuropsychological profile of patients with Parkinson's disease without dementia. *Dementia and Geriatric Cognitive Disorders, 15*, 126–131.

Jefferson, A. L., Cosentino, S. A., Ball, S. K., Bogdanoff, B., Leopold, N., Kaplan, E., & Libon, D. J. (2002). Errors produced on the Mini-Mental State Examination and neuropsychological test performance in Alzheimer's disease, ischemic vascular dementia, and Parkinson's disease. *Journal of Neuropsychiatry and Clinical Neurosciences, 14*, 311–320.

Joel, D. (2001). Open interconnected model of basal ganglia-thalamocortical circuitry and its relevance to the clinical syndrome of Huntington's disease. *Movement Disorders, 16*, 407–423.

Jurko, M. F., & Andy, O. J. (1964). Psychological aspects of diencephalotomy. *Journal of Neurology, Neurosurgery, and Psychiatry, 27*, 516–521.

Kalteis, K., Tröster, A. I., & Alesch, F. (2002). Auswirkungen der tiefen Hirnstimulation auf neuropsychologische Funktionen bei Patienten mit Morbus Parkinson. *Aktuelle Neurologie, 29*, 490–498.

Kaplan, E., Fein, D., Morris, R., & Delis, D. C. (1991). *WAIS–R as a neuropsychological instrument*. San Antonio, TX: Psychological Corporation.

Kaszniak, A. W., Trosset, M. W., Bondi, M. W., & Bayles, K. A. (1992). Procedural learning of Parkinson's disease patients in a serial rection time task. *Journal of Clinical and Experimental Neuropsychology, 14*, 51.

Katai, S., Maruyama, T., Hashimoto, T., & Ikeda, S. (2003). Event based and time based prospective memory in Parkinson's disease. *Journal of Neurology, Neurosurgery, and Psychiatry, 74*, 704–709.

Kaufer, D. I. (2002). Pharmacologic therapy of dementia with Lewy bodies. *Journal of Geriatric Psychiatry and Neurology, 15*, 224–232.

Kegl, J. A., & Poizner, H. (1998). Shifting the burden to the interlocutors: Compensating for pragmatic deficits in signers. *Journal of Neurolinguistics, 11*, 137–152.

Kensinger, E. A., Shearer, D. K., Locascio, J. J., & Growdon, J. H. (2003). Working memory in mild Alzheimer's disease and early Parkinson's disease. *Neuropsychology, 17*, 230–239.

Knight, R. G., Godfrey, H. P. D., & Shelton, E. J. (1988). The psychological deficits associated with Parkinson's disease. *Clinical Psychology Review, 8*, 391–410.

Knoke, D., Taylor, A. E., & Saint-Cyr, J. A. (1998). The differential effects of cueing on recall in Parkinson's disease and normal subjects. *Brain and Cognition, 38*, 261–274.

Knowlton, B. J., Mangels, J. A., & Squire, L. R. (1996). A neostriatal habit learning system in humans. *Science, 273*, 1399–1402.

Koenig, O., Thomas-Antérion, C., & Laurent, B. (1999). Procedural learning in Parkinson's disease: Intact and impaired cognitive components. *Neuropsychologia, 37*, 1103–1109.

Koller, W. C., Glatt, S. L., Hubble, J. P., Paolo, A., Troster, A. I., Handler, M. S., et al. (1995). Apolipoprotein E genotypes in Parkinson's disease with and without dementia. *Annals of Neurology, 37*, 242–245.

Koller, W. C., Marjama, J., & Tröster, A. I. (2002). Psychogenic movement disorders. In J. Jankovic & E. Tolosa (Eds.), *Parkinson's disease and movement disorders* (4th ed., pp. 546–552). Philadelphia: Lippincott, Williams & Wilkins.

Koller, W. C., & Montgomery, E. B. (1997). Issues in the early diagnosis of Parkinson's disease. *Neurology, 49*, S10–S25.

Kosaka, K., Matsushita, M., Oyanagi, S., & Mehraein, P. (1980). A clinicopathological study of the "Lewy body disease". *Psychiatria et Neurologia Japonica, 82*, 292–311.

Kulisevsky, J., García-Sánchez, C., Berthier, M. L., Barbanoj, M., Pascual-Sedano, B., Gironell, A., & Estevez-Gonzalez, A. (2000). Chronic effects of dopaminergic replacement on cognitive function in Parkinson's disease: A two-year follow-up study of previously untreated patients. *Movement Disorders, 15*, 613–626.

Kuopio, A. M., Marttila, R. J., Helenius, H., & Rinne, U. K. (1999b). Environmental risk factors in Parkinson's disease. *Movement Disorders, 14*, 928–939.

Kuzis, G., Sabe, L., Tiberti, C., Leiguarda, R., & Starkstein, S. E. (1997). Cognitive functions in major depression and Parkinson disease. *Archives of Neurology, 54*, 982–986.

Kuzis, G., Sabe, L., Tiberti, C., Merello, M., Leiguarda, R., & Starkstein, S. E. (1999). Explicit and implicit learning in patients with Alzheimer disease and Parkinson disease with dementia. *Neuropsychiatry, Neuropsychology, and Behavioral Neurology, 12*, 265–269.

Lange, K. W., Robbins, T. W., Marsden, C. D., James, M., Owen, A. M., & Paul, G. M. (1992). L-dopa withdrawal in Parkinson's disease selectively impairs cognitive performance in tests sensitive to frontal lobe dysfunction. *Psychopharmacology, 107*, 394–404.

Lee, A. C., Harris, J. P., & Calvert, J. E. (1998). Impairments of mental rotation in Parkinson's disease. *Neuropsychologia, 36*, 109–114.

Lee, C., Grossman, M., Morris, J., Stern, M. B., & Hurtig, H. I. (2003). Attentional resource and processing speed limitations during sentence processing in Parkinson's disease. *Brain and Language, 85*, 347–356.

Lee, S. S., Wild, K., Hollnagel, C., & Grafman, J. (1999). Selective visual attention in patients with frontal lobe lesions or Parkinson's disease. *Neuropsychologia, 37*, 595–604.

Leentjens, A. F., Verhey, F. R., Lousberg, R., Spitsbergen, H., & Wilmink, F. W. (2000). The validity of the Hamilton and Montgomery-Asberg depression rating scales as screening and diagnostic tools for depression in Parkinson's disease. *International Journal of Geriatric Psychiatry, 15*, 644–649.

Leentjens, A. F. G., Verhey, F. R. J., Luijckx, G.-J., & Troost, J. (2000). The validity of the Beck Depression Inventory as a screening and diagnostic instrument for depression in patients with Parkinson's disease. *Movement Disorders, 15*, 1221–1224.

Lees, A. J., & Smith, E. (1983). Cognitive deficits in the early stages of Parkinson's disease. *Brain*, *106*, 257–270.

Leplow, B., Dierks, C., Herrmann, P., Pieper, N., Annecke, R., & Ulm, G. (1997). Remote memory in Parkinson's disease and senile dementia. *Neuropsychologia*, *35*, 547–557.

Levin, B. E., & Katzen, H. L. (1995). Early cognitive changes and nondementing behavioral abnormalities in Parkinson's disease. In W. J. Weiner & A. E. Lang (Eds.), *Advances in meurology: Vol. 65. Behavioral neurology of movement disorders* (pp. 85–95). New York: Raven Press.

Levin, B. E., Llabre, M. M., Reisman, S., Weiner, W. J., Sanchez-Ramos, J., Singer, C., & Brown, M. C. (1991). Visuospatial impairment in Parkinson's disease. *Neurology*, *41*, 365–369.

Levin, B. E., Llabre, M. M., & Weiner, W. J. (1989). Cognitive impairments associated with early Parkinson's disease. *Neurology*, *39*, 557–561.

Lewis, F. M., Lapointe, L. L., & Murdoch, B. E. (1998). Language impairment in Parkinson's disease. *Aphasiology*, *12*, 193–206.

Lewy, F. H. (1912). Paralysis agitans I. pathologische anatomie. In M. Lewandowsky (Ed.), *Handbuch der neurologie, band 3* (pp. 920–933). Berlin: Springer-Verlag.

Lewy, F. H. (1923). *Die Lehre vom Tonus und der Bewegung. Zugleich Systmatische Untersuchungen zur Klinik, Physiologie, Pathologie und Pathogenese der Paralysis Agitans.* Berlin: Julius Springer.

Lieberman, A. (1998). Managing the neuropsychiatric symptoms of Parkinson's disease. *Neurology*, *50*(Suppl. 6), S33–S38.

Lieberman, P., Friedman, J., & Feldman, L. S. (1990). Syntax comprehension deficits in Parkinson's disease. *Journal of Nervous and Mental Disease*, *178*, 360–365.

Loftus, E. F. (1971). Memory for intentions: The effect of presence of a cue and interpolated activity. *Psychonomic Science*, *23*, 315–316.

Lund-Johansen, M., Hugdahl, K., & Wester, K. (1996). Cognitive function in patients with Parkinson's disease undergoing stereotaxic thalamotomy. *Journal of Neurology, Neurosurgery, and Psychiatry*, *60*, 564–571.

Mahieux, F., Fenelon, G., Flahault, A., Manifacier, M. J., Michelet, D., & Boller, F. (1998). Neuropsychological prediction of dementia in Parkinson's disease. *Journal of Neurology, Neurosurgery, and Psychiatry*, *64*, 178–183.

Mahieux, F., Michelet, D., Manifacier, M.-J., Boller, F., Fermanian, J., & Guillard, A. (1995). Mini-Mental Parkinson: First validation study of a new bedside test constructed for Parkinson's disease. *Behavioural Neurology*, *8*, 15–22.

Marder, K., Tang, M. X., Cote, L., Stern, Y., & Mayeux, R. (1995). The frequency and associated risk factors for dementia in patients with Parkinson's disease. *Archives of Neurology*, *52*, 695–701.

Massman, P. J., Delis, D. C., Butters, N., Levin, B. E., & Salmon, D. P. (1990). Are all subcortical dementias alike? Verbal learning and memory in Parkinson's and Huntington's disease patients. *Journal of Clinical and Experimental Neuropsychology*, *12*, 729–744.

Matison, R., Mayeux, R., Rosen, J., & Fahn, S. (1982). "Tip-of-the-tongue" phenomenon in Parkinson disease. *Neurology*, *32*, 567–570.

Mattay, V. S., Tessitore, A., Callicott, J. H., Bertolino, A., Goldberg, T. E., Chase, T. N., et al. (2002). Dopaminergic modulation of cortical function in patients with Parkinson's disease. *Annals of Neurology*, *51*, 156–164.

Mattis, S. (1988). *Dementia Rating Scale*. Odessa, FL: Psychological Assessment Resources.

Mattis, S. (2001). *Dementia Rating Scale–2*. Lutz, FL: Psychological Assessment Resources, Inc.

Mayeux, R., Chen, J., Mirabello, E., Marder, K., Bell, K., Dooneief, G., et al. (1990). An estimate of the incidence of dementia in idiopathic Parkinson's disease. *Neurology, 40*, 1513–1517.

Mayeux, R., Marder, K., Cote, L. J., Denaro, J., Hemenegildo, N., Mejia, H., et al. (1995). The frequency of idiopathic Parkinson's disease by age, ethnic group, and sex in northern Manhattan, 1988–1993. *American Journal of Epidemiology, 142*, 820–827.

Mayeux, R., Stern, Y., Cote, L., & Williams, J. B. (1984). Altered serotonin metabolism in depressed patients with Parkinson's disease. *Neurology, 34*, 642–646.

McCarter, R. J., Walton, N. H., Rowan, A. F., Gill, S. S., & Palomo, M. (2000). Cognitive functioning after subthalamic nucleotomy for refractory Parkinson's disease. *Journal of Neurology, Neurosurgery, and Psychiatry, 69*, 60–66.

McFadden, L., Sampson, M., & Mohr, E. (1994). Screening for cognitive dysfunction in neurodegenerative illness. *Journal of Neurology, Neurosurgery, and Psychiatry, 57*, 1282.

McFie, J. (1960). Psychological effects of stereotaxic operations for the relief of parkinsonian symptoms. *Journal of Mental Science, 106*, 1512–1517.

McKeith, I., Del Ser, T., Spano, P., Emre, M., Wesnes, K., Anand, R., et al. (2000). Efficacy of rivastigmine in dementia with Lewy bodies: A randomised, double-blind, placebo-controlled international study. *Lancet, 356*, 2031–2036.

McKeith, I. G., Burn, D. J., Ballard, C. G., Collerton, D., Jaros, E., Morris, C. M., et al. (2003). Dementia with Lewy bodies. *Seminars in Clinical Neuropsychiatry, 8*, 46–57.

McNamara, P., & Durso, R. (2003). Pragmatic communication skills in patients with Parkinson's disease. *Brain and Language, 84*, 414–423.

McNamara, P., Durso, R., Brown, A., & Lynch, A. (2003). Counterfactual cognitive deficit in persons with Parkinson's disease. *Journal of Neurology, Neurosurgery, and Psychiatry, 74*, 1065–1070.

Mega, M. S., & Cummings, J. L. (1994). Frontal-subcortical circuits and neuropsychiatric disorders. *Journal of Neuropsychiatry and Clinical Neuroscience, 6*, 358–370.

Mentis, M. J., McIntosh, A. R., Perrine, K., Dhawan, V., Berlin, B., Feigin, A., et al. (2002). Relationships among the metabolic patterns that correlate with mnemonic, visuospatial, and mood symptoms in Parkinson's disease. *American Journal of Psychiatry, 159*, 746–754.

Merello, M., Nouzeilles, M. I., Kuzis, G., Cammarota, A., Sabe, L., Betti, O., et al. (1999). Unilateral radiofrequency lesion versus electrostimulation of posteroventral pallidum: A prospective randomized comparison. *Movement Disorders, 14*, 50–56.

Middleton, F. A., & Strick, P. L. (2000). Basal ganglia output and cognition: Evidence from anatomical, behavioral, and clinical studies. *Brain and Cognition, 42*, 183–200.

Mohr, E., Juncos, J., Cox, C., Litvan, I., Fedio, P., & Chase, T. N. (1990). Selective deficits in cognition and memory in high-functioning parkinsonian patients. *Journal of Neurology, Neurosurgery, and Psychiatry, 53*, 603–606.

Mohr, E., Mendis, T., & Grimes, J. D. (1995). Late cognitive changes in Parkinson's disease with an emphasis on dementia. *Advances in Neurology, 65,* 97–113.

Molina, J. A., Sainz-Artiga, M. J., Fraile, A., Jimenez-Jimenez, F. J., Villanueva, C., Orti-Pareja, M., & Bermejo, F. (2000). Pathologic gambling in Parkinson's disease: A behavioral manifestation of pharmacologic treatment? *Movement Disorders, 15,* 869–872.

Montgomery, S. A., & Åsberg, M. (1979). A new depression scale designed to be sensitive to change. *British Journal of Psychiatry, 134,* 382–389.

Morris, R. G., Downes, J. J., Sahakian, B. J., Evenden, J. L., Heald, A., & Robbins, T. W. (1988). Planning and spatial working memory in Parkinson's disease. *Journal of Neurology, Neurosurgery, and Psychiatry, 51,* 757–766.

Murray, L. L. (2000). Spoken language production in Huntington's and Parkinson's diseases. *Journal of Speech, Language, and Hearing Research, 43,* 1350–1366.

Naarding, P., Leentjens, A. F., van Kooten, F., & Verhey, F. R. (2002). Disease-specific properties of the Hamilton Rating Scale for depression in patients with stroke, Alzheimer's dementia, and Parkinson's disease. *Journal of Neuropsychiatry and Clinical Neurosciences, 14,* 329–334.

Naville, F. (1922). Les complications et let sequelles mentales de l'encephalite epidemique. *Encephale, 17,* 369–375, 423–436.

Nelson, D. L., & McEvoy, C. L. (1979). Encoding context and set size. *Journal of Experimental Psychology: Human Learning and Memory, 5,* 292–314.

Norman, S., Tröster, A. I., Fields, J. A., & Brooks, R. (2002). Effects of depression and Parkinson's disease on cognitive functioning. *Journal of Neuropsychiatry and Clinical Neuroscience, 14,* 31–36.

Owen, A. M., Doyon, J., Dagher, A., Sadikot, A., & Evans, A. C. (1998). Abnormal basal ganglia outflow in Parkinson's disease identified with PET: Implications for higher cortical functions. *Brain, 121,* 949–965.

Owen, A. M., James, M., Leigh, P. N., Summers, B. A., Marsden, C. D., Quinn, N. P., et al. (1992). Fronto-striatal cognitive deficits at different stages of Parkinson's disease. *Brain, 115,* 1727–1751.

Owen, A. M., Roberts, A. C., Hodges, J. R., Summers, B. A., Polkey, C. E., & Robbins, T. W. (1993). Contrasting mechanisms of impaired attentional set-shifting in patients with frontal lobe damage or Parkinson's disease. *Brain, 116,* 1159–1175.

Owen, A. M., Sahakian, B. J., Hodges, J. R., Summers, B. A., Polkey, C. E., & Robbins, T. W. (1995). Dopamine-dependent fronto-striatal planning deficits in early Parkinson's disease. *Neuropsychology, 9,* 126–140.

Paolo, A. M., Tröster, A. I., Glatt, S. L., Hubble, J. P., & Koller, W. C. (1995). Differentiation of the dementias of Alzheimer's and Parkinson's disease with the Dementia Rating Scale. *Journal of Geriatric Psychiatry and Neurology, 8,* 184–188.

Parkinson, J. (1817). *An essay on the shaking palsy.* London: Sherwood, Neely & Jones.

Pascual-Leone, A., Grafman, J., Clark, K., Stewart, M., Massaquoi, S., Lou, J. S., & Hallett, M. (1993). Procedural learning in Parkinson's disease and cerebellar degeneration. *Annals of Neurology, 34,* 594–602.

Passafiume, D., Boller, F., & Keefe, M. C. (1986). Neuropsychological impairment in patients with Parkinson's disease. In I. Grant & K. M. Adams (Eds.), *Neuropsychological assessment of neuropsychiatric disorders* (pp. 374–383). New York: Oxford University Press.

Peavy, G. M., Salmon, D., Bear, P. I., Paulsen, J. S., Cahn, D. A., Hofstetter, C. R., et al. (2001). Detection of mild cognitive deficits in Parkinson's disease patients with the WAIS–R NI. *Journal of the International Neuropsychological Society, 7*, 535–543.

Perry, E. K., Curtis, M., Dick, D. J., Candy, J. M., Atack, J. R., Bloxham, C. A., et al. (1985). Cholinergic correlates of cognitive impairment in Parkinson's disease: Comparisons with Alzheimer's disease. *Journal of Neurology, Neurosurgery, and Psychiatry, 48*, 413–421.

Piatt, A. L., Fields, J. A., Paolo, A. M., Koller, W. C., & Tröster, A. I. (1999). Lexical, semantic, and verb fluency in Parkinson's disease with and without dementia. *Journal of Clinical and Experimental Neuropsychology, 21*, 435–443.

Piccirilli, M., D'Alessandro, P., Finali, G., Piccinin, G. L., & Agostini, L. (1989). Frontal lobe dysfunction in Parkinson's disease: Prognostic value for dementia? *European Neurology, 29*, 71–76.

Pillon, B., Ardouin, C., Damier, P., Krack, P., Houeto, J. L., Klinger, H., et al. (2000). Neuropsychological changes between "off" and "on" STN or GPi stimulation in Parkinson's disease. *Neurology, 55*, 411–418.

Pillon, B., Boller, F., Levy, R., & Dubois, B. (2001). Cognitive deficits and dementia in Parkinson's disease. In F. Boller & S. F. Cappa (Eds.), *Handbook of neuropsychology* (2nd ed., Vol. 6, pp. 311–371). Amsterdam: Elsevier.

Pillon, B., Deweer, B., Vidailhet, M., Bonnet, A. M., Hahn-Barma, V., & Dubois, B. (1998). Is impaired memory for spatial location in Parkinson's disease domain specific or dependent on "strategic" processes? *Neuropsychologia, 36*, 1–9.

Pillon, B., Dubois, B., Cusimano, G., Bonnet, A. M., Lhermitte, F., & Agid, Y. (1989). Does cognitive impairment in Parkinson's disease result from non-dopaminergic lesions? *Journal of Neurology, Neurosurgery, and Psychiatry, 52*, 201–206.

Pillon, B., Dubois, B., Lhermitte, F., & Agid, Y. (1986). Heterogeneity of cognitive impairment in progressive supranuclear palsy, Parkinson's disease, and Alzheimer's disease. *Neurology, 36*, 1179–1185.

Pillon, B., Dubois, B., Ploska, A., & Agid, Y. (1991). Severity and specificity of cognitive impairment in Alzheimer's, Huntington's, and Parkinson's diseases and progressive supranuclear palsy. *Neurology, 41*, 634–643.

Pirozzolo, F. J., Hansch, E. C., Mortimer, J. A., Webster, D. D., & Kuskowski, M. A. (1982). Dementia in Parkinson disease: A neuropsychological analysis. *Brain and Cognition, 1*, 71–83.

Pondal, M., Del Ser, T., & Bermejo, F. (1996). Anticholinergic therapy and dementia in patients with Parkinson's disease. *Journal of Neurology, 243*, 543–546.

Postle, B. R., Locascio, J. J., Corkin, S., & Growdon, J. H. (1997). The time course of spatial and object learning in Parkinson's disease. *Neuropsychologia, 35*, 1413–1422.

Psychological Corporation. (1997). *WAIS–III/WMS–III technical manual* . San Antonio, TX: Author.

Randolph, C., Braun, A. R., Goldberg, T. E., & Chase, T. N. (1993). Semantic fluency in Alzheimer's, Parkinson's, and Huntington's disease: Dissociation of storage and retrieval failures. *Neuropsychology, 7*, 82–88.

Ransmayr, G., Schmidhuber-Eiler, B., Karamat, E., Engler-Plörer, S., Poewe, W., & Leidlmair, K. (1987). Visuoperception and visuospatial and visuorotational performance in Parkinson's disease. *Journal of Neurology, 235*, 99–101.

Reading, P. J., Luce, A. K., & McKeith, I. G. (2001). Rivastigmine in the treatment of parkinsonian psychosis and cognitive impairment: Preliminary findings from an open trial. *Movement Disorders, 16,* 1171–1174.

Reber, P. J., & Squire, L. R. (1999). Intact learning of artificial grammars and intact category learning by patients with Parkinson's disease. *Behavioral Neuroscience, 113,* 235–242.

Rieger, M., Gauggel, S., & Burmeister, K. (2003). Inhibition of ongoing responses following frontal, nonfrontal, and basal ganglia lesions. *Neuropsychology, 17,* 272–282.

Riklan, M., & Levita, E. (1969). *Subcortical correlates of human behavior: A psychological study of thalamic and basal ganglia surgery.* Baltimore: Williams & Wilkins.

Robbins, T. W., Owen, A. M., & Sahakian, B. J. (1998). The neuropsychology of basal ganglia disorders: An integrative cognitive and comparative approach. In M. A. Ron & A. S. David (Eds.), *Disorders of brain and mind* (pp. 57–83). Cambridge, UK: Cambridge University Press.

Roncacci, S., Troisi, E., Carlesimo, G. A., Nocentini, U., & Caltagirone, C. (1996). Implicit memory in parkinsonian patients: Evidence for deficient skill learning. *European Neurology, 36,* 154–159.

Ross, H. F., Hughes, T. A., Boyd, J. L., Biggins, C. A., Madeley, P., Mindham, R. H., & Spokes, E. G. (1996). The evolution and profile of dementia in Parkinson's disease. In L. Battistin, G. Scarlato, T. Caraceni, & S. Ruggieri (Eds.), *Advances in neurology* (Vol. 69, pp. 343–347). Philadelphia: Lippincott-Raven Publishers.

Rothlind, J. C., & Brandt, J. (1993). A brief assessment of frontal and subcortical functions in dementia. *Journal of Neuropsychiatry and Clinical Neurosciences, 5,* 73–77.

Rouleau, I., Imbault, H., Laframboise, M., & Bedard, M. A. (2001). Pattern of intrusions in verbal recall: Comparison of Alzheimer's disease, Parkinson's disease, and frontal lobe dementia. *Brain Cognition, 46*(1–2), 244–249.

Rowe, A. D., Bullock, P. R., Polkey, C. E., & Morris, R. G. (2001). "Theory of mind" impairments and their relationship to executive functioning following frontal lobe excisions. *Brain, 124,* 600–616.

Sagar, H. J., Cohen, N. J., Sullivan, E. V., Corkin, S., & Growdon, J. H. (1988). Remote memory function in Alzheimer's disease and Parkinson's disease. *Brain, 111,* 185–206.

Sahgal, A., Galloway, P. H., McKeith, I. G., Lloyd, S., Cook, J. H., Ferrier, I. N., & Edwardson, J. A. (1992). Matching-to-sample deficits in patients with senile dementias of the Alzheimer and Lewy body types. *Archives of Neurology, 49,* 1043–1046.

Saint-Cyr, J. A. (2003). Frontal-striatal circuit functions: Context, sequence, and consequence. *Journal of the International Neuropsychological Society, 9,* 103–127.

Saint-Cyr, J. A., Taylor, A. E., & Lang, A. E. (1988). Procedural learning and neostriatal dysfunction in man. *Brain, 111,* 941–959.

Saint-Cyr, J. A., Taylor, A. E., & Lang, A. E. (1993). Neuropsychological and psychiatric side effects in the treatment of Parkinson's disease. *Neurology, 43*(Suppl. 6), S47–S52.

Saint-Cyr, J. A., & Trépanier, L. L. (2000). Neuropsychologic assessment of patients for movement disorder surgery. *Movement Disorders, 15,* 771–783.

Salmon, D. P., & Galasko, D. (1996). Neuropsychological aspects of Lewy body dementia. In R. Perry, I. McKeith, & E. Perry (Eds.), *Dementia with Lewy bodies:*

Clinical, pathological, and treatment issues (pp. 99–113). Cambridge, UK: Cambridge University Press.

Salmon, D. P., Galasko, D., Hansen, L. A., Masliah, E., Butters, N., Thal, L. J., & Katzman, R. (1996). Neuropsychological deficits associated with diffuse Lewy body disease. *Brain and Cognition*, *31*, 148–165.

Saltzman, J., Strauss, E., Hunter, M., & Archibald, S. (2000). Theory of mind and executive functions in normal human aging and Parkinson's disease. *Journal of the International Neuropsychological Society*, *6*, 781–788.

Schiller, F. (2000). Fritz Lewy and his bodies. *Journal of the History of the Neurosciences*, *9*, 148–151.

Schroeder, U., Kuehler, A., Hennenlotter, A., Haslinger, B., Tronnier, V. M., Krause, M., et al. (2004). Facial expression recognition and subthalamic nucleus stimulation. *Journal of Neurology Neurosurgery and Psychiatry*, *75*, 648–650.

Scott, R., Gregory, R., Hines, N., Carroll, C., Hyman, N., Papanasstasiou, V., et al. (1998). Neuropsychological, neurological and functional outcome following pallidotomy for Parkinson's disease: A consecutive series of eight simultaneous bilateral and twelve unilateral procedures. *Brain*, *121*, 659–675.

Scott, R. B., Harrison, J., Boulton, C., Wilson, J., Gregory, R., Parkin, S., et al. (2002). Global attentional-executive sequelae following surgical lesions to globus pallidus interna. *Brain*, *125*, 562–574.

Scott, S., Caird, F. I., & Williams, B. O. (1984). Evidence for an apparent sensory speech disorder in Parkinson's disease. *Journal of Neurology, Neurosurgery, and Psychiatry*, *47*, 840–843.

Seedat, S., Kesler, S., Niehaus, D. J., & Stein, D. J. (2000). Pathological gambling behaviour: Emergence secondary to treatment of Parkinson's disease with dopaminergic agents. *Depression and Anxiety*, *11*, 185–186.

Seidler, A., Hellenbrand, W., Robra, B. P., Vieregge, P., Nischan, P., Joerg, J., et al. (1996). Possible environmental, occupational, and other etiologic factors for Parkinson's disease: A case-control study in Germany. *Neurology*, *46*, 1275–1284.

Seltzer, B., Vasterling, J. J., Mathias, C. W., & Brennan, A. (2001). Clinical and neuropsychological correlates of impaired awareness of deficits in Alzheimer disease and Parkinson disease: A comparative study. *Neuropsychiatry, Neuropsychology, and Behavioral Neurology*, *14*, 122–129.

Shapiro, D. Y., Sadowsky, D. A., Henderson, W. G., & van Buren, J. M. (1973). An assessment of cognitive function in postthalamotomy Parkinson patients. *Confinia Neurologica*, *35*, 144–166.

Shaskin, D., Yarnell, H., & Alper, K. (1942). Physical, psychiatric, and psychometric studies of post-encephalitic parkinsonism. *Journal of Nervous and Mental Disease*, *96*, 652–662.

Shimomura, T., Mori, E., Yamashita, H., Imamura, T., Hirono, N., Hashimoto, M., et al. (1998). Cognitive loss in dementia with Lewy bodies and Alzheimer disease. *Archives of Neurology*, *55*, 1547–1552.

Siegfried, J., & Blond, S. (1997). *The neurosurgical treatment of Parkinson's disease and other movement disorders*. London: Williams & Wilkins Europe Ltd.

Skeel, R. L., Crosson, B., Nadeau, S. E., Algina, J., Bauer, R. M., & Fennell, E. B. (2001). Basal ganglia dysfunction, working memory, and sentence comprehension in patients with Parkinson's disease. *Neuropsychologia*, *39*, 962–971.

Snowden, J. S., Gibbons, Z. C., Blackshaw, A., Doubleday, E., Thompson, J., Craufurd, D., et al. (2003). Social cognition in frontotemporal dementia and Huntington's disease. *Neuropsychologia*, *41*, 688–701.

Sommer, M., Grafman, J., Clark, K., & Hallett, M. (1999). Learning in Parkinson's disease: Eyeblink conditioning, declarative learning, and procedural learning. *Journal of Neurology, Neurosurgery, and Psychiatry*, *67*, 27–34.

Spicer, K. B., Brown, G. G., & Gorell, J. M. (1994). Lexical decision in Parkinson disease: Lack of evidence for generalized bradyphrenia. *Journal of Clinical and Experimental Neuropsychology*, *16*, 457–471.

Starkstein, S. E., Bolduc, P. L., Mayberg, H. S., Preziosi, T. J., & Robinson, R. G. (1990). Cognitive impairments and depression in Parkinson's disease: A follow up study. *Journal of Neurology, Neurosurgery, and Psychiatry*, *53*, 597–602.

Starkstein, S. E., Sabe, L., Petracca, G., Chemerinski, E., Kuzis, G., Merello, M., & Leiguarda, R. (1996). Neuropsychological and psychiatric differences between Alzheimer's disease and Parkinson's disease with dementia. *Journal of Neurology, Neurosurgery, and Psychiatry*, *61*, 381–387.

Stebbins, G. T., Gabrieli, J. D., Masciari, F., Monti, L., & Goetz, C. G. (1999). Delayed recognition memory in Parkinson's disease: A role for working memory? *Neuropsychologia*, *37*, 503–510.

Stefanova, E. D., Kostic, V. S., Ziropadja, L. J., Ocic, G. G., & Markovic, M. (2001). Declarative memory in early Parkinson's disease: serial position learning effects. *Journal of Clinical and Experimental Neuropsychology*, *23*, 581–591.

Stern, Y., & Langston, J. W. (1985). Intellectual changes in patients with MPTP-induced parkinsonism. *Neurology*, *35*, 1506–1509.

Stern, Y., Mayeux, R., & Cote, L. (1984). Reaction time and vigilance in Parkinson's disease: Possible role of altered norepinephrine metabolism. *Archives of Neurology*, *41*, 1086–1089.

Stern, Y., Mayeux, R., & Rosen, J. (1984). Contribution of perceptual motor dysfunction to construction and tracing disturbances in Parkinson's disease. *Journal of Neurology, Neurosurgery, and Psychiatry*, *47*, 983–989.

Stern, Y., Tang, M. X., Jacobs, D. M., Sano, M., Marder, K., Bell, K., et al. (1998). Prospective comparative study of the evolution of probable Alzheimer's disease and Parkinson's disease dementia. *Journal of the International Neuropsychological Society*, *4*, 279–284.

Stout, J. C., Rodawalt, W. C., & Siemers, E. R. (2001). Risky decision making in Huntington's disease. *Journal of the International Neuropsychological Society*, *7*, 92–101.

Stuss, D. T., Gallup, G. G., Jr., & Alexander, M. P. (2001). The frontal lobes are necessary for "theory of mind". *Brain*, *124*, 279–286.

Suhr, J. A., & Jones, R. D. (1998). Letter and semantic fluency in Alzheimer's, Huntington's, and Parkinson's dementias. *Archives of Clinical Neuropsychology*, *13*, 447–454.

Sullivan, E. V., & Sagar, H. J. (1989). Nonverbal recognition and recency discrimination deficits in Parkinson's disease and Alzheimer's disease. *Brain*, *112*, 1503–1517.

Sullivan, E. V., Sagar, H. J., Gabrieli, J. D., Corkin, S., & Growdon, J. H. (1989). Different cognitive profiles on standard behavioral tests in Parkinson's disease and Alzheimer's disease. *Journal of Clinical and Experimental Neuropsychology*, *11*, 799–820.

Tanner, C. M. (1989). The role of environmental toxins in the etiology of Parkinson's disease. *Trends in Neurosciences*, *12*, 49–54.

Tanner, C. M., Chen, B., Wang, W. Z., Peng, M., Liu, Z., Liang, X., et al. (1987). Environmental factors in the etiology of Parkinson's disease. *Canadian Journal of Neurological Sciences*, *14*, 419–423.

Tanner, C. M., Goldman, S., & Ross, G. W. (2002). Etiology of Parkinson's disease. In J. J. Jankovic & E. Tolosa (Eds.), *Parkinson's disease & movement disorders* (pp. 90–103). Philadelphia: Lippincott, Williams & Wilkins.

Tanner, C. M., Hubble, J. P., & Chan, P. (1997). Epidemiology and genetics of Parkinson's disease. In R. L. Watts & W. C. Koller (Eds.), *Movement disorders: Neurologic principles and practice* (pp. 137–152). New York: McGraw-Hill.

Tanner, C. M., Ottman, R., Goldman, S. M., Ellenberg, J., Chan, P., Mayeux, R., & Langston, J. W. (1999). Parkinson disease in twins: An etiologic study. *Journal of the American Medical Association*, *281*, 341–346.

Taylor, A. E., & Saint-Cyr, J. A. (1995). The neuropsychology of Parkinson's disease. *Brain and Cognition*, *28*, 281–296.

Taylor, A. E., Saint-Cyr, J. A., & Lang, A. E. (1986). Frontal lobe dysfunction in Parkinson's disease: The cortical focus of neostriatal outflow. *Brain*, *109*, 845–883.

Taylor, A. E., Saint-Cyr, J. A., & Lang, A. E. (1987). Parkinson's disease: Cognitive changes in relation to treatment response. *Brain*, *110*, 35–51.

Taylor, A. E., Saint-Cyr, J. A., & Lang, A. E. (1990). Memory and learning in early Parkinson's disease: Evidence for a "frontal lobe syndrome". *Brain and Cognition*, *13*, 211–232.

Tierney, M. C., Nores, A., Snow, W. G., Fisher, R. H., Zorzitto, M. L., & Reid, D. W. (1994). Use of the Rey Auditory Verbal Learning Test in differentiating normal aging from Alzheimer's and Parkinson's dementia. *Psychological Assessment*, *6*, 129–134.

Trennerry, M. R., Crosson, B., deBoe, J., & Leber, W. R. (1990). *Visual Search and Attention Test*. Odessa, FL: Psychological Assessment Resources.

Trépanier, L. L., Kumar, R., Lozano, A. M., Lang, A. E., & Saint-Cyr, J. A. (2000). Neuropsychological outcome of GPi pallidotomy and GPi or STN deep brain stimulation in Parkinson's disease. *Brain and Cognition*, *42*, 324–347.

Tröster, A. I. (1998). Assessment of movement and demyelinating disorders. In P. J. Snyder & P. D. Nussbaum (Eds.), *Clinical neuropsychology: A pocket handbook for assessment* (pp. 266–303). Washington, DC: American Psychological Association.

Tröster, A. I. & Arnett, P. J. (in press). Assessment of movement and demyelinating disorders. In P. J. Snyder, P. D. Nussbaum, & D. L. Robins (Eds.), *Clinical neuropsychology: A pocket handbook for assessment* (2nd ed.). Washington, DC: American Psychological Association.

Tröster, A. I., & Fields, J. A. (1995). Frontal cognitive function and memory in Parkinson's disease: Toward a distinction between prospective and declarative memory impairments? *Behavioural Neurology*, *8*, 59–74.

Tröster, A. I., & Fields, J. A. (2003a). Apolipoprotein E genotype and memory in healthy elderly and Parkinson's disease [Abstract]. *Journal of the International Neuropsychological Society*, *9*, 525.

Tröster, A. I., & Fields, J. A. (2003b). The role of neuropsychological evaluation in the neurosurgical treatment of movement disorders. In D. Tarsy, J. L. Vitek, & A. M. Lozano (Eds.), *Surgical treatment of Parkinson's disease and other movement disorders* (pp. 213–240). Totowa, NJ: Humana Press.

Tröster, A. I., Fields, J. A., & Koller, W. C. (2000). Parkinson's disease and parkinsonism. In C. E. Coffey & J. L. Cummings (Eds.), *Textbook of geriatric neuropsychiatry* (2nd ed., pp. 559–600). Washington, DC: American Psychiatric Press.

Tröster, A. I., Fields, J. A., Paolo, A. M., & Koller, W. C. (1996). Performance of individuals with Parkinson's disease on the Vocabulary and Information subtests of the WAIS–R as a neuropsychological instrument. *Journal of Clinical Geropsychology, 2*, 215–223.

Tröster, A. I., Fields, J. A., Paolo, A. M., Pahwa, R., & Koller, W. C. (1996). Visual confrontation naming in Alzheimer's disease and Parkinson's disease with dementia [Abstract]. *Neurology, 46*(Suppl), A292–A293.

Tröster, A. I., Fields, J. A., Testa, J. A., Paul, R. H., Blanco, C. R., Hames, K. A., et al. (1998). Cortical and subcortical influences on clustering and switching in the performance of verbal fluency tasks. *Neuropsychologia, 36*, 295–304.

Tröster, A. I., Fields, J. A., Wilkinson, S. B., Busenbark, K., Miyawaki, E., Overman, J., et al. (1997). Neuropsychological functioning before and after unilateral thalamic stimulating electrode implantation in Parkinson's disease [Electronic version]. *Neurosurgical Focus, 2*, Article 9, 1–6.

Tröster, A. I., Fields, J. A., Wilkinson, S. B., Pahwa, R., Miyawaki, E., Lyons, K. E., & Koller, W. C. (1997). Unilateral pallidal stimulation for Parkinson's disease: Neurobehavioral functioning before and 3 months after electrode implantation. *Neurology, 49*, 1078–1083.

Tröster, A. I., & Letsch, E. A. (2004). Evaluation and treatment of anxiety and depression in Parkinson's disease. In R. Pahwa, K. E. Lyons, & W. C. Koller (Eds.), *Therapy of Parkinson's disease* (3rd ed., pp. 423–446). New York: Marcel Dekker.

Tröster, A. I., Paolo, A. M., Lyons, K. E., Glatt, S. L., Hubble, J. P., & Koller, W. C. (1995). The influence of depression on cognition in Parkinson's disease: A pattern of impairment distinguishable from Alzheimer's disease. *Neurology, 45*, 672–676.

Tröster, A. I., Stalp, L. D., Paolo, A. M., Fields, J. A., & Koller, W. C. (1995). Neuropsychological impairment in Parkinson's disease with and without depression. *Archives of Neurology, 52*, 1164–1169.

Tröster, A. I., & Woods, S. P. (2003). Neuropsychological aspects of Parkinson's disease and parkinsonian syndromes. In R. Pahwa, K. E. Lyons, & W. C. Koller (Eds.), *Handbook of Parkinson's disease* (3rd ed., pp. 127–157). New York: Marcel Dekker.

Tröster, A. I., Woods, S. P., & Fields, J. A. (2003). Verbal fluency declines after pallidotomy: An interaction between task and lesion laterality. *Applied Neuropsychology, 10*, 69–75.

Tröster, A. I., Woods, S. P., Fields, J. A., Hanisch, C., & Beatty, W. W. (2002). Declines in switching underlie verbal fluency changes after unilateral pallidal surgery in Parkinson's disease. *Brain and Cognition, 50*, 207–217.

Troyer, A. K., Moscovitch, M., & Winocur, G. (1997). Clustering and switching as two components of verbal fluency: Evidence from younger and older healthy adults. *Neuropsychology, 11*, 138–146.

Troyer, A. K., Moscovitch, M., Winocur, G., Leach, L., & Freedman, M. (1998). Clustering and switching on verbal fluency tests in Alzheimer's and Parkinson's disease. *Journal of the International Neuropsychological Society, 4*, 137–143.

Ullman, M. T., Corkin, S., Coppola, M., Hickok, G., Growdon, J. H., Koroshetz, W. J., & Pinker, S. (1997). A neural dissociation within language: Evidence that the mental dictionary is part of declarative memory, and that grammatical rules are processed by the procedural system. *Journal of Cognitive Neuroscience, 9*, 266–276.

Vakil, E., & Herishanu-Naaman, S. (1998). Declarative and procedural learning in Parkinson's disease patients having tremor or bradykinesia as the predominant symptom. *Cortex*, *34*, 611–620.

Van den Broek, M. D., Downes, J., Johnson, Z., Dayus, B., & Hilton, N. (2000). Evaluation of an electronic memory aid in the neuropsychological rehabilitation of prospective memory deficits. *Brain Injury*, *14*, 455–462.

Van Oostrom, I., Dollfus, S., Brazo, P., Abadie, P., Halbecq, I., Thery, S., & Marie, R. M. (2003). Verbal learning and memory in schizophrenic and Parkinson's disease patients. *Psychiatry Research*, *117*, 25–34.

Van Spaendonck, K. P. M., Berger, H. J. C., Horstink, M. W. I. M., Borm, G. F., & Cools, A. R. (1995). Card sorting performance in Parkinson's disease: A comparison between acquisition and shifting performance. *Journal of Clinical and Experimental Neuropsychology*, *17*, 918–925.

Venneri, A., Nichelli, P., Modonesi, G., Molinari, M. A., Russo, R., & Sardini, C. (1997). Impairment in dating and retrieving remote events in patients with early Parkinson's disease. *Journal of Neurology, Neurosurgery, and Psychiatry*, *62*, 410–413.

Vilkki, J., & Laitinen, L. V. (1974). Differential effects of left and right ventrolateral thalamotomy on receptive and expressive verbal performances and face-matching. *Neuropsychologia*, *12*, 11–19.

Vriezen, E. R., & Moscovitch, M. (1990). Memory for temporal order and conditional associative-learning in patients with Parkinson's disease. *Neuropsychologia*, *28*, 1283–1293.

Walker, M. P., Ayre, G. A., Perry, E. K., Wesnes, K., McKeith, I. G., Tovee, M., et al. (2000). Quantification and characterisation of fluctuating cognition in dementia with Lewy bodies and Alzheimer's disease. *Dementia and Geriatric Cognitive Disorders*, *11*, 327–335.

Walker, Z., Allen, R. L., Shergill, S., & Katona, C. L. (1997). Neuropsychological performance in Lewy body dementia and Alzheimer's disease. *British Journal of Psychiatry*, *170*, 156–158.

Welman, A. J. (1971). Neuropsychologische Untersuchung von Parkinsonpatienten (Vor und nach Thalomotomie). *Schweizer Archiv für Neurologie, Neurochirurgie und Psychiatrie*, *108*, 175–188.

West, R., Ergis, A. M., Winocur, G., & Saint-Cyr, J. (1998). The contribution of impaired working memory monitoring to performance of the self-ordered pointing task in normal aging and Parkinson's disease. *Neuropsychology*, *12*, 546–554.

Whittington, C. J., Podd, J., & Kan, M. M. (2000). Recognition memory impairment in Parkinson's disease: Power and meta-analyses. *Neuropsychology*, *14*, 233–246.

Witjas, T., Kaphan, E., Azulay, J. P., Blin, O., Ceccaldi, M., Pouget, J., et al. (2002). Nonmotor fluctuations in Parkinson's disease: Frequent and disabling. *Neurology*, *59*, 408–413.

Witt, K., Nuhsman, A., & Deuschl, G. (2002a). Dissociation of habit-learning in Parkinson's and cerebellar disease. *Journal of Cognitive Neuroscience*, *14*, 493–499.

Witt, K., Nuhsman, A., & Deuschl, G. (2002b). Intact artificial grammar learning in patients with cerebellar degeneration and advanced Parkinson's disease. *Neuropsychologia*, *40*, 1534–1540.

Woods, S. P., Fields, J. A., Lyons, K. E., Koller, W. C., Wilkinson, S. B., Pahwa, R., & Troster, A. I. (2001). Neuropsychological and quality of life changes following unilateral thalamic deep brain stimulation in Parkinson's disease: A 12-month follow-up. *Acta Neurochirurgica*, *143*, 1273–1278.

Woods, S. P., Fields, J. A., & Tröster. A. I. (2002). Neuropsychological sequelae of subthalamic nucleus deep brain stimulation in Parkinson's disease: A critical review. *Neuropsychology Review, 12*, 111–126.

Woods, S. P., & Tröster, A. I. (2003). Prodromal frontal/executive dysfunction predicts incident dementia in Parkinson's disease. *Journal of the International Neuropsychological Society, 9*, 17–24.

Woodward, T. S., Bub, D. N., & Hunter, M. A. (2002). Task switching deficits associated with Parkinson's disease reflect depleted attentional resources. *Neuropsychologia, 40*, 1948–1955.

Xuereb, J. H., Tomlinson, B. E., Irving, D., Perry, R. H., Blessed, G., & Perry, E. K. (1990). Cortical and subcortical pathology in Parkinson's disease: Relationship to parkinsonian dementia. *Advances in Neurology, 53*, 35–40.

Yamada, T., Izyuuinn, M., Schulzer, M., & Hirayama, K. (1990). Covert orienting attention in Parkinson's disease. *Journal of Neurology, Neurosurgery, and Psychiatry, 53*, 593–596.

Yamadori, A., Yoshida, T., Mori, E., & Yamashita, H. (1996). Neurological basis of skill learning. *Cognitive Brain Research, 5*, 49–54.

Zakzanis, K. K., & Freedman, M. (1999). A neuropsychological comparison of demented and nondemented patients with Parkinson's disease. *Applied Neuropsychology, 6*, 129–146.

Zec, R. F., Landreth, E. S., Fritz, S., Grames, E., Hasara, A., Fraizer, W., et al. (1999). A comparison of phonemic, semantic, and alternating word fluency in Parkinson's disease. *Archives of Clinical Neuropsychology, 14*, 255–264.

Zhang, Z. X., & Roman, G. C. (1993). Worldwide occurrence of Parkinson's disease: An updated review. *Neuroepidemiology, 12*, 195–208.

11 Traumatic brain injury and the older adult

Thomas A. Martin and Brick Johnstone

Traumatic brain injury (TBI) is a leading cause of death and disability in the United States with an estimated 1.5–2 million TBIs occurring annually. Each year, these injuries result in approximately one million hospital emergency room visits; 230,000 hospitalizations; and 51,000 deaths (Thurman, Alverson, Dunn, Guerrero, & Sniezek, 1999; Woo & Thoidis, 2000). Additionally, 80,000–90,000 of TBI survivors will experience the onset of long-term disability, with the National Institutes of Health (NIH) estimating that as many as 6.5 million Americans are currently living with TBI-related disabilities (NIH, 1999).

The incidence of TBI is greatest in the 15- to 24-year-old age group, with children under the age of 5 and adults older than 65 also at increased risk (Ferrell & Tanev, 2002). Among persons of all ages, males are more than twice as likely as females to incur a TBI, although this male to female ratio decreases in the elderly (Schootman, Harlan, & Fuortes, 2000; Woo & Thoidis, 2000). While motor vehicle accidents are the leading cause of TBI among all persons, falls are the leading cause of TBI in individuals over age 74 (Woo & Thoidis, 2000). TBI-related mortality rates are highest in the 15- to 24-year-old age group at 33 per 100,000, with the elderly mortality rate estimated to be 31 per 100,000 (Woo & Thoidis, 2000).

United States census figures for 2000 indicate that 35 million people, or 12.4 % of the US population, were aged 65 or older (US Census Bureau, 2000a). This segment of the population is projected to grow in the coming years, with this age group predicted to total 47 million in 2016 and 62 million in the year 2025 (US Census Bureau, 2000b). As the number of elderly Americans increases, the number affected by TBI is also expected to grow (Fife, Faich, Hollinshead, & Wentworth, 1986; Jagger, Levine, Jane, & Rimel, 1984; Klauber, Barrett-Connor, Marshall, & Bowers, 1981). The subsequent health care demands of these individuals will undoubtedly produce increasing demands on neuropsychologists for services to this population. The remaining sections of this chapter present the neuropathology and neuropsychological sequelae of TBI, before reviewing assessment, interpretation, and treatment considerations for neuropsychologists who work with geriatric populations.

Neuropathology of traumatic brain injury

A TBI is an injury to the brain arising from blunt or penetrating trauma and/or from rotational and acceleration–deceleration forces (Hardman & Manoukian, 2002). Although the majority of fatalities following head trauma are associated with open head injuries, most traumatic brain injuries result in closed head injuries in which the skull remains intact (Lezak, 1995). A traumatic insult to the brain can result in focal damage, such as cortical contusions, or diffuse pathology with widespread axonal damage (Burke & Ordia, 2000). Depth of coma, duration of coma, and length of posttraumatic amnesia are three commonly used indicators of brain injury severity. For example, the Glasgow Coma Scale (GCS; Teasdale & Jennett, 1974) is frequently used to assess depth of coma, with scores of 13–15 suggestive of mild brain injury, scores of 9–12 indicating moderate brain injury, and scores below 9 reflective of severe brain injury. Neuroimaging can enhance the clinical utility of this scale, as GCS scores of 13–15 in the presence of an intracranial lesion are suggestive of a more complicated mild or moderate brain injury (Williams, Levin, & Eisenberg, 1990).

The neuropathological consequences of TBI are the result of a dynamic process that involves both primary and secondary injuries to the brain (McAllister, 1992; NIH, 1999). Primary injuries occur at the moment of trauma and are a direct result of the contact and/or acceleration–deceleration and rotational forces that the brain encounters. Secondary injuries are the biochemical and physiological sequelae of the primary brain insult that evolve during the hours or days that follow the initial trauma (Burke & Ordia, 2000; Hardman & Manoukian, 2002). The more common primary and secondary consequences of TBI are discussed below.

Primary injury

Skull fractures

Skull fractures are classified by the configurations they display, with the pattern of the fracture sometimes helpful in identifying the direction, location, and force of the impact that produced the trauma (Hardman & Manoukian, 2002). Linear fractures, which are identified by a break in a single line, frequently result from falls and are the most common type of skull fracture. Depressed skull fractures, which occur when bone fragments are displaced inward, frequently occur in the frontal and parietal regions of the skull (Hardman & Manoukian, 2002). Basal skull fractures, which frequently occur in the cribriform plate of the ethmoid bone, may lead to cranial nerve damage or cerebrospinal fluid rhinorrhea (leakage in the nasal cavity) or otorrhea (leakage in the aural canal) (Burke & Ordia, 2000). Regarding prevalence, skull fractures appear to be as common in the elderly as they are in younger individuals (Vollmer & Eisenberg, 1990). Although the presence of a skull fracture is not a pathonomonic sign of brain damage, skull fractures are associated with an increased risk of brain injury, hematoma, cranial nerve damage, and infection (Burke & Ordia, 2000).

Contusions

Resulting from the biomechanical forces (e.g., acceleration–deceleration) associated with TBI, cortical contusions are hemorrhagic lesions that typically form at the crests of gyri on the surface of the brain (Burke & Ordia, 2000). Coup contusions form at the site of cranial impact and are often the result of acceleration of the brain. Contrecoup contusions, which are frequently more severe, develop opposite the cranial impact and are often the result of brain deceleration (Ferrell & Tanev, 2002). Bony protrusions located on the interior wall of the skull place certain cortical areas at increased risk for contusions, with the orbital surface of the frontal lobes and the tips of the temporal lobes being common contusion sites. Clinically, contusions may lead to focal neurological deficits or seizures (Burke & Ordia, 2000).

Intracranial hemorrhage

Classified by the location of the bleeding, epidural, subdural, and subarachnoid hematomas can damage the brain by exerting pressure on underlying brain structures. Epidural hematomas, which frequently result from a laceration of the middle meningeal artery, typically display an acute and rapidly developing clinical course (Hardman & Manoukian, 2002). While the incidence of epidural hematomas peaks in the second and third decades of life, epidural hematomas are uncommon in elderly individuals because the adherence of the dura mater to the wall of the skull becomes stronger with age (Vollmer & Eisenberg, 1990). Subdural hematomas, which frequently occur from injury to cortical bridging veins, are associated with a high mortality rate (Burke & Ordia, 2000). Although common following severe brain injuries, subdural hematomas can also develop following mild brain injuries. Subdural hematomas can be classified as acute, subacute, or chronic. Acute subdural hematomas typically occur in younger adults, while chronic subdural hematomas, which form in the weeks following injury, have a peak incidence in the sixth and seventh decades of life (Karnath, 2004). The propensity of falls to produce subdural hematomas, and age-related brain atrophy that stretches parasagittal bridging veins making them more vulnerable to rupture, are likely factors contributing to the increased incidence of subdural hematomas in the elderly (Vollmer & Eisenberg, 1990). Subarachnoid hemorrhages are common following TBI, frequently resulting from shearing of microvessels in the subarachnoid space. The consequences of subarachnoid hemorrhages are related to the volume and extent of the hemorrhage. When small and not associated with other structural pathology, subarachnoid hemorrhages typically have a relatively benign course (Burke & Ordia, 2000). However, larger subarachnoid hemorrhages can lead to hydrocephalus, elevated intracranial pressure, and death.

Diffuse axonal injury

Neuronal axon damage is caused by sudden angular rotation of the brain and is frequently associated with high-speed acceleration–deceleration injuries, such as motor vehicle accidents. Midline brain structures (e.g., corpus callosum, brain stem) may be particularly vulnerable to axonal shearing, with the thalamus, basal ganglia, internal capsule, and cerebellar peduncles also frequently affected (Burke & Ordia, 2000). Significant diffuse axonal injury (DAI) can lead to loss of consciousness and prolonged coma (McAllister, 1992). DAI can be viewed as a primary and secondary process, with the initial trauma to the axon leading to axonal swelling and eventual axonal rupture in the hours following injury (Ferrell & Tanev, 2002; Maxwell, Povlishock, & Graham, 1997).

Secondary injury

Ischemia and neurochemical events

Ischemic brain damage (i.e., tissue damage resulting from a lack of adequate blood flow) and the failure of physiologic autoregulatory mechanisms following TBI initiate a complex biochemical process that can cause further brain damage by affecting vascular and metabolic functioning and causing changes in intracranial pressure, heart rate, blood pressure, and nutritional state (Burke & Ordia, 2000; Fields & Coffey, 1994). Contributors to this neurotoxic cascade include increased levels of oxygen free radicals, excitatory amino acids, endogenous opioid peptides, and acetylcholine. Additionally, plaques composed of amyloid beta are known to form following TBI, with damaged axons likely contributing to this development (Smith, Chen, Iwata, & Graham, 2003). Animal research suggests that the brains of older individuals are more vulnerable to damage from the excitotoxic neurotransmitters that are released following TBI (Hamm, Jenkins, Lyeth, White-Gbadebo, & Hayes, 1991).

Edema and intracranial pressure

Cerebral edema (i.e., swelling) results from disruption of the blood–brain barrier and impairment of vasomotor autoregulation with concomitant dilation of cerebral blood vessels (Burke & Ordia, 2000). Localized or diffuse areas of brain swelling may develop and lead to collapse of the ventricular system, herniation syndromes, occlusion of intracranial vessels with secondary strokes, or increased intracranial pressure (Hardman & Manoukian, 2002). The added mass of intracranial hematomas can also lead to heightened intracranial pressure, which can subsequently compromise cerebral blood flow and tissue oxygenation. Management of intracranial pressure and maintenance of cerebral perfusion pressure are primary concerns following TBI because these conditions (i.e., elevated intracranial pressure and diminished cerebral perfusion pressure) can contribute to cerebral ischemia and are associated with poor functional outcome and increased mortality (Lezak, 1995; Ordia, 2000).

Posttraumatic epilepsy

Seizures are a common consequence of TBI, with posttraumatic epilepsy often refractory to medical treatment (Semah et al., 1998). Posttraumatic seizures are classified according to time of onset postinjury, with immediate seizures occurring within the first 24 hours, early seizures occurring between 1 and 7 days, and late seizures developing more than 7 days postinjury (Bushnik, Englander, & Duong, 2004). The incidence of late posttraumatic seizures ranges from 5–19% in civilian populations to as high as 50% in military settings where penetrating type injuries are more common (Asikainen, Kaste, & Sarna, 1999; Bushnik et al., 2004; Englander et al., 2003; Jennett, 1975; Salazar et al., 1985). Older age has been found to increase the likelihood of seizure activity following TBI. Additional risk factors include a family history of epilepsy, a history of chronic alcoholism, and injury characteristics including loss of consciousness, prolonged duration of posttraumatic amnesia, and the presence of a skull fracture or contusion with subdural hematoma (Annegers & Coan, 2000; Bushnik et al., 2004).

Additional secondary developments

Hypoxia, hydrocephalus, brain herniation syndromes, and infection may contribute to further brain damage and complicate recovery following TBI. Minimization and management of secondary injury is of great importance as ongoing tissue damage can potentiate further secondary mechanisms creating a positive feedback loop (Ordia, 2000).

Neuropsychological sequelae of traumatic brain injury in the older adult

Cognitive sequelae

Altered cognitive functioning is common following TBI, with reductions in attention and information processing the most frequent cognitive sequelae associated with mild TBI (Lucas, 1998). While the cognitive changes resulting from mild TBI are typically restricted in scope and brief in duration, severe brain injury frequently produces diffuse and persisting cognitive deficits. Although severe TBI can impact any aspect of cognition, the high incidence of orbitofrontal and anterior temporal lobe contusions associated with these injuries often produces a constellation of symptoms that includes: (a) diminished speed of cognitive processing and behavioral responding, (b) deficits in attention, (c) impaired learning and retrieval of new information, and (d) symptoms associated with frontal lobe injury (e.g., impulsivity, perseveration, anosognosia, initiation deficits, poor planning and organization) (Lucas, 1998).

Mazzucchi et al. (1992) were among the first to focus specifically on TBI in older individuals, assessing the cognitive functioning of patients with a history of mild, moderate, and severe TBI who were 50–75 years old at time of injury. Even with the inclusion of individuals with milder injuries, only one-quarter of participants demonstrated normal functioning or mild neuro-psychological decline, with generalized cognitive deterioration and dementia found in half the sample at 6 months to 3 years postinjury. Evaluating patients with mild to moderate TBI who were aged 50 years or older, Goldstein et al. (1994) noted deficits in memory, timed word fluency, and reasoning abilities at 7 months postinjury. Aharon-Peretz et al. (1997) found similar cognitive deficits up to 6 weeks postinjury in patients with a history of closed head injury who were over 60 years old. However, this study also found no significant differences in cognitive functioning between those patients with a history of TBI and a control group of orthopedic patients, suggesting that the cognitive decline may not have been related to the brain injury. Examining the early cognitive outcomes of older adults with mild and moderate TBI, Goldstein, Levin, Goldman, Clark, and Altonen (2001) found that patients with moderate brain injuries performed significantly poorer on measures of attention, memory, expressive language, and executive functioning.

Psychiatric and behavioral sequelae

Altered mood, behavior, and personality are common following TBI, with even mild TBI associated with significant affective disturbance (Borgaro, Prigatano, Kwasnica, & Rexer, 2003; Lucas, 1998). Additionally, TBI may lead to extended or even permanent vulnerability to both Axis I and II psychiatric disorders in some individuals (Koponen et al., 2002). Van Reekum, Cohen, and Wong (2000) identified the following prevalence rates of psychiatric disorders following TBI: major depression (44.3%), substance abuse or dependence (22%), posttraumatic stress disorder (14.1%), panic disorder (9.2%), generalized anxiety disorder (9.1%), obsessive-compulsive disorder (6.4%), bipolar affective disorder (4.2%), and schizophrenia (0.7%). Additionally, fatigue, diminished frustration tolerance, adjustment disorders, emotional lability, suicidality, paranoia, aggression, and impaired social skills are commonly noted following TBI (Lucas, 1998; Simpson & Tate, 2002; Tateno, Jorge, & Robinson, 2003).

Depression and anxiety also appear to be relatively common among older adults with a history of TBI. Looking at patients 50 years of age or older with a history of mild to moderate TBI, Levin, Goldstein, and MacKenzie (1997) found a depression rate of 30% 1 month postinjury, with continued or new onset depression noted in 25% of these patients at 7 months postinjury, and 12% at 13 months. This study also found that patients with depression were rated by their significant others as showing postinjury decline in social functioning and activities of daily living. Goldstein et al. (1999) also obtained independent ratings from the significant others of older adults with mild and moderate TBI which revealed a progressive deterioration of mood and the presence of restlessness and irritability. Examining the early neurobehavioral status of older adults with mild and moderate TBI, Goldstein et al. (2001) found that both groups of patients exhibited significantly greater depression and anxiety/somatic concern than controls. It was concluded that older adults with a history of mild to moderate TBI are at significant risk for early and delayed onset depression.

Outcomes for older adults with traumatic brain injury

Severity of injury is the best predictor of general outcome following TBI (Dikmen, Machamer, Savoie, & Temkin, 1996; Fields & Coffey, 1994). While a complete and relatively speedy recovery is typical following an isolated and uncomplicated mild TBI (Binder, Rohling, & Larrabee, 1997), severe TBI is associated with significant mortality and the onset of long-term disability (Mosenthal et al., 2004; Rapoport & Feinstein, 2000; Rothweiler, Temkin, & Dikmen, 1998). Age has also been found to be a significant and independent predictor of outcome (Hukkelhoven et al., 2003), with older adults experiencing an increased rate of mortality, longer hospitalizations, and less complete recovery of functioning following TBI (Cifu et al., 1996; Mosenthal et al., 2002; Susman et al., 2002). Other psychosocial factors contributing to outcome include prior history of brain injury, history of substance abuse, vocational history, and adequacy of social relationships (Sbordone & Howard, 1989). Consistent with the concept of cognitive reserve, larger brain volume and higher education level have been found to exert a positive influence on outcome (Kesler, Adams, Blasey, & Bigler, 2003). Genetic factors also play a role, with the e4 allele of apolipoprotein E (APOE4) having a negative impact on both short- and long-term recovery and neuropsychological functioning following TBI (Crawford et al., 2002; Friedman et al., 1999; Hartman et al., 2002; Liberman, Stewart, Wesnes, & Troncoso, 2002). Additionally, APOE4 status and TBI are both risk factors for Alzheimer's disease (Lye & Shores, 2000), with these factors possibly having a synergistic effect placing APOE4 positive individuals at increased risk for developing dementia after TBI (Hartman et al., 2002).

The notion that older adults uniformly fare worse than younger individuals following TBI has been challenged. Following a critical review of research studies examining the functional outcome of elderly TBI survivors, Rapoport and Feinstein (2000) concluded that while mortality and functional disability were higher in older persons following severe TBI, outcome following mild to moderate TBI was unclear. Subsequent research studies examining the outcome of older adults with mild TBI have concluded that older persons enjoy a favorable outcome, similar to younger individuals, following isolated and uncomplicated mild TBI (Goldstein et al., 2001; Mosenthal et al., 2004; Rapoport & Feinstein, 2001). Goleburn and Golden (2001) reviewed 18 studies published between 1986 and 1999 pertaining to the outcome of older adults following TBI of varying severity. They concluded that older survivors of TBI experience increased mortality and poorer functional outcome compared to younger adults with similar injury severity. Examining the association between age and outcome in 5600 patients with a history of severe TBI, Hukkelhoven et al. (2003) concluded that advancing age is associated with worsening outcome. This analysis also concluded that it was clinically disadvantageous to define the effect of age on outcome in a discrete manner, noting instead that the negative association between age and outcome is a continuous function. Overall, the literature suggests that older adults experience outcomes similar to younger persons following isolated and uncomplicated mild TBI, with advancing age associated with poorer outcome following moderate to severe TBI.

Many factors contribute to both the increased incidence and less favorable outcome of TBI among the elderly when compared to younger persons. For example, sensory deficits, chronic medical and orthopedic conditions, and medication side effects may compromise the physical functioning of older adults and lead to increased risk for falls or motor vehicle accidents (Ferrell & Tanev, 2002). Increased exposure to minor insults and a diminished capacity for repair may increase the aging brain's vulnerability to TBI (Hukkelhoven et al., 2003). Additionally, fragility of brain structures, age-related cortical atrophy and neuronal loss, and diminished cerebral blood flow may compromise the brain's ability to recover from insult (Lezak, 1995; Vollmer & Eisenberg, 1990). Furthermore, an increased incidence of post-traumatic infections, subdural hematomas, intracranial hemorrhages, and delayed neurosurgical complications among elderly TBI survivors also contributes to poorer outcome (Fields & Coffey, 1994; Howard, Gross, Dacey, & Winn, 1989).

Neuropsychological assessment of older adults with traumatic brain injury

Neuropsychological assessment following TBI can provide critical information about a patient's cognitive, behavioral, and emotional status, which can be used to facilitate treatment, assist with resumption of life activities, and monitor recovery. Identification of an appropriate referral question, a comprehensive clinical interview, astute behavioral observations, and thoughtful test selection form the foundation of a neuropsychological evaluation. As these topics are thoroughly reviewed elsewhere in this book, this section will present issues that are specific to the assessment of older adults with TBI.

Clinical interview

The clinical interview should include a thorough review of the patient's medical and psychiatric histories (including prior brain injuries), medication and controlled substance use, sensory functioning, and level of pain, as these factors can compromise testing performance and contribute to the patient's neuropsychological presentation. For example, a majority of elderly adults suffer from chronic medical illness (e.g., diabetes, hypertension; LaRue, 1992), with many of these conditions contributing to neuropsychological deficits common to TBI. Asking patients about prior episodes of altered consciousness is important because repeated head injuries can have a cumulative effect, placing patients with a history of multiple brain injuries at risk for more severe deficits after seemingly mild TBI (Lezak, 1995). Review of medication and controlled substance use is essential as these factors can contribute to cognitive dysfunction and compromise recovery. Also, assessment of sensory functioning is important as elderly persons experience an increased incidence of sensory deficits that may compromise their testing performance. Evaluation of pain is necessary because discomfort can have a negative impact on testing performance (Martelli, 2001). Lastly, the clinical interview should include discussion with family or friends about the patient's level of fatigue, awareness of deficits, frustration tolerance, personality changes, social functioning, and ability to perform activities of daily living.

Test selection

A number of important considerations influence test selection. Selected tests should provide sufficient coverage of the neuropsychological domains necessary to answer the referral question and have adequate normative data for older adults. The need to conduct brief and efficient evaluations with this population suggests that the criterion and incremental validity of measures should also be points of concern.

Neuropsychologists are frequently called upon to identify the cognitive strengths and weaknesses of patients with TBI. To this end, the sequelae commonly associated with TBI dictate that measures of attention, processing speed, memory (verbal vs. visual; immediate vs. delayed), language, executive functioning, and emotional well-being be included in the test battery. Of course tests may need to be added or removed from the battery based upon the referral question and the status of the patient. Neuropsychologists may also be called upon to assess a patient's ability to make decisions or resume life activities. Although neuropsychological measures have been found to be useful in assessing decision-making capacity (Freedman, Stuss, & Gordon, 1991; see Chapter 18 in this volume for a review of this topic) and the ability to perform certain life activities, such as driving (Reger et al., 2004), the majority of neuropsychological tests were developed to detect and differentiate brain illness and not to predict function (Lezak, 1995). Accordingly, caution must be exercised when test results are used to predict a patient's ability to perform an activity. Also, it is important to remember that cognitive testing provides complementary information that does not replace other more direct measures of functioning (e.g., a driving evaluation), and that other rehabilitation professionals (e.g., occupational, physical, and speech pathology therapists) and/or family members should be consulted to more directly evaluate the functional abilities of older adults with TBI.

Age and other demographic variables have been found to influence the test performance of neurologically intact persons (Heaton, Taylor, & Manly, 2003) and individuals with TBI (Sherrill-Pattison, Donders, & Thompson, 2000). While the most recent revisions of the Wechsler scales (WAIS–III, WMS–III; Wechsler, 1997) are consistent with the trend for new tests to include age-extended normative data, many neuropsychological measures do not have adequate reference groups for elderly individuals. In addition to choosing tests that have appropriate normative information, neuropsychologists working with older adults need to be conscious of floor and ceiling effects that may impact the reliability of a test. For example, an 80-year-old examinee who recalls none of the word pairs on the Verbal Paired Associates subtest of the WMS–III will still earn a scaled score of 7 (Lacritz & Cullum, 2003).

The neuropsychological examination of older patients with TBI should include assessment of abilities that are resistant to TBI and can serve as markers of premorbid functioning, as well as tests that assess the cognitive changes resulting from injury. For example, research examining the criterion validity of the WAIS–III has found the Processing Speed Index to be sensitive to TBI (Martin, Donders, & Thompson, 2000), while performance on the new WAIS–III subtest Matrix Reasoning is relatively unaffected by TBI (Donders, Tulsky, & Zhu, 2001). When selecting tests, caution should be exercised to avoid including a number of measures that are highly correlated with each other. This results in redundancy of measurement and limits the clinical utility of findings. Conversely, choosing tests that have a low correlation with each other, but a strong positive association with the criterion ability, increases the likelihood that convergent findings are related to actual ability and not artifact (Vanderploeg, 2000).

Battery length

Comprehensive neuropsychological testing should not be undertaken during the early stages of recovery from moderate to severe TBI, as many patients are unable to tolerate lengthy and demanding evaluation. In addition, the results of evaluations performed during the early stages of recovery may be of limited value due to rapid changes in neuropsychological status that are common during this period (Lezak, 1995). Similarly, older adults in the later stages of recovery may also have difficulty completing extended test batteries. Chronic medical conditions, pain, medication side effects, and TBI-related sequelae such as fatigue and irritability are factors that underscore the need to conduct time-limited evaluations with this population.

Review of select neuropsychological measures and batteries

Because many older individuals with TBI cannot tolerate traditional full-day neuropsychological evaluations, it is increasingly common for neuropsychologists to use briefer test batteries to identify a patient's neuropsychological status. The Repeatable Battery for the Assessment of Neuropsychological Status (RBANS; Randolph, 1998) is a brief (20–30 minute administration time) and portable test that assesses attention, language, visuospatial/constructional abilities, and immediate and delayed memory. The test has been found to be sensitive to TBI, has alternate forms, and includes normative data extending to age 89, with recent research providing age and education corrections for elderly individuals (Duff et al., 2003). The Barrow Neurological Institute Screen for Higher Cerebral Functions consists of seven subtests that can be administered in less than 25 minutes. The test has norms extending to age 84 and has been found to be useful for assessing disorientation in patients with TBI during the acute phases of recovery (Borgaro, Kwasnica, Cutter, & Alcott, 2003). In addition, the Meyers Short Battery is a collection of commonly used neuropsychological tests that can be administered in approximately 3 hours. This test battery has been found to be sensitive to varying degrees of brain injury severity and in differentiating TBI from other disorders (Meyers & Rohling, 2004; Volbrecht, Meyers, & Kaster-Bundgaard, 2000).

Short forms of several popular tests have also been found to be sensitive to TBI, including the WAIS–III–7 (Schoop, Herrman, Johnstone, Callahan, & Roudebush, 2001), a 15-item version of the Judgement of Line Orientation Test (Mount, Hogg, & Johnstone 2002), and the Wisconsin Card Sorting Test–64 (Sherer, Nick, Millis, & Novack, 2003). While the necessity to develop time efficient test batteries contributes to the appeal of shortened tests, abbreviated measures must demonstrate utility with elderly populations before being used for clinical purposes. For example, research has indicated that a seven-subtest version of the WAIS–R may not be a reliable predictor of intelligence for persons with Alzheimer's disease (Schopp, Callahan, Johnstone, & Schwake, 1998).

Assessment of emotional functioning is an essential part of a neuropsychological evaluation. However, because the majority of measures designed to assess emotional status were developed for neurologically intact populations, they may misinterpret TBI-related sequelae as symptoms of psychiatric illness. For example, the Beck Depression Inventory (BDI), Geriatric Depression Scale (GDS), and Minnesota Multiphasic Personality Inventory–2 (MMPI2) all contain neurologically based test items that patients with central nervous system impairment may endorse even in the absence of a psychiatric condition (Spreen & Straus, 1998). Moreover, the BDI was not designed to assess depression in elderly populations, with the multiple-choice format of this test possibly being confusing to older individuals (Spreen & Strauss, 1998). Similarly, the length and cognitive demands necessary to complete the

MMPI2 complicate its use with elderly and/or neurologically impaired individuals. Comparatively, the GDS is a brief measure that consists of 30 yes/no questions designed specifically to screen for depression in elderly persons. In the absence of measures developed specifically for older adults with a history of TBI, clinicians are encouraged to utilize measures that are appropriate for older persons and to incorporate a review and analysis of patient responses, as opposed to using a cutoff score, as part of their assessment of emotional status.

Interpretation of data for older adults with traumatic brain injury

The interpretation of neuropsychological data is a multistage process that involves the integration of information from several sources, including the patient's history, the clinical interview, behavioral observations, and test results. While background information and behavioral observations provide qualitative information, the interpretation of test scores is a quantitative process that begins with the use of standardized normative data against which individual performance is measured. While this comparison identifies a patient's cognitive strengths and weaknesses, findings must be considered in light of the patient's historical abilities to determine if a decline in functioning has occurred.

As prior test results documenting a patient's historical capacities are rarely available, a number of methods have been developed to estimate premorbid intellectual functioning. For example, demographic variables, reading ability, performance on select WAIS subtests, and formulas combining demographic variables and test performance have all been used to estimate premorbid functioning. While each of these approaches has merit, some considerations are warranted when assessing the premorbid functioning of older adults with TBI. For instance, educational and occupational history may be unreliable predictors of premorbid functioning in elderly individuals who may have quit school out of necessity, rather than lack of ability, and who despite having the potential may not have pursued professional careers (Koltai & Welsh-Bohmer, 2000). Also, recent research suggests that reading ability may decline following TBI, counter to previous contentions that measures of reading ability are "hold" tests, and as a result may provide an underestimate of premorbid functioning following TBI (Orme, Johnstone, Hanks, & Novack, 2004).

After comparing test results to normative data and premorbid estimates, the neuropsychologist can determine if evaluation findings are consistent with TBI. For instance, TBI is associated with the immediate onset of deficits that tend to show some degree of improvement in the months following injury. This is in contrast to the symptom profile associated with other neurological disorders (e.g., a progressive dementia) that demonstrate a gradual and progressive decline of functioning. Additionally, symptoms should be consistent with injury characteristics. For example, diffuse neuropsychological impairment would be inconsistent with TBI resulting in focal brain damage.

Likewise, severe or prolonged deficits would be uncharacteristic of isolated and uncomplicated mild TBI. When evaluating neuropsychological profiles, it is essential to determine if deficits are consistent with noted areas of brain injury. For example, orbitofrontal damage often results in a syndrome that is characterized by disinhibition, impulsivity, perseveration, affective lability, and increased distractibility. Identification of TBI-related cognitive deficits also requires consideration of neuroanatomy, as damage to underlying brain structures or intracerebral conduction pathways may lead to neuropsychological deficits that at first glance may appear unrelated to the TBI.

Distinguishing TBI-related impairments from the effects of other medical conditions may be complicated, as the cognitive sequelae associated with TBI are common to many disorders. For example, hypertension has been associated with general cognitive dysfunction, including memory impairment (Prencipe, Santini, Casini, Pezzella, Scaldaferri, & Culasso, 2003). Additionally, subclinical levels of cardiovascular disease can compromise speed of performance, attention, working memory, verbal fluency, and visuospatial abilities (Saxton et al., 2000). Congestive heart failure can contribute to a significant decline in cognitive functioning, including impaired attention (Almeida & Tamai, 2001). Deficits in cognitive processing speed, working memory, and executive functioning are common in elderly survivors of stroke (Ballard et al., 2003). Also, advancing age and history of hypertension or stroke are known risk factors for white matter lesions, which have been found to contribute to deficits in psychomotor speed, attention, working memory, and executive functioning (Swan et al., 2000).

Differentiating the cognitive effects of Alzheimer's disease from early recovery of mild to moderate TBI can also be challenging. For example, deficits in storing and retrieving new information, reduced verbal fluency, and naming impairments are common to both conditions (Goldstein et al., 1996). However, neuropsychological markers have been identified to assist with this differential diagnosis. For instance, memory (i.e., verbal recall) and semantic processing (i.e., letter and category fluency) have been found to be significantly more impaired in individuals with Alzheimer's disease (Goldstein et al., 1996). Similarly, it may be difficult to distinguish the effects of a remote TBI from symptoms associated with the onset of Alzheimer's disease. More specifically, it has been suggested that individuals with a history of TBI may be more vulnerable to the aging process, with these two factors having a synergistic effect contributing to the development of a neuropsychological profile that mimics Alzheimer's disease (Hinkebein, Martin, Callahan, & Johnstone, 2003).

Geriatric depression has also been associated with neuropsychological dysfunction, with deficits in working memory and processing speed associated with this condition. Additionally, these cognitive deficits were found to persist even after the depression remitted (Nebes et al., 2000). While assessment and treatment of psychiatric illness is a primary concern following TBI, distinguishing symptoms of depression from symptoms related to TBI can be difficult. For instance, sleep disturbance, irritability, and difficulties with concentration and memory are common to both conditions. Additionally, damage to the mesial frontal lobe or anterior cingulate gyrus can result in akinesia and apathy, which may be mistaken for symptoms of depression. Investigating a patient's outlook on the future may be helpful in clarifying etiology, as significant feelings of hopelessness would be suggestive of a depressive disorder. Additionally, assessment of executive functioning may be helpful as patients with TBI-related akinesia or apathy may also demonstrate failure of response inhibition on go/no-go tasks secondary to their brain injury.

Accidents producing TBI often result in injury to other bodily systems that may hinder a patient's testing ability and complicate the interpretation of neuropsychological findings. For example, orthopedic injury to an upper extremity may compromise a patient's grip strength or ability to complete tasks requiring fine motor skills. Likewise, peripheral neuropathy may lead to sensory deficits unrelated to central nervous system dysfunction. As TBI or accompanying trauma may require surgical intervention, it is noteworthy that neuropsychological compromise is common among elderly persons in the days following surgery, with a small proportion of patients experiencing ongoing difficulties (Peisah, 2002). Multitrauma may also contribute to chronic pain and increased medication usage, both of which can compromise neuropsychological functioning.

As this section illustrates, a number of factors complicate the interpretation of neuropsychological data of older adults with TBI. The importance of a thorough clinical interview to document symptom characteristics, comorbid medical conditions, medication usage, sensory deficits, and changes in personality cannot be overstated. Moreover, a comprehensive appreciation of geriatric issues, TBI, and brain–behavior relationships is essential. Given the symptom commonality between TBI and other medical conditions, evaluating the onset and course of symptoms is often helpful in identifying TBI-related sequelae. Additionally, identification and evaluation of confounding factors that may be contributing to the patient's neuropsychological presentation, and basing diagnostic conclusions on patterns of findings rather than single observations, will also promote diagnostic accuracy. Lastly, longitudinal testing may be helpful in sorting through particularly challenging cases in which multiple conditions may be contributing to neuropsychological dysfunction.

Treatment considerations for older adults with traumatic brain injury

Treatment following moderate to severe TBI often consists of cognitive and physical rehabilitation, social and psychotherapeutic support, and judicious use of pharmacotherapy to treat neuropsychiatric symptoms (Ferrell & Tanev, 2002). Treatment approaches during the acute phase of recovery typically include acute trauma and neurosurgical care and acute inpatient hospitalization and rehabilitation. Postacute approaches to rehabilitation include comprehensive day treatment programs, transitional living programs, home-based rehabilitation, adult day care centers, and residential treatment programs. Rehabilitation programs should be interdisciplinary, comprehensive, and tailored to the needs of the individual. Moreover, patients and their families should play an integral role in the planning and design of the program (NIH, 1999). As a group, older adults typically experience a slower rate of recovery secondary to decreased cognitive and physical reserve due to normal aging, preexisting medical problems, and a higher incidence of medical complications (Goleburn & Golden, 2001). Nonetheless, older adults benefit from rehabilitation services, with improved functional status and quality of life noted in response to treatment (Mosenthal et al., 2004).

Geriatric neuropsychologists may provide cognitive rehabilitation and psychotherapy services to promote the cognitive and emotional functioning of TBI survivors. Broadly defined, cognitive rehabilitation is a systematic program designed to modify and enhance cognitive function. Two major approaches to cognitive rehabilitation exist. Restorative approaches aim to restore a specific cognitive ability to baseline levels through a series of selectively challenging tasks; for example, exposing a patient to a progression of increasingly demanding computer-based attention tasks to promote concentration. In contrast, compensatory approaches utilize a patient's cognitive strengths and/or compensatory mechanisms to facilitate increased functioning. For instance, a patient with poor verbal memory could be taught to rely on visual memory or to routinely use a daily organizer. Overall, restorative techniques have demonstrated utility in improving fundamental abilities such as attention, mental speed, or visual scanning, while compensatory approaches have been more successful in alleviating the disability associated with the persistent memory deficits that often follow TBI (Guilmette, 1997). However, as the utilization of compensatory strategies and aids requires an adequate appreciation of one's deficits, patients with a limited awareness of their impairments may resist using these interventions.

Psychotherapy is a necessary component of rehabilitation for many older adults with TBI and their family members. In addition to addressing psychiatric disorders and behavioral disturbance, this forum can be utilized to provide education about TBI and recovery and to promote coping and problem-solving skills, self-awareness, the reestablishment of intimate and social relationships, and positive lifestyle change. Also, as substance abuse can complicate recovery following TBI and impede successful community reintegration, substance abuse treatment should be provided as warranted. Because TBI impacts the entire family system, psychotherapy services should be extended to family members and significant others as needed. Given the cognitive and behavioral manifestations of TBI, psychotherapy services may need to be modified to accommodate the patient's level of functioning. For example, the length of sessions may need to be reduced, and therapy may need to progress at a slower rate. Additionally, interventions may need to be concise and void of abstraction. Similarly, style of therapy may also need to be altered. Interpersonal, supportive, and cognitive approaches may be useful with patients whose cognitive functioning is more intact, while behavioral approaches may be more applicable to patients with significant cognitive impairment who display behavioral disruption (Fields & Coffey, 1994). For instance, promoting a structured environment with scheduled rest periods, and reinforcing intervals of cooperative behavior, may promote the safety of a confused patient who becomes physically aggressive when overly stimulated or fatigued.

Medications are used in the treatment of TBI to enhance cognitive functioning and address affective disorders and behavioral disruption. It is important to note that none of the medications used to treat TBI were developed specifically for this purpose, and that no single medication is able to treat the wide variety of cognitive and behavioral disturbances that may accompany TBI. Pharmacological interventions utilized in the treatment of TBI-related symptoms must reflect consideration of potential side affects associated with these medications, as adverse effects can compromise a patient's emotional, behavioral, or cognitive functioning. For example, medications used to treat severe agitation or behavior disturbance (e.g., Haldol) can contribute to drowsiness and confusion and impede a patients cognitive or physical functioning. Additionally, medications utilized to promote attention (e.g., Ritalin) can contribute to sleeplessness or anxiety. It is also important to appreciate that pharmacological interventions affect patients with TBI differently, depending upon their physiological injuries, stage of recovery, and personal history (see Chapter 15 in this volume for a more comprehensive review of geriatric psychopharmacology).

Depending on the reason for the referral, the neuropsychological evaluation is often most valuable when it culminates with recommendations designed to promote the patient's functioning and quality of life. While recommendations should be tailored to the patient's unique strengths and weaknesses, many TBI survivors benefit from some general suggestions to promote functioning. For instance, reduced frustration tolerance and difficulty dealing with ambiguity or excessive stimulation are common following TBI. Accordingly, encouraging patients and family members to maintain a structured, predictable, and low stress home environment may be beneficial. Additionally, advising patients to focus on a single task at a time and avoid "multitasking" when possible may promote cognitive efficiency by minimizing demands on divided attention. Likewise, encouraging patients to allow themselves appropriate time to process information and to avoid tasks with significant time restrictions may decrease cognitive difficulties related to diminished speed of processing. In addition to encouraging the use of memory strategies (e.g., organizing information) to promote recall, recommending the use of a daily organizer, prioritized checklists, or tape recorder may promote a patient's level of independence. Deficits in social skills and decreased social activity are also common following TBI. Accordingly, interventions designed to enhance social functioning and promote social activity (e.g., involvement in local organizations or volunteer work) may be beneficial. Lastly, the interdisciplinary approach to TBI rehabilitation emphasizes the need to make referrals to speech, physical, or occupational therapists; hearing or vision specialists; pain management clinics; substance abuse treatment programs; or other health care providers as needed.

In closing, treatment following TBI should be interdisciplinary, comprehensive, and tailored to the needs of the patient. Geriatric neuropsychologists are often well-positioned to provide a number of services that can enhance the functioning and quality of life of TBI survivors and their families. As there is no cure for TBI, prevention is the best treatment. Proactive interventions to decrease the risk of TBI in the elderly include, addressing sensory deficits (e.g., hearing aids, glasses) and treatable health conditions that may increase the risk of incurring a TBI, evaluating the necessity and side effects of medications, and promoting improved physical and emotional well-being.

Conclusion

TBI is a major health and socioeconomic problem in the United States, with advancing age associated with both a higher incidence of TBI and poorer outcome following moderate to severe injury. Although older adults typically experience a slower rate of recovery following more severe TBI, they benefit from rehabilitation services with improved functional outcome and quality of life noted in response to treatment. As a field, geriatric neuropsychology is in a unique position to meet a number of growing geriatric health care needs, including providing assessment and treatment services to older adults with TBI, educating the public and health care providers about TBI, and conducting research to guide the rehabilitation of elderly persons with TBI.

References

Aharon-Peretz, J., Kliot, D., Amyel-Zvi, E., Tomer, R., Rakier, A., & Feinsod, M. (1997). Neurobehavioural consequences of closed head injury in the elderly. *Brain Injury, 11*(12), 871–875.

Almeida, O. P., & Tamai, S. (2001). Congestive heart failure and cognitive functioning amongst older adults. *Arquivos de Neuro-Psiquiatria, 59*(2-B), 324–329.

Annegers, J. F., & Coan, S. P. (2000). The risks of epilepsy after traumatic brain injury. *Seizure, 9*(7), 453–457.

Asikainen, I., Kaste, M., & Sarna, S. (1999). Early and late posttraumatic seizures in traumatic brain injury rehabilitation patients: Brain injury factors causing late seizures and influence of seizures on long-term outcomes. *Epilepsia, 40*, 584–589.

Ballard, C., Stephens, S., Kenny, R., Kalaria, R., Tovee, M., & O'Brien, J. (2003). Profile of neuropsychological deficits in older stroke survivors without dementia. *Dementia and Geriatric Cognitive Disorders, 16*, 52–56.

Binder, L. M., Rohling, M. L., & Larrabee, G. J. (1997). A review of mild head trauma: Part I. Meta-analytic review of neuropsychological studies. *Journal of Clinical and Experimental Neuropsychology, 19*, 421–431.

Borgaro, S. R., Kwasnica, C., Cutter, N., & Alcott, S. (2003). The use of the BNI screen for higher cerebral functions in assessing disorientation after traumatic brain injury. *Journal of Head Trauma Rehabilitation, 18*(3), 284–291.

Borgaro, S. R., Prigatano, G. P., Kwasnica, C., & Rexer, J. L. (2003). Cognitive and affective sequelae in complicated and uncomplicated mild traumatic brain injury. *Brain Injury, 17*(3), 189–198.

Burke, D., & Ordia, J. I. (2000). Pathophysiology of traumatic brain injury. In B. Woo & S. Nesathurai (Eds.), *The rehabilitation of people with traumatic brain injury* (pp. 19–33). Malden, MA: Blackwell Science.

Bushnik, T., Englander, J., & Duong, T. (2004). Medical and social issues related to posttraumatic seizures in persons with traumatic brain injury. *Journal of Head Trauma Rehabilitation, 19*(4), 296–304.

Cifu, D. X., Kreutzer, J. S., Marwitz, J. H., Rosenthal, M., Englander, J., & High, W. (1996). Functional outcomes of older adults with traumatic brain injury: A prospective, multicenter analysis. *Archives of Physical Medicine and Rehabilitation, 77*, 883–888.

Crawford, F. C., Vanderploeg, R. D., Freeman, M. J., Singh, S., Waisman, M., Michaels, L., et al. (2002). APOE genotype influences acquisition and recall following traumatic brain injury. *Neurology, 58*, 1115–1118.

Dikmen, S., Machamer, J., Savoie, T., & Temkin, N. (1996). Life quality outcome in head injury. In I. Grant & K. Adams (Eds.), *Neuropsychological assessment of neuropsychiatric disorders* (pp. 552–576). New York: Oxford University Press.

Donders, J., Tulsky, D. S., & Zhu, J. (2001). Criterion validity of the new WAIS–III subtest scores after traumatic brain injury. *Journal of the International Neuropsychological Society, 7*(7), 892–898.

Duff, K., Patton, D., Schoenberg, M. R., Mold, J., Scott, J. G., & Adams, R. L. (2003). Age- and education-corrected independent normative data for the RBANS in a community dwelling elderly sample. *The Clinical Neuropsychologist, 17*(3), 351–366.

Englander, J., Bushnik, T., Duong, T. T., Cifu, D. X., Zafonte, R., Wright, J., et al., (2003). Analyzing risk factors for late posttraumatic seizures: A prospective, multi-center investigation. *Archives of Physical Medicine Rehabilitation, 84*(3), 365–373.

Ferrell, R. B., & Tanev, K. S. (2002). Traumatic brain injury in older adults. *Current Psychiatry Reports, 4*(5), 354–362.

Fields, R. B., & Coffey, C. E. (1994). Traumatic brain injury. In C. Coffey & J. Cummings (Eds.), *The American Psychiatric Press textbook of geriatric neuropsychiatry* (pp. 480–507). Washington, DC: American Psychiatry Press.

Fife, D., Faich, G., Hollinshead, W., & Wentworth, B. (1986). Incidence and outcome of hospital-treated head injury in Rhode Island. *American Journal of Public Health, 76*, 773–778.

Freedman, M., Stuss, D. T., & Gordon, M. (1991). Assessment of competency: The role of neurobehavioral deficits. *Annuals of Internal Medicine, 115*, 203–208.

Friedman, G., Froom, P., Sazbon, L., Grinblatt, I., Shochina, M., Tsenter, J., et al. (1999). Apolipoprotein E 4 genotype predicts a poor outcome in survivors of traumatic brain injury. *Neurology, 52*, 244–248.

Goldstein, F. C., Levin, H. S., Goldman, W. P., Clark, A. N., & Altonen, T. K. (2001). Cognitive and neurobehavioral functioning after mild versus moderate traumatic brain injury in older adults. *Journal of the International Neuropsychological Society*, *7*(3), 373–383.

Goldstein, F. C., Levin, H. S., Goldman, W. P., Kalechstein, A. S., Clark, A. N., & Kenehan-Altonen, T. (1999). Cognitive and behavioral sequelae of closed head injury in older adults according to their significant others. *Journal of Neuropsychiatry and Clinical Neurosciences*, *11*, 38–44.

Goldstein, F. C., Levin, H. S., Presley, R.M., Searcy, J., Colohan, A. R. T., Eisenberg, H. M., et al. (1994). Neurobehavioral consequences of closed head injury in older adults. *Journal of Neurology, Neurosurgery, and Psychiatry*, *57*, 961–966.

Goldstein, F. C., Levin, H. S., Roberts, V. J., Goldman, W. P., Kalechstein, A. S., Winslow, M., et al. (1996). Neuropsychological effects of closed head injury in older adults: A comparison with Alzheimer's disease. *Neuropsychology*, *10*(2), 147–154.

Goleburn, C. R., & Golden, C. J. (2001). Traumatic brain injury outcome in older adults: A critical review of the literature. *Journal of Clinical Geropsychology*, *7*(3), 161–187.

Guilmette, T. J., (1997). *Pocket guide to brain injury, cognitive, and neurobehavioral rehabilitation*. San Diego, CA: Singular Publishing Group, Inc.

Hamm, R. J., Jenkins, L. W., Lyeth, B. G., White-Gbadebo, D. M., & Hayes, R. L. (1991). The effect of age on outcome following traumatic brain injury in rats. *Journal of Neurosurgery*, *75*(6), 916–921.

Hardman, J. M., & Manoukian, A. (2002). Pathology of head trauma. *Neuroimaging Clinics of North America*, *12*(2), 175–187.

Hartman, R. E., Laurer, H., Longhi, L., Bales, K. R., Paul, S. M., McIntosh, T. K., et al. (2002). Apolipoprotein E4 influences amyloid deposition but not cell loss after traumatic brain injury in a mouse model of Alzheimer's disease. *Journal of Neuroscience*, *22*(23), 10083–10087.

Heaton, R. K., Taylor, M. J., & Manly, J. (2003). Demographic effects and use of demographically corrected norms with the WAIS–III and WMS–III. In D. S. Tulsky, D. H. Saklofske, G. J. Chelune, R. K. Heaton, R. J. Ivnik, R. Bornstein et al. (Eds.), *Clinical interpretation of the WAIS–III and WMS–III* (pp. 181–210). San Diego, CA: Academic Press.

Hinkebein, J. H., Martin, T. A., Callahan, C. D., & Johnstone, B. (2003). Traumatic brain injury and Alzheimer's: Deficit profile similarities and the impact of normal ageing. *Brain Injury*, *17*(12), 1035–1042.

Howard, M. A., Gross, A. S., Dacey, R. G., & Winn, H. R. (1989). Acute subdural hematomas: An age dependent clinical entity. *Journal of Neurosurgery*, *71*, 858–863.

Hukkelhoven, C. W., Steyerberg, E. W., Rampen, A. J., Farace, E., Habbema, J. D., Marshall, L. F., et al. (2003). Patient age and outcome following severe traumatic brain injury: An analysis of 5600 patients. *Journal of Neurosurgery*, *99*(4), 666–673.

Jagger, J., Levine, J. I., Jane, J. A., & Rimel, R. W. (1984). Epidemiologic features of head injury in a predominantly rural population. *Journal of Trauma*, *24*, 40–44.

Jennett, B. (1975). *Epilepsy after non-missile head injuries*. London: William Heinemann Medical Books.

Karnath, B. (2004). Subdural hematoma: Presentation and management in older adults. *Geriatrics*, *59*(7), 18–23.

Kesler, S. R., Adams, H. F., Blasey, C. M., & Bigler, E. D. (2003). Premorbid intellectual functioning, education, and brain size in traumatic brain injury: An investigation of the cognitive reserve hypothesis. *Applied Neuropsychology*, *10*(3), 152–162.

Klauber, M. R., Barrett-Connor, E., Marshall, L. F., & Bowers, S. A. (1981). The epidemiology of head injury: A prospective study on an entire community—San Diego County, California, 1978. *American Journal of Epidemiology*, *113*, 500–509.

Koltai, D. C., & Welsh-Bohmer, K. A. (2000). Geriatric neurological assessment. In R. D. Vanderploeg (Ed.), *Clinicians guide to neuropsychological assessment* (pp. 383–415). Mahwah, NJ: Lawrence Erlbaum Associates, Inc.

Koponen, S., Taiminen, T., Portin, R., Himanen, L., Isoniemi, H., Heinonen, H., et al. (2002). Axis I and II psychiatric disorders after traumatic brain injury: A 30-year follow-up study. *American Journal of Psychiatry*, *159*, 1315–1321.

Lacritz, L. H., & Cullum, C. M. (2003). The WAIS–III and WMS–III: Practical issues and frequently asked questions. In D. S. Tulsky, D. H. Saklofske, G. J. Chelune, R. K. Heaton, R. J. Ivnik, R. Bornstein et al. (Eds.), *Clinical interpretation of the WAIS–III and WMS–III* (pp. 491–532). San Diego, CA: Academic Press.

LaRue, A. (1992). *Aging and neuropsychological assessment*. New York: Plenum Press.

Levin, H. S., Goldstein, F. C., & MacKenzie, E. J. (1997). Depression as a secondary condition following mild and moderate traumatic brain injury. *Seminars in Clinical Neuropsychiatry*, *2*, 207–215.

Lezak, M. D. (1995). *Neuropsychological assessment* (3rd ed.). New York: Oxford University Press.

Liberman, J. N., Stewart, W. F., Wesnes, K., & Troncoso, J. (2002). Apolipoprotein E 4 and short-term recovery from predominantly mild brain injury. *Neurology*, *58*, 1038–1044.

Lucas, J. A. (1998). Traumatic brain injury and postconcussive syndrome. In P. J. Snyder & P. D. Nussbaum (Eds.), *Clinical neuropsychology* (pp. 243–265). Washington, DC: American Psychological Association.

Lye, T. C., & Shores, E. A. (2000). Traumatic brain injury as a risk factor for Alzheimer's disease: A review. *Neuropsychology Review*, *10*(2), 115–129.

Martelli, M. F. (2001). Does pain confound interpretation of neuropsychological test results? *Neurorehabilitation*, *16*, 225–230.

Martin, T. A., Donders, J., & Thompson, E. (2000). Potential of and problems with new measures of psychometric intelligence after traumatic brain injury. *Rehabilitation Psychology*, *45*(4), 402–408.

Maxwell, W. L., Povlishock, J. T., & Graham, D. L. (1997). A mechanistic analysis of nondisruptive axonal injury: A review. *Journal of Neurotrauma*, *14*, 419–440.

Mazzucchi, A., Cattelani, R., Missale, G., Gugliotta, M., Brianti, R., & Parma, M. (1992). Head-injured subjects aged over 50 years: Correlations between variables of trauma and neuropsychological follow-up. *Journal of Neurology*, *39*, 256–260.

McAllister, T. W. (1992). Neuropsychiatric sequelae of head injuries. *Psychiatric Clinics of North America*, *15*(2), 395–413.

Meyers, J. E., & Rohling, M. L. (2004). Validation of the Meyers Short Battery on mild TBI patients. *Archives of Clinical Neuropsychology*, *19*(5), 637–651.

Mosenthal, A. C., Lavery, R. F., Addis, M., Kaul, S., Ross, S., Marburger, R., et al. (2002). Isolated traumatic brain injury: Age is an independent predictor of mortality and early outcome. *Journal of Trauma—Injury, Infection, and Critical Care* *52*(5), 907–911.

Mosenthal, A. C., Livingston, D. H., Lavery, R. F., Knudson, M. M., Lee, S., Morabito, D., et al. (2004). The effect of age on functional outcome in mild traumatic brain injury: 6-month report of a prospective multicenter trial. *Journal of Trauma*, *56*(5), 1042–1048.

Mount, D. L., Hogg, J., & Johnstone, B. (2002). Applicability of the 15-item versions of the Judgement of the Line Orientation Test for individuals with traumatic brain injury. *Brain Injury*, *16*(12), 1051–1055.

National Institutes of Health Consensus Development Panel on Rehabilitation of Persons with Traumatic Brain Injury. (1999). Rehabilitation of persons with traumatic brain injury. *Journal of the American Medical Association*, *282*(10), 974–983.

Nebes, R. D., Butters, M. A., Mulsant, B. H., Pollock, B. G., Zmuda, M. D., Houck, P. R., et al. (2000). Decreased working memory and processing speed mediate cognitive impairment in geriatric depression. *Psychological Medicine*, *30*(3), 679–691.

Ordia, J. I. (2000). Surgical management of traumatic brain injury. In B. Woo & S. Nesathurai (Eds.), *The rehabilitation of people with traumatic brain injury* (pp. 35–43). Malden, MA: Blackwell Science.

Orme, D., Johnstone, B., Hanks, R., & Novack, T. (2004). The WRAT–3 reading subtest as a measure of premorbid intelligence among persons with brain injury. *Rehabilitation Psychology*, *49*(3), 250–253.

Peisah, C. (2002). Practical geriatrics: Persistent postoperative cognitive decline in an elderly woman with preexisting neuropathology. *Psychiatric Services*, *53*, 277–279.

Prencipe, M., Santini, M., Casini, A. R., Pezzella, F. R., Scaldaferri, N., & Culasso, F. (2003). Prevalence of non-dementing cognitive disturbances and their association with vascular risk factors in an elderly population. *Journal of Neurology*, *250*(8), 907–912.

Randolph, C. (1998). *Repeatable Battery for the Assessment of Neuropsychological Status (RBANS) manual*. San Antonio, TX: Psychological Corporation.

Rapoport, M. J., & Feinstein, A. (2000). Outcome following traumatic brain injury in the elderly: A critical review. *Brain Injury*, *14*(8), 749–761.

Rapoport, M. J., & Feinstein, A. (2001). Age and functioning after mild traumatic brain injury: The acute picture. *Brain Injury*, *15*(10), 857–864.

Reger, M. A., Welsh, R. K., Watson, G. S., Cholerton, B., Baker, L. D., & Craft, S. (2004). The Relationship between neuropsychological functioning and driving ability in dementia: A meta-analysis. *Neuropsychology*, *18*(1), 85–93.

Rothweiler, B., Temkin, N. R., & Dikmen, S. S. (1998). Aging effect on psychosocial outcome in traumatic brain injury. *Archives of Physical Medicine and Rehabilitation*, *79*, 881–887.

Salazar, A. M., Jabbari, B., Vance, S. C., Grafman, J., Amin, D., & Dillon, J. D. (1985). Epilepsy after penetrating head injury, I: Clinical correlates. *Neurology*, *35*(10), 1406–1414.

Saxton, J., Ratcliff, G., Newman, A., Belle, S., Fried, L., Yee, J., et al. (2000). Cognitive test performance and presence of subclinical cardiovascular disease in the cardiovascular health study. *Neuroepidemiology*, *19*, 312–319.

Sbordone, R. J., & Howard, M. (1989). *Predictors of rehabilitation potential and outcome from head trauma*. Unpublished manuscript.

Schoop, L. H., Callahan, C. D., Johnstone, B., & Schwake, C. J. (1998). Utility of a seven subtest version of the WAIS–R among an Alzheimer's disease sample. *Archives of Clinical Neuropsychology*, *13*(7), 637–643.

Schoop, L. H., Herrman, T. D., Johnstone, B., Callahan, C. D., & Roudebush, I. S. (2001). Two abbreviated versions of the Wechsler Adult Intelligence Scale–III: Validation among persons with traumatic brain injury. *Rehabilitation Psychology*, *46*(3), 279–287.

Schootman, M., Harlan, M., & Fuortes, L. J. (2000). Epidemiology of severe traumatic brain injuries in Iowa: The use of the capture–recapture method. *Journal of Trauma*, *48*, 70–75.

Semah, F., Picot, M. C., Adam, C., Broglin, D., Arzimanoglou, A., Bazin, B., et al. (1998). Is the underlying cause of epilepsy a major prognostic factor for recurrence? *Neurology*, *51*, 1256–1262.

Sherer, M., Nick, T. G., Millis, S. R., & Novack, T. A. (2003). Use of the WCST and the WCST-64 in the assessment of traumatic brain injury. *Journal of Clinical and Experimental Neuropsychology*, *25*(4), 512–520.

Sherrill-Pattison, S., Donders, J., & Thompson, E. (2000). Influence of demographic variables on neuropsychological test performance after traumatic brain injury. *The Clinical Neuropsychologist*, *14*, 496–503.

Simpson, G., & Tate, R. (2002). Suicidality after traumatic brain injury: Demographic, injury, and clinical correlates. *Psychological Medicine*, *32*(4), 687–697.

Smith, D. H., Chen, X. H., Iwata, A., & Graham, D. I. (2003). Amyloid beta accumulation in axons after traumatic brain injury in humans. *Journal of Neurosurgery*, *98*(5), 1072–1077.

Spreen, O., & Strauss, E. (1998). *A compendium of neuropsychological tests* (2nd ed.). New York: Oxford University Press.

Susman, M., DiRusso, S. M., Sullivan, T., Risucci, D., Nealon, P., Cuff, S., et al. (2002). Traumatic brain injury in the elderly: Increased mortality and worse functional outcome at discharge despite lower injury severity. *Journal of Trauma— Injury, Infection, and Critical Care 53*(2), 219–223.

Swan, G. E., DeCarli, C., Miller, B. L., Reed, T., Wolf, P. A., & Carmelli, D. (2000). Biobehavioral characteristics of nondemented older adults with subclinical brain atrophy. *Neurology*, *54*, 2108–2114.

Tateno, A., Jorge, R. E., & Robinson, R. G. (2003). Clinical correlates of aggressive behavior after traumatic brain injury. *Journal of Neuropsychiatry and Clinical Neuroscience*, *15*, 155–160.

Teasdale, G., & Jennett, B. (1974). Assessment of coma and impaired consciousness: A practical scale. *Lancet*, *2*, 81–83.

Thurman, D. J., Alverson, C., Dunn, K. A., Guerrero, J., & Sniezek, J. E. (1999). Traumatic brain injury in the United States: A public health perspective. *Journal of Head Trauma Rehabilitation*, *14*(6), 602–615.

US Census Bureau. (2000a). *Census 2000*. Washington, DC: Author.

US Census Bureau. (2000b). *Populations Projections Program, Population Division*. Washington, DC: Author.

Van Reekum, R., Cohen, T., & Wong, J. (2000). Can traumatic brain injury cause psychiatric disorders? *Journal of Neuropsychiatry and Clinical Neuroscience*, *12*, 316–327.

Vanderploeg, R. D. (2000). Interview and testing: The data collection phase of neuropsychological evaluations. In R. D. Vanderploeg (Ed.), *Clinicians' guide to neuropsychological assessment* (pp. 3–38). Mahwah, NJ: Lawrence Erlbaum Associates, Inc.

Volbrecht, M. E., Meyers, J. E., & Kaster-Bundgaard, J. (2000). Neuropsychological outcome of head injury using a short battery. *Archives of Clinical Neuropsychology*, *15*(3), 251–265.

Vollmer, D. G., & Eisenberg, H. M. (1990). Head injury (including subdural hematoma). In W. R. Hazzard, R. Andres, E. L. Bierman, & J. P. Blass (Eds.), *Principles of geriatric medicine and gerontology* (2nd ed., pp. 990–998). New York: McGraw-Hill.

Wechsler, D. (1997). *WAIS–III and WMS–III technical manual*. San Antonio, TX: Psychological Corporation.

Williams, D. H., Levin, H. S., & Eisenberg, H. M. (1990). Mild head injury classification. *Neurosurgery*, *27*, 422–428.

Woo, B. H., & Thoidis, G. (2000). Epidemiology of traumatic brain injury. In B. Woo & S. Nesathurai (Eds.), *The rehabilitation of people with traumatic brain injury* (pp. 13–17). Malden, MA: Blackwell Science.

Section IV

Clinical considerations

12 Co-occurring psychiatric and neurological impairments in older adults

Mary R. Hibbard, Sabrina Breed, Teresa Ashman, and Julie Williams

With the "graying" of America (US Department of Health and Human Services, 1999), the number of older adults referred for psychological evaluations will only continue to expand. Specialists in geropsychology will be called upon to differentiate concerns of older adults about normal aging from symptoms reflective of incipient cognitive impairments or late onset psychiatric diagnoses. Such challenges are further compounded when individuals with known neurological disease or injury present for clinical evaluation and treatment planning. In the present chapter, the frequency of major depression, anxiety disorders, and psychosis in older adults will be reviewed and contrasted with the incidence of these psychiatric disorders in older adults with acquired neurological impairments. Traditional psychological interventions in older adults will be summarized, with modifications of these approaches to enhance treatment effectiveness for older adults with co-occurring psychiatric and neurological disorders suggested. This chapter will not focus on issues related to medication management of psychiatric disorders nor on substance abuse disorders in older adults since those topics are covered in detail in Chapters 15 and 16 of this volume.

Unique diagnostic issues in older adults

Approximately 20% of individuals aged 55 and older will experience the disabling symptoms of a psychiatric disorder (US Department of Health and Human Services, 1999). This significant proportion of older adults comprises both individuals who have experienced mental illness throughout their life span and now have aged with these psychiatric challenges as well as individuals who are experiencing new onset psychiatric illness for the first time in their later years. Despite these high prevalence rates, psychiatric illnesses in older adults remain both underdiagnosed and undertreated. Unfortunately, treating clinicians and older adults themselves often erroneously view psychiatric symptoms as a "normal" part of growing older (National Institutes of Health, 1991). The failure to treat a primary psychiatric illness in older adults is potentially dangerous for patients, especially given the fairly good response of older adults to a wide variety of treatments (Benedict & Nacoste, 1990; Koenig & Blazer, 1992).

In part, underdiagnosis and nontreatment of psychiatric disorders are reflective of the often complex challenges confronting older adults across medical, biological, and developmental spheres. For example, psychiatric symptoms, particularly anxiety and depression, often present in older adults within the context of a physical illness (US Department of Health and Human Services, 1999). Illness in older adults can precipitate psychiatric disorders secondary to either a direct biological mechanism (for example, depression secondary to stroke) or as a result of stress associated with either coping with the illness itself or its resultant increase in physical disability and increased dependence. Further, older adults often focus solely on the acquired health problems, ignoring the psychiatric symptoms themselves (National Institutes of Health, 1991). Alternatively, psychiatric symptoms in older adults tend to coexist with decreased cognitive abilities, making it difficult for clinicians to recognize the psychiatric symptomatology (National Institutes of Health, 1991). Coexisting cognitive deficits can further complicate treatment initiation and/or treatment compliance by older adults. Aging itself may present a major developmental challenge for older individuals; that is, completing a life review during the later ages. The outcome of this review is facing the end of life with "integrity" or succumbing to "despair" (Erikson, 1964), and the process itself may herald emergence of late onset psychiatric symptoms.

Specific psychosocial changes inherent in the process of aging can result in underdiagnosis of psychiatric pathology. For example, the onset of retirement is typically accompanied by decreased functional expectations that may mask reduced levels of cognitive abilities and/or emerging emotional impairments. Limited support networks may result in older adults becoming increasingly isolated. Older adults, especially the oldest old, often outlive spouses, siblings, and friends, leaving them increasingly vulnerable to development of psychiatric illnesses as they age. Increased physical and cognitive disability associated with normal aging typically result in greater reliance on family members, other support systems, and caregivers. These family/care providers often become the referrers of older adults for needed psychological assessment and treatment.

Prevalence and patterns of psychiatric challenges in older adults vary from those observed in younger adults. The prevalence of depression, anxiety disorders, and psychosis in older adults will be summarized and then contrasted with patterns of psychiatric challenges observed in neurologically impaired older adults. Consideration of substance abuse is essential to psychological and neuropsychological evaluation of older adults (see Chapter 16 of this volume).

Depression in older adults

The Surgeon General, in a report on mental illness in older adults (US Department of Health and Human Services, 1999), estimated that 4.4% of older adults met DSM-IV (American Psychiatric Association, 1994) diagnosis of a major depressive disorder. Approximately 2% of the older adult population has a dysthymic disorder, and 4% have an adjustment disorder with depressed mood (Koenig & Blazer, 1992). However, depressive symptoms that fail to meet full diagnosis for a major depression are more prevalent in older adults. An additional 8–10% of community-dwelling older adults and 17–35% of primary care patients present with depressive symptomatology that fail to meet DSM-IV diagnostic criteria (Koenig & Blazer, 1992). These factors may have contributed to the popular misconception that major depression is more common in older than younger adults (US Department of Health and Human Services, 1999). In contrast, major depression in older adults often remains underrecognized due to another misconception, namely that depression is a normal feature of aging (Katona, 2000).

The incidence of a major depressive disorder in older adults is lower than in younger adults. One year prevalence rates for depression for adults age 65 and older were reported to be 0.9%, in contrast to rates of 2.9% for those aged 18–29 and 3.9% in those aged 30–44 (Weissman, Bruce, Leaf, Florio, & Holzer, 1991). Further, rates of depression vary significantly by setting. While the prevalence of major depression among community-dwelling older adults is generally thought to be less than 3%, 13% of nursing home residents develop a new major depression over a 1-year period, with rates of depressive symptomatology even higher (National Institutes of Health, 1991). Factors associated with depression in older adults include female gender, use of pharmaceuticals, family history, medical conditions (e.g., stroke, Alzheimer's disease, cancer, and heart disease), and alcohol and substance abuse histories (Mulsant & Ganguli, 1999). Mania or hypomania constitutes 5–10% of the psychiatric diagnoses for older adult patients (Young & Klerman, 1992). Studies of first hospital admissions suggest that the risk of mania declines with age. However, there is some evidence that first admissions for mania increase after the age of 60, especially in men (Alexopoulos, 1990).

Prevalence rates of major depression in older adults need to be reviewed in light of whether the older adults are experiencing a new onset depression as contrasted with those who have a prior history of a depressive illness. Given that major depression typically follows a relapsing and remitting course, many older adults with depression experience a relapse of an illness that initially presented in young adulthood. In contrast, new onset depression, beginning after age 60, has many distinguishing features. Older individuals with a new onset depression demonstrate less lifetime personality dysfunction and less family history of depression than individuals with a prior history of depression (US Department of Health and Human Services, 1999). Risk factors for new onset depression in older adults include physical illness, low educational attainment, impaired functional status, heavy alcohol intake, and widowhood (US Department of Health and Human Services, 1999). Cognitive deficits are more prominent, particularly decreased memory, executive dysfunction, and apathy.

New onset depression is associated with greater medial temporal abnormalities on MRI (US Department of Health and Human Services, 1999).

Alexopoulos, Meyers, Young, Silbersweig, and Charlson (1997) proposed a vascular theory of small, but numerous, cerebrovascular events causing damage to the prefrontal regions of the brain as the underlying etiology of these new onset depressions in older adults. Older adults with a new onset depression also appear to be at increased risk for later onset dementia (Alexoupoulos, Young, & Meyers, 1993). The relationship between depression and cognitive impairment in older adults is further complicated by the fact that individuals with depression can also present with a "pseudodementia," a constellation of cognitive impairments, particularly decreased attention and memory, which remit as the depressive episode remits. Mania can also occur in older adults; one study reports estimated prevalence rates between 6% and 19% in older patients consecutively admitted to psychiatric settings with the diagnosis of an affective disorder (Post, 1984).

The vital importance of accurate diagnosis and treatment of depression in older adults is highlighted by the devastating effects that major depression can have on individuals recovering from physical illness. More specifically, the presence of depression elevates mortality rates in individuals with both myocardial infarction (US Department of Health and Human Services, 1999) and cancer (Pennix et al., 1998). Depression in nursing home patients increased their mortality by 59% (Rovner, 1993). The Department of Health and Human Services reports that the effects of depression on mortality are comparable in potency to smoking, obesity, or hypertension (Pearson, 2003). Furthermore, major depression is a risk factor for decreased physical strength and increased disability (Lenze et al., 2001; Pennix, Deeg, van Eijk, Beekman, & Guralnik, 2000; Pennix, Leveille, Ferrucci, van Eijk, & Guralnik, 1999).

By far, the most devastating outcome of major depression in older adults is suicide. Suicide is more frequent in older adults than in any other age group, with those 65 years old and older committing 18% of all reported suicides in 2000, despite the fact that older adults made up only 13% of the population (National Institute of Mental Health, 2003). Passive suicidal behaviors in older adults, such as cutting down on food or noncompliance with medications, are difficult to quantify; therefore, the actual frequency of suicide in older adults may be underestimated. Significant demographic differences in suicide rates among older adults have been noted, with white males at the greatest risk. In 2000, white males over age 85 had the highest rates of suicide of any age group at 59 per 100,000 or six times the national rate (National Institute of Mental Health, 2003). In contrast, suicide rates are much lower for African Americans, particularly African-American women (Pearson, 2003).

When an older adult presents with depressive symptoms, it is important to parse out the possible contribution of bereavement. Because of their age, many older adults have experienced the deaths of people who made up their support network, including spouses, siblings, friends, and sometimes children. While bereavement, which is typically characterized by feelings of sadness that the person regards as "normal," is not considered a mental illness, it may well become a focus of treatment if symptoms are severe or persistent. Bereavement, widowhood, and a reduced social support network increase an individual's vulnerability to experiencing a major depressive episode. For example, one-third of widows and widowers meet criteria for major depression 1 month after losing a spouse, though only half of these individuals remain depressed after 1 year (National Institutes of Health, 1991).

Co-occurring depression in older adults with neurological diseases

The frequency and nature of depressive disorders shift considerably in older adults when faced with a comorbid neurological injury or diagnosis. Prevalence rates are far greater than would be expected in either community-based samples of adults in general (American Psychiatric Association, 1994) or older adults specifically (Weissman et al., 1991), with major depression the most prevalent co-occurring psychiatric diagnosis. Specific issues related to co-occurring depression in select acquired neurological illnesses are highlighted below.

Traumatic brain injury

Individuals over the age of 65 are at increased risk of traumatic brain injury (TBI), with increased incidence rates of TBI noted after age 60 (Kraus & Sorenson, 1994). Falls are the second leading cause of brain injury and associated most frequently with old age (Kraus & Sorenson, 1994). Older adults are more likely to experience complicated TBIs, to have longer hospitalizations, and to be more severely disabled at the time of acute hospital discharge (Whiteneck et al., 2001). Because of the unique pathophysiology of the older brain (Ellis, 1990), older adults are at greater risk of subdural hematomas post TBI. Enlargement of the subdural spaces that occurs with advanced age allows for a relatively large volume of fluid to accumulate before creating a significant mass effect on the brain. As a result, older adults may experience subdural hemorrhages after seemingly trivial injuries resulting in indirect trauma to the brain (Rozzelle, Wofford, & Branch, 1995). Because the common clinical presentation of a subdural hematoma is a gradual decline in mental state, the effects of a mild TBI may be mistaken for the onset of a dementia process (Jones & Kafetz, 1999). Subdural hematomas may also result in the development of normal pressure hydrocephalus secondary to obstruction of central spinal fluid flow (Cummings & Benson, 1992), which presents with a similar clinical picture of gradual cognitive decline.

Major depression is the most common co-occurring psychiatric disorder post TBI (Fann, Katon, Uomoto, & Esselman, 1995; Hibbard, Uysal, Kepler, Bogdany, & Silver, 1998; van Reekum, Bolago, Finlayson, Gardner, & Links, 1996). Prevalence rates of post-TBI depression are significantly higher than the 0.9% found in community-based older adults (Weissman et al., 1991). Age has been independent of onset of post-TBI depression (Ashman et al., 2004; Fedoroff et al., 1992; Hibbard et al., 1998, 2004); therefore, findings regarding the prevalence of post-TBI depression are applicable to older individuals who experience a TBI. At 1-year post TBI, 26% of individuals met criteria for major depression (Jorge, Robinson, Starkstein, & Arndt, 1994). Major depression appears to increase over time post TBI. For example, in cross-sectional studies completed 3–8 years after injury, prevalence rates of major depression ranged from 30% to 77% (Fann et al., 1995; Hibbard et al., 1998; van Reekum et al., 1996; Varney, Martzke, & Robert, 1987). Robust rates of resolution of Major Depressive Disorder (MDD) have been reported (Ashman et al., 2004; Fann et al., 1995; Hibbard et al., 1998; van Reekum et al., 1996), suggesting a time-limited nature of depressive episodes. Unfortunately, a significant number (approximately 25%) of individuals who experience major depression post TBI remain chronically depressed over time (Hibbard et al., 2004).

Across studies, expected demographic factors of marital status, education, socioeconomic status, diversity, and TBI-related characteristics (e.g., TBI severity or duration post TBI) were unrelated to onset of depression after injury (Ashman et al., 2004; Fedoroff et al., 1992; Hibbard et al., 1998, 2004). Two risk factors have been identified—being female and having a prior history of depression or another pre-TBI psychiatric disorder (Ashman et al., 2004; Hibbard et al., 1998). The risk of development of major depression remains elevated for decades following TBI and appears to be highest in those with more severe TBI (Holsinger et al., 2002).

The additive impact of major depression on the cognitive, physical, and behavioral challenges associated with TBI can significantly limit the older individual's ability to successfully reintegrate into the community. Acquired emotional disabilities post TBI have been viewed as more seriously handicapping than either the cognitive or physical challenges of the TBI itself (Lezak, 1983). Individuals with co-occurring TBI and depression have poorer rehabilitation outcomes (Brooks, Campsie, Symington, Beattie, & McKinlay, 1987; Thomsen, 1984), increased functional disability (Fann et al., 1995), and increased family dysfunction (Carnevale, Anselmi, Busichio, & Millis, 2002).

In a New Haven NIMH Epidemiological Catchment Area Study focused on mental health in the community, individuals with a reported loss of consciousness (and therefore a high probability of a prior TBI) and a psychiatric disorder were at heightened risk of suicide (Silver, Kramer, Greenwood, & Weissman, 2001). This statistic is particularly important for older adults given their already elevated rates of suicide (National Institute of Mental Health, 2003). The risk of suicide increases with the length of time since injury and the degree of disruptions in the individual's relationships and occupational functioning (Yudofsky & Hales, 1992). When combining documented poorer outcomes post TBI with the known prevalence of depression after TBI in older adults, older individuals can be seen to be at heightened risk of suicide after TBI.

Secondary manic or hypomanic states have been reported in individuals who have experienced a TBI (Shukla, Cook, Mukherjee, Godwin, & Miller,

1987), with prevalence rates of approximately 9% (Robinson & Jorge, 1994). Secondary mania has been associated with posttraumatic partial complex seizures (Shukla et al., 1987) and right hemisphere lesions (Starkstein et al., 1990). Neither family history of a bipolar disorder (Shukla et al., 1987) nor severity of TBI (Robinson & Jorge, 1994) was related to development of mania after TBI.

Seizure disorders post TBI have been related to increased psychopathology, ranging from changes in personality characteristics to frank psychosis with either episodic or chronic courses, post TBI (McKenna, Kane, & Parrish, 1985; Trimble, 1991). The most problematic seizure disorders are those accompanied by depressive manifestations with suicidal thoughts and/or actual suicidal attempts (Fedoroff et al., 1992; Shukla et al., 1987).

Cerebrovascular accidents

A cerebrovascular accident (stroke) is a devastating vascular event with a high mortality rate. Those who survive strokes are often left with severe handicaps and are at significant risk of developing a psychiatric disorder. Similar to TBI, the most common mental health disorder post stroke is major depression. Estimated prevalence rates range between 20% and 50% for stroke survivors admitted to either a hospital or rehabilitation setting (Kramer & Reifler, 1992; Stevens, Merikangas, & Merikangas, 1995). Individuals with cortical and lacunar infarcts or more anterior left hemisphere lesions have the highest comorbidity with depression (Starkstein, Robinson, & Price, 1988). Slightly lower rates of major depression after a stroke are reported in community settings (Beekman et al., 1998). Thus, the prevalence of depression among individuals who have experienced a stroke, regardless of whether the individuals reside in the community or a hospital, remains substantially higher than expected in either healthy community samples (Burvill et al., 1995) or healthy older adults (Weissman et al., 1991).

Both psychosocial variables and characteristics of the stroke itself have been suggested as predictors of depression after stroke. Biological pathways for poststroke depression have been suggested by prior studies of brain lesion localization (Robinson, Kubos, Starr, Rao, & Price, 1984; Starkstein et al., 1988) and by studies documenting the depletion of select neurotransmitters (Bryer et al., 1992). However, not all authors agree with these findings (Andersen, Vestergaard, Ingemann-Nielsen, & Lauritzen, 1995; House, Dennis, & Mogridge, 1991). Similar to the TBI literature, stroke-related variables such as previous strokes, duration of time since the stroke, and comorbid illnesses were unrelated to the emergence of poststroke depression. Several risk factors predictive of depression in the general population have been identified as predictive of depression following a stroke. These risk factors include being female, the absence of a close relationship, inadequate social supports, and select personality characteristics (Morris, Robinson, Andrzejewski, Samuels, & Prince, 1993; Sharpe et al., 1994). Specific predictors of poststroke depression include extent of functional limitations, extent of cognitive and speech impairments, lack of perceived support from spouse caregivers (Morris, Robinson, Rapheal, & Bishop, 1991), spousal overprotectiveness (Thompson, Sobolew-Shubin, Graham, & Janigian, 1989), and an external locus of control (Beekman et al., 1998).

Poststroke depression has been associated with poorer rehabilitation outcomes (Krauhanen et al., 1999), reduced quality of life for patients (Astrom, Asplund, & Astrom, 1992; Fruhwald, Loeffler, Eher, Saletu, & Bauhackl, 2001; King, 1996; Suenkeler et al., 2002) and their caregivers (Kotila, Numminen, Waltimo, & Kaste, 1998), increased suicidal ideation, and increased risk of mortality (Andersen, Vestergaard, & Lauritzen, 1994; Angeleri, Angeleri, Foschi, Giaquinto, & Nolfe, 1993; Astrom et al., 1992; Morris et al., 1993). Depression significantly worsens between 6 and 12 months post stroke (Suenkeler et al., 2002). Despite stability of neurological functioning, reductions in quality of life and decline in life satisfaction have been documented 1 year post stroke (Suenkeler et al., 2002).

Dementia

Multiple subtypes of dementia have been delineated in the DSM-IV (American Psychiatric Association, 1994). For the purposes of this chapter, our review will be limited to the most common dementias referred for clinical neuropsychological interventions in older adults: Alzheimer's disease (AD), vascular dementia (VD), and Parkinson's disease (PD). Dementia has been diagnosed in approximately 8–15% of the general population over the age of 65 (Green & Davis, 1993; Ritchie & Kildea, 1995). The prevalence of dementia is higher in women, although this may reflect women's longer lifespan, since studies fail to show gender differences in overall incidence rates. Incidence rates reveal age-related increases of dementia (Aevarsson & Skoog, 1996; Paykel et al., 1994). For example, while prevalence rates of 1% have been reported for individuals between 60 and 64 years old, prevalence rates increase to between 30% and 45% in those aged 85 and older (Evans et al., 1989; Jorm, Korten, & Henderson, 1987). Patients with dementia develop depression at a rate higher than that of the general population. Depressive manifestations of varying intensity occur in approximately 50% of patients with dementia (Alexopoulos, 1990).

Alzheimer's disease is a dementing disorder of pivotal importance in older adults (Ritchie & Kildea, 1995), with both genetic and environmental factors attributed to its etiology. Genetic factors, such as mutations of select chromosomes, specifically ApoE-e4 allele, excessive plaques of B-amyloid, the loss of acetylcholine, and a history of a prior head injury have all been related to the subsequent development of AD (Corder et al., 1993; Mayeux et al., 1998; Twamley & Bondi, 2004). Family history is also a strong predictor of AD, with approximately 50% of individuals with a positive family history developing the disorder (Mohs, Breitner, Sliverman, & Davis, 1987).

A growing number of studies suggest depression to be a common psychiatric disturbance in AD, both in its early preclinical stages (Berger, Fratiglioni, Forsell, Winblad, & Backman, 1999) and after a full diagnosis of AD is made. Research on the comorbidity of depression and AD has suggested a wide variety of familial (Pearlson et al., 1990), clinical (Pearlson, Teri, Reifler, & Raskind, 1989; Rovner, Broadhead, Spencer, Carson, & Folstein, 1989) and neuropathological (Zubenko & Moossy, 1988; Zweig et al., 1988) correlates. Psychiatric and behavioral symptoms vary as AD advances. For example, depression and anxiety occur most frequently during the early stages of AD, whereas psychotic symptoms and aggressive behaviors occur during the later stages of the disease (Alexopoulos & Abrams, 1991; Devanand et al., 1997).

Early research on the prevalence of depression and AD was limited by a lack of established procedures to ascertain depressive symptoms in severely cognitively impaired individuals. As a result, wide variability (15–86%) in the prevalence rates of major depressive disorders in individuals diagnosed with AD were initially reported (Merriam, Aronso, Gaston, Wey, & Katz, 1988; Reding, Haycox, & Blass, 1985; Rovner et al., 1989). A series of studies have highlighted the potential insensitivity of assessments that rely solely on the self-report of individuals with AD and have stressed the need for a more comprehensive assessment, including the use of collateral informants (Gilley et al., 1995; Teri & Wagner, 1991). Expected predictors of depression (i.e., age, gender, marital status, extent of cognitive or functional impairments, history of prior alcohol use, coexisting medical conditions) are poor predictors of depression after a diagnosis of AD (Harwood et al., 2000). Gender differences in symptom presentation have been suggested, in that men report more somatic symptoms. Mood symptoms have been found to be inversely related to age (Gilley, Wilson, Bienias, Bennett, & Evans, 2004).

Vascular dementia includes dementia due to a single cerebrovascular infarct or dementia due to more diffuse infarcts of small or medium size vessels (Twamley & Bondi, 2004). VD is more frequent in men than women, with onset typically after age 70. Medical conditions such as hypertension, atrial fibrillation, smoking, diabetes, and coronary artery disease are significant risk factors for VD. As cerebrovascular damage accrues, most often in a stepwise fashion, cognitive impairments associated with the disease increase. Affective disturbances have been commonly observed in patients with VD, particularly depression (Twamley & Bondi, 2004). Prevalence rates for depression in individuals with VD are greater than those with AD: 19% and 8%, respectively (Ballard et al., 2000).

Parkinson's disease is a progressive, neurodegenerative disease affecting the basal ganglia. Typically, onset is between the ages of 40 and 70, with diagnosis more likely in men. Most individuals with PD have significant motor and cognitive deficits that worsen over time. In addition, a substantial proportion (estimated between 20% and 40%) develop dementia (Twamley & Bondi, 2004), often from the use of dopaminergic medications that can put patients at risk of developing delirium or psychosis (Reynaud, von Gunten, & Kung, 2001).

Emotional and behavioral changes are prominent in PD. Cross-sectional studies estimate rates of depression in individuals with PD, varying from a low of 4% to a high of 70% (Cummings & Benson, 1992; Gotham, Brown, & Marsden, 1986; Huber, Paulson, & Shuttleworth, 1988; Mayeux et al., 1986; Sano et al., 1989; Santamaria, Tolosa, & Valles, 1986). Unlike TBI and stroke, the majority of the depressive disorders observed after PD are minor depressive episodes, with only 4–6% meeting full criteria for a DSM-IV diagnosis of a major depressive disorder (Tandberg, Laarsen, Aarsland, & Cummings, 1996). When depression is diagnosed in an individual with PD, predominant symptoms include anxiety, somatic symptoms, sleep disturbances, anhedonia, and loss of initiation, with infrequent reports of guilt or suicidal ideation (Girotti & Soliveri, 2003; Poewe & Seppi, 2001). Although depression after PD has been found to be unrelated to severity of motor symptoms, prevalence tends to peak during the early phase of the disease (Mayeux, Stern, Cote, & Williams, 1984; Mayeux et al., 1986). Depression symptoms of mild to moderate severity have been diagnosed in 30% of patients with incipient PD (Santamaria et al., 1986). Depressive symptoms are also frequent features of advancing PD (Mayeux et al., 1984, 1986), with severity of depression the single most important factor associated with severity of cognitive impairment (Sano et al., 1989).

Mechanisms underlying depression emergence in PD have been linked to a variety of neurotransmitter abnormalities, such as dopamine deficiency in mesocorticolimbic projections (Javoy-Agid & Agid, 1980), neuroadrenergic cortical deficiency (Hornykiewicz, 1982), and loss of serotonin neurons in the midbrain (Hornykiewicz, 1982; Huber et al., 1988). Other researchers have viewed depression as more of a reactive response to the disabling and progressive nature of the disease itself (Bieliauskas & Glantz, 1989; Bieliauskas, Klawans, & Glantz, 1986; Taylor, Saint-Cyr, Lang, & Kenny, 1986).

Depression is a potential source of error variance when completing cognitive testing of individuals with PD, and can easily result in an overestimation of cognitive deterioration (Raskin, Borod, & Tweedy, 1990; Youngjohn, Beck, Jogerst, & Caine, 1992). Depression in PD is also viewed as a risk factor for later development of dementia (Marder, Tang, Cote, & Stern, 1995). Because of this, a common referral question is the differentiation of cognitive dysfunction caused by the PD from a "pseudodementia" attributable to depression (Salzman & Gutfreund, 1986; Youngjohn et al., 1992).

Anxiety disorders in older adults

Although depression has been the most frequently researched psychiatric illness in older adults, anxiety disorders are by far the most prevalent of all psychiatric disorders in this age group (Sheikh & Salzman, 1995). Overall prevalence rates for anxiety disorders are 11.4% (Flint, 1994), with older adults being more than twice as likely to suffer from an anxiety disorder as major depression. As with major depression, the prevalence of anxiety disorders in older adults is lower than in younger adults (Flint, 1994). Epidemiological data suggesting that most anxiety syndromes typically present during a young age, only to reoccur or worsen as a person ages (Lang & Stein, 2001). For example, most phobic disorders emerge between childhood and the mid-twenties, and the mean age of onset of panic disorders is the mid-thirties (Weissman et al., 1991). In older adults, anxiety disorders often coexist with major depression (Alexopoulos, 1991; Leckman, Merikangas, Pauls, Prusoff, & Weissman, 1983). Important risk indicators for anxiety in older adults include being female, the presence of a comorbid depression, lack of social support, poor physical health, and functional and cognitive impairments (Smalbrugge, Pot, Jongenelis, Beekman, & Efsting, 2003).

It should be noted that an additional 17–21% of older adults experience significant symptoms of anxiety, but their symptoms fail to meet DSM-IV criteria for a specific disorder (US Department of Health and Human Services, 1999). Further, the diagnosis of anxiety in older adults can be complicated by the fact that many older adults experience concomitant physical illnesses that include anxiety symptoms that are often related to the medical diagnoses themselves (e.g., cardiovascular problems or pulmonary disorders) (Sheikh, 1990).

Epidemiological rates for new or recurrent anxiety disorders in older adults are difficult to determine since different subgroups in different settings across studies have been evaluated. In the Epidemiological Catchment Area Survey (Eaton, Dryman, & Weissman, 1991), 1-year prevalence rates of anxiety disorders for adults age 65 and older were unexpectedly highest for simple phobia (8.8% for women and 4.9% for men), and agoraphobia was equally prevalent in late life and childhood–early adulthood (Anthony & Aboraya, 1992; Flint, 1994). The presentation of simple phobias in older adults is reportedly similar to that in younger adults (Lindesay, 1991), suggesting that many of the common fears (such as of animals or heights) may have been present in younger adulthood and subsequently exacerbated in later age. Late onset agoraphobia tends to be associated with a physical illness or a traumatic event, such as a fall or mugging, while in younger adults it is more likely to be associated with panic attacks (Lindesay, 1991). Generalized Anxiety Disorder (GAD) is cited as the second most common anxiety disorder in older adults (Flint, 1994; Weissman et al., 1991), with 1-year prevalence rates between 2.2% (Blazer, Hughes, George, Swartz, & Boyer, 1991) and 7.1% for older adults (Flint, 1994). Panic disorder in older adults (0.4% women and 0.04% men) tends to occur infrequently (Eaton et al., 1991; Karno & Golding, 1991) and is typically characterized by fewer panic symptoms, less avoidance, and lower scores on somatization measures (Sheikh, 1990). While Obsessive Compulsive Disorders (OCD) are diagnosed in less than 1% of older adults (Eaton et al., 1991; Karno & Golding, 1991), the incidence rates of OCD increase in women around the age of 75. Anthony and Aboraya (1992) hypothesize that this OCD peak may be due to changes in biologic amines related to age, neurological illness, and associated cognitive decline.

Finally, Posttraumatic Stress Disorder (PTSD), while typically sustained in young or middle adulthood, often persists into late life (Flint, 1994). The Surgeon General's report on mental health in older adults notes that while there has been little research on PTSD in older adults to date, its importance is expected to rise as veterans of the Vietnam War age (US Department of Health and Human Services, 1999). Unfortunately, ongoing global terrorism attacks will likely increase the number of individuals with PTSD who will need future services as they age.

Co-occurring anxiety disorders in older adults with neurological disorders

In contrast to depression, anxiety has been less frequently investigated in individuals with acquired neurological disease, particularly when using DSM-IV criteria to determine prevalence of anxiety disorders. Most research in this area has been completed in the area of TBI.

Traumatic brain injury

Anxiety disorders are the second most prevalent psychiatric disorder post-TBI. Prevalence rates using DSM-IV criteria are significantly higher for individuals post TBI than for community samples, with ranges between 2% and 15% depending on type of anxiety disorder criteria. Unlike depression, there is minimal resolution of post-TBI anxiety disorders over time (Hibbard et al., 1998). Expected demographic predictors of anxiety disorders (e.g., marital status, age, socioeconomic status) and TBI-related variables (e.g., severity of TBI, time since injury) were unrelated to prevalence of anxiety disorders after injury. Two factors were predictive of anxiety post TBI—being female and coming from Hispanic origins (Ashman et al., 2004).

Across anxiety disorders, individuals with TBI experience significantly greater anxiety than expected in either community samples or in a population of healthy older adults (Weissman et al., 1991). The most frequent anxiety disorder following TBI is PTSD. Estimates range from 19% in a cross-sectional sample of individuals who were on average 8 years post injury (Hibbard et al., 1998) to 33% in a cross-sectional sample of individuals who were 1–4 years post TBI (Ashman et al., 2004). Individuals with mild TBI tend to have higher prevalence rates of PTSD, varying between 20% and 30% (Ohry, Rattok, & Solomon, 1996; Rattock, 1996; Silver, Rattok, & Anderson, 1997). Typically, PTSD symptoms are related to the traumatic situation that led to the TBI (Blanchard et al., 1995; Green, McFarlane, Hunter, & Griggs, 1993). For example, a person who was involved in a car crash will have repeated nightmares about car crashes and avoid driving or riding in a car.

Generalized anxiety disorder has been diagnosed in 11% of individuals at 1 year post TBI (Jorge et al., 1994), and 20% in individuals who are on average 3–5 years post injury (Ashman et al., 2004; Fann et al., 1995; van Reekum et al., 1996). Panic disorder has been diagnosed in 4–6% of individuals averaging 3–5 years post injury (Ashman et al., 2004; Fann et al., 1995; van Reekum et al., 1996) and 14% of individuals who are on average 8 years post TBI (Hibbard et al., 1998). Obsessive compulsive disorder was diagnosed in 15% and phobia in 10% of individuals who were on average 8 years post TBI (Hibbard et al., 1998). Pre-TBI anxiety disorders have been found to be predictive of post-TBI anxiety disorders, reflecting the chronic nature of these anxiety disorders (Hibbard et al., 1998).

The comorbidity of depression and anxiety has been well established in the general population (US Department of Health and Human Services, 1999) and in individuals with TBI (Ashman et al., 2004; Deb, Lyons, Koutzoukis, Ali, & McCarthy, 1999; Hibbard et al., 1998; Levin et al., 2001; McCauley, Boake, Levin, Contant, & Song, 2001; van Reekum et al., 1996). As with depression alone, a comorbid diagnosis of depression and anxiety post TBI creates additional psychosocial stresses (Hibbard et al., 2004), decreasing quality of life, increasing pain, and creating poor community integration, and greater physical, cognitive, and behavioral complaints.

Cerebrovascular accident

Anxiety disorders have been infrequently examined in individuals post stroke, in part due to the difficulties in differentiating anxiety from a coexisting depressive disorder and cognitive impairments in older adult patients (Katona, 2000). Only one study of 294 stroke survivors examined anxiety disorders following stroke onset (Burvill et al., 1995). The study found that 12% of men and 28% of women were diagnosed with an anxiety disorder, agoraphobia being most common. However, when the prevalence of prestroke anxiety disorders was factored in, prevalence rates of anxiety post stroke declined to 9% of men and 20% of women. Additional studies are clearly indicated in this area.

Dementia

Anxiety symptoms have been more thoroughly studied in individuals with dementia than acquired brain injuries. In community-based samples of individuals with probable AD, anxiety symptoms were present in the majority of patients, with reported anxiety symptoms noted in 56% (McCurry, Gibbons, Logsdon, & Teri, 2004) and 70% (Teri et al., 1999) of individuals. Furthermore, most patients with AD exhibited symptoms of both anxiety and depression (Teri et al., 1999), with anxiety symptoms most often expressed as motor agitation (Goudemand & Thomas, 1994). While anxiety symptoms are prevalent in AD, only 5–6% of individuals meet full criteria for

GAD (Chemerinski, Petracca, Manes, Leiguarda, & Starkstein, 1998; Ferretti, McCurry, Logsdon, Gibbons, & Teri, 2001). Patients with AD and GAD were found to exhibit significantly more irritability, overt aggression, mania, and pathological crying (Chemerinski et al., 1998) than patients without the comorbid diagnosis. Anxiety symptoms have also been associated with onset of VD (Porter et al., 2003). In fact, one study contrasting individuals with VD and those with AD found more anxiety symptoms in VD (72% vs. 38%; Ballard et al., 2000). Furthermore, VD patients with the most severe dementia (94%) were the most likely to be anxious.

PD has also been associated with comorbid onset of anxiety disorders. Upward of 40% of patients with PD have been diagnosed with an anxiety disorder, the most prevalent being GAD, panic, and social phobias (Richard, Schiffer, & Jurlan, 1996; Sadavoy & LeClair, 1997). The presence of anxiety has been linked to the neurobiological disease process rather than being understood as a purely psychological reaction to the illness itself (Richard et al., 1996).

Psychotic disorders in older adults

One-year prevalence rates of schizophrenia among individuals age 65 and older are 0.6%, about half of the rates of adults aged 18–54 (US Department of Health and Human Services, 1999). Schizophrenia in older adults is distinguished on the basis of age of onset. Because schizophrenia is viewed as a lifelong disease, many adults who first experienced schizophrenia in their youth will grow old with the disease. However, there is growing evidence to suggest that the symptom burden both changes and lessens with age. In particular, older adults with lifelong schizophrenia experience fewer symptoms than middle-aged individuals with schizophrenia, with positive symptoms less prominent than negative symptoms (US Department of Health and Human Services, 1999).

Individuals with early onset schizophrenia often experience a worsening of their preexisting cognitive impairments as they age (Dahlman, Ashman, & Mohs, 2000). In addition, among older adults with schizophrenia there is a subgroup that can still be encountered in clinical practice who are old enough to have undergone elective brain surgery as a treatment for the disease in their youth. While these surgeries may have been effective in reducing the psychotic symptoms, they were undertaken at cost to the individual who was left with lifelong neuropsychological dysfunction, the most dominant being poor initiation.

In contrast, there is a small number of people who present with schizophrenia for the first time in later life. Those with late-onset schizophrenia are more likely to be female, with presentation of paranoia a prominent symptom and with fewer cognitive impairments. Competing theories about late-onset schizophrenia exist. One theory posits that late-onset schizophrenia is a less severe form of the illness that was delayed in its presentation due to the presence of protective factors. Another theory posits that late-onset schizophrenia is a distinct neurobiological subtype of the illness (US Department of Health and Human Services, 1999).

Although schizophrenia may be uncommon in older adults, psychotic symptoms can appear in older adults who are experiencing the effects of a dementia. A common psychotic presentation is a nonbizarre paranoia, which upon careful examination, can be seen as a byproduct of decreased memory functioning. For example, older adults who cannot remember where they have placed valuable items may believe that aides or family members are stealing from them. These beliefs can be heightened by the anxiety and vulnerability experienced by many individuals with dementia. Psychotic symptoms can also present in the course of progressive dementing illness (e.g., advanced Alzheimer's disease) secondary to biostructural and biochemical changes in the brain (Rabins, 1992).

Finally, older adults may present with new-onset psychotic symptoms secondary to delirium. Typically the delirium represents an acute change in mental status for the older adult secondary to an underlying medical condition. Approximately 18% of general hospital patients are delirious (Trezpacz, 1994), with higher incidences of delirium in select surgical populations. Most delirium is reversible once the underlying medical disorder is treated. However, dementia is a risk factor for delirium; thus, the presence of a delirium (in the absence of a known medical condition) may be the first indication that an individual has been experiencing a previously undiagnosed dementia (Rabins, 1992). Psychotic depression can also occur. Between 20% and 45% of hospitalized older adults with major depression (Meyers, 1992) and 3.6% of older adults living in the community with major depression (Kivela, Pahkala, & Laippala, 1988) will experience psychotic depression with delusions, with hallucinations less frequent. Typical themes of delusions include guilt, hypochrondriasis, nihilism, persecution, and sometimes jealousy (Alexopoulos, 1996).

Psychiatric interventions with older adults

As in younger individuals, treatment of psychiatric disorders in older adults typically encompasses a variety of pharmacological and psychosocial interventions, alone or in combination. A primary role of geropsychologists is to determine which interventions are most appropriate to address the psychiatric challenges of older adult patients, while interfacing knowledge of the patients' ability to comply with recommended interventions. Such treatment considerations must be based on appropriate evaluation. For a comprehensive review of assessment methods and procedures, the reader is referred to Chapters 2 and 3 in this volume.

When considering medications for treatment of either mood or anxiety disorders in older adults, detailed evaluation of the current and prediagnosis medication history is necessary. It is not uncommon for older individuals to have been prescribed numerous medications from a variety of specialists, with little concern for potential drug–drug interactions. Many older adults remain on standing doses of medications with no clear indication as to why continuation of the drugs is necessary. Assessment of necessary medications to treat coexisting medical conditions is required, and such medications may limit the choice of the pharmacology used to address the affective disorders.

Medication compliance presents as potentially more complicated in older adults. Individuals may cease taking prescribed medications due to unpleasant side effects long before therapeutic levels of the medication have been attained. Memory impairment may limit the ability of older adults to follow the recommended medication regime. Medication noncompliance may also present as overuse or abuse, or alternately, underuse due to cost of the prescribed medication. As a result, careful selection of psychiatric medications, close monitoring of drug dosage and side effects, and ensuring medication compliance are key aspects of effective pharmacological management in older adults with neurological impairments. The reader is referred to the coverage of medication issues relevant to older adults provided by Gonzales and colleagues in Chapter 15 of this volume.

In select situations, severely depressed older adults fail to respond to medications. In such situations, electroconvulsive therapy (ECT) has been viewed as an effective intervention (Sackheim, 1994; Weiner & Krystal, 1994), especially for older adults with melancholic depression (Rudorfer, Henry, & Sackheim, 1997). NIH and NIMH practice guidelines suggest ECT to be used only in the case of severe depression with active suicidal risk or psychosis, in patients who are unresponsive to medications, and in patients who cannot tolerate medication (National Institutes of Health and National Institute of Mental Health, 1985). Specific concerns in the use of ECT with older adults focus on the long-term memory losses associated with the time period surrounding the use of ECT and reports of persistent memory loss following ECT (US Department of Health and Human Services, 1999). Following completion of a course of ECT, use of antidepressants for maintenance treatment is typically necessary to prevent relapse (Rudorfer et al., 1997).

In the following sections, individual and group psychological interventions for depression and anxiety disorders in older adults with and without neurological disorders will be addressed.

Psychotherapeutic interventions with older adults

The type and intensity of the psychotherapeutic interventions selected for older adults may differ from those chosen for younger adults. Mental health services have been underutilized by the older adults, with cohort- and age-related discomfort in acknowledging psychological problems and the need for treatment a barrier to engaging older adults in beneficial treatment interventions (Newton & Lazarus, 1992). Thus, issues such as the willingness of an older adult patient to participate in any psychological modality, be it individual or group, must be assessed. The older adult's ability to cognitively profit from these interventions, and their physical agility and independence to attend sessions on a consistent basis, must all be considered in light of the aging process itself.

Interest in adapting psychotherapy for older adults from theoretical, research, and service delivery perspectives is a relatively recent phenomenon, with the last two decades witnessing a significant interest in the applications of a variety of treatment modalities to older adults. In general there are very few differences in insight oriented psychotherapeutic approaches and treatment objectives between young and older adults. Combining psychosocial interventions with adjunct pharmacology has been found to be most effective in the treatment of depression and anxiety in older adults, with response rates of approximately 80% (Reynolds et al., 1996).

Empirical studies of the efficacy of individual and group psychosocial interventions in the treatment of mood and anxiety disorders in older adults are few. Despite this lack of firm empirical support, psychosocial interventions are often the preferred treatment modality for older individuals. This is especially true for older adults who have been unable to tolerate antidepressant medications, prefer not to take medications to address their mood disorders, are confronting current stressful life situations, or are socially isolated and lack adequate social support (Lebowitz et al., 1997). Psychotherapy not only has been shown to help relieve the symptoms of a variety of psychiatric disorders but also has demonstrated the added benefit of strengthening coping mechanisms, encouraging medication compliance, and promoting healthy behavior in older adults. Ultimately, psychosocial interventions are likely to assume greater prominence in the treatment of mental health issues in older adults as a result of population demographics which will result in increased need for mental health treatment for older adults, especially for the very old (US Department of Health and Human Services, 1999).

Mood disorders in older adults

Traditional psychotherapeutic techniques require minor modifications in order to maximally engage older individuals. Modifications are often directed at building therapeutic alliance, such as maintaining less formal relationship with the patient, assuming a more active stance in providing direction within sessions, and directed exploration of conflicts (Newton & Lazarus, 1992). Treatment approaches should also incorporate a time perspective of the past, the present, and the future in order to maximize overall treatment efficacy (Fuchs, Kurz, & Lauter, 1991).

Several forms of psychotherapy have been found to be effective in treating late-life depression. These forms include cognitive behavioral therapy (Gallagher & Thompson, 1982; Newton & Lazarus, 1992; Steuer & Hammen, 1983), interpersonal psychotherapy (Klerman, Weissman, Rounsaville, & Sherron, 1984), problem-solving therapy (Hawton & Kirk,

1989), brief psychodynamic psychotherapy (Gallagher & Thompson, 1982), and reminiscence therapy (Butler, Lewis, & Sunderland, 1991). These psychotherapies, regardless of type, were found to be more effective than a no treatment control group in the treatment of depression in older adults (Scogin & McElreath, 1994).

Cognitive behavioral therapy (CBT), designed to challenge and restructure automatic thought patterns into more rational self-statements, improve skills, and alter affect states that perpetuate depressive thoughts (Beck, Rush, Shaw, & Emery, 1979), has demonstrated effectiveness in the treatment of late-life depression (Gallagher & Thompson, 1982), anxiety disorders (Beck & Stanley, 1997; Kocsis, 2000; McGinn, 2000; Stanley, Beck, & Glassco, 1996; Thase et al., 2000), and depression secondary to a wide variety of health conditions (Boyce, Gilchrist, Talley, & Rose, 2000; Cuijpers, 1998; Kole-Snijders et al., 1999; Lustman, Freedland, Griffith, & Clouses, 1998; Markowitz et al., 1995). Specific modifications of CBT in the treatment of older adults have been proposed. Specifically, Thompson et al. (1991) suggested greater flexibility and activity on the part of the therapist, keeping the patient focused on the "here and now," proceeding at a slower pace, and adopting the patient's own language when addressing certain topics. Puentes (2004) suggested the need to integrate life review techniques within CBT sessions.

Problem-solving therapy, designed to address deficiencies in social problem-solving skills and provide coping skills to address life stressors, has been effective in reducing symptoms of depression in older adults (Arean et al., 1993; Hawton & Kirk, 1989). Interpersonal therapy, designed to address grief, role disputes, role transitions, and interpersonal deficits (Klerman et al., 1984), either alone or in combination with pharmacological interventions, was found to be effective in addressing all phases of late life depression (Reynolds et al., 1992; Schneider, 1995). Interpersonal therapy has also been found to be particularly effective in the treatment of depression following bereavement (Pasternak et al., 1997).

Brief psychodynamic therapy, designed primarily to address adjustment to medical health issues, facilitates mourning of physical limitations, addresses fears of dependency, and promotes resolution of interpersonal difficulties (Lazarus & Sadavoy, 1990). In one of the few studies that compared differing psychotherapeutic approaches, brief psychodynamic therapy yielded higher relapse and recurrence rates than did cognitive or behavioral therapies (Gallagher & Thompson, 1982).

Anxiety disorders in older adults

Psychotherapeutic interventions are also beneficial in treating anxiety disorders in older adults. Cognitive-behavioral therapy is viewed as the first choice of interventions for several anxiety disorders. CBT has been found to be beneficial in the treatment of generalized anxiety in both younger (Beck, 1988) and older adults (Fishel, 1998; Stanley & Novy, 2000), and in panic disorders in younger (Barlow & Cerny, 1988) and older adults (Beck & Stanley, 1997; Fishel, 1998). Alternative approaches for anxiety management with older adults include biofeedback (Zeichner & Boczkowski, 1986), systematic desensitization (Haden, 1991; Thomas & Gafner, 1993), stress inoculation (Hussian, 1982), and relaxation techniques (Scogin, Richard, Keith, Wilson, & McElreath, 1992).

CBT and relaxation training, in combination with antidepressant medications, appear to be most effective in addressing other anxiety disorders of older adults (Lang & Stein, 2001; Sheikh, 1990). Selective Serotonin Reuptake Inhibitors (SSRIs) are the pharmacological interventions of choice for obsessive compulsive disorders, for example, while the combination of an SSRI and CBT has been shown to decrease OCD behaviors in both younger (Sheikh, 1990) and older individuals (Marks, 1981). Likewise, CBT in combination with pharmacological agents has been proven efficacious in the treatment of phobias (Hocking & Koenig, 1995; Marks, 1987).

Mood and anxiety disorders in older adults with neurological impairments

Older individuals with acquired neurological impairments and comorbid depression or anxiety disorders present additional challenges when selecting a psychotherapeutic approach to address affective disorders. Despite the known prevalence of depression in both TBI (Rosenthal Christensen, & Ross, 1998) and stroke (Gordon & Hibbard, 1997; Kneebone & Dunmore, 2001; Palmer & Glass, 2003), surprisingly little research has focused on psychotherapeutic outcome methods to date. Case descriptions suggesting the efficacy of psychotherapy for affective disturbances in individuals with neurological impairments exist (Birkett, 1996; Langenbahn, Sherr, Simon, & Hanig, 1999). Across neurological impairments, the most frequently recommended psychotherapeutic approach is the use of CBT, with most approaches utilizing modified approaches to CBT to better address the additive challenges of cognitive deficits in individuals with neurological impairments (see below for details of these modifications). Modified CBT has been effective in case studies of individuals poststroke depression (Hibbard, Grober, Gorden, Aletta, & Friedman, 1990; Hibbard, Grober, Stein, & Gordon, 1992), with the approach reported to be well suited to working with families of stroke survivors (Palmer & Glass, 2003). Other researchers have validated the efficacy of CBT in the treatment of TBI-related depression (Payne, 2000), anger management (Medd & Tate, 2000), and co-occurring anxiety disorders (Hibbard, Gordon, & Kothera, 2000).

CBT has also been reported to be the psychotherapeutic modality of choice for individuals in the early phases of AD (Teri & Gallagher-Thompson, 1991; Teri & Uomoto, 1991), although other psychotherapy approaches have also been recommended (Cheston, Jones, & Gilliard, 2003). In early phase AD, the focus of CBT is to assist the patient in coping with depression by reducing cognitive distortions and fostering more adaptive perceptions. As AD progresses, behavioral interventions are emphasized to a greater extent (Teri, Logsdon, Uomoto, & McCurry, 1997), such as actively involving family members in increasing pleasant activities for the patient (Teri & Gallagher-Thompson, 1991). In addition to psychosocial interventions, timely assessment and treatment of coexisting anxiety using pharmacological interventions may well improve the patient's overall quality of life (Qazi, Shankar, & Orrell, 2003; Shankar, Walker, Frost, & Orrell, 1999). As the behavioral symptoms of dementia advance, antipsychotic, antidepressant, and anticonvulsant medications are used more aggressively (Poewe & Seppi, 2001).

Hibbard and colleagues (Hibbard, Grobner, Gorden, & Atetta, 1990; Hibbard et al., 1992) have modified CBT (Beck, 1972; Beck et al., 1979) to address the often shifting cognitive and behavioral challenges of individuals post stroke. This approach is applicable for addressing the varied emotional, cognitive, and behavioral challenges that emerge in older adults with both stable (e.g., TBI, stroke) and shifting (e.g. vascular dementia, PD, AD) neurological disorders. CBT offers several advantages over traditional insight-oriented therapies. It provides a flexible approach that permits individualized interventions necessary to address specific cognitive and behavioral issues as they emerge during the course of the neurological disorder; it incorporates a high level of structure necessary for an individual's maximal functioning secondary to acquired cognitive limitations; and it is factual in nature and deals with current and important situations for the individual. To maximize its efficacy, CBT should be considered for use in conjunction with antidepressant and anxiolytic medications.

Principles of CBT, originally modified for treatment of poststroke depression (Hibbard, Grober, Gordon, & Aletta, 1990; Hibbard, Grober, Gordon, Aletta, & Freeman, 1990), have been expanded to address the affective symptoms of individuals with both stable and declining neurological conditions:

- *Cognitive functioning moderates treatment strategies utilized*: Individuals with greater neurological damage (e.g., severe TBI, extensive stroke, or moderate to severe dementia) often present with significant cognitive deficits. As a general guideline, the more severe the cognitive deficits, the greater the emphasis on behavioral and pharmacological approaches utilized; the less severe the cognitive deficits, the greater the emphasis on traditional psychotherapeutic or cognitive approaches utilized.
- *Cognitive remediation enhances the individual's ability to profit from therapy*: To maximize psychotherapeutic efficacy, the clinician needs to understand the nature and severity of an individual's cognitive, physical, and behavioral challenges as well as the individual's awareness of how these acquired challenges impact their mood. Since acquired cognitive deficits typically present as the most significant challenge for the individual, accommodations for these deficits are needed within treatment

sessions. Left unaddressed, these cognitive deficits will only thwart treatment success.

- *New learning and generalization are difficult for individuals with neurological impairment*: Following any neurological disability, new learning and generalization become more difficult. Since psychotherapeutic interventions involve new learning, new concepts must be introduced slowly and in a stepwise fashion within sessions. Additional repetition is needed across sessions to ensure competency of skill development. Once novel concepts are learned and practiced to competency within sessions, additional assistance will be required to help the individual generalize learned skills outside of sessions.

- *Patient's awareness of depressive symptomatology moderates therapeutic strategy*: Individuals with neurological impairments present with varied levels of awareness of the extent of their cognitive and behavioral changes and how these changes impact on mood and functioning. The greater the unawareness, the more likely that a behavioral intervention will be the best choice of treatment.

- *Mourning is an important component of treatment*: An individual's "real" physical and cognitive losses, as well as anticipated future loss secondary to a neurological impairment, need to be mourned. Grieving multiple losses is an essential first step towards acceptance of a "new self" and gradual readjustment to an "altered self."

- *Premorbid lifestyle and interests provide a context for understanding current behaviors*: Careful exploration of abilities and traits that were valued pre-illness/disability often sheds clinical light on areas of greatest losses for an individual post onset of neurological impairment.

- *Understanding the discrepancy between actual and perceived losses is essential to treatment*: Following an acute neurological event (e.g., stroke, TBI), an individual typically experiences an "abrupt" loss in cognitive, physical, and behavioral abilities. Cognitive, physical, and behavioral losses secondary to a gradual onset of dementia can be equally devastating. The extent of the person's actual and perceived losses and their meaning will vary from individual to individual, and from family to family. Cognitive distortions will further intensify any "real" losses for an individual and his/her family. Corroboration by family members as to the extent of changes pre- and postneurological insult is often helpful in creating a realistic understanding of the person's real vs. perceived functional losses. The greater the "self-perceived" discrepancy between who the individual was "before" and who the individual is "now" (and in dementia, who the individual "will be"), the greater the affective distress to be addressed in treatment.

- *Reinforcing even small therapeutic gains improves mood*: Following neurological impairment, gains tend to be slow due to reduced learning capacity. Hence, reinforcement of gains, no matter how small, should be stressed in treatment.

- *Emphasis on the collaborative nature of the therapeutic relationship facilitates a working alliance*: The clinician is encouraged to engage the individual in a collaborative partnership: The individual becomes empowered to be the "expert in living with a neurological disorder" and the therapist "the expert in learning to cope with cognitive distortions." In this manner, the therapist and individual can create a working alliance, which has been found to be beneficial to the treatment process with older adults.
- *To ensure continuity of treatment, session flexibility is essential*: Oftentimes, treatment of older adults is interrupted due to medical set backs, inclement weather, or transportation difficulties. Such disruptions should be viewed as a normal part of therapy with older adults.
- *Fluctuations in medical status impact the course of treatment*: Changes in the older person's internal state (secondary to medication change, new illness, etc.) and the person's environment (living arrangement, death of a friend, etc.) may significantly impact the overall course of treatment, often resulting in a temporary halt or regression in treatment progress.
- *The distortions of family members must be addressed in therapy*: Family members often hold unrealistic expectations for their loved ones, either minimizing their potential or exaggerating their current abilities. When identified, these distortions need to be addressed with family members, since they are often counterproductive to the therapy.
- *Family members' mourning must be addressed*: Family members, like the older individual, must be allowed to mourn the former person and the loss of a former relationship before building a new foundation of mutual support.
- *Family members are important therapeutic helpers*: Family members are valuable additions to the therapeutic team. They can assist the therapist by providing feedback about pain or current functional abilities, and they can assist in helping the patient generalize and practice strategies learned in treatment to the home and community setting.

Psychotherapeutic group interventions for older adults

Group psychotherapy has been used with success equal to that of individual therapy with older adults. Supportive group psychotherapy provides additive benefits for older adults, including an opportunity to build relationships with peers with similar experiences while confronting similar psychological issues and enhancing self-esteem (Newton & Lazarus, 1992). Group modalities may also create a social support network, serve as a means of diminishing social isolation, and help promote social engagement (Wong, 1991) in a structure that may be more acceptable to many older individuals (Newton & Lazarus, 1992). Not all older adults are well suited for group participation, with group therapy contraindicated in older patients who are suicidal or have active drug or alcohol abuse, paranoid ideations, or cognitive impairments that will limit their ability to participate (Leszcz, 1990). Group therapy may be employed as the sole treatment or as adjunctive treatment to either pharmacology or individual treatment.

Few empirical studies of group psychotherapy outcomes with older adults can be found. CBT in a group modality has been demonstrated to be effective in the treatment of late life depression (Beutler et al., 1987) and anxiety disorders (Stanley et al., 1996). Reminiscence or life review groups (Poulton & Strassberg, 1986) have been embedded in several psychotherapy group modalities and are often used to enhance initial group cohesiveness (Leszcz, 1990). The majority of these groups do not include individuals with neurological conditions such as stroke or TBI.

The literature on psychotherapeutic interventions for older individuals with dementia suggests that group therapy, rather than individual modalities, is most beneficial for patients and their caregivers. Group interventions are traditionally part of a larger holistic approach that includes pharmacological interventions to enhance cognition and address the affective disturbances associated with the progressive nature of dementia. Structured psychotherapy groups for individuals with mild to moderate levels of dementia were found to reduce levels of depression and anxiety (Cheston et al., 2003).

Individualized cognitive remediation sessions that focused on teaching mnemonic strategies were also beneficial for both reducing affective distress of the individuals with AD and reducing caregiver burden (Clare, Wilson, Carter, & Hodges, 2003). Innovative psychotherapeutic approaches such as validation therapy (Neil & Briggs, 2003) are being evaluated in groups of individuals with mild to moderate dementia. As the dementia progresses, group modalities shift from a "talk therapy" focus to one that emphasizes sensation. For example, alternative group modalities such as reminiscence music therapy (Ashida, 2000) and art therapy (Bonder, 1994) have shown promise of reducing depressive symptoms and minimizing problematic behaviors in patients with more severe dementia. Caregiver interventions have been demonstrated to be effective in indirectly decreasing depression, agitation, and anxiety in patients with AD, while decreasing the perceived burdens and positively impacting motivation for care providers (Chang, 1999; Haupt, Karger, & Janner, 2000).

Conclusions

Older adults are vulnerable to a variety of psychiatric and neurological disorders. As a result, neuropsychologists working with older adults and their support systems must understand the ways in which these disorders may, individually and in combination, affect the neuropsychological presentations of older adults. The meaning that cognitive and psychiatric symptoms have for each patient and the people involved in the patient's life must be appreciated in order for interventions to be appropriately designed and implemented. This chapter has attempted to provide an overview of such issues in order to facilitate neuropsychological evaluation and treatment of older adults with co-occurring psychiatric and neurologic disorders.

Acknowledgements

This work was supported by the Research and Training Center on the Community Integration for Individuals with Traumatic Brain Injury (Grant No. H133B9080013) and the TBI Model System Program (Grant No. H133A020501) from the National Institute of Disability and Rehabilitation Research, US Department of Education to the Department of Rehabilitation Medicine, The Mount Sinai School of Medicine, New York.

References

Aevarsson, O., & Skoog, I. (1996). A population-based study on the incident of dementia disorders between 85 and 88 years of age. *Journal of the American Geriatrics Society, 44*, 1455–1460.

Alexopoulos, G. S. (1990). Affective disorders. In J. Sadavoy, L. Lazarus, L. Jarvik, & G. Grossman (Eds.), *Comprehensive review of geriatric psychiatry II* (2nd ed., pp. 563–592). Washington, DC: American Psychiatric Press.

Alexopoulos, G. S. (1991). Anxiety and depression in the elderly. In C. Salzman & B. D. Lebowitz (Eds.), *Anxiety in the elderly* (pp. 63–77). New York: Springer Publishing Company.

Alexopoulos, G. S. (1996). The treatment of depressed demented patients. *Journal of Clinical Psychiatry, 57*, 12–22.

Alexopoulos, G. S., & Abrams, R. C. (1991). Depression in Alzheimer's disease. *Psychiatric Clinics of North America, 14*, 327–340.

Alexopoulos, G. S., Meyers, B. S, Young, R. C., Silbersweig, D., & Charlson, M. (1997). "Vascular depression" hypothesis. *Archives of General Psychiatry, 54*, 915–922.

Alexopoulos, G. S., Young, R. C., & Meyers, B. S. (1993). Geriatric depression: Age of onset and dementia. *Biological Psychiatry, 34*, 141–145.

American Psychiatric Association. (1994). *Diagnostic and statistical manual of mental disorders* (4th ed.). Washington, DC: American Psychiatric Press.

Andersen, G., Vestergaard, K., Ingemann-Nielsen, M., & Lauritzen, L. (1995). Risk factors for post-stroke depression. *Acta Psychiatrica Scandanavica, 92*, 193–198.

Andersen, G., Vestergaard, K., & Lauritzen, L. (1994). Effective treatment of post-stroke depression with the selective serotonin re-uptake inhibitor citalopram. *Stroke, 25*, 1099–1104.

Angeleri, R., Angeleri, V. A., Foschi, N., Giaquinto, S., & Nolfe, G. (1993). The influence of depression, social activity and family stress on functional outcomes after stroke. *Stroke, 24*, 1478–1483.

Anthony, J. C., & Aboraya, A. (1992). The epidemiology of selected mental disorders in later life. In J. E. Birren, R. B. Sloane, & G. D. Cohen (Eds.), *Handbook of mental health and aging* (pp. 27–73). New York: Academic Press.

Arean, P. A., Perri, M. G., Nezu, A. M., Schein, R. L., Christopher, F., & Josephs, T. X. (1993). Comparative effectiveness of social problem-solving therapy and reminiscence therapy as treatments for depression in older adults. *Journal of Consulting and Clinical Psychology*, *61*, 1003–1010.

Ashida, S. (2000). The effect of reminiscence music therapy on change in depressive symptoms in elderly with dementia. *Journal of Music Therapy*, *37*(3), 170–182.

Ashman, T., Speilman, L. A, Hibbard, M. R., Silver, J. M., Chandar, T., & Gordon, W. G. (2004). Psychiatric challenges in the first six years after traumatic brain injury: Cross-sequential analyses of axis I disorders. *Archives of Physical Medicine and Rehabilitation*, *85*(Suppl. 2), 36–42.

Astrom, M., Asplund, K., & Astrom, T. (1992). Psychosocial function and life satisfaction after stroke. *Stroke*, *23*, 527–531.

Ballard, C., Neill, D., O'Brien, J., McKeith, I. G., Ince, P., & Perry, R. (2000). Anxiety, depression and psychosis in vascular dementia: Prevalence and associations. *Journal of Affective Disorders*, *59*(2) 97–106.

Barlow, D. H., & Cerny, J. A. (1988). *Psychological treatment of panic*. New York: Guilford Press.

Beck, A. T. (1972). *Depression: Cause and treatment*. Philadelphia: University of Pennsylvania Press.

Beck, A. T. (1988). Cognitive approaches to panic disorder: Theory and therapy. In S. Rachman & J. D. Maser (Eds.), *Panic: Psychological perspectives* (pp. 91–110). Hillsdale, NJ: Lawrence Erlbaum Associates, Inc.

Beck, A. T., Rush, A. J., Shaw, B. F., & Emery, G. (1979). *Cognitive therapy for depression*. New York: Guilford Press.

Beck, J. G., & Stanley, M. A. (1997). Anxiety disorder in the elderly: The emerging role of behavioral therapy. *Behavior Therapy*, *28*, 83–100.

Beekman, A. T. F., Pennix, B. H., Deeg, D. H., Ormel, J., Smit, J. H., Braam, A. W., et al. (1998). Depression in survivors of stroke: A community-based study of prevalence, risk factors and consequences. *Social Psychiatry and Psychiatric Epidemiology*, *33*, 463–470.

Benedict, K. B., & Nacoste, D. B. (1990). Dementia and depression: A framework for addressing difficulties in differential diagnosis. *Clinical Psychology Review*, *10*, 513–537.

Berger, A. K., Fratiglioni, L., Forsell, Y., Winblad, B., & Backman, L. (1999). The occurrence of depressive symptoms in the preclinical phase of AD. *Neurology*, *53*, 1998–2002.

Beutler, L. E., Scogin, F., Kirkish, P., Schretlen, D., Corbishley, A., Hamblin, D., et al. (1987). Group cognitive therapy and alprozalam in the treatment of depression in older adults. *Journal of Consulting and Clinical Psychology*, *55*, 550–556.

Bieliauskas, F. A., & Glantz, R. H. (1989). Depression type in Parkinson's disease. *Journal of Clinical and Experimental Neuropsychology*, *11*, 597–604.

Bieliauskas, F. A., Klawans, L., & Glantz, R. H., (1986). Depression and cognitive changes in Parkinson's disease: A review. *Advances in Neurology*, *45*, 437–438.

Birkett, D. P. (1996). *The psychiatry of stroke*. Washington, DC: American Psychiatric Press.

Blanchard, E. B., Hickling, E. J., Taylor, A. E., Loos, W. R., Forneris, C. A., & Jaccard, J. (1995). Who develops PTSD from motor vehicle accidents? *Behavior Research and Therapy*, *34*(1), 1–10.

Blazer, D. G., Hughes, D., George, L. K., Swartz, M., & Boyer, R. (1991). Generalized anxiety disorder. In L. N. Robins & D. A. Reigier (Eds.), *Psychiatric disorders in America* (pp. 180–203). New York: Free Press.

Bonder, B. R. (1994). Psychotherapy for individuals with Alzheimer's disease. *Alzheimer's Disease and Associated Disorders, 8*(Suppl. 3), 75–81.

Boyce, P., Gilchrist, J., Talley, N. J., & Rose, D. (2000). Cognitive and behavioral therapy as a treatment for irritable bowel syndrome: A pilot study. *Australian and New Zealand Journal of Psychiatry, 34*(2), 300–309.

Brooks, N., Campsie, L., Symington, C., Beattie, A., & McKinlay, W. (1987). The effects of head injury on patients and relatives within seven years of injury. *Journal of Head Trauma Rehabilitation, 2*, 1–13.

Bryer, J. B., Starkstein, S. E., Votypka, V., Parikh, R. M., Price, T. R., & Robinston, R. G. (1992). Reduction of SCF monamine metabolism in post-stroke depression: A preliminary report. *Journal of Neuropsychiatry and Clinical Neurosciences, 4*, 440–442.

Burvill, P. W., Johnson, G. A., Jamrozik, K. D., Anderson, C. S., Stewart-Wynne, E. G., & Chakera, T. M. (1995). Anxiety disorders after stroke: Results from the Perth Community Stroke Study. *British Journal of Psychiatry, 166*(3), 328–332.

Butler, R. N., Lewis, M. I., & Sunderland, T. (1991). *Aging and mental health: Positive psychosocial and biomedical approaches.* Columbus, OH: Charles E. Merrill.

Carnevale, G. J., Anselmi, V., Busichio, K., & Millis, S. R. (2002). Changes in ratings of caregiver burden following community based behavioral management program for persons with traumatic brain injury. *Journal of Head Trauma Rehabilitation, 17*(2), 83–95.

Chang, B. L. (1999). Cognitive-behavioral intervention for homebound caregivers of persons with dementia. *Nursing Research, 48*(3), 173–183.

Chemerinski, E., Petracca, G., Manes, F., Leiguarda, R., & Starkstein, S. E. (1998). Prevalence and correlates of anxiety in Alzheimer's disease. *Depression and Anxiety, 7*(4), 166–170.

Cheston, R., Jones, K., & Gilliard, J. (2003). Group psychotherapy and people with dementia. *Aging and Mental Health, 7*(6), 452–461.

Clare, L., Wilson, B. A., Carter, G., & Hodges, J. R. (2003). Cognitive rehabilitation as a component of early interventions in Alzheimer's disease: A single case study. *Aging and Mental Health, 7*(1), 15–21.

Corder, E. H., Saunders, A. M., Strittmatter, W. J., Schmechel, D. E., Gaskell, P. C., Small, G. Y., et al. (1993). Gene dose of apoliprotein E type 4 allele and the risk of Alzheimer's disease in late onset families. *Science, 261*, 921–923.

Cuijpers, P. (1998). Prevention of depression in chronic general medical disorders: A pilot study. *Psychological Reports, 82*, 735–738.

Cummings, J. L., & Benson, D. F. (1992). *Dementia: A clinical approach* (2nd ed.). Boston: Butterworth-Heinemann.

Dahlman, K. L., Ashman, T. A., & Mohs, R. C. (2000). Psychological assessment of the elderly. In G. Goldstein & M. Hersen (Eds.), *Handbook of psychological assessment* (pp. 553–578). New York: Pergamon.

Deb, S., Lyons, I., Koutzoukis, C., Ali, I., & McCarthy, G. (1999). Rate of psychiatric illness 1 year after traumatic brain injury. *American Journal of Psychiatry, 156*(3), 374–378.

Devanand, D. P., Jacobs, D. M., Tang, M. X., Del Castillo-Castaneda, C., Sano, M., Marder, K., et al. (1997). The course of psychopathologic features in mild to moderate Alzheimer's disease. *Archives of General Psychiatry, 54*, 257–263.

Eaton, W. W., Dryman, A., & Weissman, M. M. (1991). Panic and phobia. In L. N. Robins & D. A. Reigier (Eds.), *Psychiatric disorders in America* (pp. 155–179). New York: Free Press.

Ellis, G. L. (1990). Subdural hematoma in the elderly. *Emergency Medicine Clinics of North America, 8*, 281–294.

Erikson, E. H. (1964). *Insight and responsibility*. New York: W. W. Norton.

Evans, D. A., Funkenstein, H. H., Albert, M. S., Scherr, P. A., Cook, N. R., Chown, J. M., et al. (1989). Prevalence of Alzheimer's disease in a community population of older persons: Higher than previously reported. *Journal of the American Medical Association, 262*, 2551–2556.

Fann, J., Katon, W., Uomoto, J., & Esselman, P. (1995). Psychiatric disorders and functional disability in outpatient treatment with traumatic brain injury. *American Journal of Psychiatry, 152*, 1493–1499.

Fedoroff, J. P., Starkstein, S. E., Forrester, A. W., Geisler, F. H., Jorge, R. E., Arndt, S. V., et al. (1992). Depression in patients with acute traumatic brain injury. *American Journal of Psychiatry, 149*, 918–923.

Ferretti, L., McCurry, S. M., Logsdon, R., Gibbons, L., & Teri, L. (2001). Anxiety and Alzheimer's disease. *Journal of Geriatric Psychiatry and Neurology, 14*(1), 52–58.

Fishel, A. H. (1998). Nursing management of anxiety and panic. *Nursing Clinics of North America, 33*(1), 135–151.

Flint, A. J. (1994). Epidemiology and comorbidity of anxiety disorders in the elderly. *American Journal of Psychiatry, 151*(5), 640–649.

Fruhwald, S., Loeffler, H., Eher, R., Saletu, B., & Bauhackl, U. (2001). The relationship between depression, anxiety and quality of life: A study of stroke patients compared to chronic low back pain and myocardial ischemia patients. *Psychopathology, 34*, 50–56.

Fuchs, T., Kurz, A., & Lauter, H. (1991). Time perspective in the treatment of elderly depressed patients. *Der Nervenarzt, 62*(5), 313–317.

Gallagher, D., & Thompson, L. (1982). Treatment of major depressive disorder in older adult outpatients with brief psychotherapies. *Psychotherapy Theory, Research, and Practice, 19*, 482–490.

Gilley, D. W., Wilson, R. S., Bienias, J. L., Bennett, S. A., & Evans, D. A. (2004). Predictors of depressive symptoms in persons with Alzheimer's disease. *Journals of Gerontology: Series B. Psychological and Social Sciences, 59*, 75–83.

Gilley, D. W., Wilson, R. S., Fleishman, D. A., Harrison, S. W., Goetz, C. G., & Tanner, C. M. (1995). Impact of Alzheimer's-type dementia and information source on the assessment of depression. *Psychological Assessment, 7*(1), 42–48.

Girotti, F., & Soliveri, P. (2003). Cognitive and behavioral disturbances in Parkinson's disease. *Neurological Science, 24*, S30–S31.

Gordon, W. A., & Hibbard, M. R. (1997). Post stroke depression: An examination of the literature. *Archives of Physical Medicine and Rehabilitation, 78*, 658–663.

Gotham, A. M., Brown, R. G., & Marsden, C. D. (1986). Depression in Parkinson's disease: A quantitative and qualitative analysis. *Journal of Neurology, Neurosurgery, and Psychiatry, 49*, 381–389.

Goudemand, M., & Thomas, P. (1994). Anxiety, depression and dementia. *La Revue du Praticien, 44*(1), 1448–1452.

Green, C. R., & Davis, K. L. (1993). Clinical assessment of Alzheimer's type dementia and related disorders. *Human Psychopharmacology, 4*, 53–71.

Green, M. M., McFarlane, A. C., Hunter, C. E., & Griggs, W. M. (1993). Undiagnosed post traumatic stress disorder following motor vehicle accidents. *Medical Journal of Australia, 159*, 529–534.

Haden, B. (1991). Stress and stress management with the elderly. In P. Wisock (Ed.), *Handbook of clinical behavior therapy with the elderly client* (pp. 169–183). New York: Plenum.

Harwood, D. G., Barker, W. W., Ownby, R. L., Bravo, M., Aguero, H., & Duara, R. (2000). Depressive symptoms in Alzheimer's disease: An examination among community-dwelling Cuban American patients. *American Journal of Geriatric Psychiatry, 8*, 84–91.

Haupt, M., Karger, A., & Janner, M. (2000). Improvement of agitation and anxiety in demented patients after psychoeducation group intervention with their caregivers. *International Journal of Geriatric Psychiatry, 15*(12), 1125–1129.

Hawton, K., & Kirk, J. (1989). Problem solving. In K. Hawton, P. M. Salkovskis, J. Kirk, & D. M. Clark (Eds.), *Cognitive behaviour therapy for psychiatric patients: A practical guide* (pp. 406–426). Oxford, UK: Oxford University Press.

Hibbard, M. R., Ashman, T. A., Spielman, L. A., Chun, D., Charatz, H. J., & Melvin, S. (2004). Relationship between depression and psychosocial functioning after traumatic brain injury. *Archives of Physical Medicine and rehabilitation, 85*(Suppl. 2), S43–S53.

Hibbard, M. R., Gordon, W. A., & Kothera, L. (2000). Traumatic brain injury. In F. M. Dattilio & A. Freeman (Eds.), *Cognitive-behavioral approaches to crisis interventions* (4th ed., pp. 219–242). New York: Guilford Press.

Hibbard, M. R., Grober, S. E., Gordon, W. A., & Aletta, E. G. (1990). Modification of cognitive psychotherapy for the treatment of post stroke depression. *The Behavior Therapist, 1*, 15–17.

Hibbard, M. R., Grober, S. E., Gordon, W. A., Aletta, E. G., & Freeman, A. (1990). Cognitive therapy and the treatment of post stroke depression. *Topics in Geriatric Rehabilitation, 5*(3), 43–55.

Hibbard, M. R., Grober, S. E., Stein, P. N., & Gordon, W. A. (1992). Post stroke depression. In A. Freeman & F. M. Datillio (Eds.), *Comprehensive casebook of cognitive therapy* (pp. 303–310). New York: Plenum Press.

Hibbard, M. R., Uysal, S., Kepler, K., Bogdany, J., & Silver, J. (1998). Axis I psychopathology in individuals with TBI. *Journal of Head Trauma Rehabilitation, 13*(4), 24–39.

Hocking, L. B., & Koenig, H. G. (1995). Anxiety in medically ill older patients: A review and update. *International Journal of Psychiatry and Medicine, 25*, 221–238.

Holsinger, T., Steffens, D. C., Phillips, C., Helms, M. J., Havlik, R. J., Breitner, J. C., et al. (2002). Head injury in early adulthood and the lifetime risk of depression. *Archives of General Psychiatry, 59*, 17–24.

Hornykiewicz, O. (1982). Imbalance of brain monoamines and clinical disorders. *Progress in Brain Research, 55*, 419–429.

House, A., Dennis, M., & Mogridge, L. (1991). Mood disorders in the year after first stroke. *British Journal of Psychiatry, 158*, 83–92.

Huber, S. J., Paulson, G. W., & Shuttleworth, E. C. (1988). Relationship of motor symptoms, intellectual impairment, and depression in Parkinson's disease. *Journal of Neurology, Neurosurgery, and Psychiatry, 51*, 855–858.

Hussian, R. A. (1982). *Geriatric psychology: A behavioral perspective*. New York: Van Nostrand.

Javoy-Agid, R., & Agid, Y. (1980). Is the mesocortical dopaminergic system involved in Parkinson's disease? *Neurology, 30*, 1326–1330.

Jones, S., & Kafetz, K. (1999). A prospective study of chronic subdural hematoma in elderly patients. *Age and Ageing, 28*, 519–521.

Jorge, R. E., Robinson, R. G., Starkstein, S. E., & Arndt, S. V. (1994). Influence of major depression on 1-year outcome in patients with traumatic brain injury. *Journal of Neurosurgery, 81*, 726–733.

Jorm, A. F., Korten, A. E., & Henderson, A. S. (1987). The prevalence of dementia: A quantitative integration of the literature. *Acta Psychiatrica Scandinavica, 76*, 465–479.

Karno, M., & Golding, J. M. (1991). Obsessive compulsive disorder. In L. N. Robins & D. A. Reigier (Eds.), *Psychiatric disorders in America* (pp. 204–219). New York: Free Press.

Katona, C. (2000). Managing depression and anxiety in the elderly patient. *European Neuropsychopharmacology: The Journal of the European College of Neuropsycho-pharmacology, 10*(Suppl. 4), S427–S432.

King, R. B. (1996). Quality of life after stroke. *Stroke, 27*, 1467–1472.

Kivela, S. L., Pahkala, K., & Laippala, P. (1988). Prevalence of depression in an elderly Finnish population. *Acta Psychiatrica Scandanavica, 78*, 401–413.

Klerman, G. L., Weissman, M. M., Rounsaville, B. J., & Sherron, E. S. (1984). *Interpersonal psychotherapy of depression*. New York: Basic Books.

Kneebone, I. I., & Dunmore, E. (2001). Psychological management of post-stroke depression. *British Journal of Clinical Psychology, 39*(1), 53–65.

Kocsis, J. H. (2000). New strategies for treating chronic depression. *Journal of Clinical Psychiatry, 61*(11), 42–45.

Koenig, H. G., & Blazer, D. G. (1992). Epidemiology of geriatric affective disorders. *Clinical Geriatric Medicine, 8*, 235–251.

Kole-Snijders, A. M., Vlaeyen, J. W., Goossens, M. E., Rutten-van Molken, M. R., Heuts, P. H., van Breukelen, G., et al. (1999). Chronic low-back pain: What does cognitive coping skills training add to operant behavioral treatment? Results of a randomized clinical trial. *Journal of Consulting and Clinical Psychology, 67*(6), 931–944.

Kotila, M., Numminen, H., Waltimo, O., & Kaste, M. (1998). Depression after stroke: Results of the Finnstroke Study. *Stroke, 29*, 368–372.

Kramer, S. I., & Reifler, B. V. (1992). Depression, dementia and reversible dementia. *Archives in Geriatric Medicine, 8*, 289–297.

Krauhanen, M., Korpelainen, J. T., Hiltunen, P., Brusin, E., Mononen, H., Maatta, R., et al. (1999). Post stroke depression correlates with cognitive impairment and neurological deficits. *Stroke, 30*, 1857–1880.

Kraus, J. F., & Sorenson, S. B. (1994). Epidemiology. In J. Sadavoy, L. Lazarus, L. Jarvik, & G. Grossman (Eds.), *Comprehensive review of geriatric psychiatry II* (2nd ed., pp. 3–41). Washington, DC: American Psychiatric Press.

Lang, A. J., & Stein, M. B. (2001). Anxiety disorders: How to recognize and treat the medical symptoms of emotional illness. *Geriatrics, 56*(5), 24–27, 31–34.

Langenbahn, D. M., Sherr, R. L., Simon, D., & Hanig, B. (1999). Group psychotherapy. In K. G. Langer, L. Lastsch, & L. Lewis (Eds.), *Psychotherapeutic interventions for adults with brain injury or stroke: A clinician's treatment resource* (pp. 167–189). Madison, CT: Psychosocial Press.

Lazarus, L. W., & Sadavoy, J. (1996). Individual psychotherapy. In J. Sadavoy, L. W. Lazarus, L. F. Jarvik, & G. T. Grossberg (Eds.), *Comprehensive review of geriatric psychiatry* (2nd ed., pp. 819–826). Washington, DC: American Psychiatric Press.

Lebowitz, B. D., Pearson, J. L., Schneider, L. S., Reynolds, C. F., Alexopoulos, G. S., Bruce, M. L., et al. (1997). Diagnosis and treatment of depression in late life: Consensus statement update. *Journal of the American Medical Association, 278,* 1186–1190.

Leckman, J. F., Merikangas, K. R., Pauls, D. L., Prusoff, B. A., & Weissman, M. M. (1983). Anxiety disorders and depression: Contradictions between family study data and DSM III conventions. *American Journal of Psychiatry, 140,* 880–882.

Lenze, E. J., Rofer, J. C., Martire, L. M., Mulsant, B. H., Rollman, B. L., Dew, M. A., et al. (2001). The association of late-life depression and anxiety with physical disability: A review of the literature and prospectus for future research. *American Journal of Geriatric Psychiatry, 9,* 113–135.

Leszcz, M. (1990). Group therapy. In J. Sadavoy, L. W. Lazarus, L. F. Jarvik, & G. T. Grossberg (Eds.), *Comprehensive review of geriatric psychiatry* (2nd ed., pp. 851–879). Washington, DC: American Psychiatric Press.

Levin, H. S., Brown, S. A., Song, J. X., McCauley, S. R., Boake, C., & Contant, C. F. (2001). Depression and post traumatic stress disorder at three months after mild to moderate traumatic brain injury. *Journal of Clinical and Experimental Neuropsychology, 23*(6), 754–769.

Lezak, M. D. (1983). *Neuropsychological assessment* (2nd ed.). New York: Oxford University Press.

Lindesay, J. (1991). Phobic disorders in the elderly. *British Journal of Psychiatry, 159,* 531–541.

Lustman, P. J., Freedland, K. E., Griffith, L. S., & Clouses, R. E. (1998). Predicting response to cognitive behavior therapy of depression in type 2 diabetes. *General Hospital Psychiatry, 20*(5), 302–306.

Marder, K., Tang, M., Cote, L., & Stern, Y. (1995). The frequency and associated risk factors for dementia in patients with Parkinson's disease. *Archives of Neurology, 52,* 695–701.

Markowitz, J. C., Klerman, G. L., Clougherty, K. F., Spielman, L. A., Jacobsen, L. B., Fishman, B., et al. (1995). Individual psychotherapies for depressed HIV-positive patients. *American Journal of Psychiatry, 152*(10), 1504–1509.

Marks, I. M. (1981). Behavioral psychotherapy for anxiety disorders. *Psychiatric Clinics of North America, 5,* 25–31.

Marks, I. M. (1987). Flooding (implosion) and allied treatments. In W. S. Agras (Ed.), *Behavior modification: Principles and clinical applications* (pp. 151–213). Boston: Little, Brown.

Mayeux, R., Saunders, A. M., Shea, S., Mirra, S., Evans, D., Roses, A. D., et al. (1998). Utility of the apolipoprotein E genotype in the diagnosis of Alzheimer's disease: Alzheimer's Disease Center Consortium on Apolipoprotein E and Alzheimer's Disease. *New England Journal of Medicine, 338,* 506–511.

Mayeux, R., Stern, Y., Cote, L., & Williams, J. B. (1984). Altered serotonin metabolism in depressed patients with Parkinson's disease. *Neurology, 31,* 645–650.

Mayeux, R., Stern, Y., Williams, J. B., Cote, L., Frantz, A., & Dyrenfurht, I. (1986). Clinical and biochemical features of depression in Parkinson's disease. *American Journal of Psychiatry, 143,* 756–759.

McCauley, S. R., Boake, C., Levin, H. A., Contant, C. F., & Song, J. X. (2001). Postconcussional disorder following mild to moderate traumatic brain injury: Anxiety depression and social support as risk factors and comorbidities. *Journal of Clinical and Experimental Neuropsychology, 23*(6), 792–808.

McCurry, S. M., Gibbons, L. E., Logsdon, R. G., & Teri, L. (2004). Anxiety and nighttime behavioral disturbances: Awakenings in patients with Alzheimer's disease. *Journal of Gerontological Nursing*, *30*(1), 12–20.

McGinn, L. K. (2000). Cognitive behavioral therapy of depression: Theory, treatment and empirical status. *American Journal of Psychotherapy*, *54*(2), 257–262.

McKenna, P. J., Kane, J. M., & Parrish, K. (1985). Psychotic syndromes in epilepsy. *American Journal of Psychiatry*, *142*, 895–904.

Medd, J., & Tate, R. L. (2000). Evaluation of an anger management therapy programme following acquired brain injury: A preliminary study. *Neuropsychological Rehabilitation*, *10*(2), 185–201.

Merriam, A. E., Aronso, M. K., Gaston, P., Wey, S. L., & Katz, K. (1988) The psychiatric symptoms of Alzheimer's disease. *Journal of the American Geriatrics Society*, *36*, 7–12.

Meyers, B. S. (1992). Geriatric delusional depression. *Clinical Geriatric Medicine*, *8*, 299–308.

Mohs, R. C., Breitner, J. C., Silverman, J. M., & Davis, K. I. (1987). Alzheimer's disease: Morbid risk among first degree relatives approximates 50% by 90 years of age. *Archives of General Psychiatry*, *44*, 405–408.

Morris, P. L., Robinson, R. G., Andrzejewski, P., Samuels, J., & Price, T. R. (1993). Association of depression with 10-year poststroke mortality. *American Journal of Psychiatry*, *150*, 124–129.

Morris, P. L., Robinson, R. G., Rapheal, B., & Bishop, D. (1991). The relationship between the perception of social support and post-stroke depression in hospitalized patients. *Psychiatry*, *54*, 306–316.

Mulsant, B. H., & Ganguli, M. (1999). Epidemiology and diagnosis of depression in late life. *Journal of Clinical Psychiatry*, *60*(Suppl. 20), 9–15.

National Institutes of Health. (1991). Diagnosis and treatment of depression in late life. *NIH Consensus Statement Online*, *9*(3), 1–27.

National Institutes of Health and National Institute of Mental Health. (1985). Consensus conference: Electroconvulsive therapy. *Journal of the American Medical Association*, *254*, 2103–2108.

National Institute of Mental Health. (2003). *Older adults: Depression and suicide facts* [NIH Publication No. 03–4593]. Bethesda, MD: Author. Retrieved June 6, 2005, from http://www.nimh.nih.gov/publicat/elderlydepsuicide.cfm

Neil, M., & Briggs, M. (2003). Validation therapy for dementia. *Cochrane Database of Systematic Reviews*, *2*, CD001394. Retrieved June 6, 2005, from http://www.cochrane.org/cochrane/revabstr/AB001394.htm

Newton, N. A., & Lazarus, L. W. (1992). Behavioral and psychotherapeutic interventions. In J. E. Birren, R. B. Sloane, G. D. Cohen, N. R. Hooyman, B. D. Lebowitz, M. Wykle, & D. E. Deutchman (Eds.), *Handbook of mental health and aging* (2nd ed., pp. 699–720). New York: Academic Press.

Ohry, A., Rattok, J., & Solomon, Z. (1996). Post-traumatic stress disorder in brain injury patients. *Brain Injury*, *10*(9), 687–695.

Palmer, S., & Glass, T. A. (2003). Family function and stroke recovery: A review. *Rehabilitation Psychology*, *48*(4), 255–265.

Pasternak, R. E., Prigerson, H., Hall, M., Miller, M. D., Fasiczka, A., Mazumdar, S., et al. (1997). The posttreatment illness course of depression in bereaved elders: High relapse/recurrence rates. *American Journal of Geriatric Psychiatry*, *5*, 54–59.

Paykel, E. S., Brayne, C., Huppert, F. A., Gill, C., Barkley, C., Gehlhaar, E., et al. (1994) Incidence of dementia in a population older than 75 years in the United Kingdom. *Archives of General Psychiatry, 51*, 325–332.

Payne, H. C. (2000). Traumatic brain injury, depressions and cannabis use: Assessing their effects on cognitive performance. *Brain Injury, 5*, 479–489.

Pearlson, G. D., Ross, C. A., Lohr, W. D., Rovner, B. W., Chase, G. A., & Folstein, M. R. (1990). Association between family history of affective disorder and the depressive syndrome of Alzheimer's disease. *American Journal of Psychiatry, 147*, 452–456.

Pearlson, G. D., Teri, L., Reifler, B., & Raskind, M. (1989). Functional status and cognitive impairments in Alzheimer's disease patients with and without depression. *Journal of the American Geriatrics Society, 37*, 1117–1121.

Pearson, J. L. (2003). *NIMH research on geriatric depression and suicide.* Paper presented as part of Senior depression: Life saving mental health treatments for older adults. Hearing before the Special Committee on Aging, United States Senate, 108th Congress, 1st session, Washington, DC, July 18, 2003, serial number 108-17 (pp. 48–52). Washington, DC: US Government Printing Office. Retrieved June 6, 2005, from http://frwebgate.access.gpo.gov/cgi-bin/getdoc.cgi?dbname=108_senate_hearings&docid=f:90051.pdf

Pennix, B. W., Deeg, D. J., van Eijk, J. T., Beekman, A. T., & Guralnik, J. M. (2000). Changes in depression and physical decline in older adults: A longitudinal perspective. *Journal of Affective Disorders, 61*, 1–12.

Pennix, B. W., Guralnik, J., Pahor, M., Ferrucci, L., Cerhan, J. R., Wallace, R. B., et al. (1998). Chronically depressed mood and cancer risk in older persons. *Journal of the National Cancer Institute, 90*, 1888–1893.

Pennix, B. W., Leveille, S., Ferrucci, L., van Eijk, J. T., & Guralnik, J. M. (1999). Exploring the effect of depression on physical disability: Longitudinal evidence from the established populations for epidemiologic studies of the elderly. *American Journal of Public Health, 89*, 1346–1352.

Poewe, W., & Seppi, K. (2001). Treatment options for depression and psychosis in Parkinson's disease. *Journal of Neurology, 248*(Suppl. 3), 111/12–111/21.

Porter, V. R., Buxton, W. G., Fairbanks, L. A., Strickland, T., O'Connor, S. M., & Rosenberg-Thompson, S. (2003). Frequency and characteristics of anxiety among patients with Alzheimer's disease and related dementias. *Journal of Neuropsychiatry and Clinical Neurosciences, 15*, 180–186.

Post, F. (1984). Affective disorders in old age. In E. S. Paykel (Ed.), *Handbook of affective disorders* (pp. 393–401). New York: Guilford Press.

Poulton, J. L., & Strassberg, D. S. (1986). The therapeutic use of reminiscence. *International Journal of Group Psychotherapy*, 36, 381–398.

Puentes, W. J. (2004). Cognitive therapy integrated with life review techniques: An eclectic treatment approach for affective symptoms in older adults. *Journal of Clinical Nursing, 13*(1), 84–89.

Qazi, A., Shankar, K., & Orrell, M. (2003). Managing anxiety in people with dementia: A case study. *Journal of Affective Disorders, 76*(1–3), 261–265.

Rabins, P. V. (1992). Schizophrenia and psychotic states. In J. E. Birren, R. B. Sloane, & G. D. Cohen (Eds.), *Handbook of mental health and aging* (pp. 464–473). San Diego, CA: Academic Press.

Raskin, S. A., Borod, J. C., & Tweedy, J. R. (1990). Neuropsychological aspects of Parkinson's disease. *Neuropsychological Review, 1*, 185–221.

Rattock, J. (1996). Do patients with mild brain injuries have post traumatic stress disorder too? *Journal of Head Trauma Rehabilitation, 11*(1), 95–96.

Reding, M., Haycox, J., & Blass, J. (1985). Depression in patients referred to a dementia clinic. *Archives of Neurology, 42*, 894–898.

Reynaud, G., von Gunten, A., & Kung, A. (2001). Psychiatric disorders in elderly patients with Parkinson's disease and their treatment. *Revue Medicale de la Suisse Romande, 121*(2), 145–151.

Reynolds, C. F., Frank, E., Kupfer, D. J., Thase, M. E., Perel, J. M., Mazumdar, S., et al. (1996). Treatment outcome in recurrent major depression: A post hoc comparison of elderly ("young old") and midlife patients. *American Journal of Psychiatry, 153*, 1288–1292.

Reynolds, C. F., Frank, E., Perel, J. M., Imber, S. D., Cornes, C., Morycz, R. K., et al. (1992). Combined pharmocotherapy and psychotherapy in the acute and continuation treatment of elderly patients with recurrent major depression: A preliminary report. *American Journal of Psychiatry, 149*, 1687–1692.

Richard, I. H., Schiffer, R. B., & Jurlan, R. (1996). Anxiety and Parkinson's disease. *Journal of Neuropsychiatry and Clinical Neurosciences, 8*(4), 383–392.

Ritchie, R., & Kildea, D. (1995). Is senile dementia "age-related" or ageing-related"? Evidence from meta-analysis of dementia prevalence in the oldest old. *Lancet, 346*, 931–934.

Robinson, R. G., & Jorge, R. (1994). Mood disorders. In J. M. Silver, S. C. Yudofsky, & R. Hales (Eds.), *Neuropsychiatry of traumatic brain injury* (pp. 219–250). Washington, DC: American Psychiatric Press.

Robinson, R. G., Kubos, K. L., Starr, L. B., Rao, K., & Price, T. R. (1984). Mood disorders in stroke patients: Importance of location of lesion. *Brain, 107*, 81–93.

Rosenthal, M., Christensen, B. K., & Ross, T. P. (1998). Depression following traumatic brain injury. *Archives of Physical Medicine and Rehabilitation, 79*, 90–103.

Rovner, B. W. (1993). Depression and increased risk of mortality in the nursing home patient. *American Journal of Medicine, 94*, 19S–22S.

Rovner, B. W., Broadhead, J., Spencer, M., Carson, K., & Folstein, M. F. (1989). Depression and Alzheimer's disease. *American Journal of Psychiatry, 146*, 350–353.

Rozzelle, C. J., Wofford, J. L., & Branch, C. L. (1995). Predictors of hospital mortality in older patients with subdural hematoma. *Journal of the American Geriatrics Society, 43*, 241–244.

Rudorfer, M. V., Henry, M. E., & Sackheim, H. A. (1997). Electroconvulsive therapy. In A. Tasman, J. Kay, & J. Lieberman (Eds.), *Psychiatry* (pp. 1535–1556). Philadelphia: W. B. Saunders.

Sackheim, H. A. (1994). Use of electroconvulsive therapy in late life depression. In L. S. Schneider, C. F. Reynolds, B. D. Lebowitz, & A. J. Friedhoff (Eds.), *Diagnosis and treatment of depression in late life* (pp. 259–277). Washington, DC: American Psychiatric Press.

Sadavoy, J., & LeClair, J. K. (1997). Treatment of anxiety disorders in late life. *Canadian Journal of Psychiatry, 42*(1), 28S–34S.

Salzman, C., & Gutfreund, M. J. (1986). Clinical techniques and research strategies for studying depression and memory. In L. W. Poon, T. Cook, K. Davis, C. Eisdorfer, B. Gurland, A. Kaszniak, & L. Thompson (Eds.), *Clinical memory assessment of older adults* (pp. 257–267). Washington, DC: American Psychological Association.

Sano, M., Stern, Y., Williams, J., Cote, L., Rosenstein, R., & Mayeux, R. (1989). Coexisting dementia and depression in Parkinson's disease. *Archives of Neurology*, *46*, 1284–1286.

Santamaria, J., Tolosa, E., & Valles, A. (1986). Parkinson's disease with depression: A possible subgroup of idiopathic parkinsonism. *Neurology*, *36*, 1130–1133.

Schneider, L. S. (1995). Efficacy of clinical treatment for mental disorders among older persons. In M. Gatz (Ed.), *Emerging issues in mental health and aging* (pp. 19–71). Washington, DC: American Psychiatric Press.

Scogin, F., & McElreath, L. (1994). Efficacy of psychosocial treatments for geriatric depression: A quantitative review. *Journal of Consulting and Clinical Psychology*, *62*, 69–74.

Scogin, F., Richard, H., Keith, S., Wilson, J., & McElreath, L. (1992). Progressive and imaginal relaxation training with elderly persons with subjective anxiety. *Psychology and Aging*, *7*, 419–424.

Shankar, K. K., Walker, M., Frost, D., & Orrell, M. W. (1999). The development of a valid and reliable scale for rating anxiety in dementia (RAID). *Aging and Mental Health*, *3*(1), 39–49.

Sharpe, M., Hawton, K., Seagroatt, V., Bamford, J., House, A., Molyneus, A., et al. (1994). Depressive disorders in long term survivors of stroke. *British Journal of Psychiatry*, *164*, 380–386.

Sheikh, J. L. (1990). Anxiety disorders. In J. Sadavoy, L. Lazarus, L. Jarvik, & G. Grossman (Eds.), *Comprehensive review of geriatric psychiatry II* (2nd ed., pp. 615–636). Washington, DC: American Psychiatric Press.

Sheikh, J. I., & Salzman, C. (1995). Anxiety in the elderly: Course and treatment. *Psychiatric Clinics of North America*, *18*(4), 871–883.

Shukla, S., Cook, B. L. Mukherjee, S., Godwin, C., & Miller, M. G. (1987). Mania following head trauma. *American Journal of Psychiatry*, *144*, 93–96.

Silver, J. M., Kramer, R., Greenwood, S., & Weissman, M. (2001). The association between head injuries and psychiatric disorders: Findings from the New Haven NIMH epidemiologic catchment area study. *Brain Injury*, *15*(11), 935–945.

Silver, J. M., Rattok, J., & Anderson, K. (1997). Post traumatic stress disorder and traumatic brain injury. *Neurocase*, *3*, 1–7.

Smalbrugge, M., Pot, A. M., Jongenelis, K., Beekman, A. T., & Efsting, J. A. (2003). Anxiety disorders in nursing homes: A literature review of prevalence, course and risk indicators. *Tijdschrift Voor Gerontologie en Geriatrie*, *34*(5), 215–221.

Stanley, M. A., Beck, J. G., & Glassco, J. D. (1996). Treatment of generalized anxiety in older adults: A preliminary comparison of cognitive-behavioral and supportive approaches. *Behavioral Therapy*, *27*, 565–581.

Stanley, M. A., & Novy, D. M. (2000). Cognitive-behavior therapy for generalized anxiety in later life: An evaluative overview. *Journal of Anxiety Disorders*, *14*, 191–207.

Starkstein, S. E., Mayberg, H. D., Berthier, M. L. Fedoroff, P., Price, T. R., Dannals, R. F., et al. (1990). Mania after brain injury: Neuroradiological and metabolic findings. *Annals of Neurology*, *27*, 652–659.

Starkstein, S. E., Robinson, R. G., & Price, T. R. (1988). Comparison of patients with and without post stroke major depression matched for size and location of lesion. *Archives of General Psychiatry*, *45*, 247–252.

Steuer, J. L., & Hammen, C. L. (1983). Cognitive-behavioral group therapy for the depressed elderly: Issues and adaptations. *Cognitive Therapy and Research*, *7*(4), 285–296.

Stevens, D. E., Merikangas, K. R., & Merikangas, J. R. (1995). Comorbidity of depression with other medical conditions. In E. E. Beckham & W. R. Leber (Eds.), *Handbook of depression* (pp. 147–199). New York: Guilford Press.

Suenkelei, I. C. H., Nowak, M., Misselwitz, B., Kugler, C., Schreibler, W., Oertel, W. H., et al. (2002). Timecourse of health-related quality of life as determined 3, 6, and 12 months after stroke-relationship to neurological deficit, disability and depression. *Journal of Neurology, 249,* 1160–1167.

Tandberg, E., Laarsen, J. P., Aarsland, D., & Cummings, J. L. (1996). The occurrence of depression in Parkinson's disease: A community based study. *Archives of Neurology, 53,* 175–179.

Taylor, A. E., Saint-Cyr, J. A., Lang, A. E., & Kenny, F. T. (1986). Parkinson's disease and depression: A critical re-evaluation of the brain. *Brain, 109,* 279–292.

Teri, L., Ferretti, L. E., Gibbons, L. E., Logsdon, R. G., McCurry, S. M., Kukull, W. A., et al. (1999). Anxiety of Alzheimer's disease: Prevalence and comorbidity. *Journal of Gerontology and Biological Sciences, 54*(7), 348–352.

Teri, K., & Gallagher-Thompson, D. (1991). Cognitive-behavioral interventions for treatment of depression in Alzheimer's patients. *The Gerontologist, 31,* 413–416.

Teri, L., Logsdon, R. G., Uomoto, J., & McCurry, S. M. (1997). Behavioral treatment of depression in dementia patients: A controlled clinical trial. *Journals of Gerontology: Series B. Psychological Sciences and Social Sciences, 52,* 156–166.

Teri, L., & Utomoto, J. (1991). Reducing excess disability in dementia patients: Training caregivers to manage patient depression. *Clinical Gerontologist, 10,* 49–63.

Teri, L., & Wagner, A. W. (1991). Assessment of depression in patients with Alzheimer's Disease: Concordence among informants. *Psychology and Aging, 6*(2), 280–285.

Thase, M. E., Freidman, E. S., Fasiczka, A. L., Berman, S. R., Frank, E., Nofzinger, E. A., et al. (2000). Treatment of men with major depression: A comparison of sequential cohorts treated with either cognitive-behavioral therapy or newer generation antidepressants. *Journal of Clinical Psychiatry, 61*(7), 466–472.

Thomas, R., & Gafner, G. (1993). PTSD in an elderly male: Treatment with eye movement desensitization and reprocessing. *Clinical Gerontologist, 14,* 57–59.

Thompson, L. W., Ganz, F., Florsheim, M., DelMaestro, S., Rodman, J., Gallagher-Thompson, D., et al. (1991). Cognitive-behavioral therapy for affective disorders. In W. S. Myers (Ed.), *New techniques in the psychotherapy of older patients* (pp. 3–20). Washington, DC: American Psychiatric Press.

Thompson, S. C., Sobolew-Shubin, A., Graham, M. A., & Janigian, A. S. (1989). Psychosocial adjustment following stroke. *Social Science and Medicine, 28,* 239–247.

Thomsen, I. V. (1984). Late outcome of very severe blunt head trauma: A 10–15 year second followup. *Journal of Neurology, Neurosurgery, and Psychiatry, 47,* 260–268.

Trimble, M. R. (1991). *The psychosis of epilepsy.* New York: Rover.

Trezpacz, P. T. (1994). Delirium. In J. M. Silver, S. C. Yudofsky, & R. Hales (Eds.), *Neuropsychiatry of traumatic brain injury* (pp. 189–218). Washington, DC: American Psychiatric Press.

Twamley, E. W., & Bondi, M. W. (2004). The differential diagnosis of dementia. In J. Ricker (Ed.), *Differential diagnosis in adults neuropsychological assessment* (pp. 276–326). New York: Springer Publishing Company.

US Department of Health and Human Services. (1999). Older adults and mental health. In *Mental Health: A Report of the Surgeon General—Executive Summary.*

Rockville, MD: US Department of Health and Human Services, Substance Abuse and Mental Health Services Administration, Center for Mental Health Services, National Institutes of Health, National Institute of Mental Health.

Van Reekum, R., Bolago, I., Finlayson, M., Gardner, S., & Links, P. (1996). Psychiatric disorders after traumatic brain injury. *Brain Injury*, *10*, 319–327.

Varney, N., Martzke, J., & Robert, R. (1987). Major depression in patients with closed head injury. *Neuropsychology*, *1*, 7–8.

Weiner, R. D., & Krystal, A. D. (1994). The present use of electroconvulsive therapy. *Annual Review of Medicine*, *45*, 273–281.

Weissman, M. A., Bruce, M., Leaf, P. J., Florio, L. P., & Holzer, C. (1991). Affective disorders. In L. N. Robins & D. A. Regier (Eds.), *Psychiatric disorders in America: The Epidemiologic Catchment Area Study* (pp. 53–80). New York: Free Press.

Whiteneck, G., Mellick, D., Brooks, C. A., Harrison-Felix, C., Terill, M. S., & Noble, K. (2001). *Colorado traumatic brain injury registry and follow up system—datebook*. Denver, CO: Craig Hospital.

Wong, P. (1991). Social support functions of group reminiscence. *Canadian Journal of Community Mental Health*, *10*, 151–161.

Young, R. C., & Klerman, G. L. (1992). Mania in late life: Focus on age of onset. *American Journal of Psychiatry*, *149*, 867–876.

Youngjohn, J. R., Beck, J., Jogerst, G., & Caine, C. (1992). Neuropsychological impairment, depression and Parkinson's disease. *Neuropsychology*, *6*(2), 1429–1458.

Yudofsky, S. C., & Hales, R. E. (1992). *Textbook of neuropsychology*. Washington, DC: American Psychiatric Press.

Zeichner, A., & Boczkowski, J. (1986). Clinical application of biofeedback techniques for the elderly. *Clinical Gerontologist*, *5*, 457–473.

Zubenko, G. S., & Moossy, J. (1988). Major depression in primary dementia: Clinical and neuropathologic correlates. *Archives of Neurology*, *45*, 1182–1186.

Zweig, R. M., Ross, C. A., Hedreen, J. C., Steele, C., Cardillo, S. E., Whitehouse, P. J., et al. (1988). The neuropathology of aminergic nuclei in Alzheimer's disease. *Annals of Neurology*, *24*, 233–242.

13 Sleep disorders and geriatric neuropsychology

Manfred F. Greiffenstein

Sleep medicine and clinical neuropsychology are highly complementary fields. Specialization in one field provides a knowledge base accelerating specialization in the other (Greiffenstein, 2001). Both require (a) knowledge of the neurosciences and measurement theory, (b) integration of much multimodal data into a diagnostic theory, and (c) assessment of dual sleep and cognitive complaints. In the individual patient, it is not clear whether sleep and cognitive complaints have a causal relationship, share the same underlying syndrome, or are completely independent of each other. The interaction of sleep and aging has many controversies that have yet to be settled, and some of these controversies are of great interest to neuropsychologists. The purpose of this chapter is to provide an overview of basic sleep concepts, the sleep and aging literature, and neuropsychological studies in sleep disordered older persons.

Basic sleep terminology

The geriatric neuropsychologist does not need a comprehensive in-depth understanding of sleep, but the ubiquity of sleep laboratories and routine sleep study referral requires some understanding of sleep terminology. Much about sleep disorders can be learned through understanding how to read a diagnostic sleep report. Table 13.1 displays the format of a typical sleep report.

A sleep report is divided into standard sections. There is a sleep summary providing quantification of key electroencephalogram (EEG) variables. This includes *sleep efficiency* (percentage of "dark time" spent asleep). Next, total sleep time (hours) is subdivided into percentage of time spent in rapid eye movement (REM) sleep, stages 1 and 2 (collectively referred to as non-REM percentage), and stages 3 and 4 (collectively termed "slow-wave sleep"). An increased stage 1 percentage may indicate an abnormal arousal pattern associated with sleep apnea or some other sleep disruptive event that does not fully awaken the patient. Key latency measures include minutes to first sleep period (sleep latency) and *REM latency* (minutes to enter REM after sleep onset). Prolonged stage 1 latency (> 30 min) may be evidence for insomnia while a short REM latency (< 20 min) may be evidence for narcolepsy or chronic sleep deprivation.

Table 13.1 Sample sleep report

Monroe Sleep Disorders Laboratory

Name: GONIFF, Ira *Age*: 67 *Gender*: Male *Education*: High School
Doctor: Helmut Smith MD

HISTORY

This 5'8'', 67 year old, married, retired male trucker driver with a body mass index of 34 comes to the sleep laboratory with chief complaints of snoring, unrefreshing sleep, memory complaints, and daytime somnolence. His wife reports she no longer sleeps in the same room because of snoring, so is unable to comment on breath stoppage. Patient believes sleep problem worsened with weight gain over last 5 years. He rates daytime somnolence as severe and naps are unrefreshing, but he otherwise denies signs of the narcoleptic tetrad. Past medical history indicates hypertension; SOB with exertion and recent car accident with unclear injury characteristics. Current medications include Lipitor, Vasotec, and vitamin supplement. Current social habits include 2–3 drinks in the evening, ½ pack of cigarettes and "a pot of coffee" during the day. Family history is strong for snoring but no psychiatric problems in first rank relatives.

TECHNICAL SUMMARY

Method: Standard apnea montage with total dark time of 7 h 58 min. This is a reliable sleep sample.

EEG: The sleep efficiency of 72% is below the customary range for this age. The patient fell asleep in a brisk 1 min and entered REM 187 min later. Stage 1 is an excessive 58%, evidence for an abnormal arousal pattern. Stage 2 = 38%, stage 3–4 = 0%, REM = 4%. Wakefulness of 28% is explained by two major awakenings in the second half of the night.

Respiration: The apnea index is 15/hr, the hypopnea index is 69, and the combined respiratory distress index is 84/hr. He produced events at a rate of 100/hr in the supine versus 68/hr in the lateral. The REM RDI is 68, and the NREM RDI is 112. Pulse oximetry showed 128 hypoxic events with a nadir of 63% in association with a long apnea during brief REM.

EKG: Normal sinus rhythm in wake, bradytachycardia pattern associated with apneas and frequent PVCs.

EMG: The PLM index is an unremarkable 3.4/hr and the PLM arousal index = 1.6/hr; increased tone with respiratory events.

MSLT: The mean latency to stage 1 sleep during four systematic naps is 4.8 min with one SOREMP.

Other: The snoring channel shows moderate to heroic snoring in the supine. The Epworth Sleepiness Scale is 26, consistent with severe subjective daytime sleepiness. The MMPI-2 shows elevations on scales 1 and 8, indicating unusual focus on health and a perception of cognitive inefficiency.

INTERPRETIVE SUMMARY

Impressions: This sleep study is abnormal and documents severe disruption of sleep secondary to repetitive obstructive respiratory events of severe proportions. OSAS may be worsened by evening ETOH consumption.
Functionally, his OSAS causes pathological daytime sleepiness, nervous preoccupation with health, and mistrust in his cognition. He may be a driving risk.

Table 13.1 (contd.)

Diagnoses: 780.53-0, Severe obstructive sleep apnea syndrome; 780.53-4, primary snoring, severe.

Recommendations:

1. Weight loss
2. Nasal CPAP trial in the sleep laboratory
3. Driving and power tools advisory
4. Referral to ENT, correlate otolaryngology features with sleep findings.

M. Frank Greiffenstein, PhD, ACP, ABPP-CN
Certified, American Board of Clinical Neuropsychology
Certified, American Board of Sleep Medicine

The respiratory summary addresses sleep disorder breathing. *Apneas* are defined as cessations of airflow greater than 10 seconds in the context of normal respiratory effort; *hypopneas* are defined as diminished cessation of airflow with intact respiratory effort, and *central apneas* mean cessation of airflow with absent respiratory effort. Two indicia of abnormal respiration are usually calculated: The apnea index (AI; total apneas per sleep time) and the respiratory distress index (RDI; sum of apneas and hypopneas divided by total sleep time). Positional and stage-specific RDIs are also calculated (e.g., events per hour of supine or REM sleep). Generally accepted cutting scores for diagnosis of sleep disorder breathing are AI $\geq$ 5 and RDI $\geq$ 10. Pulse oximetry data shows the number of *hypoxic* events (< 90% oxyhemoglobin saturation) and the magnitude of the hypoxia (the nadir).

The electromyogram (EMG) documents any rhythmic burst activity from the legs meeting criteria for *periodic leg movements*, which are repetitive stereotyped leg jerks. The PLM index is the number of these undesirable movements per hour of sleep, while the *PLM arousal index* is the number of movements associated with EEG arousal. The EKG records heart rhythms, and the polysomnographer is alert for cardiac patterns associated with disturbed breathing. The MSLT (Multiple Sleep Latency Tests; see Measurement section) is an objective measure of daytime sleepiness. Two scores are derived: *Mean latency* to stage 1 sleep and number of *sleep onset REM periods* (SOREMP). MSLT scores < 5 minutes indicate pathological daytime sleepiness. Other sleep variables include snoring, the Epworth Sleepiness Scale score, and the MMPI-2.

Measurement issues in sleep medicine

Nosology and classification

The International Classification of Sleep Disorders Revised (ICSD-R; American Sleep Disorders Association, 1997) is the generally accepted diagnostic classification system for disturbances of sleep and wakefulness. This sleep nosology is a hybrid of symptomatic and etiological classification criteria containing two major groupings: *Primary* and *secondary* sleep disorders. In the primary sleep disorders, a sleep complaint is the focus of clinical concern. These are further subdivided into the *dyssomnias* and the *parasomnias*. The dyssomnias are disorders that produce primary complaints of insomnia or somnolence. The parasomnias are disorders that intrude into or occur during sleep without necessarily causing insomnia or hypersomnolence complaints. The secondary sleep disorders refer to sleep problems caused or aggravated by primary medical, psychiatric, and neurologic problems.

The dyssomnias

These are clinical disorders signaled by complaints of insomnia, somnolence, or both. The dyssomnias are further subdivided intro three groupings. The *intrinsic* dyssomnias are disorders in which the sleep disorder is caused by an internal somatic problem. The 13 specific intrinsic diagnoses include obstructive sleep apnea syndrome (OSAS), narcolepsy, and periodic leg movement disorder. The *extrinsic* dyssomnias are disorders in which external factors disturb sleep in otherwise healthy persons. Included here are adjustment sleep disorder (e.g., insomnia related to psychosocial stressors), insufficient sleep (voluntary restriction of time in bed), environmental sleep disorder (e.g., noisy environments), altitude insomnia (hypoxia in mountain climbers), and hypnotic dependent disorder (e.g., tolerance to Xanax). The third intrinsic subdivision, *circadian-rhythm disorders*, refers to a misalignment between a patient's sleep pattern and the socially conventional sleep pattern. This category can include both intrinsic and extrinsic etiologies. Examples include shift work sleep disorder (externally imposed), and non-24 hour sleep–wake disorder (probable dysfunction of hypothalamic nuclei).

The parasomnias

The parasomnias consist of clinical disorders that are not abnormalities of the sleep process itself, but represent that intrusion of undesirable physical phenomenon into sleep. Most of these disorders represent a combination of autonomic nervous system and skeletal-muscle activation occurring during sleep. The parasomnias include problems in which impaired arousal is postulated as etiology. This includes sleepwalking, sleep terrors, and confusional arousals. Other parasomnias are associated with REM sleep (nightmares, REM-sleep behavior disorder) and other parasomnias (enuresis, snoring).

Sleep disorders in medical conditions

A large number of sleep problems are associated with medical, neurologic, and psychiatric diagnoses. An exhaustive list of medical disorders causing sleep problems is not provided in the ICSD-R, but a list of the most common medical diagnoses associated with sleep disturbance is. This major category is divided into psychiatric, neurologic, and medical disorders. Psychiatric diagnoses most likely associated with sleep disturbance include psychoses, mood disorders, anxiety disorders, and alcoholism. Neurologic diagnoses associated with sleep problems include dementia, cerebral degenerative disorders, fatal familial insomnia, sleep-related epilepsy, and sleep-related headaches. Medical disorders commonly associated with sleep complaints include chronic obstructive pulmonary disease.

Physiological recording

Polysomnographic recording.

The generally accepted approach to measuring normal and abnormal sleep processes is the polysomnograph (PSG). The PSG provides a simultaneous recording of multiple biological signals during sleep. The minimum multi-channel montage includes EEG, electrooculogram (EOG), surface EMG of the chin and legs, respiration effort, airflow, and pulse oximetry. These recordings can be saved on compact media such as optical disks. This data is used to assess sleep, sleep stage, wakefulness, and abnormal intrusions into the sleep process.

Only the EEG, EOG, and submentalis (chin) EMG channels are used to score sleep and wakefulness per generally accepted criteria proposed by Rechtschaffen and Kales (1973). Sleep stage scoring requires at least two monopolar (referential) EEG leads at the occipital and supraparietal (vertex) regions. These brain regions were selected because the alpha rhythm is most prominent in the occipital region, and both excitatory and inhibitory potentials (K-complexes and spindles respectively) necessary for stage 2 scoring are most prominent in the parietal regions. Scoring is based on patterns dominating ($> 50\%$) each 30-second interval (called an "epoch"). Stage 1 (drowsiness) is scored when the posterior alpha rhythm slows or disappears and is replaced by the mixed voltage and frequency pattern known as theta (3–7 cps). The EOG may show slow rolling eye movements. The appearance of K-complexes and spindles in the parietal region defines stage 2 sleep. K-complex morphology includes a sharp negative amplitude up to several hundred microvolts followed by a lower voltage positive wave and this sequence is at least 0.5 seconds in duration. K-complexes are excitatory, considered evoked responses, and can be elicited by auditory stimuli. Spindles are brief bursts of 12–16 Hz activity lasting from 0.5 to several seconds. Stages 3 and 4 are often termed "synchronized" sleep because delta waves (≤ 2 Hz and amplitude of ≥ 75 mV) dominate at least 20% of an epoch. REM sleep scoring is complicated because of many embedded rules, but in general, REM is scored with the (a) appearance of sharp eye movements, (b) EEG shows faster frequencies similar to that of stage 1, and (c) EMG shows resting chin muscular activity dropping to the lowest level of the night. This latter feature is termed "muscle atonia of REM."

Daytime sleepiness

The polygraphic recording described above is used to classify nocturnal sleep. Of considerable interest is measurement of daytime alertness and sleepiness. Many patients complain of excessive daytime sleepiness (EDS), and there are methods to objectively quantify their problems. The Multiple Sleep Latency Tests (MSLT) is designed to measure daytime sleepiness. The MSLT consists of four or five brief naps separated by 2 hours beginning at 10 a.m. and ending at 4 or 6 p.m. Two measures are derived: mean latency to stage 1 sleep and number of sleep onset REM periods (SOREMPs). Mean latencies ≤ 5 minutes is evidence for pathological daytime sleepiness. Scores between 5 and 10 minutes indicate unusual sleepiness, and scores above 10 minutes are negative for daytime sleepiness. The occurrence of REM during brief naps is helpful in the diagnosis of narcolepsy, especially if they occur in the later naps. A related measure is Maintenance of Wakefulness Test (MWT). The MSLT is a measure of vulnerability to daytime sleepiness in a sleep promoting setting, but the MWT measures *resistance* to sleepiness. Patients are asked to stay awake and remain seated in a darkened room for four or five 20-minute intervals. Reliability and validity studies have shown mixed results. The MSLT shows excellent validity in the detection of narcolepsy. The MWT is rarely used. The MWT does not correlate very well with the MSLT, probably because the MWT is more motivation dependent. It is easier to welcome sleepiness during an MSLT than resist it in the MWT.

Behavioral methods

Checklists

Some paper-and-pencil measures are given as standard in sleep laboratories, each with a different application. The Epworth Sleepiness Scale (ESS) is a measure of subjective sleepiness. The patient rates degree of sleepiness associated with eight common activities. Scores range from 0 to 32 with higher scores indicating greater perceived sleepiness. While the ESS is a global measure of subjective sleepiness, the Stanford Sleepiness Scale (SSS) provides point estimates of sleepiness. The patient circles one of seven categories that best describe current level of alertness. The SSS is intended for real-time, repeated estimates in experimental settings, while the ESS is a better clinical measure meant to capture customary alertness levels.

Johns (1992) reported the ESS showing a 5-month test–retest reliability of .82 and internal consistency (Cronbach alpha) of .88 when given to medical students. Chen et al. (2002) reported a 1-month test–retest reliability of .72 and internal consistency of .81. Validity as a measure of sleepiness is acceptable, as

ESS scores correlate positively with number of nocturnal awakenings, apneic events, and sedentary lifestyle (Whitney et al., 1998). As would be predicted, the ESS correlates negatively with MSLT latencies: (Chung, 2000) reported $r = -.42$ in a large series of Chinese patients with apnea. It also correlates positively with snoring indices (Gliklich & Wang, 2002). Reductions in ESS scores follow successful interventions for narcolepsy and sleep apnea syndrome (Weaver, 2001). The SSS also shows acceptable reliability (Glenville & Broughton, 1978). It shows validity to the extent it correlates with clinical diagnosis, e.g., narcolepsy status (Newman & Broughton, 1991) and circadian phase (Taub, 1981).

Wrist actigraph

Self-report has many limitations. Self-report is subject to bias, poor insight and frame of reference. Ambulatory monitoring of rest/activity periods in operational environments can be easily recorded with the wrist actigraph. This wrist-worn device records the duration and timing of active and passive periods in patients and research participants. Some inference is required, as the absence of movement can denote either rest or sleep. Brooks, Friedman, Bliwise, and Yesavage (1993), Friedman et al. (2000), and Redeker and Wykpisz (1999) demonstrated actigraph recordings to have higher correlations with PSG total sleep time than sleep logs filled out by older insomnia patients. In a double-blind study, Singer et al. (2003) used actigraphy to determine the effects of Melatonin versus placebo on Alzheimer patients selected for insomnia. They found no significant differences in sleep time as defined by actigraphic recording.

Sleep and aging

Consideration of age's role in sleep is relatively new. The index of Birren's (1959) classic textbook on the psychology of aging shows only one page devoted to the issue. The second edition devoted a whole chapter (Woodruff, 1985). One of the great achievements of neurobiology is a demonstration of a reliable sleep ontogeny from 27 weeks' conceptional age to the eighth decade (Aldrich, 1999), and it is now accepted that age is the best predictor of EEG confirmed sleep patterns (Carskadon & Dement, 1997). The increasing prevalence of sleep complaints and problems after middle age is beyond dispute, although the causes and correlates remain a matter of controversy. It is tempting to divide this section into sleep patterns associated with "normal" and "abnormal" aging subsections. The term "normal aging" may be oxymoronic and creates confusion because of its many senses (Bliwise, 1997). The complexities of defining normal aging are beyond the scope of this chapter and the reader should note that few sleep studies rely on exhaustive diagnostic workups to rule out all possible medical and psychiatric problems in older persons. The general criteria for examining sleep patterns in "normal" aging rely on nondemented, community-residing persons. For this reason, this section simply focuses on the sleep correlates of aging.

Prevalence of sleep complaints

Subjective evidence in the form of large scale surveys documents increasing sleep complaints after age 50 with acceleration after 65. General sleep complaints ("Do you regularly have difficulties going to or staying asleep?") are strongly associated with age. McGhie and Russel (1962) reported less than 10% of men and less than 15% of women aged 15–64 years complained of disturbed sleep, but this rose to 25% in men aged 65–74 years and 43% in women of that age. Bixler, Kales, Soldatos, Kales, and Healey (1979) reported insomnia prevalence rate of 43% in 1006 Los Angeles County residents, with more frequent complaints in older persons, especially females. Klink, Quan, Kaltenborn, and Lebowitz (1992) identified female gender and age as the highest risk factors for general insomnia complaints. Sutton, Moldofsky, and Bradley (2001) examined age-specific Canadian cohorts and reported insomnia prevalence of 20% in 15- to 20-year-olds versus 36% in 75- to 99-year-olds. Investigation of specific sleep complaints also shows greater frequency among older adults. This includes increased frequency of early morning awakenings, nocturnal awakenings, and estimates of less refreshing sleep (Dement, Miles, & Carskadon, 1982; Karacan et al., 1976; Rosekind, 1992).

Cultural, psychosocial, and demographic variables moderate the association of age and sleep complaints. Sutton et al. (2001) reported low income persons four times more likely to complain of insomnia than well-to-do Canadians, and women were 1.6 times more likely to complain than men. Covariate removal attenuates the relation between age and insomnia complaints, sometimes to the point of disappearance (Roberts, Shema, & Kaplan, 1999). Roberts, Shema, Kaplan, and Strawbridge (2000) found the association between age and insomnia weakened with removal of depressive symptoms.

Changes in sleep architecture

By the end of the first year of life, infant's non-REM (NREM) sleep shows all the adult characteristics such as K-complexes, spindles, and delta waves, although REM sleep continues to dominate. REM continues to decline as a percentage of total sleep time until age 5 when it reaches the adult proportion of 20–25%. From that point on, REM percentage shows a mean of 25% of total sleep time, although absolute time spent in REM decreases dramatically.

Many studies have shown age-related changes in the EEG architecture of sleep, and one consistent finding is a decrease in slow-wave, or delta sleep (stages 3 and 4), and it is generally accepted that the most prominent sign of adult aging is the steady decrease in delta wave amplitude (Miles & Dement,

1980; Woodruff, 1985). Some studies have shown deepest sleep, stage 4, to be almost absent in senescence (Foret & Webb, 1980; Hayashi & Endo, 1982). The Rechtschaffen and Kales (1973) scoring criteria demand delta sleep be scored only if waveforms have amplitude > 75 mV, so age-related declines in the amplitude of delta sleep means stages 3 and 4 can not be scored. Some have argued the elderly still show the same prevalence of delta sleep if one relies on frequency criteria only (Webb & Dreblow, 1982). Some studies have shown delta sleep better preserved in older women (Reynolds et al., 1985), although skull thickness may be a confounding variable. Decreased synaptic density, dendritic pruning, and declining cortical metabolism have been offered as explanations for decreased delta amplitude (Feinberg, 1982). A related EEG finding is changes in spindle activity. Guazzelli et al. (1986) reported inverse correlations between radiologists' ratings of sulcal atrophy and sleep spindle amplitude.

Other age-related EEG changes include increases in stage 1 sleep as a percentage of total sleep, awakenings, brief arousals, and wakefulness. One universal finding across studies is a reduction in sleep efficiency into the 70–80% range while stage 1 increases to 8–15% of total sleep time. There is also an age-related increase in spontaneous transient arousals (Carskadon, Brown, & Dement, 1982). Hence, older persons spend more time awake while in bed and show more abnormal arousal patterns. Gender is a moderator variable, and it appears older women show objectively better sleep than men (Rediehs, Reis, & Creason, 1990), although subjectively women report more sleep problems than men (Klink et al., 1992). Objectively, polysomnographic studies confirm the subjective complaints, showing an increase in awakenings, especially in the second half of the night (Webb, 1982a). The inability to maintain sleep is particularly noteworthy in older men (Webb, 1982b). Similarly, Webb and Campbell (1980) showed individuals 50–60 years old took longer to fall asleep when awakened than did participants in their early 20s.

Another finding is the temporal ordering of sleep and distribution of sleep across a 24-hour day. This research addresses the common belief that older people "need less sleep." Although it is clear the elderly get less sleep at night, if one includes nap time in sleep quota calculations, net sleep times may not change with aging, indicating a redistribution but not reduction of sleep need (Bliwise, 1997). Studies have shown that experimentally sleep-deprived geriatric insomniacs and geriatric "normal" sleepers show larger sleep gains on recovery nights than young controls, proving sleep need or homeostatic response to sleep loss is not affected by age (Bonnet & Rosa, 1987). Other data also challenges the neurobiological basis of age-related sleep changes by noting the elderly spend more time in bed for various reasons, and hence, the quality of sleep diminishes. Carskadon (1982) showed marked improvement in stages 3–4 sleep during recovery nights following sleep deprivation in older persons. She predicted improved sleep parameters if the elderly spent only 6 hours rather than the typical 10–12 hours in bed.

Medication use and sleep

Medication use in general and specific hypnotic use increases with age in almost every industrialized nation. Because of mounting medical problems faced by the elderly, persons over 60 receive a disproportionate number of prescription medications. National and international prevalence studies over the past two decades have consistently shown high rates of hypnotic use in persons over 60. In a national survey, Mellinger, Balter, and Uhlenhuth (1985) found 69% of persons taking prescription medications for sleep were in the 50- to 79-year-old group. Roehrs, Hollebeek, Drake, and Roth (2002) conducted a telephone survey and found prescription and over the counter sleep aides most common in older females with insomnia complaints, while self-medication with alcohol was more common in younger males reporting daytime somnolence. In Germany, Englert and Linden (1998) reported hypnotic use in 19% of persons over 70, while Linden and Thiels (2001) reported half the neuroleptic prescriptions per annum were written for persons over 65. In Spain, Rayon et al. (1996) reported the elderly three times more likely to receive a hypnotic than younger persons with the same level of sleep complaint. In France, Ohayon, Caulet, and Lemoine (1996) reported 33% of persons over 75 receiving some form of psychotropic for sleep complaints, compared to 24% for those aged 65–74.

Main theories of age-related sleep decline

There are two major theories of age-related sleep decline. Neuronal/homeostatic degeneration theories hold that damage to neuronal populations controlling sleep is responsible for increasing sleep problems of the elderly. These theories derive from well-established observations: dampened amplitude of circadian rhythms (e.g., temperature cycle), altered periodicity (e.g., early evening onset of sleepiness after 65), and age-related decreases in hypothalamic nuclei known to control temporal organization of body processes (Hofman, Fliers, Goudsmit, & Swaab, 1988). Czeisler et al. (1992) showed the amplitude of the endogenous circadian rhythm for temperature is 40% attenuated in older relative to younger men. They hypothesized age-related deterioration of hypothalamic nuclei controlling the circadian rhythm. Dijk, Duffy, Riel, Shanahan, and Czeisler (1999) also demonstrated decreased homeostatic drive for sleep in the elderly. The suprachiasmatic nucleus (SCN) of the hypothalamus is widely believed to be the circadian rhythm pacemaker. Viswanathan and Davis (1995) observed a shortening of the activity/rest cycle in aging Syrian hamsters. They ablated the oldest hamsters' SCN and replaced it with fetal SCN tissue. This lengthened the circadian period to the levels of younger hamsters. Van Someren (2000) reviewed the literature and theorized that decreased sensory input to the suprachiasmatic nucleus causes sleep problems in the elderly.

The other major theoretical trend may be termed the "health burden theory." This idea posits the steady accumulation of medical and psychosocial disturbances with age as responsible for sleep disturbance. The decreased amplitude and altered periodicity of circadian rhythms may simply reflect various medical problems or altered environmental conditions (e.g., more time in bed) that decrease or alter sensory input to homeostatic mechanisms. Aldrich (1999) noted that conditions considered a normal part of aging could have dramatic impact on sleep continuity, such as prostatic hypertrophy (causing nocturia) and osteoarthritis (subthreshold pain causing arousals). About one-fourth of community-residing persons over 65 have more than 5 apneas per hour and 60% have more than 10 respiratory events per hour, the generally accepted threshold between normal and sleep-disordered breathing (Ancoli-Israel et al., 1991). Coleman et al. (1981) argued that sleep complaints in the elderly could be explained by a higher prevalence of specific sleep disorders; one-third of their sample showed OSAS. Examining a large cohort of Swedish males, Gislason and Almqvist (1987) found fewest sleep complaints in those without hypertension, diabetes, or pulmonary disease. Vitiello, Moe, and Prinz (2002) provided powerful evidence for cosegregation of sleep problems and medical issues. They performed health screenings on nearly 3000 older volunteers, eliminating those with major medical, psychiatric, or medication use issues. Only 2.25% of the remaining volunteers showed sleep complaints. The findings of striking improvement in sleep quality following sleep deprivation are also evidence against neuronal/homeostatic degradation theories (Bonnet & Rosa, 1987; Carskadon, 1982).

Neurologically based sleep disorders

Advancing age is a risk factor for many sleep disorders, with some disorders seen exclusively after the fifth decade, and others showing accelerated incidence. This subsection focuses on age-related sleep disorders with a known neurological basis.

Periodic leg movement disorder

Periodic leg movement disorder (PLMD) is a transient involuntary movement disorder associated with NREM sleep. It is a common abnormal polysomnographic finding in persons over 60 years. Coleman et al. (1981) reported finding PLMD in 18% of older persons, although some estimates run as high as 34% (Partinen, 1994). A related finding of restless legs may be seen in up to 30% of persons with rheumatoid arthritis. Mosko and Nudleman (1986) found normal brainstem evoked responses in older established PLMD patients, ruling out deafferentiation as a cause. This indirectly supports the notion that descending inhibitory motor pathways may be defective.

REM sleep behavior disorder

REM sleep behavior disorder (RBD) is of great relevance to neurologists and neuropsychologists. A syndrome first identified in the 1980s, RBD's essential characteristic is polysomnographic and behavioral evidence for emergence of complex behavior during REM sleep (Schenck & Mahowald, 1996). Normally, an activated brain with inhibition of skeletal muscle characterizes REM sleep. The latter, referred to as muscle atonia, is believed necessary to avoid acting on intense dream imagery. Cells in the locus coerelus activate the giant cells of the medullar reticular formation that in turn send descending inhibitory volleys to spinal alpha motorneurons. In RBD, the descending inhibition of skeletal muscle is lost and the patient shows overt motor expression of dreams. These behaviors are either aggressive or exploratory but never appetitive and occur within REM sleep, not during arousals from it. Interestingly, the dreams of RBD patients are unusually aggressive, suggesting RBD also involves altered dream generation mechanisms. Advanced age appears to be a risk factor, as men in their eighties predominate among idiopathic cases. RBD in younger men appears to be symptomatic and more likely to be associated with neurodegenerative disorders such as Parkinson's disease.

Dementia

The family of dementias is often associated with sleep problems, some of them creating safety risks and caregiver burdens greater than those of other diagnostic features. Alzheimer's disease (AD) is the most common of the dementias, and the putative cholinergic dysfunction affects brain areas associated with sleep. There is no distinctive sleep disorder associated with AD, and the many manifestations are badly confounded with medication status and other disorders of aging such as periodic leg movements and apnea. Polysomnographic studies have identified a core of findings which include reduced sleep spindles and K-complexes, decreased REM sleep, and sleep–wake rhythm disturbances relative to age matched controls.

The ICSD-R recognizes that Irregular Sleep–Wake Pattern (ISWP) is a type of circadian disturbance associated with dementia. This diagnosis consists of temporally irregular sleep and waking with near-normal average amounts of total sleep time. Sleep consists of short naps never longer than 4 hours during any 24-hour period. This disorder is considered the basis for "sundowning," referring to increased confusion and agitated behavior after nightfall. This sleep–wake pattern is reminiscent of newborn sleep, although net sleep per day is much lower. Although this pattern can be seen in cognitively intact, schizoid persons completely indifferent to social conventions, it is often seen in demented individuals (Bliwise, 1994). Neurologically, ISWP may reflect disruption of hypothalamic centers controlling circadian rest/activity cycles. Stopa et al. (1999) examined the SCN of 30 dementia patients and found higher astrocyte to neuron ratios relative to matched controls, indicating greater degeneration. However, SCN cell loss was relatively less than in other brain areas, meaning the SCN finding may not be the specific reasons for sleep changes in persons with dementia.

Neuropsychological studies

Neurocognitive findings in sleep disorders

An important diagnostic question is whether sleep disturbance or sleepiness impacts cognitive performance. If neurocognitive abnormalities are detected in the geriatric patients, sleep complaints may be viewed as a confounding variable, competing with a hypothesis of neuronal dysfunction. Geriatric neuropsychologists should be aware of the pertinent literature.

REM behavior disorder

Ferman et al. (1999) compared neurocognitive performance between 31 patients with dementia and PSG-confirmed RBD and 31 patients with probable Alzheimer's disease with no brainstem Lewy body pathology later detected at autopsy. Both groups were naturally matched on overall dementia severity but the RBD/dementia group showed significantly worse attention, perceptual organization, letter fluency, and visual memory, while the AD group showed worse visual naming and verbal memory. Based on these findings and additional evidence for more extrapyramidal signs, Ferman et al. concluded dual diagnosis of RBD and dementia likely reflects Lewy body disease. Ferman et al. (2002) showed persons with combined RBD/dementia but without prodromal extrapyramidal signs still show the same pattern of poor perceptual organization with relatively intact naming in comparison to Alzheimer patients. They concluded that RBD/dementia is the earliest manifestation of Lewy body dementia.

Sleep apnea in the aged

Sleep-disordered breathing is a natural area of inquiry for neuropsychologists. It is reasonable to speculate whether recurrent disruptions of blood-gas dynamics and attendant sleep disruption affects daytime cognitive function (Decary, Rouleau, & Montplaisir, 2000; Montplaisir, Bedard, Richer, & Rouleau, 1992). Beebe, Groesz, Wells, Nichols, and McGee (2003) conducted a meta-analysis of 25 studies representing neuropsychological functioning in 1092 OSAS patients and 899 controls. They reported reliable associations of untreated OSAS with lower performance in vigilance and executive functioning, mixed associations with motor and visual-perceptual functioning and no association with intellectual or verbal function. However, Beebe et al. did not examine age as a moderator, despite their meta-analyzed sample showing sample mean ages ranging from 44 to 63 years.

Inspection of the OSAS and neuropsychological functioning literature indicates only a few studies containing older samples. In an uncontrolled pilot study of neuropsychological performance in a single group of 41 older apneic patients, Yesavage, Bliwise, Guilleminault, Carskadon, and Dement (1985) described performance deficits on various tasks, based on historical norms. In a between-groups design, Findley, Presty, Barth, and Suratt (1991) compared older apneics (mean = 46 obstructive events per hour) with non-apneic age-matched controls on nine cognitive measures. They found no differences on seven of the nine measures, but reported poorer performance on Paced Auditory Serial Addition Test (PASAT) and the "Steer Clear" vigilance task, a long driving simulation task. Nevertheless, they did not explore within-group variation; for example, they did not correlate vigilance performance with respiratory parameters.

In contrast to the above findings, subsequent controlled quasiexperimental research has repeatedly failed to show any reliable association between neurocognitive scores and sleep respiratory parameters in older patients. Ingram, Henke, Levin, Ingram, and Kuna (1994) were unable to replicate Findley et al.'s (1991) findings in their investigation of driving simulation in persons aged 61–75 years. They found no vigilance score differences between the − OSAS and + OSAS groups. When subdivided into good and poor vigilance groups, they found age accounted for 31% of the variance, but there was no association with other abnormal sleep indices such as periodic leg movements. Further, a demonstration of within-group correlations is necessary for proving a link between OSAS and neurocognitive deficits. Lojander, Kajaste, Maasilta, and Partinen (1999) explored within group variation and also could not find any association between attention/memory scores, measures of daytime sleepiness, and OSAS severity in a group of middle-aged men. Verstraeten, Cluydts, Verbraecken, and de Roeck (1996) were unable to detect neuropsychological differences between middle-aged insomniacs and moderate–severe OSAS patients (mean age = 53 years, range 29–73 years). Only Greenberg, Watson, and Deptula (1987) reported significant correlations between hypoxemia and performance in apneic patients on seven out of fourteen cognitive measures. However, this result likely represents Type I error, as the number of measures was almost the same as the number of subjects. Davies et al. (2001) assessed brain MRI evidence for "silent" cerebrovascular disease in + OSAS and − OSAS patients. They reported a overall base rate 34% periventricular abnormalities but no apparent excess of MRI-evident brain vascular disease in the + OSAS group.

The Honolulu-Asia Aging study (Foley et al., 1999) is providing substantial data on issues of aging, sleep, and cognitive decline. This is a large-scale, prospective longitudinal examination of the relations between sleep, aging, health, neurological status, and cognitive decline. Foley et al. (2003) examined the relations between nocturnal sleep, sleep-disordered breathing, and daytime cognitive function in a large cohort of aging Japanese-American males between 79 and 97 years of age. They reported sleep apnea syndrome in 70% of the sample, and apnea-hypopnea counts correlated with ESS scores. However, they found no correlation between apnea counts and cognitive function as measured by the Cognitive Abilities Scale.

Insomnia

Szelenberger and Niemcewicz (2000) examined learning and memory in chronic insomniacs. They found no correlation between MSLT and the Buschke Selective Reminding Test. Stone, Morin, Hart, Remsberg, and Mercer (1994) examined psychomotor performances in older insomnia patients with and without PSG-confirmed OSAS. The results showed few differences on cognitive and psychomotor performance between individuals with sleep disruptions alone compared with those whose insomnia was associated with sleep-disordered breathing and blood-gas disturbances. There were also no significant relationships between nocturnal sleep and respiratory variables and daytime functioning. Stone et al. also reported no mean differences between both group performances and historical age-matched data.

Neurocognitive findings in sleep-related variables

Daytime sleepiness and neurocognitive function

Bliwise, Carskadon, Seidel, Nekich, and Dement (1991) obtained reliable MSLT scores from neurologically normal elderly persons and reported inter-subject variability in daytime sleepiness scores sufficient for a good correlational study. However, they failed to find any significant correlations between MSLT scores and various neuropsychological measures.

Foley et al. (2001) showed that cognitive decline and daytime somnolence were associated only in older men with dementia. Hence, cerebral dysfunction associated with brain disease determines both cognitive impairment and alertness, and there is no direct causal link between alertness and impairment. The APOE e4 alleli is commonly believed to be a genetic marker for Alzheimer's disease. Caselli et al. (2002) administered the ESS and a memory battery (e.g., Rey Auditory Verbal Learning Test) to three groups varying in APOE c4 penetrance: homozygotes, heterozygotes, and noncarriers. They reported high within-group correlations between all memory tests and ESS (higher ESS predicted lower memory) in the homozygotic group, a smaller negative correlation in the heterozygotic group, and no association in the noncarriers. Again, as in the study by Foley et al. (2001), somnolence and cognitive decline may both be mediated by underlying neuronal loss but have no causal link with each other. Whitney et al. (1998) administered cognitive screening batteries and the ESS, obtained brain MRIs, and collected neuro-medical survey data from over 4000 Medicare recipients over 65 years of age. There were no correlations between subjective sleepiness (the ESS) and cognitive scores or brain MRI findings.

The studies suggest EDS by itself has minimal impact on standardized neurocognitive measures. Although sleepiness may not necessarily affect the behavioral endpoint represented by a single score, normal scores may be achieved only at the price of increased effort. Starbuck, Kay, Platenberg, Lin, and Zielinski (2000) performed fMRI on sedated and nonsedated subjects performing the PASAT. The fMRI showed increased metabolism in the sedated group despite lack of group differences in PASAT accuracy. This suggests increased mental effort may be necessary to overcome the negative impact of sleepiness on performance.

Lichtor, Alessi, and Lane (2002) investigated the impact of drug-induced sleepiness on cognitive function. Volunteers received powerful sedative medications (e.g., Fentanyl) and then underwent MSLT and psychomotor evaluation at 2-hour intervals. The psychomotor battery included a digit symbol substitution test and simple auditory and visual reaction time. Lichtor et al. reported cognitive impairment only at the first 2-hour interval but residual sleepiness up to 4 hours post injection. These findings suggest that cognitive impairment is related to the direct effect of drugs on brain substrate and not related to sleepiness. Alternatively, this data could indicate critical thresholds for determining impact on cognitive function: Mild sleepiness may not impact cognitive function but severe EDS does.

Concluding comments

Sleep and cognitive complaints rise dramatically in older patients, and neuropsychologists are often faced with questions of sleep's impact on neurocognitive function. There are two major theories of sleep changes in the elderly, but the evidentiary arrow points at cumulative health burdens rather than nuclei-specific neuronal loss as the best explanation for most sleep complaints. This could change with new research.

The main implication for geriatric neuropsychological practice is that most sleep problems of older patients do not represent a confounding variable that complicates differential diagnosis. Objective daytime sleepiness, insomnia complaints, brief hypoxic episodes associated with OSAS, and disrupted nocturnal sleep do not impact the neuropsychological measures typically given during examinations in otherwise neurologically normal older persons. Somnolence and cognitive dysfunction may be associated in groups with underlying neuropathology of the brain, indicating sleep problems are only coincidental and cognitive deficits may be interpreted as directly related to neuronal loss. The types of medication taken by the elderly may simultaneously impact daytime alertness and neurocognitive performance, but the common mechanism is impaired cortical function, not excessive sleepiness. Somnolence may potentially impact performance on longer vigilance tasks, although this type of testing is usually impractical in clinical settings. That is not to say that sleep disturbance has no implications for neurocognitive testing. Good evidence suggests REM behavior disorder may be a precursor of Lewy body dementia.

References

Aldrich, M. (1999). Ontogeny of sleep. In M. S. Aldrich, *Sleep medicine* (pp. 70–81). New York: Oxford University Press.

American Sleep Disorders Association. (1997). *The international classification of sleep disorders, revised: Diagnostic and coding manual.* Rochester, MN: Author.

Ancoli-Israel, S., Kripke, D. F., Klauber, M. R., Mason, W. J., Fell, R., & Kaplan, O. (1991). Sleep-disordered breathing in community-dwelling elderly. *Sleep, 14*(6), 486–495.

Beebe, D. W., Groesz, L., Wells, C., Nichols, A., & McGee, K. (2003). The neuropsychological effects of obstructive sleep apnea: A meta-analysis of norm-referenced and case-controlled data. *Sleep, 26*, 298–307.

Birren, J. E. (1959). *Handbook of normal aging and the individual.* Chicago: University of Chicago Press.

Bixler, E. O., Kales, A., Soldatos, C. R., Kales, J. D., & Healey, S. (1979). Prevalence of sleep disorders in the Los Angeles metropolitan area. *American Journal of Psychiatry, 136*, 1257–1262.

Bliwise, D. (1994). What is sundowning? *Journal of the American Geriatric Society, 42*, 1009–1011.

Bliwise, D. L. (1997). Normal aging. In M. H Kryger, T. Roth, & W. Dement (Eds.), *Principles and practice of sleep medicine (*pp. 26–39). New York: W. B. Saunders.

Bliwise, D. L., Carskadon, M. A., Seidel, W. F., Nekich, J. C., & Dement, W. C. (1991). MSLT-defined sleepiness and neuropsychological test performance do not correlate in the elderly. *Neurobiology and Aging, 12*, 463–468.

Bonnet, M. H., & Rosa, R. R. (1987). Sleep and performance in young adults and older normals and insomniacs during acute sleep loss and recovery. *Biological Psychology, 25*, 153–172.

Brooks, J. O., III, Friedman, L., Bliwise, D. L., & Yesavage, J. A. (1993). Use of the wrist actigraph to study insomnia in older adults. *Sleep, 16*, 151–155.

Carskadon, M. (1982). Sleep fragmentation, sleep loss and sleep need in the elderly. *The Gerontologist, 22*, 187.

Carskadon, M., & Dement, W. (1997). Normal human sleep: An overview. In M. Kryger, T. Roth, & W. Dement (Eds.), *Principles and practice of sleep medicine* (pp. 16–25). New York: W. B. Saunders.

Carskadon, M. A., Brown, E. D., & Dement, W. C. (1982). Sleep fragmentation in the elderly: Relationship to daytime sleep tendency. *Neurobiology of Aging, 3*, 321–327

Caselli, R. J., Reiman, E. M., Hentz, J. G., Osborne, D., Alexander, G. E., & Boeve, B. F. (2002). A distinctive interaction between memory and chronic daytime somnolence in asymptomatic APOE e4 homozygotes. *Sleep, 25*, 447–453.

Chen, N. H., Johns, M. W., Li, H. Y., Chu, C. C., Liang, S. C., Shu, Y. H., et al. (2002). Validation of a Chinese version of the Epworth Sleepiness Scale. *Quality of Life Research, 11*, 817–821.

Chung, K. F. (2000). Use of the Epworth Sleepiness Scale in Chinese patients with obstructive sleep apnea and normal hospital employees. *Journal of Psychosomatic Research, 49*(5), 367–372.

Coleman, R. M., Miles, L. E., Guilleminault, C. C., Zarcone, V. P., Jr., van den Hoed, J., & Dement, W. C. (1981). Sleep–wake disorders in the elderly: Polysomnographic analysis. *Journal of the American Geriatrics Society, 29*, 289–296.

Czeisler, C. A., Dumont, M., Duffy, J. F., Steinberg, J. D., Richardson, G. S., Brown, E. N., et al. (1992). Association of sleep–wake habits in older people with changes in output of circadian pacemaker. *Lancet, 340*, 933–936.

Davies, C. W., Crosby, J. H., Mullins, R. L., Traill, Z. C., Anslow, P., Davies, R. J., & Strandling, J. R. (2001). Case control study of cerebrovascular damage defined by magnetic resonance imaging in patients with OSA and normal matched control subjects. *Sleep, 24*, 715–720.

Decary, A., Rouleau, I., & Montplaisir, J. (2000). Cognitive deficits associated with sleep apnea syndrome: A proposed neuropsychological test battery. *Sleep, 23*, 369–381.

Dement, W. C., Miles, L. E., & Carskadon, M. A. (1982). "White paper" on sleep and aging. *Journal of the American Geriatrics Society, 30*(1), 25–50.

Dijk, D. J., Duffy, J. F., Riel, E., Shanahan, T. L., & Czeisler, C. A. (1999). Ageing and the circadian and homeostatic regulation of human sleep during forced desynchrony of rest, melatonin and temperature rhythms. *Journal of Physiology, 516*(Pt. 2), 611–627.

Englert, S., & Linden, M. (1998). Differences in self-reported sleep complaints in elderly persons living in the community who do or do not take sleep medication. *Journal of Clinical Psychiatry, 59*(3), 137–144; quiz 145.

Feinberg, I. (1982). Schizophrenia: Caused by a fault in programmed synaptic elimination during adolescence? *Journal of Psychiatric Research, 17*, 319–334.

Ferman, T. J., Boeve, B. F., Smith, G. E., Silber, M. H., Kokmen, E., Petersen, R. C., et al. (1999). REM sleep behavior disorder and dementia: Cognitive differences when compared with AD. *Neurology, 52*, 951–957.

Ferman, T. J., Boeve, B. F., Smith, G. E., Silber, M. H., Lucas, J. A., Graff-Radford, N. R., et al. (2002). Dementia with Lewy bodies may present as dementia and REM sleep behavior disorder without parkinsonism or hallucinations. *Journal of the International Neuropsychological Society, 8*(7), 907–914.

Findley, L. J., Presty, S. K., Barth, J. T., & Suratt, P. M. (1991). Impaired cognition and vigilance in elderly subjects with sleep apnea. In S. T. Kuna, P. M. Suratt, & J. E. Remmers (Eds.), *Sleep and respiration in aging adults* (pp. 259–263). New York: Elsevier Publishing.

Foley, D. J., Masaki, K., White, L., Larkin, E. K., Monjan, A., & Redline, S. (2003). Sleep-disordered breathing and cognitive impairment in elderly Japanese-American men. *Sleep, 26*(5), 596–599.

Foley, D. J., Monjan, A. A., Masaki, K. H., Enright, P. L., Quan, S. F., & White, L. R. (1999). Associations of symptoms of sleep apnea with cardiovascular disease, cognitive impairment, and mortality among older Japanese-American men. *Journal of the American Geriatrics Society, 47*(5), 524–528.

Foley, D., Monjan, A., Masaki, K., Ross, W., Havlik, R., White, L., et al. (2001). Daytime sleepiness is associated with 3-year incident dementia and cognitive decline in older Japanese-American men. *Journal of the American Geriatrics Society, 49*(12), 1628–1632.

Foret, J., & Webb, W. B. (1980). Changes in temporal organization of sleep stages in man aged from 20 to 70 years. *Revue d'Electroencephalographie et de Neurophysiolie Clinique, 10*, 171–176.

Friedman, L., Benson, K., Noda, A., Zarcone, V., Wicks, D. A., O'Connell, K., et al. (2000). An actigraphic comparison of sleep restriction and sleep hygiene treatments for insomnia in older adults. *Journal of Geriatric Psychiatry and Neurology, 13*(1), 17–27.

Gislason, T., & Almqvist, M. (1987). Somatic diseases and sleep complaints: An epidemiological study of 3,201 Swedish men. *Acta Medica Scandinavica, 221*(5), 475–481.

Glenville, M., & Broughton, R. (1978). Reliability of the Stanford Sleepiness Scale compared to short duration performance tests and the Wilkinson Auditory Vigilance Task. *Advances in the Biosciences*, *21*, 235–244.

Gliklich, R. E., & Wang, P. C. (2002). Validation of the snore outcomes survey for patients with sleep-disordered breathing. *Archives of Otolaryngology: Head and Neck Surgery*, *128*(7), 819–824.

Greenberg, G. D., Watson, R. K., & Deptula, D. (1987). Neuropsychological dysfunction in sleep apnea. *Sleep*, *10*, 254–262.

Greiffenstein, M. F. (2001, February). *Sleep disorders for the neuropsychologist*. Workshop presented at the 29th annual meeting of the International Neuropsychological Society, Chicago.

Guazzelli, M., Feinberg, I., Aminoff, M., Fein, G., Floyd, T. C., & Maggini, C. (1986). Sleep spindles in normal elderly: Comparison with young adult patterns and relation to nocturnal awakening, cognitive function and brain atrophy. *Electroencephalography and Clinical Neurophysiology*, *63*, 526–539.

Hayashi, Y., & Endo, S. (1982). All-night sleep polygraphic recordings of healthy aged persons: REM and slow-wave sleep. *Sleep*, *5*, 277–283.

Hofman, M. A., Fliers, E., Goudsmit, E., & Swaab, D. F. (1988). Morphometric analysis of the suprachiasmatic and paraventricular nuclei in the human brain: Sex differences and age-dependent changes. *Journal of Anatomy*, *160*, 127–143.

Ingram, F., Henke, K. G., Levin, H. S., Ingram, P. T., & Kuna, S. T. (1994). Sleep apnea and vigilance performance in a community-dwelling older sample. *Sleep*, *17*, 248–252.

Johns, M. W. (1992). Reliability and factor analysis of the Epworth Sleepiness Scale. *Sleep*, *15*, 376–381.

Karacan, I., Thornby, J. I., Anch, M., Holzer, C. E., Warheit, G. J., Schwab, J. J., et al. (1976). Prevalence of sleep disturbance in a primarily urban Florida County. *Society for Science and Medicine*, *10*, 239–244.

Klink, M. E., Quan, S. F., Kaltenborn, W. T., & Lebowitz, M. D. (1992). Risk factors associated with complaints of insomnia in a general adult population: Influence of previous complaints of insomnia. *Archives of Internal Medicine*, *152*, 1634–1637.

Lichtor, J. L., Alessi, R., & Lane, B. S. (2002). Sleep tendency as a measure of recovery after drugs used for ambulatory surgery. *Anesthesiology*, *96*, 878–883.

Linden, M., & Thiels, C. (2001). Epidemiology of prescriptions for neuroleptic drugs: Tranquilizers rather than antipsychotics. *Pharmacopsychiatry*, *34*, 150–154.

Lojander, J., Kajaste, S., Maasilta, P., & Partinen, M. (1999). Cognitive function and treatment of obstructive sleep apnea syndrome. *Journal of Sleep Research*, *8*, 71–76.

McGhie, A., & Russel, S. N. (1962). The subjective assessment of normal sleep patterns. *Journal of Mental Science*, *108*, 642–654.

Mellinger, G. D., Balter, M. B., & Uhlenhuth, E. H. (1985). Insomnia and its treatment: Prevalence and correlates. *Archives of General Psychiatry*, *42*, 225–232.

Miles, L. E., & Dement, W. C. (1980). Sleep and aging. *Sleep*, *3*, 1–220.

Montplaisir, J., Bedard, M. A., Richer, F., & Rouleau, I. (1992). Neurobehavioral manifestations in obstructive sleep apnea syndrome before and after treatment with continuous positive airway pressure. *Sleep*, *15*(6 Suppl.), S17–S19.

Mosko, S. S., & Nudleman, K. L. (1986). Somatosensory and brainstem auditory evoked responses in sleep-related periodic leg movements. *Sleep*, *9*, 399–404.

Newman, J., & Broughton, R. (1991). Pupillometric assessment of excessive daytime sleepiness in narcolepsy-cataplexy. *Sleep*, *14*, 121–129.

Ohayon, M., Caulet, M., & Lemoine, P. (1996). The elderly, sleep habits and use of psychotropic drugs by the French population. *L'Encephale, 22*, 337–350.

Partinen, M. (1994). Epidemiology of sleep disorders. In M. H. Kryger, T. Roth, & W. C. Dement (Eds.), *Principles and practice of sleep medicine* (pp. 437–445). New York: W. B. Saunders.

Rayon, P., Serrano-Castro, M., del Barrio, H., Alvarez, C., Montero, D., Madurga, M., et al. (1996). Hypnotic drug use in Spain: A cross-sectional study based on a network of community pharmacies. Spanish Group for the Study of Hypnotic Drug Utilization. *Annals of Pharmacotherapy, 30*, 1092–1100.

Rechtschaffen, A., & Kales, A. (1973). *A manual of standardized terminology, techniques and scoring system for sleep stages of human subjects.* Los Angeles: Brain Research Institute of University of California at Los Angeles.

Redeker, N. S., & Wykpisz, E. (1999). Effects of age on activity patterns after coronary artery bypass surgery. *Heart and Lung, 28*(1), 5–14.

Rediehs, M. H., Reis, J. S., & Creason, N. S. (1990). Sleep in old age: Focus on gender differences. *Sleep, 13*, 410–424.

Reynolds, C. F., III, Kupfer, D. J., Taska, L. S., Hoch, C. C., Sewitch, D. E., & Spiker, D. G. (1985). Sleep of healthy seniors: A revisit. *Sleep, 8*(1), 20–29.

Roberts, R. E., Shema, S. J., & Kaplan, G. A. (1999). Prospective data on sleep complaints and associated risk factors in an older cohort. *Psychosomatic Medicine, 61*(2), 188–196.

Roberts, R. E., Shema, S. J., Kaplan, G. A., & Strawbridge, W. J. (2000). Sleep complaints and depression in an aging cohort: A prospective perspective. *American Journal of Psychiatry, 157*(1), 81–88.

Roehrs, T., Hollebeek, E., Drake, C., & Roth, T. (2002). Substance use for insomnia in metropolitan Detroit. *Journal of Psychosomatic Research, 53*(1), 571–576.

Rosekind, M. R. (1992). The epidemiology and occurrence of insomnia. *Journal of Clinical Psychiatry, 53*(Suppl.), 4–6.

Schenck, C. H., & Mahowald, M. W. (1996). REM sleep parasomnias. In M. S. Aldrich (Ed.), *Neurologic clinics: Sleep disorders II* (pp. 697–720). Philadelphia: Saunders.

Singer, C., Tractenberg, R. E., Kaye, J., Schafer, K., Gamst, A., Grundman, M., et al. (2003). A multicenter, placebo-controlled trial of melatonin for sleep disturbance in Alzheimer's disease. *Sleep, 26*(7), 893–901.

Starbuck, V. N., Kay, G. G., Platenberg, R. C., Lin, C. S., & Zielinski, B. A. (2000). Functional magnetic resonance imaging reflects changes in brain functioning with sedation. *Human Psychopharmacology, 15*, 613–618.

Stone, J., Morin, C. M., Hart, R. P., Remsberg, S., & Mercer, J. (1994). Neuropsychological functioning in older insomniacs with or without obstructive sleep apnea. *Psychology and Aging, 9*(2), 231–236.

Stopa, E. G., Volicer, L., Kuo-Leblanc, V., Harper, D., Lathi, D., Tate, B., & Satlin, A. (1999). Pathologic evaluation of the human suprachiasmatic nucleus in severe dementia. *Journal of Neuropathology and Experimental Neurology, 58*, 29–39.

Sutton, D. A., Moldofsky, H., & Bradley, E. M. (2001). Insomnia and health problems in Canadians. *Sleep, 24*(6), 665–670.

Szelenberger, W., & Niemcewicz, S. (2000). Severity of insomnia correlates with cognitive impairment. *Acta Neurobiologiae Experimentalis, 60*(3), 373.

Taub, J. M. (1981). Disturbances in diurnal rhythms following a night of reduced sleep. *International Journal of Neuroscience, 14*(3–4), 239–245.

Van Someren, E. J. (2000). Circadian and sleep disturbances in the elderly. *Experimental Gerontology*, *35*(9–10), 1229–1237.

Verstraeten, E., Cluydts, R., Verbraecken, J., & de Roeck, J. (1996). Neuropsychological functioning and determinants of morning alertness in patients with obstructive sleep apnea syndrome. *Journal of the International Neuropsychological Society*, *2*, 306–314.

Viswanathan, N., & Davis, F. C. (1995). Suprachiasmatic nucleus grafts restore circadian function in aged hamsters. *Brain Research*, *686*(1), 10–16.

Vitiello, M. V., Moe, K. E., & Prinz, P. N. (2002). Sleep complaints cosegregate with illness in older adults: Clinical research informed by and informing epidemiological studies of sleep. *Journal of Psychosomatic Research*, *53*(1), 555–559.

Weaver, T. E. (2001). Outcome measurement in sleep medicine practice and research. Part 1: Assessment of symptoms, subjective and objective daytime sleepiness, health-related quality of life and functional status. *Sleep Medicine Reviews*, *5*(2), 103–128.

Webb, W. B. (1982a). The sleep of older subjects fifteen years later. *Psychological Reports*, *50*(1), 11–14.

Webb, W. B. (1982b). The measurement and characteristics of sleep in older persons. *Neurobiology of Aging*, *3*(4), 311–319.

Webb, W. B., & Campbell, S. S. (1980). Awakenings and the return to sleep in an older population. *Sleep*, *3*(1), 41–46.

Webb, W. B., & Dreblow, L. M. (1982). A modified method for scoring slow wave sleep of older subjects. *Sleep*, *5*, 195–199.

Whitney, C. W., Enright, P. L., Newman, A. B., Bonekat, W., Foley, D., & Quan, S. F. (1998). Correlates of daytime sleepiness in 4578 elderly persons: The Cardiovascular Health Study. *Sleep*, *21*, 27–36.

Woodruff, D. S. (1985). Arousal, sleep, and aging. In J. E. Birren & K. W. Schaie (Eds.), *Handbook of the psychology of aging* (2nd ed., pp. 261–295). New York: Van Nostrand & Reinhold.

Yesavage, J., Bliwise, D., Guilleminault, C., Carskadon, M., & Dement, W. (1985). Preliminary communication: Intellectual deficit and sleep-related respiratory disturbance in the elderly. *Sleep*, *8*, 30–33.

14 Geriatric pain and neuropsychological assessment

Felicia Hill-Briggs, Jennifer Jacobson Kirk, and Stephen T. Wegener

Pain is a significant problem for the older person, and prevalence increases with age. It is a complex phenomenon involving multiple biological, psychological, and social/environmental determinants. Impact of pain on the functioning and quality of life of older adults can be high due to associations of pain with impaired physical function (Khana, Khana, Namazi, Kercher, & Stange, 1997; Scudds & Robertson, 2000), depression (Khana et al., 1997; Magni, Marchetti, Moreschi, Merskey, & Luchini, 1993), increased sleep disturbance (Ferrell, Ferrell, & Osterweil, 1990; Magni et al., 1993), and increased health care utilization and costs (Gallagher, Verma, & Mossey, 2000). Older adults with pain are three times more likely to become disabled than those without pain, controlling for age, number of chronic conditions, depressive symptoms, and sleep quality (Scudds & Robertson, 1998). Severe pain that interferes with function is not part of the natural aging process and should not be accepted as "part of growing old;" it is a health problem that requires vigorous assessment and management.

The understanding of pain in older adults is complicated by a number of factors unique to the aging process that have a major impact on the experience of pain, its assessment and management, and its influence on neuropsychological function. This chapter will provide an overview of key issues relevant to pain and neuropsychology in older adults. These issues include pain classification and prevalence, neurological mechanisms affecting pain perception, pain assessment methods in cognitively intact and impaired older adults, and relationships between pain and neuropsychological functioning. The chapter concludes with clinical recommendations for assessing and interpreting the role of pain in the neuropsychological evaluation of older adults.

Pain classification, prevalence, and underdiagnosis

Aging is associated with increased physical illness (e.g., musculoskeletal problems, cancer, stroke, diabetes) and medical treatments that can lead to pain. Geriatric pain may be classified as acute, postoperative, or persistent (Gagliese, Katz, & Melzack, 1999). Acute pain refers to pain that is brief in duration and related to a specific pathological process, such as tissue damage.

Postoperative pain is common in elderly persons as this age group has the highest incidence of surgery (Politser & Schneidman, 1990). Although evidence is contradictory regarding age-related differences in reporting of postoperative pain levels (Oberle, Paul, Wry, & Grace, 1990), consistently reported is the inadequate treatment of postoperative pain in older adults in spite of the availability of effective treatments (see Pasero & McCaffery, 1996, for a review). Persistent or chronic pain continues beyond the expected time frame for healing and is operationally defined as pain that persists for greater than 6 months. The term *persistent pain* may be more helpful than *chronic pain*, as the latter is a label often associated with negative stereotypes and expectations by clinicians and patients. Due to the prolonged nature of persistent chronic pain, psychological, interpersonal, and environmental variables have greater potential to influence the pain experience.

The problem of underdiagnosis and undertreatment of pain among older adults has been well-documented (Herr & Garand, 2001; Kamel, Phlavan, Malekgoudarzi, Gogel, & Morley, 2001; Yonan & Wegener, 2003). Epidemiologic investigations have found that older adults are more likely than younger adults to have persistent pain (Magni et al., 1993) and are more likely to have multiple pain sites (Andersson, Ejlertsson, Leden, & Rosenberg, 1993). It is estimated that 25–50% of community-dwelling older adults experience significant pain at least some of the time (American Geriatric Society [AGS] Panel on Persistent Pain in Older Adults, 2002). The prevalence of pain in nursing home populations is even higher, with rates ranging from 49% to 83% (Fox, Raina, & Jadad, 1999). In spite of the fact that 40–50% of nursing home residents are using analgesic medication (Sengstaken & King, 1993), older age appears to be a risk factor for inadequate pain management (Cleeland et al., 1994).

Risk for underdiagnosis and undertreatment may be higher for cognitively impaired patients. In a study of pain assessment in nursing home residents, Cohen-Mansfied and Lipson (2002) found that physicians consistently perceived lower levels of pain in patients with severe cognitive impairment as compared to those with mild or moderate impairment, regardless of pain-related medical diagnoses. It has been shown that elderly patients with Alzheimer's disease (AD) are administered fewer doses of nonsteroidal anti-inflammatory drugs (NSAIDs) and other analgesic medications than patients not diagnosed with dementia (Frampton, 2003). Challenges with regard to pain perception and reliability of assessment in cognitively impaired older adults may also contribute to undertreatment.

Neurological mechanisms of pain in aging and dementia

Pain can be characterized as having sensory-discriminative, cognitive/evaluative, and motivational-affective dimensions (Melzack & Casey, 1968). The sensory-discriminative dimension refers to the detection of nociception and the processing of the stimulus. Although brain systems contribute to more than one pathway, the lateral pain system (spinothalamic tract projecting through the lateral thalamus to the primary and secondary somatosensory cortex, parietal operculum and insula) is particularly involved in the sensory-discriminative dimension.

The cognitive/evaluative dimension of pain refers to the central processing, labeling, memory, and assigning of meaning to the stimulus. The motivational-affective dimension refers to the negative, unpleasant aspect of pain that motivates the organism to act, including the related emotional response. The medial pain system (intralaminar/medial thalamic nuclei, reticular formation, mesencephalon, thalamic ventral caudal parvocellular/portea nuclei [VCPC, VCPOR], the parisylvian area, anterior cingulate cortex, amygdala, hippocampus, and hypothalamus) plays a central role in the cognitive-evaluative and motivational-affective dimensions of pain. These brain structures and pain dimensions may be variably impacted by developmental or pathological changes found in older persons.

Changes in sensory and cognitive processes and a reluctance to report pain make it more difficult to assess and treat pain in older adults. Researchers have speculated that older adults may be willing to accept a certain level of pain and discomfort as part of growing old, a hypothesis that is consistent with the finding that older adults report less emotional response (depression, anxiety, anger, and fear) to pain and exhibit less pain behavior than younger adults (Riley, Wade, Robinson, & Price, 2000).

As pain perception is dependent on integrated cognitive processes, it may be expected that individuals with dementia will have alterations in pain experience. These alterations may vary based on the type of dementia, physiological and functional changes associated with the dementia, and the degree to which pain-related brain pathways are impacted. In general, there is a consistent finding of decreased pain experience in persons with AD. Changes in pain processing systems, diminished capacity to report pain (dysphasia), or decreased pain experience related to reduced comorbidities, specifically osteoarthritis (Farrell, Katz, & Helme, 1996), may underlie findings of reduced pain experience in AD patients. Data do not support poor memory as a factor in reduced pain reporting (Scherder et al., 2001).

Experimental pain studies of persons with AD and matched controls (Benedetti et al., 1999; Gibson, Voukelatos, Ames, Flicker, & Helme, 2001; Rainero, Vighetti, Bergamasco, Pinessi, & Benedetti, 2000) indicate that there appears to be no difference in pain threshold (level at which the person reports stimulus as painful), suggesting that the sensory-discriminative aspect of pain is retained, but this group may be less reliable in detecting differences in pain stimuli due to slower cortical processing. Increased pain tolerance (level at which the person requests to terminate the pain stimulus) suggests that the motivational-affective dimension of pain is altered in this population.

Scherder, Sergeant, and Swaab (2003) reported evidence that in frontotemporal dementia, perhaps to a greater extent than in AD, there is a decrease in the motivational-affective dimension of pain, which may account for the increased pain tolerance observed. While the influence of vascular dementia might be expected to vary more from person to person, there is evidence of a general increase in motivational-affective pain experience, which may lead to greater suffering associated with painful stimuli in persons with vascular dementia. In addition to the neurological exam, neuropsychological testing has been posited as a means of detecting whether the medial and lateral pain systems are intact (Scherder et al., 2003). For example, normal, age-related scores on tactile object recognition and on the Stroop interference task can be used to indicate integrity of brain areas associated with pain processing and cognition (e.g., the parietal operculum and secondary somatosensory cortex, and the anterior cingulate cortex, respectively, using these two tests).

Pain assessment in older adults

Because of the prevalence of pain in older adults and the impact of pain on functional status, basic pain assessment should be part of the initial evaluation of all older persons who present for evaluation or treatment. The goals of the assessment should be to identify the impact of pain on cognitive, psychosocial, and physical functioning and to target areas for intervention. Issues related to pain perception and sensory abilities in older adults necessitate careful attention to assessment methods. Adequate pain assessment emphasizes the use of interview, chart review, and established measures for pain, function, and mood, with appropriate modifications for persons with significant cognitive impairments.

Pain interview and chart review

Interviews with the patient, and caregivers when indicated, provide unique and critical information. Interview questions focus on the following: (a) pain experience, including location, intensity, quality, frequency, and exacerbating and relieving factors; (b) pain impact on functioning, mood, and sleep quality; (c) pain management, including medications, modalities, activity and exercise, family/caregiver response, adaptive equipment, coping skills, spirituality, and alternative medicine; and (d) beliefs and attitudes, including pain-related fears, knowledge of pain and management strategies, satisfaction with pain management, and expectations for pain relief.

For individuals who are cognitively intact or who have mild–moderate cognitive impairment, patient self-report should be the primary source of these interview data, and alternative sources (others' report) should not be used as substitutes. Interviews with caregivers can be useful in providing the clinician an opportunity to assess caregiver and family member responses to the patient's pain behavior. For institutionalized patients or those with significant medical histories, careful chart review provides information regarding current health status and history of illness, presence of comorbidities that may impact treatment, prior and current treatments, pain medications, and level of pain relief from medication.

Pain scales

A number of tools are available to assess pain intensity, experience, and impact. Patient self-report is generally considered the most accurate and reliable indicator of pain intensity and experience (AGS Panel on Persistent Pain in Older Persons, 2002); consequently, unidimensional, self-report pain scales have been widely used to assess pain severity in the general population.

Visual analog scales (VAS) consist of a horizontal or vertical line (10 cm long) that is anchored by descriptions of pain intensity ranging from 0 "no pain" to 10 "the worst pain I can imagine." Participants are asked to make a mark on the line to indicate the intensity of their current pain. Verbal descriptor scales (VDS) offer the participants verbal labels to describe their pain, such as "no pain," "slight pain," "mild pain," "moderate pain," "severe pain," "extreme pain," or "pain as bad as it could be." Respondents choose one of the descriptors to indicate their current level of pain. Evidence suggests that the VDS may be preferable to the VAS when assessing pain in older adults and that the typical horizontal orientation of the VAS is rated as the most difficult to use (Gagliese & Melzack, 1997; Herr & Garand, 2001). One difficulty associated with verbal descriptor scales is that patients may not identify their pain experience with any of the descriptors listed along the continuum (DeWaters, Popovich, & Faut-Callahan, 2003). The Faces Pain Scale (FPS) consists of a series of six simple drawings of faces with expressions that range from neutral to very distressed. Participants are asked to indicate which face most accurately represents the severity of their current pain. The FPS is easy to administer and has shown good construct validity and test–retest reliability with cognitively intact older adults (Herr, Mobily, Kohout, & Wagenaar, 1998; Krulewitch et al., 2000).

Due to their relative simplicity, these unidimensional scales are thought to be helpful when assessing pain in cognitively impaired older adults. Chibnall and Tait (2001) compared the accuracy, reliability, and validity of the following four unidimensional scales in cognitively impaired older adults: A 5-point verbal descriptor scale, a faces pain scale, a 21-point horizontal box scale, and a 21-point vertical box scale. The horizontal box scale (a row of 21 boxes labeled from 0 "no pain" to 100 "pain as bad as it could be" in 5-point increments) had superior psychometric properties and validity for both the communicative cognitively impaired and unimpaired participants. This study and others provide evidence that communicative older adults with mild to moderate cognitive impairment can complete one of the established pain scales and that these scales should be a primary source of pain assessment.

In addition to unidimensional pain scales are multidimensional scales such as the McGill Pain Questionnaire (MPQ), a frequently used pain measure that yields a pain index from ratings of sensory, affective, and evaluative aspects of pain (Melzack, 1975). Although older adults who are cognitively intact can complete this questionnaire, older individuals tend to have difficulty with the word choices on the pain descriptor/adjective selection section. Its clinical use outside of centers focused on pain management is limited due to its length;

however, a short form exists for easier use, and psychometric properties are reasonably well established (Melzack, 1987).

Pain assessment in populations with severe cognitive impairment

Assessment of pain in persons who have severe cognitive impairment or who are uncommunicative poses significant challenges (Bachino, Snow, Kunik, Cody, & Wristers, 2001; Herr & Garand, 2001). Alternative pain assessment options are available, including behavioral observation, clinician rating scales, and chart data. Behavioral indicators such as changes in facial expression, pain vocalizations, body movements, activity patterns/routines, or interpersonal responses in a person with severe cognitive impairment or dementia should raise the question of pain as a potential underlying factor (AGS Panel on Persistent Pain in Older Persons, 2002). Observation of facial expression in noncommunicative, older adults may be adequate for determining the presence of pain but not level of pain intensity (Manfredi, Breuer, Meier, & Lebow, 2003). Agitation and aggression may be indicators of pain in the very old (> 85 years) with severe cognitive impairment (Manfredi, Breuer, Wallenstein, Stegmann, Bottomley, & Libow, 2003).

To address reduced reliability and validity of standard pain scales in adults with moderate to severe cognitive impairment, several behavior observation tools have been developed specifically for the evaluation of pain in this population (see Table 14.1). Initial psychometric data on these scales are promising for persons with advanced dementia or aphasia.

Neuropsychological functioning in chronic pain patients

Development of alternative scales for assessing pain in specific older adult populations resulted from a growing body of research on the influence of neuropsychological impairment on altered pain perception, experience, and self-report in older adults. In contrast, the influence of pain on the neuropsychological functioning of older adults with pain has received relatively little attention. The relationships between pain and neuropsychological functioning in older populations are complex and are subject to confounding by several factors, including: (a) the role of comorbid conditions including depression, anxiety, fatigue, sleep disturbance, and chronic disease in patients with chronic pain; (b) the potential influence of pain experience at the time of testing on cognitive performance; and (c) the potential impact of chronic pain medication use on neuropsychological performance.

Comorbidity in chronic pain

Depression is often associated with pain, and this is true in the older adult as well. Significant relationships have been found between depression and pain in older persons even after controlling for physical health and functional status

Table 14.1 Observation scales for pain assessment in persons with severe cognitive impairment

Instrument	Behaviors assessed	Scoring
Abbey Pain Scale (Abbey et al., 2004)	(6 items) Vocalization, facial expression, change in body language, behavioral change, physiological change, physical changes	Each behavior rated as: Absent/0, Mild/1, Moderate/2, Severe/3. Total ratings classify pain status as: No Pain/0–2, Mild Pain/3–7, Moderate Pain/8–13, or Severe Pain/14+
Discomfort in Dementia of the Alzheimer's Type (DS-DAT; Hurley, Volicer, Hanrahan, Houde, & Volicer, 1992)	(9 items) Noisy breathing, negative vocalizations, content facial expression, sad facial expression, frightened facial expression, frown, relaxed body language, tense body language, fidgeting	Each behavior rated on a 100 mm scale from 0 (absent) to 100 (extreme) following a 5-minute observation period to account for their number, intensity, and duration. Pain rating is scored as 0 (0), 1 (1–33 mm), 2 (34–66 mm), or 3 (67–100 mm), with higher scores indicating higher levels of observed discomfort
Pain Assessment in Advanced Dementia (PAINAD; Warden, Hurley, & Volicer, 2003)	(5 items) Breathing independent of vocalization, negative vocalization, facial expression, body language, consolability	Each behavior rated on a 3-point scale: 0 = absence/normal, 1 = mild to moderate, and 2 = severe. Total ratings yield a pain score between 0 (no pain) and 10 (severe pain) that can be compared with other commonly used pain scales
Checklist of Nonverbal Pain Indicators (CNPI; Feldt, 2000)	(6 items) Nonverbal vocalizations, grimaces, bracing, rubbing, restlessness, verbal complaint. Used as a clinical intervention tool	Presence of any pain-associated behavior indicates presence of pain and indication for treatment
Assessment of Discomfort in Dementia (ADD; Kovach, Noonan, Griffie, Muchka, & Weissman, 2002)	(5 areas): Facial expression, mood, body language, voice and behavior. Used as a clinical intervention tool	Each area evaluated for presence of pain-related behaviors. Behaviors observed must be a change in behavior. Observation of behavior leads to a four-step protocol of determining cause of pain and initiating interventions to validate pain behavior observation

(Parmelee, Katz, & Lawton, 1991; Wang, Liu, Fuh, Wang, & Lu, 1999). Older individuals who have both pain and depression appear to be particularly vulnerable to physical disability (Reid, Williams, Concato, Tinetti, & Gill, 2003; Williamson & Schulz, 1992). Moreover, the presentation of cognitive impairment in depressed older adults can result in difficulty differentiating a primary neuropsychological deficit from a dementia syndrome of depression (Kaszniak & Christenson, 1994). A depression screening scale designed specifically for older adults (the Geriatric Depression Scale; Yesavage et al., 1983) can be used to determine whether further evaluation for depression is necessary.

Several studies have examined pain, depression, and cognitive impairment as interrelated conditions. In a population of nursing home and senior apartment residents with cognitive impairment, pain, and depression, Parmelee (1996) found that the association of pain with depression was strongest in persons with severe, rather than mild or moderate, cognitive impairment. Cohen-Mansfield and Taylor (1998) reported a curvilinear relationship of pain and cognitive impairment with depression; depression was higher in nursing home residents who had pain and moderate cognitive impairment than in residents who had pain and either mild or severe cognitive impairment. In analyses of a nursing home and a day care sample, significant main effects of cognitive function on depression, and pain on depression, were found, with failure to find a significant interaction of cognitive function and pain (Cohen-Mansfield & Taylor, 1998). In at least one study, no associations were found among the comorbidities of pain, cognitive functioning, and depression. In a population-based sample of 70-year-olds living in the community, Bergh et al. (2003) reported that neither performance on a brief neuropsychological battery nor depressive symptoms scores were associated with report of pain during the previous 14 days or level of pain severity, which was rated as "mild" to "discomforting" (1–2 on a 0–5 scale).

In addition to depression, older adults have high rates of comorbid medical conditions (e.g. diabetes, hypertension, lung disease) with known associations with cognitive impairment and increased incidence of dementia. This is particularly the case in samples drawn from settings such as nursing homes and day care centers. These co-occurring medical conditions, which are often not exclusion criteria, can confound scientific and clinical understanding of the relationship of chronic pain with neuropsychological performance.

Effects of comorbidity observed in younger adult pain samples may be present in older populations as well. Hart, Martelli, and Zasler (2000) reviewed 23 studies of neuropsychological functioning in young to middle-aged chronic pain patients without history of head trauma or neurological disorder. The majority of studies compared persons with history of chronic pain (e.g. musculoskeletal, fibromyalgia) to other diagnostic groups (e.g., mild TBI), normal controls, or neuropsychological test normative data. While, overall, studies reported reduced attentional skills, processing speed, and psychomotor speed in some chronic pain groups, several methodological limitations, including nonexamination of multiple comorbid variables in a majority of studies, made it difficult to draw firm conclusions.

More specific analyses suggest that comorbid factors may account for a portion of the association of pain with neuropsychological performance (Hart et al., 2000). For example, when psychological distress variables were also included in analyses, several studies found that observed neuropsychological deficits were primarily accounted for by presence of depression or anxiety rather than pain *per se* (Eccleston, Crombez, Aldrich, & Stannard, 1997; Grace, Nielson, Hopkins, & Berg, 1999; Iezzi, Archibald, Barnett, Klinck, & Duckworth, 1999; Pincus, Fraser, & Pierce, 1998). Few studies that assessed mood reported no correlation between emotional distress and test performance in chronic pain samples (e.g., Dick, Eccleston, & Crombez, 2002). Comorbid fatigue and sleep disturbance, when assessed, have been found to be significantly associated with neuropsychological test performance (Cote & Moldofsky, 1997), and improved cognitive performance has followed sleep and improvement in disordered serotonergic projections in chronic headache patients (Meyer, Thornby, Crawford, & Rauch, 2000).

In order to investigate the influence of pain on neuropsychological test performance in older adults, future studies will need to employ rigorous study designs that address the multiple comorbidities that are known to alter neuropsychological test performance or have potential to influence the relationship. Such comorbidities include older age, education, depression, sleep disturbance, fatigue, chronic illness or disease, history of brain injury, and neurological disease.

Pain at time of testing

Pain at time of testing has seldom been investigated, especially in older adults. Two studies involving primarily middle-aged adults with history of posttraumatic headache found that headache severity at the time of testing did not alter neuropsychological test scores. Tsushima and Newbill (1996), for example, found that patients who self-reported severe headache, mild headache, or no headache at the beginning of testing did not differ on any of 11 Luria Nebraska Neuropsychological Battery scores. Similarly, Lake, Branca, Lutz, and Saper (1999) reported that performance on neuropsychological tests of verbal and visual memory, language, attention, and cognitive shift was not associated with mild headache intensity (rated as 1–2/5), or moderate/severe intensity (rated as 3–5/5). Moreover, during the course of the 4-hour testing, headache pain tended to increase without a resulting neuropsychological performance decrement. In a population-based sample of 70-year-olds, presence or absence of pain at the time of testing was not associated with performance on neuropsychological tests of verbal ability, perceptual speed, inductive reasoning, psychomotor speed, memory, and cognitive flexibility (Bergh et al., 2003). Because the majority of persons in the sample reported average pain over the past 14 days as mild (rated as 1/5) or discomforting (rated as 2/5), pain intensity during testing may have also been minimal.

Eccleston (1995) provided evidence that during a complex attention task requiring high demand, patients reporting "high pain" at the time of testing (defined as above a group median VAS score of 39.6 and above a group median score of 66 on a 0–100 numerical pain rating scale) had performance decrements as compared to patients with "low pain" (defined as below the median scores), or no pain. This series of experiments further demonstrated that, for the group experiencing low levels of pain during testing, the attention task served as a distraction from pain and was maintained for the duration of the task. The attention task appeared to provide *distractional psychoanalgesia*, allowing patients to complete the task based on their actual cognitive ability (Eccleston, 1995). Collectively, these studies suggest that in patients with chronic pain, mild–moderate intensity of pain during testing may not impede neuropsychological test performance.

Long-term opioid analgesic use

Opioid medications are gaining increased use in treatment of noncancer chronic pain. Opioids can lead to increased sedation and acute, transient decline in mental status for a short period immediately after therapy has begun, requiring initiation of low dosages administered at spaced intervals for older adults. For older patients receiving insufficient pain relief from acetaminophen or tramadol, opioids may be safer with regard to risk of toxicity than are NSAIDs (Podichetty, Mazanec, & Biscup, 2003).

Concerns regarding impairment in cognition have resulted in studies of neuropsychological functioning with chronic use of opioids such as morphine and oxycodone in samples of middle-aged to older adults. These studies consistently demonstrate that once patients have been stabilized on an opioid regimen, long-term use does not result in decline from baseline preopioid therapy abilities in psychomotor function (Digit Symbol, Grooved Pegboard, Trail Making Test Part B), information processing speed (Stroop interference), or verbal learning skills (Jamison et al., 2003; Raja et al., 2002; Tassain et al., 2003). Treatment with long-acting opioid therapy has also been found to improve skills such as psychomotor speed, sustained attention, and vigilance from baseline, preopioid therapy performance (Haythornthwaite, Menefee, Quatrano-Piacentini, & Pappagallo, 1998; Lorenz, Beck, & Bromm, 1997). Improved pain control and decreased pain-related emotional distress are associated with preservation of neuropsychological performance with long-term opioid use. Neurophysiological studies utilizing evoked cerebral potentials and measuring vigilance, cognitive performance, sedation, and pain during trials of morphine analgesia have provided further evidence that opioids appear to improve cognitive performance by removing pain and enhancing mood (Lorenz et al., 1997).

Clinical recommendations

Pain is an important and pervasive issue in older adult populations. Changes in pain perception, issues of reliability in pain assessment, and tendencies toward underdiagnosis and undertreatment are challenges in older adult populations with chronic pain. Because of the impact of pain on mood and adjustment, functional status, disability, and quality of life, pain assessment should be included in a comprehensive evaluation. The impact of pain on overall functional status and neuropsychological performance should be considered.

The literature is relatively silent on what level of pain precludes accurate neuropsychological assessment. Mild to moderate pain at the time of testing has been demonstrated not to result in poorer performance. As part of the interview prior to comprehensive neuropsychological assessment, the clinician should ascertain if pain is present and if so have the client rate current, highest, lowest, and usual level of pain over the past week. Pain may be classified as mild (1–3/10), moderate (4–7/10), or severe (7–10/10) using a standard written or verbal VAS (Jensen, Turner, Turner, & Romano, 1996). Whenever possible, clients reporting moderate to severe levels of pain, particularly if this is unusual for them, should be asked if they wish to defer assessment to a period of better pain control. For individuals reporting severe levels of pain, assessment should be deferred assuming periods of lower levels of pain control do occur. Levels of pain should be included in the assessment report, and any potential confounding impact on test results should be noted. Furthermore, due to the potential for emotional distress to adversely impact neuropsychological testing performance in person with chronic pain, mood assessment findings should be incorporated into interpretation and reporting of neuropsychological test results.

The relatively small body of literature to date is consistent with regard to absence of a decline in neuropsychological functioning in middle-aged to older adults whose chronic pain is managed with long-term opioid therapy. Reduction in pain severity and improvement in pain-related emotional distress appear in some cases to lead to selected improvement in neuropsychological functioning. Adequate pain control using these medications, therefore, may be an effective strategy for improving mood disturbance, quality of life, and functioning, without loss of neuropsychological capacity. Cautious regimens are recommended for initiation of these analgesics in older adults.

Finally, clinicians and researchers are often quick to identify the challenges and barriers faced by older adults in pain. There is a need to avoid negative bias and consider both the barriers and the resources of geriatric pain patients that impact prevention or management of pain in this population. The aging process may provide older adults with certain resources or assets that may help them cope with multiple losses and pain. Personal (financial, self-esteem, and sense of coherence), social, and cognitive resources do not always diminish with age and can be assets in pain management (Bengston, Reedy, & Gordon, 1985; Erikson, Erikson, & Kivnick, 1986). The belief that older adults can be as adaptive as younger adults in coping with pain is consistent with the finding that older adults appear to use similar and equally effective coping strategies as younger adults (Keefe & Williams, 1990). Accurate pain assessment and treatment hold promise for maintenance of functional and neuropsychological ability in older adults with chronic pain.

References

Abbey, J., Piller, N., de Bellis, A., Esterman, A., Parker, D., Giles, L., & Lowcay, B. (2004). The Abbey Pain Scale: A 1-minute numerical indicator for people with end-stage dementia. *International Journal of Palliative Nursing, 10*(1), 6–13.

American Geriatric Society Panel on Persistent Pain in Older Persons. (2002). The management of persistent pain in older persons. *Journal of the American Geriatrics Society, 50*(6 Suppl.), S205–S224.

Andersson, H. I., Ejlertsson, G., Leden, I., & Rosenberg, C. (1993). Chronic pain in a geographically defined general population: Studies of differences in age, gender, social class, and pain localization. *Clinical Journal of Pain, 9*, 174–182.

Bachino, C., Snow, A. L., Kunik, M. E., Cody, M., & Wristers, K. (2001). Principles of pain assessment and treatment in non-comunicative demented patients. *Clinical Gerontologist, 23*, 97–115.

Benedetti, F., Vighetti, S., Ricco, C., Lagna, E., Bergamasco, B., Pinessi, L., & Rainero, I. (1999). Pain threshold and tolerance in Alzheimer's disease. *Pain, 80*(1–2), 377–382.

Bengston, V. L., Reedy, M. N., & Gordon, C. (1985). Aging and self-conceptions: Personality processes and social contexts. In J. E. Birren & K. W. Schale (Eds.), *Handbook of the psychology of aging* (pp. 544–593). New York: Van Nostrand Reinhold.

Bergh, I., Steen, G., Waern, M., Johansson, B., Oden, A., Sjostrom, B., & Steen, B. (2003). Pain and its relation to cognitive function and depressive symptoms: A Swedish population study of 70-year-old men and women. *Journal of Pain and Symptom Management, 26*(4), 903–912.

Chibnall, J. T., & Tait, R. C. (2001). Pain assessment in cognitively impaired and unimpaired older adults: A comparison of four scales. *Pain, 92*, 173–186.

Cleeland, C. S., Gonin, R., Hatfield, A. K., Edmonson, J. H., Blum, R. H., Stewart, J. A., & Pandya, K. J. (1994). Pain and its treatment in outpatients with metastatic cancer. *New England Journal of Medicine, 330*, 592–596.

Cohen-Mansfield, J., & Lipson, S. (2002). Pain in cognitively impaired nursing home residents: How well are physicians diagnosing it? *Journal of the American Geriatrics Society, 50*(6), 1039–1044.

Cohen-Mansfield, J., & Taylor, L. (1998). The relationship between depressed affect, pain, and cognitive function: A cross-sectional analysis of two elderly populations. *Aging and Mental Health, 2*(4), 313–318.

Cote, K. A., & Moldofsky, H. (1997). Sleep, daytime symptoms, and cognitive performance in patients with fibromyalgia. *Journal of Rheumatology, 24*, 14–23.

DeWaters, T., Popovich, J., & Faut-Callahan, M. (2003). An evaluation of clinical tools to measure pain in older people with cognitive impairment. *British Journal of Community Nursing, 8*(5), 226–234.

Dick, B., Eccleston, C., & Crombez, G. (2002). Attentional functioning in fibromyalgia, rheumatoid arthritis, and musculoskeletal pain patients. *Arthritis and Rheumatism, 47*(6), 639–644.

Eccleston, C. (1995). Chronic pain and distraction: An experimental investigation into the role of sustained and shifting attention in the processing of chronic persistent pain. *Behavior Research and Therapy, 33*(4), 391–405.

Eccleston, C., Crombez, G., Aldrich, S., & Stannard, C. (1997). Attention and somatic awareness in chronic pain. *Pain, 72,* 209–215.

Erikson, E. H., Erikson, J. M., & Kivnick, H. Q. (1986). *Vital involvement in old age: The experience of old age in our time.* New York: W. W. Norton & Company.

Farrell, M. J., Katz, B., & Helme, R. D. (1996). The impact of dementia on the pain experience. *Pain, 67*(1), 7–15.

Feldt, K. S. (2000). The Checklist of Nonverbal Pain Indicators (CNPI). *Pain Management Nursing, 1*(1), 13–21.

Ferrell, B. A., Ferrell, B. R., & Osterweil, D. (1990). Pain in the nursing home. *Journal of the American Geriatrics Society, 38,* 409–414.

Fox, P. L., Raina, P., & Jadad, A. R. (1999). Prevalence and treatment of pain in older adults in nursing homes and other long-term care institutions: A systematic review. *Canadian Medical Association Journal, 160,* 329–333.

Frampton, M. (2003). Experience assessment and management of pain in people with dementia. *Age and Aging, 32*(3), 248–251.

Gagliese, L., Katz, J., & Melzack, R. (1999). Pain in the elderly. In R. Melzack & P. D. Wall (Eds.), *Textbook of pain* (pp. 991–1006). Edinburgh, UK: Churchill Livingstone.

Gagliese, L., & Melzack, R. (1997). Age differences in the quality of chronic pain: A preliminary study. *Pain Research and Management, 2,* 157–162.

Gallagher, R. M., Verma, S., & Mossey, J. (2000). Chronic pain: Sources of late-life pain and risk factors for disability. *Geriatrics, 55,* 40–45.

Gibson, S. J., Voukelatos, X., Ames, D., Flicker, L., & Helme, R. D. (2001). An examination of pain perception and cerebral event-related potentials following carbon dioxide laser stimulation in patients with Alzheimer's disease and age-matched control volunteers. *Pain Research Management, 6*(3), 126–132.

Grace, G. M., Nielson, W. R., Hopkins, M., & Berg, M. A. (1999). Concentration and memory deficits in patients with fibromyalgia syndrome. *Journal of Clinical and Experimental Neuropsychology, 21,* 477–487.

Hart, R. P., Martelli, M. F., & Zasler, N. D. (2000). Chronic pain and neuropsychological functioning. *Neuropsychology Review, 10*(3), 131–149.

Haythornthwaite, J. A., Menefee, L. A., Quatrano-Piacentini, A. L., & Pappagallo, M. (1998). Outcome of chronic opioid therapy for non-cancer pain. *Journal of Pain and Symptom Management, 15*(3), 185–194.

Herr, K. A., & Garand, L. (2001). Assessment and measurement of pain in older adults. *Clinics in Geriatric Medicine, 17*(3), 457–478.

Herr, K. A., Mobily, P. R., Kohout, F. J., & Wagenaar, D. (1998). Evaluation of the faces pain scale for use with the elderly. *Clinical Journal of Pain, 14,* 29–38.

Hurley, A. C., Volicer, B. J., Hanrahan, P. A., Houde, S., & Volicer, L. (1992). Assessment of discomfort in advanced Alzheimer's patients. *Research in Nursing and Health, 15,* 369–377.

Iezzi, T., Archibald, Y., Barnett, P., Klinck, A., & Duckworth, M. (1999). Neurocognitive performance and emotional status in chronic pain patients. *Journal of Behavioral Medicine, 22*(3), 205–216.

Jamison, R. N., Schein, J. R., Vallow, S., Ascher, S., Vorsanger, G. J., & Katz, N. P. (2003). Neuropsychological effects of long-term opioid use in chronic pain patients. *Journal of Pain Symptom Management, 26*(4), 913–921.

Jensen, M. P., Turner, L. R., Turner, J. A., & Romano, J. M. (1996). The use of multiple-item scales for pain intensity measurement in chronic pain patients. *Pain*, *67*(1), 35–40.

Kamel, H. K., Phlavan, M., Malekgoudarzi, B., Gogel, P., & Morley, J. E. (2001). Utilizing pain assessment scales increases the frequency of diagnosing pain among elderly nursing home residents. *Journal of Pain and Symptom Management*, *21*(6), 450–455.

Kaszniak, A. W., & Christenson, G. D. (1994). Differential diagnosis of dementia and depression. In M. Storandt & G. R. Vandenbos (Eds.), *Neuropsychological assessment of dementia and depression in older adults: A clinician's guide* (pp. 81–118). Washington, DC: American Psychological Association.

Keefe, F., & Williams, D. A. (1990). A comparison of coping strategies in chronic pain patients in different age groups. *Journals of Gerontology: Psychological Sciences*, *45*, 161–165.

Khana, B., Khana, E., Namazi, K., Kercher, K., & Stange, K. (1997). The role of pain in the cascade from chronic illness to social disability and psychological distress in late life. In D. I. Mostofsky & J. Lomranz (Eds.), *Handbook of pain and aging* (pp. 185–206). New York: Plenum Press.

Kovach, C. R., Noonan, P. E., Griffie, J., Muchka, S., & Weissman, D. E. (2002). The assessment of discomfort in dementia protocol. *Pain Management Nursing*, *3*(1), 16–27.

Krulewitch, H., London, M. R., Skakel, V. J., Lundstedt, G. J., Thomason, H., & Brummel-Smith, K. (2000). Assessment of pain in cognitively impaired older adults: A comparison of pain assessment tools and their use by nonprofessional caregivers. *Journal of the American Geriatrics Society*, *48*(12), 1607–1611.

Lake, A., Branca, B., Lutz, T. E., & Saper, J. R. (1999). Headache level during neuro-psychological testing and test performance in patients with chronic posttraumatic headache. *Journal of Head Trauma Rehabilitation*, *14*(1), 70–80.

Lorenz, J., Beck, H., & Bromm, B. (1997). Cognitive performance, mood and experimental pain before and during morphine-induced analgesia in patients with chronic non-malignant pain. *Pain*, *73*(3), 369–375.

Magni, G., Marchetti, M., Moreschi, C., Merskey, H., & Luchini, S. R. (1993). Chronic musculoskeletal pain and depressive symptoms in the National Health and Nutrition Examination I. Epidemiologic follow-up study. *Pain*, *53*, 163–168.

Manfredi, P. L., Breuer, B., Meier, D. E., & Libow, L. (2003). Pain assessment in elderly patients with severe dementia. *Journal of Pain Symptoms and Management*, *25*(1), 48–52.

Manfredi, P. L., Breuer, B., Wallenstein, S., Stegmann, M., Bottomley, G., & Libow, L. (2003). Opioid treatment for agitation in patients with advanced dementia. *International Journal of Geriatric Psychiatry*, *18*(8), 700–705.

Melzack, R. (1975). The McGill Pain Questionnaire: Major properties and scoring methods. *Pain*, *1*, 277–299.

Melzack, R. (1987). The short-form McGill Pain Questionnaire. *Pain*, *30*, 191–197.

Melzack, R., & Casey, K. L. (1968). Sensory, motivational and central control determinants of pain: A new conceptual model. In D. R. Kenshalo (Ed.), *The skin senses* (pp. 423–443). Springfield, IL: Thomas.

Meyer, J. S., Thornby, J., Crawford, K., & Rauch, G. M. (2000). Reversible cognitive decline accompanies migraine and cluster headaches. *Headache*, *40*, 638–646.

Oberle, K., Paul, P., Wry, J., & Grace, M. (1990). Pain, anxiety and analgesics: A comparative study of elderly and younger surgical patients. *Canadian Journal on Aging*, *9*, 13–22.

Parmelee, P. (1996). Pain in cognitively impaired older persons. *Pain Management, 12*, 473–487.

Parmelee, P. A., Katz, I. R., & Lawton, M. P. (1991). The relation of pain to depression among institutionalized aged. *Journals of Gerontology: Psychological Sciences, 46*, 15–21.

Pasero, C., & McCaffrey, M. (1996). Postoperative pain management in the elderly. In B. R. Ferrell & B. A. Ferrell (Eds.), *Pain in the elderly* (pp. 45–68). Seattle, WA: International Association for the Study of Pain.

Pincus, T., Fraser, L., & Pearce, S. (1998). Do chronic pain patients "Stroop" on pain stimuli? *British Journal of Clinical Psychology, 37*, 49–58.

Podichetty, V. K., Mazanec, D. J., & Biscup, R. S. (2003). Chronic non-malignant musculoskeletal pain in older adults: Clinical issues and opioid intervention. *Postgraduate Medical Journal, 79*, 627–633.

Polister, P., & Schneidman, D. (1990). *American College of Surgeons: Socioeconomic factbook for surgery 1990*. Chicago: American College of Surgeons.

Rainero, I., Vighetti, S., Bergamasco, B., Pinessi, L., & Benedetti, F. (2000). Autonomic responses and pain perception in Alzheimer's disease. *European Journal of Pain, 4*(3), 267–274.

Raja, S. N., Haythornthwaite, J. A., Pappagallo, M., Clark, M. R., Travison, T. G., Sabeen, S., et al. (2002). Opioids versus antidepressants in postherapeutic neuralgia: A randomized, placebo-controlled trial. *Neurology, 59*, 1015–1021.

Reid, M. C., Williams, C. S., Concato, J., Tinetti, M. E., & Gill, T. M. (2003). Depressive symptoms as a risk factor for disabling back pain in community-dwelling older persons. *Journal of the American Geriatrics Society, 51*, 1710–1717.

Riley, J. L., Wade, J. B., Robinson, M. E., & Price, D. D. (2000). The stages of pain processing across the adult lifespan. *Journal of Pain, 1*, 162–170.

Scherder, E., Bouma, A., Slaets, J., Ooms, M., Ribbe, M., Blok, A., & Sergeant, J. (2001). Repeated pain assessment in Alzheimer's disease. *Dementia and Geriatric Cognitive Disorders, 12*(6), 400–407.

Scherder, E. J., Sergeant, J. A., & Swaab, D. F. (2003). Pain processing in dementia and its relation to neuropathology. *Lancet: Neurology, 2*(11), 677–686.

Scudds, R. J., & Robertson, J. M. (1998). Empirical evidence of the association between the presence of musculoskeletal pain and physical disability in community-dwelling senior citizens. *Pain, 75*, 229–235.

Scudds, R. J., & Robertson, J. M. (2000). Pain factors associated with physical disability in a sample of community-dwelling senior citizens. *Journals of Gerontology: Medical Sciences, 55*, 393–399.

Sengstaken, E., & King, S. A. (1993). The problem of pain and its detection among geriatric nursing home residents. *Journal of the American Geriatrics Society, 41*, 541–544.

Tassain, V., Attal, N., Fletcher, D., Brasseur, L., Degieux, P., Chauvin, M., & Bouhassira, D. (2003). Long term effects of oral sustained release morphine on neuropsychological performance in patients with chronic non-cancer pain. *Pain, 104*, 389–400.

Tsushima, W. T., & Newbill, B. A. (1996). Effects of headaches during neuropsychological testing of mid head injury patients. *Headache, 36*, 613–615.

Wang, S.-J., Liu, H.-C., Fuh, C.-Y., Wang, P.-N., & Lu, S.-R. (1999). Comorbidity of headaches and depression in the elderly. *Pain, 82*, 239–243.

Warden, V., Hurley, A. C., & Volicer, L. (2003). Development and psychometric evaluation of the pain assessment in advanced dementia (PAINAD) scale. *Journal of the American Medical Directors Association, 4*(1), 9–15.

Williamson, G. M., & Schulz, R. (1992). Pain, activity restriction, and symptoms of depression among community-residing elderly adults. *Journals of Gerontology: Psychological Sciences, 47,* 367–372.

Yesavage, J. A., Brink, T. L., Rose, T. L., Lum, O., Huang, V., Adey, M., & Leirer, V. O. (1983). Development and validation of a geriatric depression screening scale: A preliminary report. *Journal of Psychiatric Research, 17,* 37–49.

Yonan, C. A., & Wegener, S. T. (2003). Assessment and management of pain in the older adult. *Rehabilitation Psychology, 28*(1), 4–13.

15 Geriatric psychopharmacology

Efrain A. Gonzalez, Margaret M. Mustelier, and Jose A. Rey

Advancing age is associated with increased use of medication, with adults age 65 years and older consuming 30% of all prescription drugs and 40% of all non-prescription drugs (Dharmarajan & Ugalino, 2001). On average, older adults use three or more medications at any given time, with this polypharmacy associated with an increased incidence of adverse drug reactions (ADR). Other factors contributing to the increased incidence of ADR among older adults include age-related changes in pharmacokinetics and pharmacodynamics and a lack of dosing guidelines for elderly populations. Despite the increased use of medication and incidence of ADR among older adults, geriatric psychopharmacology has historically been a neglected area of medicine and research (Naranjo, Herrmann, Mittmann, & Bremner, 1995). This chapter reviews (a) the pharmacodynamics and pharmacokinetics of pharmacological treatment, (b) the pharmacological treatment of common geriatric disorders, (c) the side effects and neuropsychological consequences of compounds frequently used to treat the elderly, (d) the use of dietary supplements, and (e) polypharmacy considerations.

Pharmacodynamics and pharmacokinetics

Pharmacodynamics

Pharmacodynamics is the study of the biochemical and physiologic effects of a drug. Stated simply, it is "what the drug does to the body." When a medication is used for the treatment, cure, prevention, or management of a disease state, it is the pharmacological mechanisms of action that the medication is utilizing that produce its beneficial and harmful effects. The pharmacodynamics of a drug encompasses its mechanisms of action, adverse effects, and other physiological changes that are brought about due to a drug's presence at both its intended and unintended sites of action. As the body ages, physiological changes that alter the response to medication may occur. For instance, with older adults, changes in neurotransmitter production (usually decreased) and certain neurotransmitter receptor sensitivities (increased or decreased) may lead to a level of unpredictability in medication effects, and increase the risk of ADR (Hardman & Limbird, 1996).

Pharmacokinetics

Pharmacokinetics involves the absorption, distribution, metabolism, and excretion of a drug. Stated simply, it is "what the body does to the drug." Age-related changes that can decrease the rate of absorption of a drug include the following: decreased swallowing, increased gastric pH (decrease in acid production), decreased gastric emptying, decreased intestinal motility, and decreased mesenteric blood flow. The absorption of a drug can also be influenced by certain medications, such as anticholinergics, antacids, and other agents affecting gastric pH. Distribution of a drug may be compromised in older adults as a result of reduced plasma protein binding (in response to a decrease in plasma albumin concentrations), decreased cardiac output, and anatomical changes (especially an increase in the percentage of body weight that is fat, and a decrease in lean muscle mass). Decreased liver blood flow, drug interactions, disease states common in the elderly (e.g., congestive heart failure), and drug-induced metabolic changes may affect the metabolism of a drug. Lastly, age-related decline in renal function can compromise the excretion of a drug and contribute to the increased half-life of drugs in the elderly.

Pharmacological treatment of common geriatric disorders

Alzheimer's disease

Overview

Alzheimer's disease (AD) is the leading cause of dementia in the United States, with advancing age associated with an increased incidence of this disorder (Evans et al., 1989). The pathophysiology of AD consists of the accumulation of amyloid plaques and neurofibrillary tangles, which lead to neuronal cell death (Zec, 1993). Additionally, there is a decrease in the production of acetylcholine, likely due to a reduction in the activity of choline acetyltransferase. The reader is referred to Chapter 8 in this volume for a thorough review of the neuropathology of AD.

Pharmacological treatment

The pharmacological interventions utilized to treat AD have shown limited, but measurable, efficacy in treating the cognitive and behavioral symptoms associated with this disorder. Currently, there are no marketed medications that have been shown to stop the decline or reverse the effects of AD. While a small percentage of patients may demonstrate improvements in cognitive functioning following pharmacological intervention, a positive treatment outcome is noted if a patient's mental status does not deteriorate for at least 6 months. Acetylcholinesterase inhibitors are indicated for the treatment of mild to moderate AD, and one glutamate antagonist is currently indicated for patients in the moderate to severe stages of the disease. Table 15.1 presents the current medications used to treat AD, the proposed mechanism of action, starting and target doses, and general comments specific to each medication (Cummings, Frank, & Cherry, 2002).

Adverse effects of pharmacologic treatment

Common adverse effects that occur in patients taking acetylcholinesterase inhibitors include gastrointestinal (GI) distress (e.g., nausea, vomiting, and diarrhea) and anorexia. In placebo-controlled trials used for approval of the acetylcholinesterase inhibitors in the United States, rivastigmine (Exelon) demonstrated a higher incidence of GI distress than donepezil (Aricept) or galantamine (Reminyl). Slow titration and consumption of these medications with food minimizes the risk for GI disturbance. Other adverse effects associated with this class of medications include: fatigue, muscle cramps, insomnia, dizziness, sleep disturbances, syncope, bradycardia, and tremors.

Depression

Overview

Clinical depression among elderly persons is a major health problem that is commonly underdiagnosed and undertreated (Salzman, 1992). Additionally, a significant number of older adults fall into a "subsyndromal" category, whereby they exhibit symptoms of depression without meeting the full criteria for the disorder. Suicide rates are considered to be the highest in late life, with men aged 85 years and older having six times the rate of suicide of the general population (Lavretsky, Kim, Kumar, & Reynolds, 2003; Salzman, 1992). Interestingly, the majority of older adults who commit suicide have seen their primary care physician in the weeks preceding the event (Navarro, Gasto, Torres, Marcos, & Pintor, 2001). Chronicity and vulnerability to relapse appear to characterize depressive syndromes among elderly persons. For instance, treatment of the elderly often does not result in complete remission of depression, with many patients experiencing a recurrence of symptoms within 2 years of treatment (Zis, Grof, & Webster, 1980). The reader is referred to Chapter 12 in this volume for a thorough review of psychiatric disorders common to elderly persons.

Pathophysiology

Neurobiological research indicates that depressive disorders result from the interaction between the Biogenic Amine Hypothesis and increased receptor sensitivity; that is, the depletion of serotonin and/or norepinephrine results in the upregulation of postsynaptic receptors. Low levels of these neurotransmitters in the brain appear to cause an increase in the number and sensitivity

Table 15.1 Medications used to treat Alzheimer's disease

Generic medication	Brand name	Proposed mechanisms of action	Starting doses	Target doses	Comments
Tacrine	Cognex	Acetylcholinesterase and butarylcholinesterase inhibition	10 mg po QID	40 mg po QID	Monitor liver function due to high incidence of hepatotoxicity; rarely used due to ADRs
Donepezil	Aricept	Acetylcholinesterase inhibition	5 mg po QD	10 mg po QD	Sleep disturbances and usual class ADRs
Rivastigmine	Exelon	Acetylcholinesterase and butarylcholinesterase inhibition	1.5 mg po BID	3–6 mg po BID	Slow titration necessary to minimize GI disturbances. Usual class ADRs
Galantamine	Reminyl	Acetylcholinesterase inhibition and nicotinic receptor modulation	4 mg po BID	8–12 mg po BID	Decrease dose in patients with hepatic and renal impairment. Usual class ADRs
Memantine	Namenda	Glutamate antagonist	5 mg po QD	10 mg po BID	Well tolerated. Best results when combined with acetylcholinesterase inhibitors. ADRs: dizziness, agitation, confusion, headache, constipation

of postsynaptic receptors, a process that may take up to several weeks due to DNA involvement in the synthesis of new proteins. This phenomenon is thought to be one of the primary factors in the biological development of depressive illness, and possibly the primary reason that it takes several weeks for most antidepressants to have an effect on ameliorating depressive symptomatology. Therefore, the majority of these classes of medications involve the "downregulation" (decrease in the amount and sensitivity) of these receptors by initially elevating the amount of available neurotransmitter in the brain.

Pharmacologic treatment

Antidepressant medications increase the concentration of selected neurotransmitters in a variety of ways. For example, the mechanism of action of monoamine oxidase inhibitors (MAOIs) occurs by the irreversible binding of these compounds to the monoamine oxidase enzyme, which is the enzyme responsible for deactivating catecholamine neurotransmitters such as dopamine, norepinephrine, and serotonin in the central and autonomic nervous system. By binding to the monoamine oxidase enzyme, the metabolism of catecholamines decreases, allowing for more available neurotransmitter in the presynaptic cell and, consequently, for synaptic transmission. Given that tyramine is structurally related to norepinephrine and has a similar effect on blood pressure, caution should be taken to avoid tyramine-containing foods due to the possibility of a hypertensive crisis, particularly with older adults who may have difficulty understanding or adhering to a strict tyramine-free diet.

The mechanism of action of tricyclic antidepressants (TCAs) involves the augmentation of serotonin and norepinephrine neurotransmitters by the blockade of their respective reuptake transporter proteins. Unfortunately, many of these medications are considered to be "dirty" drugs due to their effect on other receptors that have the potential to produce a number of untoward side effects. For example, TCAs block, or are antagonist of, alpha 1 receptors. The stimulation of alpha 1 produces vasoconstriction, whereas the antagonism produces vasodilation. Consequently, this blockade may result in dizziness and orthostasis. With elderly patients, these side effects can lead to falls and other serious medical consequences requiring hospitalization and surgery. TCAs also block histamine 1 receptors both peripherally and centrally. The histaminergic pathways in the hypothalamus play a primary role in wakefulness and alertness. Therefore, central blockade of histamine may result in sedation, and possibly confusion and disorientation. Weight gain, another potential side effect of histamine blockade, is poorly understood, although some literature suggests an association between decreased metabolic rate and histamine 2 receptors (Sacchetti, Guarneri, & Bravi, 2000). TCAs, by blocking the parasympathetic muscarinic receptor of the autonomic nervous system, also have anticholinergic side effects. In addition, TCAs can also have cardiotoxic effects, and elderly patients with a history of cardiac problems should be carefully screened prior to the utilization of such medications.

Selective serotonin reuptake inhibitors (SSRIs) block the reuptake of serotonin by binding to specific neurotransmitter transporter proteins, whose normal function is to bind with the neurotransmitter and carry it back to the presynaptic neuron. This process, which is similar to the reuptake inhibition of TCAs, results in decreased sensitivity and downregulation of serotonin receptors, resulting in an antidepressant effect.

SSRIs are preferred over TCAs and MAOIs because they have fewer, and less severe, side effects, while still demonstrating efficacy with older adults. For example, studies of SSRIs, such as sertraline (Zoloft) and paroxetine (Paxil), have yielded results of 60–80% efficacy among geriatric patients (Naranjo et al., 1995). In addition, SSRIs are not believed to cause or exacerbate cognitive impairment in the elderly. The most commonly reported adverse effects with SSRIs are gastrointestinal symptoms, such as nausea, although insomnia and sexual dysfunction are noted frequently as well. Weight loss during the initial stages of treatment has also been reported, and this possibility should be considered when treating patients who are malnourished (Naranjo et al., 1995).

The abrupt increase of serotonin on certain serotonergic pathways and receptors may explain some of the adverse effects of this class of medications. For example, SSRIs may cause or exacerbate anxiety due to sudden serotonergic increase in the raphe/limbic pathway. In these cases, initial dosing with SSRIs should start low, with gradual titration depending on response. Naranjo et al. (1995) also recommended the use of one-half or one-quarter dose with the elderly, especially those individuals who are frail or medically ill. The stimulation of the 5-HT3/4 receptors in the brainstem and gastrointestinal tract are thought to be responsible for the gastrointestinal side effects associated with this medication. Extrapyramidal side effects, such as akathesia and bradycardia, have also been reported due to basal ganglia involvement (Georgotas, McCue, & Hapworth, 1986).

SSRIs in general, and fluoxetine (Prozac) in particular, can also result in the inappropriate secretion of vasopressin from neurohypophysis, which is known as the syndrome of inappropriate antidiuretic hormone secretion (SIADH). Therefore, sodium levels should be monitored when administering fluoxetine to elderly patients (Flint, 1994). Moreover, hyponatremia associated with SSRIs and the SNRI (serotonin-norepinephrine reuptake inhibitor) venlafaxine (Effexor) was also found in a study controlling for age, sex, depression status, and illnesses or prescribed medications (Kirby, Harrigan, & Ames, 2002). The mechanisms involved differed in the development of hyponatremia in that thiazide diuretics induced hyponatremia by impairment of urinary dilution, renal loss of sodium and potassium, and stimulation of antidiuretic hormone. SSRIs, on the other hand, caused hyponatremia through inappropriate ADH release. Controlling for thiazide status did not reduce the odds of these patients having hyponatremia. Kirby and colleagues cautioned that elderly patients on SSRIs or venlafaxine should have sodium levels checked before and after commencement of antidepressant treatment regardless of thiazide involvement. Rosner (2004) stated that because thiazide diuretics and SSRIs are among the most commonly prescribed medications for the elderly, there is a strong possibility of a synergistic effect in impairment of renal free water clearance when both medications are given.

Of all the SSRIs, fluoxetine (Prozac) has the longest half life, which is 3 days for the parent compound, and approximately 7–15 days for its active metabolite, norfluoxetine. Therefore, the washout period for fluoxetine is 5 weeks, as compared to 2 weeks with other SSRIs. SSRIs should not be coadministered with MAOIs due to the possibility of the development of serotonin syndrome, a potentially fatal hyperserotonergic state characterized by anxiety, restlessness, confusion, chills, incoordination, and insomnia (Naranjo et al., 1995). Similarly, a careful history of over-the-counter preparations (OTCs) should be taken, as some of these compounds, such as St. John's wort, are also known to increase serotonergic levels and possibly augment the effects of SSRIs and antidepressants in other classes that also elevate the level of serotonin.

Most SSRIs inhibit the hepatic isoenzyme CYP-450-2D6, increasing the blood concentration of any coadministered drugs that are also metabolized by this enzyme. Paroxetine (Paxil) and fluoxetine (Prozac) appear to be much more potent inhibitors, and toxicity may occur when these drugs are administered with certain medications, such as metoprolol, quinidine, some antipsychotics (haloperidol, thioridazine), and some TCAs (desipramine, amitriptyline) (Naranjo et al., 1995).

Citalopram (Celexa) is reported to be more selective than other SSRIs, as this drug has minimal effect on other receptors such as dopamine and norepinephrine. Given its higher selectivity, citalopram is believed to have fewer side effects, and a better drug interaction profile, which are important considerations due to the high number of medications that many elderly persons are prescribed. When compared to nortriptyline (Pamelor) in a randomized 12-week flexible dose treatment of moderate to severe depression, the remission rate to a therapeutic plasma level of nortriptyline was higher than the remission rate to a standard dose of citalopram, especially for individuals with endogenous or psychotic features. However, citalopram appears to be better tolerated (Gasto et al., 2003).

Sertraline (Zoloft) has also proven to be relatively safe and efficacious and has well-established antidepressant and anxiolytic activity. According to Muijsers, Plosker, and Noble (2002), sertraline is generally well tolerated in elderly patients with major depressive disorder, and it has a low potential for drug interactions.

Pooled data from two double-blind studies was used to compare the cognitive performance of older adults with major depression treated with sertraline, fluoxetine (Prozac), or nortriptyline (Pamelor) (Doraiswamy et al., 2003). A cognitive battery was administered pretreatment and posttreatment. Tests included the Shopping List Task (SLT), which measures short-term memory and long-term storage and retrieval, and the Digit Symbol Substitution Test (DSST), which measures visual tracking, motor performance, and coding ability. Results revealed that older age, male gender, higher systolic blood pressure, and higher illness severity were associated with lower performance on specific cognitive measures at baseline. For the entire group, improved depression, and a lower anticholinergic side effect severity were associated with statistically significant improvement on the SLT and DSST. The correlations between improvements in depression and cognitive function were highest for sertraline, followed by nortiptyline and then fluoxetine.

Venlafaxine (Effexor) blocks both serotonin and norepinephrine reuptake and has some anticholinergic effects. The most common adverse effects associated with this drug include nausea, somnolence, insomnia, dry mouth, dizziness, anxiety, and constipation, and a possible sustained increase in blood pressure. While some authors have concluded that venlafaxine is a relatively safe and efficacious medication for the elderly (Gasto et al., 2003; Staab & Evans, 2000), Oslin et al. (2003) concluded that venlafaxine was less well tolerated and, possibly, less safe than sertraline, without evidence of an increase in efficacy among frail elderly patients.

Buproprion (Wellbutrin), a unicyclic aminoketone, is believed to exert its effects through noradrenergic systems, and may have weak dopaminergic activity (Steffens, Doraiswamy, & McQuoid, 2001). Due to this probable mechanism of action, clinicians commonly prescribe bupropion as a single agent, or in combination with SSRIs to augment response (Nelson, Kennedy, & Pollock, 1999). According to Navarro et al. (2001), bupropion is well tolerated by the elderly because of its lack of anticholinergic side effects, orthostasis, and sedation. These authors also state that it may be prescribed in divided doses to reduce adverse effects, of which insomnia and headache are most common. Both the immediate release and sustained release versions of this drug are frequently used to treat geriatric depression, primarily due to the favorable side-effect profile. The major concern of this medication is that it can cause seizures in persons who are bulimic, have had head trauma, or have a personal or family history of seizures.

Mirtazepine (Remeron) has a tetracyclic chemical structure unrelated to SSRIs, TCAs, or MAOIs. A piperazino-azepine compound, it is thought to have therapeutic action mainly mediated through its alpha 2 presynaptic autoreceptor antagonism. The primary mechanism of action is the antagonism of alpha 2 receptors, thus disinhibiting both serotonin and norepinephrine release (Stahl, 2000). In addition to the antagonism of adrenergic alpha 2 autoreceptors and alpha 2 heteroreceptors, it is also antagonistic for 5-HT-2A and 5-HT-3 receptors. The release of norepinephrine and 5-HT-2 mediated serotonergic activity may explain the rapid onset of action of this compound. Due to histaminergic blockade, dry mouth, sedation, and increased appetite and body weight are common side effects. Mirtazapine has well-established efficacy, and appears to be useful in patients suffering from depression with concomitant anxiety and sleep disturbance (Anttila & Leinonen, 2001). A study by Florkowski, Gruszczynski, and Zboralski (2002) revealed improvement in mood, sleep, and anxiety among 75% of the sample treated with this medication. When compared with paroxetine (Paxil), there was comparable efficacy, although patients taking paroxetine were more likely to discontinue therapy in the acute phase of treatment because of adverse effects (Schatzberg, Kremer, Rodrigues, & Murphy, 2002). The authors concluded that mirtazapine has an earlier onset of action and a better tolerability profile, and is a valuable option for the treatment of depression in elderly patients. In a study using mirtazapine for difficult-to-treat patients who were resistant to SSRIs, Hirschfeld (2002) found that mirtazapine had a more rapid onset of action than sertraline and that mirtazapine was more effective and had a faster onset of action than paroxetine. However, a case report of serotonin syndrome in a 75-year-old man led the authors to conclude that even though mirtazapine has strong efficacy and good safety, elderly patients with underlying chronic conditions should be started at lower doses (Hernandez, Ramos, Infante, Rebollo, & Gonzalez-Macias, 2002).

Nefazodone (Serzone) selectively inhibits serotonin reuptake and is a potent serotonin 5-HT2 receptor antagonist. Nefazodone has beneficial effects on sleep and sleep architecture. Dry mouth, blurred vision, constipation, weakness, and nausea are the most common adverse effects (Navarro et al., 2001). Caution is indicated with this medication due to the potential for hepatic toxicity. Due to the risk of liver problems, this agent may be removed from the US market.

Trazodone (Desyrel) is an antidepressant with 5-HT-2 antagonism and weak serotonin reuptake inhibition as its proposed mechanisms of action. While this drug has no anticholinergic side effects, it has the potential to cause orthostasis due to alpha 1 antagonism. Trazodone has a very short half-life (3–9 hours) and has strong sedating effects, which may limit its use at higher doses. However, subtherapeutic doses of this medication are frequently utilized to facilitate sleep and sedation. Trazodone has also been used to treat agitation associated with dementia and may be used in conjunction with an antidepressant that has stimulating effects (Navarro et al., 2001).

An accelerated antidepressant response may be particularly beneficial for older patients. Naranjo et al. (1995) reported that methylphenidate (Ritalin) may be used to accelerate the antidepressant response to citalopram (Celexa). These authors further stated that psychostimulants have been shown to be effective in treating elderly, depressed, medically ill, demented, withdrawn, and apathetic patients (Naranjo et al., 1995). They added that the administration of Ritalin led to notable improvement in mood within days, compared to weeks with antidepressants alone. However, long-term research is still limited, and the chronic or frequent use of psychostimulants for depression, either as monotherapy or as adjunctive treatment, should be done with caution and regular follow-up.

Because depression in old age often follows a relapsing and chronic course, it has been recommended that treatment focus on minimization of relapse, recurrence, and residual symptoms to reduce the likelihood of chronicity (Cole & Dendukuri, 2003). The current recommended first-line antidepressant medications are the SSRIs. TCAs, MAOIs, and the atypical, non-SSRI antidepressants all appear to have prophylactic efficacy in geriatric depression and are considered second-line treatment in the elderly. The National Institutes of Health (NIH) consensus panel on the diagnosis and treatment of depression in later life recommends that geriatric patients with depression be continued on antidepressant medication for at least 6 months for the first episode, with treatment maintained for at least 1 year for recurrent episodes (NIH, 2004).

Anxiety disorders

Overview

Anxiety is a normal adaptive response to anticipated noxious events; however, it is considered pathologic when it becomes excessive and maladaptive (Sheikh, 2003). Anxiety is the most commonly observed psychiatric disorder for adults, with a prevalence rate twice as great for anxiety as depression (Flint, 1994). There are three common presentations of anxiety in older adults seen in health care settings: (a) anxiety associated with illness or medications, (b) mixed anxiety and depression, and (c) anxiety associated with dementia (Sheikh, 2003). Pharmacologic treatment options for these three presentations follow.

Pharmacologic treatment

Anxiety-related cognitive, behavioral, and physical symptoms associated with medical illness or medications are among the most common manifestations of anxiety in older adults (Sheikh, 2003). Prior to beginning psychopharmacologic treatment, attempts should be made to identify and treat the underlying cause. Often, a long-standing history of an anxiety disorder is detected. In such cases, SSRIs or SNRIs are the first-line treatment, with concurrent short-term use of benzodiazepines for immediate relief of severe symptoms until the therapeutic effects of the SSRI or SNRI are observed (Sheikh & Cassidy, 2000). Similarly, when anxiety emerges in response to initiation of an antidepressant, the symptoms tend to be transient, resolving spontaneously within 2–3 weeks. In the interim, sedating medications can be given at bedtime to facilitate sleep.

Mixed anxiety and depression is also common among older adults (Copeland, Davidson, & Dewey, 1987). Due to overlapping symptoms and the frequent co-occurrence of both disorders, attempts to distinguish between them may prove difficult. Because the same classes of medications (SSRIs and SNRIs) are used to treat both disorders, attempts to distinguish between them may be academic (Doraiswamy, 2001; Sheikh, 2003). To provide short-term management of anxiety during the 2–4 weeks that these medications may require to demonstrate therapeutic effect, judicious augmentation with a short half-life benzodiazepine may be indicated (Sheikh & Cassidy, 2000).

Symptoms of anxiety (e.g., subjective apprehension) and agitation (e.g., motor restlessness) are frequently observed, individually or together, in older adults with dementia. While anxiety is more commonly experienced by those with mild-to-moderate dementia, agitation is more frequently evidenced by those with moderate-to-severe dementia. Initial interventions should include attempts to identify triggers, such as environmental stimuli, medication side effects, and communication difficulties (Sheikh, 2003). Traditionally, high potency neuroleptics (e.g., haloperidol and fluphenazine) were used, with some benefit. However, due to their potential for adverse reactions, their use seems to be increasingly limited to acute situations. Newer, atypical antipsychotics (e.g., risperidone and quetiapine), with their lower incidence of adverse effects, are now considered treatments of choice (Sheikh & Cassidy, 2000). Short-term use of benzodiazepines and use of newer anticonvulsants (e.g., gabapentin and lamotrigine) may also play a role in the treatment of anxiety and agitation in individuals with dementia (Sheikh, 2003).

Psychotic disorders

Overview

The incidence of psychotic disorders ranges from 0.2% to 4.7% in community-based elderly populations to as high as 63% for elderly persons living in nursing homes (Hoeh, Gyulai, Weintraub, & Streim, 2003). Psychotic disorders affecting the elderly include delirium; dementia with psychotic features; schizophrenia; brief reactive psychosis; schizophreniform disorder; schizoaffective disorder; delusional disorder; mania; and secondary psychotic states, including alcohol/drug intoxication or withdrawal, hyperthyroidism, cerebrovascular disease, and Parkinson's disease. Antipsychotic medications are indicated for management of psychotic symptoms including delusions, hallucinations, thought disorders, and impaired reality testing.

Pharmacologic treatment

Dopaminergic antagonism, through its apparent action in mesolimbic pathways, reduces the positive symptoms of psychosis. Prior to beginning treatment with antipsychotic medications (see Table 15.2), it is recommended that elderly patients have a white blood cell (WBC) count, liver function panel, and an electrocardiogram (Salzman, 1998). Patients being considered for treatment with clozapine (Clozaril) or olanzapine (Zyprexa) should also have baseline levels of fasting blood sugar and serum triglyceride (Gaulin, Markowitz, & Caley, 1999; Osser, Najarian, & Dufresne, 1999). The general rule of "start low and go slow" is imperative for this population. Antipsychotic therapy should be initiated at the lowest recommended dose,

Table 15.2 Typical and atypical antipsychotic medications

Generic name	Brand name
Typical antipsychotics:	
Chlorpromazine	Thorazine
Fluphenazine	Prolixin
Haloperidol	Haldol
Loxapine	Loxitane
Mesoridazine	Serentil
Molindone	Moban
Perphenazine	Trilafon
Pimozide	Orap
Thioridazine	Mellaril
Thiothixene	Navane
Trifluoperazine	Stelazine
Atypical antipsychotics:	
Aripiprazole	Abilify
Clozapine	Clozaril
Olanzapine	Zyprexa
Quetiapine	Seroquel
Risperidone	Risperdal
Ziprasidone	Geodon

and dose titration should include regular monitoring of vital signs, including temperature, orthostatic blood pressure, pulse, weight, and assessment for abnormal movements. Daily dosing of antipsychotic medications in the elderly should not exceed twice the "relative potency" value. "Treatment resistance" is observed more often in the elderly population and is often resolved by switching from typical to atypical neuroleptic agents. When antipsychotic medications are prescribed, interactions with other medications must be considered.

Maintenance treatment of schizophrenia involves regular reassessment in order to determine the lowest effective dose. Excessive motor behaviors can be treated with a benzodiazepine; however, benzodiazepine use should be minimized and carefully monitored in the geriatric population due to the potential for cognitive impairment and physical dependence with these agents. Long-term treatment ideally involves utilizing an atypical antipsychotic for its less severe side-effect profile. Delusional disorder is treated similarly to schizophrenia, except in lower doses due to a lower incidence of acute agitation; atypical antipsychotics are often recommended. Treatment of schizoaffective disorder is also similar to treatment of schizophrenia, combined with a mood stabilizer or antidepressant.

Risperidone (Risperdal) and olanzipine (Zyprexa) are reported to improve cognitive function in elderly patients with schizoaffective disorder and schizophrenia (Harvey, Napolitano, Mao, & Gharabawi, 2003). These atypical agents are also associated with improvements in core symptoms of schizophrenia and are associated with overall improvements in motor side effects (Ritchie et al., 2003). Olanzipine is also associated with improvements in psychological well-being (Ritchie et al., 2003). Both risperidone (for positive and negative symptoms) and olanzapine (for negative symptoms) have proven themselves superior to haloperidol in the treatment of psychotic symptoms in the adult population (Kennedy et al. 2003; Madhusoodanan, Sidhartha, Brenner, Gupta, & Bogunovic, 2001).

Treatment of delirium and other secondary psychotic syndromes should focus on addressing the underlying cause of the disorder, with adjunctive treatment of symptoms as necessary. Most forms of dementia are associated with psychotic symptoms. The most important consideration is accurate diagnosis of the cause of dementia to minimize potentially dangerous side effects from the chosen drug.

Psychotic symptoms associated with depression are best treated with olanzapine (Zyprexa) or risperidone (Risperdal) in conjunction with an antidepressant. Mania is covered later in this chapter, but treatment usually involves an antipsychotic in combination with a mood stabilizer and possibly a benzodiazepine.

Parkinson's disease may produce psychosis as part of the degenerative process, but medications used for treatment can also induce psychotic symptoms. Low dose atypical antipsychotics are recommended due to a decreased risk of interaction with the prodopaminergic effects of drugs commonly used to treat Parkinson's disease. Clozapine (Clozaril) has proven effective in the treatment of psychosis associated with Parkinson's disease (Friedman, Max, & Swift, 1987; Ostergaard & Dupont, 1988; Pfeiffer, Kang, & Graber, 1990). The main concerns associated with this medication, however, are: the frequent monitoring for agranulocytosis, a potentially fatal condition; a higher risk for seizures; the risk for orthostasis; and excessive sedation. Given the potential ADRs associated with clozapine, current treatment recommendations for this patient population favor the use of quetiapine (Seroquel) over the other atypical agents, due to its proven efficacy and its low risk for movement disorders. Research suggests that Clozapine (Clozaril) holds promise for treating patients who do not respond to typical neuroleptics (Chengappa, Baker, Kreinbrook, & Adair, 1995; Friedman et al., 1987; Kane, Honingfeld, & Singer, 1988).

Adverse effects of antipsychotic medications

Antipsychotics produce a number of different side effects due to the multiple receptors on which they are antagonistic. For example, in addition to dopaminergic antagonism, antipsychotic medications also have antagonism on the muscarinic, histaminergic, and alpha 1 noradrenergic receptors. As a result, anticholinergic side effects, sedation, weight gain, and orthostasis can occur.

In the case of typical neuroleptics, dopaminergic blockade in the nigrostriatal, tuberoinfundibular, and mesocortical pathways are responsible for extrapyramidal side effects, hyperprolactinemia, and possible exacerbation of negative symptoms, respectively. Other adverse reactions include cardiovascular effects, such as orthostatic hypotension, changes in cardiac conduction, and, very rarely, venous thromboembolism. Endocrinological effects include diabetes mellitus, hyperprolactinemia, and the syndrome of inappropriate antidiuretic hormone secretion. Gastrointestinal effects include antiemetic effects and sialorrhea, dermatological reactions, urinary retention, decline in WBC count, hepatic effects, and musculoskeletal changes. Neuropsychiatric effects include cognitive impairments; extrapyramidal symptoms, such as dystonias; akathisia; parkinsonism; neuroleptic malignant syndrome; and tardive dyskinesia. Other common side effects include sedation and weight gain, and, rarely, ocular abnormalities or seizures.

The rate of titration has a strong influence on the occurrence of side effects. While there is often variability, high potency antipsychotics generally have a high risk of extrapyramidal reactions and a lower rate of seizures. Low potency antipsychotics are associated with higher risk for hypotension, sedation, peripheral autonomic and anticholinergic effects, and increased risk of seizures.

The most significant and common side effects observed in the elderly are the anticholinergic, extrapyramidal, and orthostasis effects. Typical antipsychotics with the highest risk for anticholinergic effects include chlorpromazine (Thorazine) and thioridazine (Mellaril); the atypical antipsychotic most associated with these effects is clozapine (Clozaril). Typical antipsychotics that are most associated with extrapyramidal effects include fluphenazine (Prolixin), haloperidol (Haldol), pimozide (Orap), thiothixene (Navane), and trifluoperazine (Stelazine). Atypical agents have a low risk, similar to placebo in the controlled studies, with the highest incidence associated with high dose risperidone (Risperdal), though the risk in the higher doses is still only moderate compared to the older conventional agents. Orthostasis is a substantial risk with chlorpromazine (Thorazine) and thioridazine (Mellaril) use. Conversely, most atypical antipsychotics pose greater risks for orthostasis than for the previously mentioned side effects; among antipsychotics with the highest risk of orthostasis are clozapine (Clozaril) and quetiapine (Seroquel).

Sedation is a side effect that may or may not be desirable, depending on the individual's health profile and symptoms. Most atypical antipsychotics are associated with mild to moderate sedation, with risperidone (Risperdal) posing the lowest risk. Typical antipsychotics most associated with sedation include chlorpromazine (Thorazine), mesoridazine (Serentil), and thioridazine (Mellaril).

Due to evidence of superior efficacy and a relatively better tolerability profile, atypical antipsychotics are considered to be first line agents for the treatment of schizophrenia and other psychotic disorders. Recently, however, there has been significant concern over the weight gain that can result from the use of these medications. According to Kroeze et al. (2003), weight gain is a common side effect, which has the potential for serious consequences, such as hyperlipidemia, hypertension, hyperglycemia, and diabetic ketoacidosis in the most severe of cases. There are several neurotransmitter receptors that are believed to be related to the molecular mechanisms responsible for this adverse effect; namely, 5-HT (2A), 5-HT (2C) serotonin receptors, H(1) histamine receptors, alpha (1) and alpha (2) adrenergic receptors, and M(3) muscarinic receptors (acetylcholine). Interestingly, risperidone has not shown significant antagonism on H(1) receptors, and weight gain is not a major side effect of this medication.

Bipolar disorder

Overview

The incidence of bipolar disorder remains controversial in the literature. Mellow (2003) stated that the range of bipolar disorder among the elderly is 0.1–0.4%, and that this disorder accounts for 5–12% of geriatric psychiatric hospitalizations. Mellow also reported that even though most manic episodes are experienced at younger ages, the onset of mania in the ninth and tenth decades of life have been reported. In the latter cases, there was evidence of greater medical and neurological comorbidity, episodes of longer duration or greater frequency, and at least half of the late onset patients had a depressive episode with a long latency period before the first manic episode (Mellow, 2003). Shulman and Hermann (2002) pointed out that the clinical features of mania in older people do not differ from those in young people, except for a higher prevalence of cognitive dysfunction.

Pharmacologic treatment

Lithium, valproate, and carbamazepine (Tegretol) are the preferred treatments for bipolar disorder (Bowden, Brugger, & Swann, 1994; Katona & Livingston, 2002). Lithium may be less effective for bipolar patients who are "rapid cyclers" (Naranjo et al., 1995), with anticonvulsants demonstrating greater efficacy with these patients (Elphick, 1989; McElroy, Keck, Pope, & Hudson, 1992). Valproic acid has proven to be effective for acute mania and for patients with rapid cycling and mixed affective features (McElroy et al., 1992). Additionally, valproic acid tends to be well-tolerated by geriatric individuals with bipolar disorder (McFarland, Miller, & Straumfjord, 1990; Risinger, Risby, & Risch, 1994). Mood stabilizers, including valproic acid, lithium, and carbamazepine (Tegretol), are the first-line treatment for bipolar depression. Patients who are nonresponsive to monotherapy with these agents or who have a history of rapid cycling may be candidates to receive a second mood stabilizer for combination therapy. Severely depressed patients without a history of rapid cycling may benefit from the addition of an SSRI. In the case of psychotic symptoms, adjunctive antipsychotic treatment may be used. Antidepressants and antipsychotics should be tapered and eventually discontinued after 2–6 months. The atypical antipsychotics, risperidone

(Resperdal) and olanzapine (Zyprexa), and the mood stabilizer valproic acid are considered first-line treatments for bipolar mania and bipolar mixed states.

Atypical antipsychotics also have mood stabilizing properties, with olanzapine (Zyprexa), quetiapine (Seroquel), and risperidone (Resperdal) favored because of their established efficacy and better side-effect profile than the traditional neuroleptics. Benzodiazepines may also be useful, particularly when there is a delay in reaction to the mood stabilizer. Anticonvulsants are another option; among these, valproic acid has been determined to be well-tolerated by the elderly (Sajatovic, 2002). Depakote (valproic acid + valproate), the first anticonvulsant to be approved by the FDA for the treatment of mania (Rivas-Vasquez, Johnson, Rey, Blais, & Rivas-Vasquez, 2002), is one of the first choices for the treatment for bipolar disorder. The drug's mechanism of action is thought to cause an increase of gamma-aminobutyric acid (GABA) in the brain, or it may enhance or mimic the action of GABA in postsynaptic receptor sites. In addition, it can also inhibit GABA's catabolism. Although data suggests that gabapentin has minimal drug–drug interactions and few side effects (Salzman, 2001), which may make it attractive as an augmentation agent, its efficacy in the treatment of bipolar disorder is questionable and remains unproven in controlled trials (Rivas-Vasquez et al., 2002).

Adverse effects of mood stabilizers

Lithium is associated with some drug interactions, and there are dietary considerations involving sodium. Cardiovascular side effects are the most commonly observed ADRs with lithium and carbamazepine (Tegretol). Dermatological effects have been observed in patients using lamotrigine (Lamictal) and carbamazepine; lithium and valproic acid are also associated with these. Endocrine effects, such as hypothyroidism, can occur and are most often associated with lithium. Gastrointestinal effects can occur with all of the older mood stabilizers, and it is recommended that patients take these medications with food to minimize nausea. Hematological effects, including leukopenia and thrombocytopenia, are associated primarily with carbamazepine but may occur with agents such as valproic acid and lamotrigine. Hepatic effects are associated with carbamazepine and valproic acid (Gerner & Stanton, 1992). Neuropsychiatric effects include sedation, cognitive impairment, extrapyramidal effects, and cerebellar dysfunction. The risk for drug interactions among mood stabilizers and anticonvulsants has decreased with some of the newer agents.

Pretreatment laboratory tests should include renal, thyroid, and cardiac function, CBC, electrolytes, BUN, creatine, TSH, urinalysis, and ECG. Lithium needs to be carefully monitored, including 12-hour trough serum lithium levels measured 5–7 days after beginning treatment or following any change in dosage. Drug levels should also be checked routinely when carbamazepine or valproic acid have been prescribed. The majority of patients with bipolar disorder require long-term treatment.

Drug-related cognitive impairment

The medications covered to this point are active in the central nervous system (CNS), and they have the potential to exert a variety of positive and negative effects on CNS functioning. These effects may be caused by multiple pharmacological mechanisms such as effects on histamine receptors, serotonergic activity, dopaminergic activity, adrenergic activity, opioids, gamma-amino butyric acid activity, or the cholinergic system. Some classes of medications that may cause a cognitive impairment include benzodiazepines, opiates, antihistamines, antidepressants, antipsychotics, muscle relaxants, centrally acting adrenergic agonists and antagonists, anticonvulsants, and hypnotic agents. It is not within the scope of this chapter to discuss each class of medications previously listed. Because acetylcholine is the major neurotransmitter involved in AD, medications with anticholinergic properties are reviewed.

Medications with anticholinergic properties

Acetylcholine is important for many central nervous system functions, including memory and cognition. It is also important for a variety of other physiological processes, including cardiac rhythm, gastrointestinal motility, and genitourinary and bladder control. Many medications have the ability to antagonize or block acetylcholine at its receptor sites. This pharmacological property is, at times, a desired pharmacological outcome, such as in the treatment of incontinence or Parkinson's disease. On the other hand, the anticholinergic property of a medication may result in a variety of adverse effects. Common adverse effects of medications with strong anticholinergic properties include the following: blurred vision, dry mouth, constipation, urinary retention, tachycardia, confusion, and delirium.

The anticholinergic quality of a medication has the potential to interfere with the effectiveness of dementia treatments and may induce cognitive impairments, even in healthy individuals. While a medication with very low anticholinergic properties is not expected to have a negative effect on cognition, the cumulative effects of multiple mild anticholinergic medications could lead to cognitive dysfunction.

Therapeutic interventions to consider when encountering anticholinergic medications, or persons with altered mental status, include the following: (a) recognize and discontinue potentially offending agents; (b) maintain a level of suspicion for medications; (c) optimize overall health, including nutrition and exercise; (d) treat underlying medical conditions; (e) avoid unnecessary medications; (f) use nonpharmacological interventions when possible; (g) beware of unreported drugs; (h) use the fewest drugs possible; and (i) avoid polypharmacy (the use of multiple drugs) and therapeutic duplication when possible. Also, when possible, use medications that are the least likely to cause delirium or other cognitive impairment (Stahl, 2000; Tune, Carr, & Hoag, 1992). Table 15.3 lists relatively common medications with anticholinergic properties.

Table 15.3 Selected medications with anticholinergic properties

Amitriptyline (Elavil, various)
Benztropine (Cogentin, various)
Captopril (Capoten, various)
Chlorpromazine (Thorazine, various)
Cimetidine (Tagament, various)
Clomipramine (Anafranil)
Clozapine (Clozaril, various)
Codeine
Cyclobenzaprine (Flexeril, various)
Desipramine (Norpramin, various)
Digoxin (Lanoxin, various)
Dimenhydrinate (Dramamine, various)
Diphenhydramine (Benadryl, various)
Dipyridamole (Persantine, various)
Doxepin (Adapin, Sinequan, various)
Doxylamine (Unisom, various)
Fluphenazine (Prolixin, various)
Furosemide (Lasix, various)
Hydroxyzine (Atarax, Vistaril, various)
Imipramine (Tofranil, various)
Loxapine (Loxitane, various)
Meclizine (Antivert, Bonine, various)
Mesoridazine (Serentil, various)
Nifedipine (Procardia, various)
Nortriptyline (Pamelor, Aventyl, various)
Olanzapine (Zyprexa)
Orphenadrine (Norflex, various)
Oxybutinin (Ditropan, Oxytrol, various)
Perphenazine (Trilafon, various)
Prednisolone
Prochlorperazine (Compazine, various)
Procyclidine (Kemadrin)
Promethazine (Phenergan, various)
Protriptyline (Vivactil)

Table 15.3 (contd.)

Quinidine
Ranitidine (Zantac, various)
Scopolamine (Scopace, Transderm Scop Patch)
Theophylline (Theo-Dur, various)
Thioridazine (Mellaril, various)
Thiothixene (Navane, various)
Trifluoperazine (Stelazine, various)
Warfarin (Coumadin, various)

Neurocognitive effects of select medications commonly prescribed to older adults

Estrogen

Some research indicated that postmenopausal women receiving estrogen replacement therapy have increased cerebral metabolism and a lower incidence of Alzheimer's disease (Baldereschi et al. 1998; Maki & Resnick, 2001). Although neuroprotective benefits may exist, research has not indicated that estrogen improves cognition or function in women diagnosed with Alzheimer's disease (Mulnard et al., 2000). In addition, combining estrogen and progestin has been found to increase the risk of stroke and dementia (Shumaker et al., 2003; Wassertheil-Smoller et al., 2003).

Anti-inflammatory drugs

Inflammation surrounding B-amyloid plaques appears to destroy neurons and play a role in the pathogenesis in Alzheimer's disease (Akiyama et al., 2000; in t' Veld et al., 2001). Regular use of nonsteroidal anti-inflammatory drugs has been found to reduce the risk of developing Alzheimer's disease (in t' Veld et al., 2001), and anti-inflammatory treatments may play a role in slowing the progression of the disease (Akiyama et al., 2000). However, the safety of non-steroidal anti-inflammatory drugs (COX-2 inhibitors), studied for their potential prophylactic effect for individuals at risk for Alzheimer's disease (Etminan, Gill, & Samii, 2003), has recently been questioned due to reported unexpected adverse cardiovascular effects (Drazen, 2005; Topol, 2005).

Lipid-lowering agents

The use of lipid-lowering agents (statins) is associated with reduced risk of dementia, and specifically of Alzheimer's disease (Rockwood et al., 2002), thus suggesting an apparent neuroprotective effect. However, research to date has not indicated that statins are of value in the treatment of individuals with

AD. Furthermore, AD patients have been found to be particularly susceptible to the adverse effects of statins due to aberrations in signal transduction and neuronal energy metabolism and perturbed cerebral cholesterol metabolism (Algotsson & Winblad, 2004). Overall, the evidence at this time suggests that while statins may offer a protective effect against the development of AD, the literature does not lend credence to the use of statins in the general non-demented population without hyperlipidemia (Miller & Chacko, 2004).

Neurocognitive effects of dietary supplements

Complementary pharmacotherapy is the use of botanical products for the attainment or maintenance of health (Ciocon, Ciocon, & Galindo, 2004). These botanical products are considered dietary supplements (Dietary Supplement Health and Education Act, 1994), are available over-the-counter, and are unregulated. Lacking regulation, the active ingredients in these products may vary considerably from one batch to another. Yet, despite the lack of regulation, the use of complementary pharmacotherapy is common, with approximately 60–70 million Americans using dietary supplements regularly (Eisenberg et al., 1993). Awareness by geriatric neuropsychologists of commonly used dietary supplements and their potential effects may contribute to more informed neuropsychological evaluations and recommendations.

Ginkgo biloba

Intended therapeutic effects of ginkgo biloba include memory enhancement, lowering of tinnitus levels, and treatment of complications from peripheral vascular disease (Chung et al., 1987). However, bleeding, including intracranial hemorrhaging, has been associated with regular use of this supplement.

*Ginseng (*Panax ginseng*)*

Used to counter fatigue and lower blood glucose levels, ginseng, like ginko biloba, has been found to inhibit platelet function and increase the risk of bleeding.

*Kava (*Piper methysticum*)*

Through its action on the GABA neurotransmission system in the amygdala and its effect on benzodiazepine receptors, kava is commonly used as an anxiolytic and sedative (Pittler & Edzard, 2000). After exposure to sunlight, individuals taking kava may develop a dermatopathologic condition, which worsens with alcohol use. When combined with benzodiazepines, kava has been associated with the onset of coma. Toxic liver damage has also been observed. Interactions with sedative-hypnotic drugs may result in depression, delirium, somnolence, and prolonged sleep.

St. John's wort *(*Hypericum perforatum*)*

Commonly used for short-term treatment of depression, St. John's wort acts by inhibiting serotonin, norepinephrine, and dopamine reuptake (Shelton et al., 2001). As with kava, St. John's wort may cause photosensitivity. In addition, it may lead to uncontrolled hypertension in patients treated with calcium channel blockers.

Valerian *(*Valeriana officinalis*)*

Valerian is a sedative mediated through the GABA neurotransmission system. It may potentiate the sedative effects of anesthetics, resulting in prolonged sedation. Abrupt withdrawal mimics withdrawal from benzodiazepines, which may include delirium (Garges, Varia, & Doraiswamy, 1998).

Antioxidants

Free radicals are atoms that are present in air, food, and water; they also can be produced by the body. In normal amounts, they perform useful functions, such as serving the immune system to combat viruses or bacteria. However, excessive amounts can damage cells, proteins, and DNA. Accumulated damage from oxygen free radicals in the brain disrupts normal cell functioning and can lead to cell death, thus promoting age-related problems, such as memory loss.

Some nutrients are considered antioxidants because they help defend the body from the oxidative stress caused by free radicals. Examples of antioxidants include vitamins C and E, beta carotene, and flavonoids. Sources of vitamin C include citrus fruits, kiwi, sprouts, broccoli, and cabbage; sources of vitamin E include grain, nuts, milk, and egg yolk; sources of beta carotene include carrots, broccoli, spinach, and types of cabbage; and sources of flavonoids include cranberries and green and black tea.

Early research on the potential benefits of vitamin E for Alzheimer's disease patients indicated that vitamin E mitigates the inflammatory effects of B-amyloid plaque formation, making it an appealing option for patients with Alzheimer's disease (Sano et al., 1997). However, a Cochrane review of that research, adjusting for differences between patient groups, concluded that there was insufficient evidence to justify recommending vitamin E for the treatment of Alzheimer's disease (Tabet, Birks, & Grimley-Evans, 2000). In addition, some evidence indicates that long-term supplementation with high doses (≥ 400 IU/d) of vitamin E is associated with increased risk of cardiac problems and mortality among some patient groups (Lonn et al., 2005; Miller et al., 2005).

Two recent studies of the relationship between antioxidant consumption and Alzheimer's disease (AD) risk were published in the *Journal of the American Medical Association*. Morris et al. (2002), with the Chicago Health and Aging Project, evaluated 815 community-residing adults, aged 65 and older, and monitored their status for an average of nearly 4 years. These researchers found that vitamin E intake from food had a significant protective effect, with people in the top 20% of vitamin E intake being 67% less likely to develop AD than people in the lowest 20% of intake. However, this protective association was not found for people who were genetically at risk for AD. In addition, vitamin E supplement use, vitamin C intake in any form, and beta carotene use were not associated with a significantly decreased risk of AD.

Engelhart et al. (2002), with The Rotterdam Study, evaluated 5395 community-residing adults, aged 55 and older, and monitored their status for an average of 6 years. These researchers found that individuals in the top one-third of vitamin E intake from food had a significant reduction in risk of AD, 43% lower risk compared to individuals in the lowest one-third of vitamin E intake. A higher intake of vitamin C had a borderline significant association with lower risk of AD. Beta carotene and flavonoids were not associated with AD risk. The relationship between vitamin intake and AD risk varied with other variables assessed, such as education, smoking, and genetic risk. For example, high vitamin C intake was related to lower risk of AD for participants with an intermediate level of education. Also, higher intake of each of the four of antioxidants was associated with lower risk of AD in current smokers; however, the association between antioxidants and AD was not significant for nonsmokers. Additionally, higher intake of three of the four antioxidants (except flavonoids) was associated with somewhat lower risk of AD for those at genetic risk for AD. As with the study by Morris et al. (2002), the association between vitamin supplement use and risk of AD was not significant. As part of the Honolulu-Asia Aging Study, Laurin et al. (2004) found that midlife dietary intake of antioxidants did not reduce the risk of late-life dementia.

Together, these studies suggest that a high intake of antioxidants from food may be associated with a lower incidence of AD for some individuals. Although final answers regarding the neuroprotective effects of antioxidants have yet to be determined, the potential benefits of antioxidant consumption on the pathology underlying Alzheimer's disease appear to substantiate their use, particularly since it is unlikely that antioxidant-rich foods would adversely affect brain health (Foley & White, 2002).

Polypharmacy

Polypharmacy—the administration of multiple medications—is justified for the treatment of concurrent or severe illnesses. However, unnecessary polypharmacy may contribute to the development of "geriatric syndromes," which include cognitive impairment, delirium, falls, incontinence, and decreased functional status (American Medical Association Council on Scientific Affairs, 2002). Patients contribute to inappropriate polypharmacy by failing to reveal all of the medications (including over-the-counter medications) they take. Approximately 70% of dietary supplement users do not inform their doctors of their use of these over-the-counter medications (Kessler et al., 2001). Geriatric neuropsychologists should, during review of patient medication use, directly question patients about their use of dietary supplements. Such information may be of considerable value when planning evaluations or treatment, interpreting test results, or making recommendations. With appropriate consent, conveying such information to the patient's treating physicians may further facilitate understanding and treatment of the patient.

Conclusions

Neuropsychologists working with older adults benefit from a basic understanding of geriatric pharmacology. Potential adverse effects of medication use should be considered when evaluating and treating older adults, given the possible impact of commonly prescribed medications on cognitive functioning.

References

Akiyama, H., Barger, S., Barnum, S., Bradt, B., Bauer, J., & Cole, G. M. (2000). Inflammation and Alzheimer's disease. *Neurobiology of Aging, 21*(3), 383–421.

Algotsson, A., & Winblad, B. (2004). Patients with Alzheimer's disease may be particularly susceptible to adverse effects of statins. *Dementia and Geriatric Cognitive Disorders, 17*(3), 109–116.

American Medical Association Council on Scientific Affairs. (2002). *Featured CSA report: Improving the quality of geriatric pharmacotherapy.* Retrieved June 8, 2004, from http://www.ama-assn.org/ama/pub/category/13592.html

Anttila, S. A., & Leinonen, E. V. (2001). A review of the pharmacological and clinical profile of mirtazapine. *CNS Drug Reviews, 7*(3), 249–264.

Baldereschi, M., Di Carlo, A., Lepore, V., Bracco, L., Maggi, S., Grigoletto, F., et al. (1998). Estrogen-replacement therapy and Alzheimer's disease in the Italian Longitudinal Study on Aging. *Neurology, 50*, 996–1002.

Bowden, C. L., Brugger, A. M., & Swann, A. C. (1994). Efficacy of divalproex vs lithium and placebo in the treatment of mania: The Depakote Mania Study Group. *Journal of the American Medical Association, 271*, 918–924.

Chengappa, K. N., Baker, R. W., Kreinbrook, S. B., & Adair, D. (1995). Clozapine use in female geriatric patients with psychoses. *Journal of Geriatric Psychiatry and Neurology, 8*, 12–15.

Chung, K. F., Dent, G., McCusker, M., Guinot, P., Page, C. P., & Barnes, P. J. (1987). Effect of a ginkgolide mixture (BN 52063) in antagonizing skin and platelet responses to platelet activating factor in man. *Lancet, 1*(8527), 248–251.

Ciocon, J. O., Ciocon, D. G., & Galindo, D. J. (2004). Dietary supplements in primary care: Botanicals can affect surgical outcomes and follow-up. *Geriatrics, 58*(9), 20–24.

Cole, M. G., & Dendukuri, N. (2003). Risk factors for depression among elderly community subjects: A systematic review and meta-analysis. *American Journal of Psychiatry, 160*(6), 1147–1156.

Copeland, J. R., Davidson, L. A., & Dewey, M. E. (1987). The prevalence and outcome of anxious depression in elderly people aged 65 and over living in the community. In

G. Racagnia & E. Smeraldi (Eds.), *Anxious depression: Assessment and treatment* (pp. 43–47). New York: Raven Press.

Cummings, J. L., Frank, J. C., & Cherry, D. (2002). Guidelines for managing Alzheimer's disease: Part II. Treatment. *American Family Physician, 65,* 2525–2534.

Dharmarajan, T. S., & Ugalino, J. A. (2001). Understanding the pharmacology of aging. *Geriatric Medicine, 1*(4), 2–11.

Dietary Supplement Health and Education Act of 1994, Pub. L. No. 103-417, 180 Stat. 2126.

Doraiswamy, P. M. (2001). Contemporary management of comorbid anxiety and depression in geriatric patients. *Journal of Clinical Psychiatry, 62*(Suppl. 12), 30–35.

Doraiswamy, P. M., Krishnan, K. R., Oxman, T., Jenkyn, L. R., Coffey, D. J., Burt, T., et al. (2003). Does antidepressant therapy improve cognition in elderly depressed patients? *Journals of Gerontology: Series A, Biological Sciences and Medical Science, 58*(12), 1137–1144.

Drazen, J. M. (2005). COX-2 inhibitors: A lesson in unexpected problems. *New England Journal of Medicine, 352*(11), 1131–1132.

Eisenberg, D. M., Kessler, R. C., Foster, C., Norlock, F. E., Calkis, D. R., & Delbanco, T. L. (1993). Unconventional medicine in the United States: Prevalence, costs, and patterns of use. *New England Journal of Medicine, 328*(4), 246–252.

Elphick, M. (1989). Clinical issues in the use of carbamazepine in psychiatry: a review. *Psychological Medicine, 19*(3), 591–604.

Engelhart, M. J., Geerlings, M. I., Ruitenberg, A., van Swieten, J. C., Hofman, A., Witteman, J. C., & Breteler, M. M. (2002). Dietary intake of antioxidants and risk of Alzheimer's disease. *Journal of the American Medical Association, 287*(24), 3223–3229.

Etminan, M., Gill, S., & Samii, A. (2003). Effect of non-steroidal anti-inflammatory drugs on risk of Alzheimer's disease: Systematic review and meta-analysis of observational studies. *British Medical Journal, 327,* 128–132.

Evans, D. A., Funkenstein, H. H., Albert, M. S., Scherr, P. A., Cook, N. R., Chown, M. J., et al. (1989). Prevalence of Alzheimer's disease in a community population of older persons: Higher than previously reported. *Journal of the American Medical Association, 262,* 2551–2556.

Flint, A. J. (1994). Recent developments in geriatric psychopharmacology. *Canadian Journal of Psychiatry, 39*(8), 9–18.

Florkowski, A., Gruszczynski, W., & Zboralski, K. (2002). Efficacy and tolerance assessment of mirtazepine in the treatment of depression in the elderly: Preliminary report. *Psychiatria Polska, 36*(6 Suppl.), 143–146.

Foley, D. J., & White, L. R. (2002). Dietary intake of antioxidants and risk of Alzheimer's disease. *Journal of the American Medical Association, 287*(24), 3261–3263.

Friedman, J. H., Max, J., & Swift, R., (1987). Idiopathic Parkinson's disease in a chronic schizophrenic patient: Long-tern treatment with clozapine and L-DOPA. *Clinical Neuropharmacology, 10,* 470–475.

Garges, H. P., Varia, I., & Doraiswamy, P. M. (1998). Cardiac complications and delirium associated with valerian root withdrawal. *Journal of the American Medical Association, 280*(18), 1566–1567.

Gasto, C., Navarro, V., Marcos, T., Portella, M. J., Torra, M., & Rodamilans, M. (2003). Single-blind comparison of venlafaxine and nortriptyline in elderly major depression. *Journal of Clinical Psychopharmacology, 23*(1), 21–26.

Gaulin, B. D., Markowitz, J. S., & Caley, C. F. (1999). Clozapine-associated elevation in serum triglycerides. *American Journal of Psychiatry, 156*, 1270–1272.

Georgotas, A., McCue, R. E., & Hapworth, W. (1986). Comparative efficacy and safety of MAOI's versus TCA's in treating depression in the elderly. *Biological Psychiatry, 21*, 1155–1166.

Gerner, R. H., & Stanton, A. (1992). Algorithm for patient management of acute manic states: Lithium, valproate, or carbamazepine? *Journal of Clinical Psychopharmacology, 12*(1 Suppl.), 57S–63S.

Hardman, J. G., & Limbird, L. E. (1996). *Goodman & Gilman's the pharmacological basis of therapeutics* (9th ed.). New York: McGraw-Hill.

Harvey, P., Napolitano, J., Mao, L., & Gharabawi, G. (2003). Comparative effects of risperidone and olanzapine on cognition in elderly patients with schizophrenia or schizoaffective disorder. *International Journal of Geriatric Psychiatry, 18*, 820–829.

Hernandez, J. L., Ramos, F. J., Infante, J., Rebollo, M., & Gonzalez-Macias, J. (2002). Severe serotonin syndrome induced by mirtazapine monotherapy. *Annals of Pharmacotherapy, 3*(4), 641–643.

Hirschfeld, R. M. (2002). The use of mirtazapine in difficult-to-treat patient populations. *Human Psychopharmacology, 17*(1), S33–S36.

Hoeh, N., Gyulai, L., Weintraub, D., & Streim, J. (2003). Pharmacologic management of psychosis in the elderly: A critical review. *Journal of Geriatric Psychiatry and Neurology, 16*(4), 213–217.

in t' Veld, B. A., Ruitenberg, A., Hofman, A., Launer, L. J., van Duijn, C. M., Stijnen, T., et al. (2001). Nonsteroidal antiinflammatory drugs and the risk of Alzheimer's disease. *New England Journal of Medicine, 345*, 1515–1521.

Kane, J., Honingfeld, K., & Singer, J. (1988). Clozapine for the treatment resistant schizophrenic: A double-blind comparison with chlorpromazine. *Archives of General Psychiatry, 45*, 789–796.

Katona, C., & Livingston, G. (2002). *Drug treatment in old age psychiatry.* Trowbridge, UK: Cromwell Press.

Kennedy, J. S., Jeste, D., Kaiser, C. J., Golshan, G. A., Maguire, G. A., Tollefson, G., et al. (2003). Olanzipine vs haloperidol in geriatric schizophrenia: Analysis of data from a double blind controlled trial. *International Journal of Geriatric Psychiatry, 18*, 1013–1020.

Kessler, R. C., Davis, R. B., Foster, D. F., van Rompay, M. I., Walters, E. E., Wilkey, S. A., et al. (2001). Long term trends in the use of complementary and alternative medical therapies in the United States. *Annals of Internal Medicine, 135*(4), 262–268.

Kirby, D., Harrigan, S., & Ames, D. (2002). Hyponatremia in elderly psychiatric patients treated with selective serotonin reuptake inhibitors and venlafaxine: A retrospective controlled study in an impatient unit. *International Journal of Geriatric Psychiatry, 17*(3), 231–237.

Kroeze, W. K., Hufeisen, S. J., Popadak, B. A., Renock, S. M., Steinberg, S., Ernsberger, P., et al. (2003). H1-histamine receptor affinity predicts short-term weight gain for typical and atypical antipsychotic drugs. *Neuropsychopharmacology, 28*(3), 519–526.

Laurin, D., Kamal, H. Masaki, K. M., Foley, D. J., White, L. R., & Launer, L. J. (2004). Midlife dietary intake of antioxidants and risk of late-life incident dementia: The Honolulu-Asia Aging Study. *American Journal of Epidemiology, 159*, 959–967.

Lavretsky, H., Kim, M. D., Kumar, A., & Reynolds, C. F. (2003). Combined treatment with methylphenidate and citalopram for accelerated response in the elderly: An open trial. *Journal of Clinical Psychiatry, 64*(12), 1410–1414.

Lonn, E., Bosch, J., Yusuf, S., Sheridan, P., Pogue, J., Arnold, J. M. O., et al. (2005). Effects of long-term vitamin E supplementation on cardiovascular events and cancer. *Journal of the American Medical Association, 293*, 1338–1347.

Madhusoodanan, S., Sidhartha, S., Brenner, R., Gupta, S., & Bogunovic, O. (2001). Use of olanzipine for elderly patients with psychotic disorders: A review. *Annals of Clinical Psychiatry, 13*(4), 201–211.

Maki, P. M., & Resnick, S. M. (2001). Effects of estrogen on patterns of brain activity at rest and during cognitive activity: A review of neuroimaging studies. *Neuroimage, 14*, 789–801.

McElroy, S. L., Keck, P. E., Jr., Pope, H. G., Jr., & Hudson, J. I. (1992). Valproate in the treatment of bipolar disorders: Literature review and clinical guidelines. *Journal of Clinical Psychopharmacology, 12*(1), 42S–52S.

McFarland, B. H., Miller, M. R., & Straumfjord, A. A. (1990). Valproate use in the older manic patient. *Journal of Clinical Psychiatry, 51*, 479–481.

Mellow, A. M. (Ed.). (2003). *Geriatric psychiatry.* Arlington, VA: American Psychiatric Association.

Miller, E. R., Pastor-Barriuso, R., Dalal, D., Riemersma, R. A., Appel, L. J., & Guallar, E. (2005). Meta-analysis: High-dosage vitamin E supplementation may increase all-cause mortality. *Annals of Internal Medicine, 142*(1), 37–46.

Miller, L. J., & Chacko, R. (2004). The role of cholesterol and statins in Alzheimer's disease. *Annals of Pharmacotherapy, 38*(1), 91–98.

Morris, M. C., Evans, D. A., Bienias, J. L., Tangney, C. C., Bennett, D. A., Aggarwal, N., et al. (2002). Dietary intake of antioxidant nutrients and the risk of incident Alzheimer's disease in a biracial community study. *Journal of the American Medical Association, 287*(24), 3230–3237.

Muijsers, R. B., Plosker, G. L., & Noble, S. (2002). Spotlight on sertraline in the management of major depressive disorder in elderly patients. *CNS Drugs, 16*(11), 789–794.

Mulnard, R. A., Cotman, C. W., Kawas, C., van Dyck, C. H., Sano, M., Doody, R., et al. (2000). Estrogen replacement therapy for treatment of mild to moderate Alzheimer's disease: A randomized controlled trial: Alzheimer's Disease Cooperative Study. *Journal of the American Medical Association, 283*, 1007–1015.

Naranjo, C., Herrmann, N., Mittmann, N., & Bremner, K. (1995). Recent advances in geriatric psychopharmacology. *Drugs and Aging, 7*(3), 184–202.

National Institute of Mental Health. (2004). Depression and suicide acts. Retrieved March 5, 2004, from http://www.nimh.nih/gov/

Navarro, V., Gasto, C., Torres, X., Marcos, T., & Pintor, L. (2001). Citalopram versus nortriptyline in late-life depression: A 12-week randomized single-blind study. *Acta Psychiatrica Scandinavica, 103*(6), 435–440.

Nelson, J. C., Kennedy, J. S., & Pollock, B. G. (1999). Treatment of major depression with nortiptyline and paroxetine in patients with ischemic heart disease. *American Journal of Psychiatry, 156*(7), 1024–1028.

Oslin, D. W., Ten Have, T. R., Streim, J. E., Datto, C. J., Weintraub, D., DiFilippo, S., et al. (2003). Probing the safety of medications in the frail elderly: Evidence from a randomized clinical trial of sertraline and venlafaxine in depressed nursing home residents. *Journal of Clinical Psychiatry, 64*(8), 875–882.

Osser, D. N., Najarian, D. M., & Dufresne, R. L. (1999). Olanzipine increases weight and serum triglyceride levels. *Journal of Clinical Psychiatry, 60*, 767–770.

Ostergaard, K., & Dupont, E. (1988). Clozapine treatment of drug-induced psychotic symptoms in late stages of Parkinson's disease. *Acta Neurologica Scandinavica, 18*, 349–350.

Pfeiffer, R. F., Kang, J., & Graber, B. (1990). Clozapine for psychosis in Parkinson's disease. *Movement Disorders, 5*, 239–242.

Pittler, M. H., & Edzard, E. (2000). Efficacy of Kava extract for treating anxiety: Systematic review and meta-analysis. *Journal of Clinical Psychopharmacology, 20*(1), 84–49.

Risinger, R. C., Risby, E. D., & Risch, S. (1994). Safety and efficacy of divalproex sodium in elderly bipolar patients. *Journal of Clinical Psychiatry, 55*, 215.

Ritchie, C., Chiu, E., Harrigan, S., Hall, K., Hassett, A., Macfarlane, S., et al. (2003). The impact upon extra-pyramidal side effects, clinical symptoms and quality of life of a switch from conventional to atypical antipsychotics (risperidone and olanzipine) in elderly patients with schizophrenia. *International Journal of Geriatric Psychiatry, 18*, 432–440.

Rivas-Vasquez, R. A., Johnson, S. L., Rey, G. J., Blais, M. A., & Rivas-Vasquez, A. (2002). Current treatments for bipolar disorder: A review and update for psychologists. *Professional Psychology: Research and Practice, 33*(2), 212–223.

Rockwood, K., Kirkland, S., Hogan, D. B., MacKnight, C., Merry, H., Verreault, R., et al. (2002). Use of lipid-lowering agents, indication bias, and the risk of dementia in community-dwelling elderly people. *Archives of Neurology, 59*(2), 223–227.

Rosner, M. H. (2004). Severe hyponatremia associated with the combined use of thiazide diuretics and selective serotonin reuptake inhibitors. *American Journal of the Medical Sciences, 327*(2), 109–111.

Sacchetti, E., Guarneri, L., & Bravi, D. (2000). H(2) antagonist nizatidine may control olanzapine-associated weight gain in schizophrenic patients. *Biological Psychiatry, 48*(2), 167–168.

Sajatovic, M. (2002). Treatment of bipolar disorder in older adults. *International Journal of Geriatric Psychiatry, 17*, 865–873.

Salzman, C. (1992). *Clinical geriatric psychopharmacology* (2nd ed.). Baltimore: Williams & Wilkins.

Salzman, C. (1998). *Psychiatric medications for older adults: The concise guide.* New York: Guilford Press.

Salzman, C. (2001). Treatment of the agitation of late-life psychosis and Alzheimer's disease. *European Psychiatry, 16*, 25–28.

Sano, M., Ernesto, C., Thomas, R. G., Klauber, M. R., Schafer, K., Grundman, M., et al. (1997). A controlled study of selegiline, alpha-tocopherol, or both as treatment for Alzheimer's disease: The Alzheimer's Disease Cooperative Study. *New England Journal of Medicine, 336*, 1216–1222.

Schatzberg, A. F., Kremer, C., Rodrigues, H. E., & Murphy, G. M. (2002). Double-blind, randomized comparison of mirtazapine and paroxetine in elderly depressed patients. *American Journal of Geriatric Psychiatry, 10*(5), 541–550.

Sheikh, J. I. (2003). Anxiety in older adults: Assessment and management of three common presentations. *Geriatrics, 58*(5), 44–45.

Sheikh, J. I., & Cassidy, E. L. (2000). Treatment of anxiety disorders in the elderly: Issues and strategies. *Journal of Anxiety Disorders, 14*(2), 173–190.

Shelton, R. C., Keller, M. B., Gelenberg, A., Dunner, D. L., Hirschfeld, R., Thase, M. E., et al. (2001). Effectiveness of St. John's wort in major depression: A randomized controlled trial. *Journal of the American Medical Association, 285*(15), 1978–1986.

Shulman, K. I., & Hermann, N. (2002). Manic syndromes in old age. In R. Jacoby & C. Oppenheimer (Eds.), *Psychiatry in the elderly* (3rd ed., pp. 683–695). New York: Oxford University Press.

Shumaker, S. A., Legault, C., Thal, L., Wallace, R. B., Ockene, J. K., Hendrix, S. L., et al. (2003). Estrogen plus progestin and the incidence of dementia and mild cognitive impairment in postmenopausal women: The Women's Health Initiative Memory Study: A randomized controlled trial. *Journal of the American Medical Association, 289*, 2651–2662.

Staab, J. P., & Evans, D. L. (2000). Efficacy of venlafaxine in geriatric depression. *Depression and Anxiety, 12*(1), 63–68.

Stahl, S. M. (2000). *Essential psychopharmacology: Neuroscientific basis and practical applications* (2nd ed.). New York: Cambridge University Press.

Steffens, D. C., Doraiswamy, P. M., & McQuoid, D. R. (2001). Bupropion SR in the naturalistic treatment of elderly patients with major depression. *International Journal of Geriatric Psychiatry, 16*(9), 862–865.

Tabet, N., Birks, J., & Grimley-Evans, J. (2000). Vitamin E for Alzheimer's disease. Cochrane Database of Systematic Reviews (CD002854). Retrieved June 6, 2005, from http://www.cochrane.org/cochrane/revabstr/AB002854.htm

Topol, E. J. (2005). Arthritis medicines and cardiovascular events—"house of coxibs". *Journal of the American Medical Association, 293*, 336–338.

Tune, L., Carr, S., & Hoag, E., (1992). Anticholinergic effects of drugs commonly prescribed for the elderly: Potential means for assessing risk of delirium. *American Journal of Psychiatry, 149*, 1393–1394.

Wassertheil-Smoller, S., Hendrix, S., Limacher, M., Heiss, G., Kooperberg, C., Baird, A., et al. (2003). Effect of estrogen plus progestin on stroke in postmenopausal women: The Women's Health Initiative: A randomized trial. *Journal of the American Medical Association, 289*, 2673–2684.

Zec, R. F. (1993). Neuropsychological functioning in Alzheimer's disease. In R. W. Parks, R. F. Zec, & R. S. Wilson (Eds.), *Neuropsychology of Alzheimer disease and other dementias* (pp. 1–80). New York: Oxford University Press.

Zis, A. P., Grof, P., & Webster, M. (1980). Predictors of relapse in recurrent affective disorders. *Psychopharmacology Bulletin, 16*, 47–49.

16 Substance abuse in older adults

Doug Johnson-Greene and Anjeli B. Inscore

Older adults now comprise the fastest growing segment of the population. In 1995 there were approximately 34 million persons over the age of 65, but by 2030 this number is expected to double (Bernstein, 1995; Hobbs, 1995). Advancing age can be associated with negative financial, social, and medical consequences, resulting in higher levels of perceived stress. It is recognized that many of the life changes experienced by older adults, such as retirement, loss of a spouse, and development of chronic medical conditions, can contribute to the onset and severity of substance abuse. In turn, substance abuse can have adverse effects on well-being by depleting available financial resources, alienating family and friends, and causing or contributing to medical ailments. Thus, it is apparent that there is a reciprocal and synergistic relationship between substance abuse and life changes experienced by the elderly, which for some may represent an obstacle to the management of increasing medical and social needs.

Unless significant changes are made in health care delivery, problems with identification and treatment of substance misuse and abuse in the elderly will continue to grow as the population of the United States advances in age. The issue of substance abuse is unique in elderly patients, with direct implications for neuropsychological assessment and treatment. Differences in substances abused, increased utilization of prescribed and non-prescribed medication, and physiological and cognitive changes that occur with aging all combine to make the problem of substance abuse distinct in the elderly. In this chapter we review the literature pertaining to the epidemiology, causes, and consequences of alcohol and drug abuse in the elderly and their relevance to neuropsychological functioning.

Alcohol abuse

Epidemiological and diagnostic considerations

One in ten Americans has significant problems with alcohol (Miller & Brown, 1997). While there is general agreement that the incidence of alcohol abuse and dependence decreases with age, recent epidemiological studies suggest that the extent of alcohol abuse in the elderly is significantly greater than previously reported (Adams, Barry, & Fleming, 1996; Clay, 1997; Holroyd & Duryee, 1997; Oslin, Streim, Parmelee, Boyce, & Katz, 1997; Reid & Anderson, 1997). It has been estimated that up to 10% of the elderly population are "problem" drinkers. Within this population, alcohol misuse is much more common in men than in women (Adams & Cox, 1995; Bucholz, Sheline, & Helzer, 1995), and there is reason to believe that African-Americans may be more vulnerable to problem drinking in later life (Gomberg, 1995).

For large numbers of the elderly, alcohol abuse goes undiagnosed and untreated. Alcohol problems are largely unrecognized in the elderly because a number of factors complicate assessment and diagnosis in this population. One factor contributing to under recognition of alcohol problems in the elderly is that current classification schemes used for diagnosis of alcohol abuse and dependence may have limited applicability to elderly populations. For example, the fourth edition of the *Diagnostic and Statistical Manual of Mental Disorders* (DSM-IV; American Psychiatric Association, 1994) requires impairment in major life domains related to alcohol use, which may be difficult to demonstrate in elderly persons who are retired and living alone. An alternative classification scheme has been proposed in the Treatment Improvement Protocol Series on Substance Abuse Among Older Adults by the Substance Abuse and Mental Health Services Administration (SAMHSA, 1998). SAMHSA recommend that the terms alcohol abuse and dependence in the elderly be replaced by the categories of "at risk" and "problem drinkers" to more accurately reflect alcohol misuse categories in this population. At risk drinkers are defined as those whose patterns of alcohol use, although not currently causing problems, may bring about adverse consequences to the drinker or others. Problem drinkers are signified by their hazardous levels of consumption and drinking-related consequences. In general, advancing age lowers the threshold for at risk and problem drinking because of heightened sensitivity to the effects of alcohol and the presence of comorbid illnesses or functional limitations.

A second factor related to under recognition of problem drinking in the elderly that is frequently cited in the literature includes difficulties with recognition of the problem and attitudes about the elderly. Problem drinking in the elderly can mimic other medical and behavioral disorders common in this population. Somatic complaints, apathy, and emotional dysphoria are symptoms that are often erroneously associated with normal aging. However, for a portion of individuals, these complaints are actually signs of alcohol misuse. Increased efforts to educate health practitioners about common signs of alcohol misuse in the elderly have resulted in reasonable success in increasing identification of problem drinking, particularly in general medical settings and emergency departments.

Lastly, there is a general reluctance to report problem drinking in this cohort by both the problem drinkers themselves and those with whom they interact. Family members may be too ashamed or may simply choose to rationalize the behavior. Alcohol use may be viewed by some families to be a legitimate

Table 16.1 Possible characteristics of problem drinking in elderly patients

Physical and cognitive signs
- Sleep complaints and change in sleeping patterns
- Change in eating habits and gastrointestinal complaints
- Cognitive complaints including confusion, mental fatigue, impaired concentration
- Tremor, unexplained restlessness, unsteady gait or incoordination
- Persistent irritability, anxiousness, or depression

Psychosocial issues
- Inability to care for self as evidenced by self-neglect of hygiene, cleanliness of home
- Estrangement from most or all of family members
- Irritability and altered mood (depression or anxiety)

Health and safety
- Liver function abnormalities, seizures, malnutrition
- Gastrointestinal problems such as esophagitis and bleeding ulcer
- History of unexplained falls or bruising
- Recent history of car accidents

method of coping for the elderly. A list of common signs of problem drinking in the elderly can be found in Table 16.1, and a list of brief measures frequently utilized to screen for problem drinking is provided in Table 16.2.

Chronic illness and alcohol abuse in older adults

Recent research suggests that the prevalence of problem drinking in persons with chronic disabling conditions is higher than in the general population. This has led to concern that alcohol may not only contribute to the development of a number of chronic conditions, but may also slow rates of recovery

Table 16.2 Screening instruments for assessment of problem drinking in the elderly

Measure	Items	Max. score	Impaired range	Format
CAGE (Ewing, 1984)	4	4	2 or more	Yes/no
AUDIT (Babor, de la Fuenta, Saunders, & Grant, 1992)	10	40	8 or more	5-point description
MAST-G (Blow et al., 1992)	24	24	5 or more	Yes/no

Notes: CAGE = an acronym for alcohol-related thoughts and feelings that comprise the measure's four questions; AUDIT = Alcohol Use Disorders Identification Test; MAST-G = Michigan Alcohol Screening Test—Geriatric version.

and produce secondary complications in persons who already have chronic conditions. This is particularly relevant to older adults, as the prevalence of chronic disease is known to increase with age. It has been estimated that 80% of persons 65 years and over have at least one chronic disease (US Senate Special Committee on Aging, 1987–1988). Not surprisingly, many experts now believe that the major health problems facing Americans are chronic, disabling conditions (Kemp, Brumel-Smith, & Ramsdell, 1990). It is projected that the population in the years to come will be significantly older and that elderly individuals will more likely than not have at least one chronic illness. It is also well known that the risk of substance abuse increases with higher levels of stress, as is frequently seen in persons coping with chronic illness. In turn, many chronic illnesses can be worsened by behaviors associated with substance abuse, such as limited compliance with health regimens, decreased access to health care, and increased self-neglect. Exploration of the relationships between chronic illness and substance abuse is still in its infancy, but the prevalence of chronic illness in the elderly population highlights the increased potential for substance abuse in this population, given the research findings to date.

Other medical ailments that have been linked to alcohol abuse in the elderly include delirium (Elie, Cole, & Primeau, 1998), various forms of cancer (Smith, 1995), liver disease, peripheral neuropathy, poor nutrition, and late-onset seizures (Fink, Hays, Moore, & Beck, 1996). Alcohol abuse in the elderly is also associated with significantly more adverse events, including emergency room visits and hospital admissions (Holroyd & Currie, 1997).

Alcohol, traumatic injury, and disability

The relationship between alcohol and traumatic injuries resulting in disability has been well documented. The rate for alcohol problems in consecutive trauma admissions has been as high as 44%, and up to 28% of all trauma admissions meet criteria for alcohol dependence (Rivara et al., 1993; Soderstrom et al., 1997). Acquired conditions such as traumatic brain injury (TBI) have long been associated with a high rate of premorbid and postinjury alcohol-related problems (Corrigan, 1995; Corrigan, Rust, & Lamb-Hart, 1995). Studies have found alcohol to be a significant contributing factor in more than 50% of all cases of motor vehicle-related TBI, and alcohol use has also been linked specifically to motor vehicle crashes in the elderly (Higgins, Wright, & Wrenn, 1996). Similar percentages have been found for alcohol and falls, which is a common cause of traumatic brain injury in the elderly (Brennan, Kagay, Geppert, & Moos, 2000). Other conditions that have been associated with alcohol abuse include spinal cord injury (Bombardier & Rimmele, 1998; Heinemann, Keen, Donohue, & Schnoll, 1988; Kiwerski & Krasuski, 1992) and burn injury (Bassett, Chase, Folstein, & Reiger, 1998). The conclusion that can be drawn from the literature is that there is an association between problem drinking and trauma-related disability in the elderly.

Alcohol problems have also been shown to have an adverse impact on outcome from trauma-related disabling conditions. Not surprisingly, many post-traumatic injury patients continue to abuse alcohol, complicating their recovery and long-term rehabilitation. Alcohol abuse increases complications from, and mortality during, the acute phase of recovery in patients with traumatic brain injury (Dikmen, Donovan, Loberg, Machmer, & Temkin, 1993), severe burn injury (Grobmyer, Maniscalco, Purdue, & Hunt, 1996; Kelley & Lynch, 1992), and in general trauma populations (Jurkovich et al., 1992). Alcohol may also affect postinjury outcome in persons with disability across a broad range of functional measures, including resumption of employment (Faucrbach, Engrav, & Kowalske, 2001), neurological complications (Kaplan & Corrigan, 1992), decreased activity level, and rehabilitation participation (Heinemann, Goranson, Ginsburg, & Schnoll, 1989), and may also contribute to higher rates of suicide (Charlifue & Gerhart, 1991). Though alcohol has been shown to play a counterproductive role in positive outcomes following trauma-related disability, more research is needed to determine if patient age moderates the effect of problem drinking.

Neuropathological changes and neuropsychological functioning

There is a rather large body of literature indicating that even in the absence of distinctive syndromes, such as Wernicke-Korsakoff syndrome, severe chronic alcoholism damages the central nervous system. Consumption of excessive amounts of alcohol produces major morphological changes in the aging human cerebral cortex (Courville, 1955; Harper & Kril, 1989, 1991; Kril & Harper, 1989), with correlated disorders of higher cerebral function, particularly in the areas of rule and concept formation, selective attention, and the capacity to shift strategies in problem solving (Adams et al., 1993, 1995; Johnson-Greene, Adams, Gilman, Koeppe et al., 1997). The extent of the relationship among cognition, alcohol, and aging has not been fully explored because of methodological complexities. However, there has been some limited support to suggest that alcohol may accelerate site-specific neuronal loss in the elderly (Freund, 1982; Pfefferbaum et al., 1992; Wiggins et al., 1988), which has been shown to correlate with cognitive impairment (Freund, 1982; Wiggins et al., 1988). The frontal lobes appear to be the most susceptible to neuronal loss related to alcohol abuse (Harper et al., 1998; Leuchter et al., 1994; Pfefferbaum et al., 1992), which is consistent with histological changes observed in normal aging. Acceleration of neuronal loss similar to patterns seen in elderly persons in response to chronic repeated alcohol exposure has led to development of a paradigm termed premature aging. However, this paradigm is not well validated because a clear dose response relationship between alcohol intake, neuronal loss, and cognitive dysfunction has not been established (Christian et al., 1995). Thus, the interaction between alcohol and aging as it relates to neuropathology for now must be considered inconclusive.

The role of alcohol abuse in the development of alcoholic cerebellar degeneration has also been well documented (Jernigan et al., 1991; Jernigan, Schafer, Butters & Cermak, 1991). Studies of neuropathological changes in the brains of persons with chronic alcoholism have shown asymptomatic degeneration of the cerebellum in up to 27% of chronic alcoholics, particularly neurons in the anterior superior vermis (Coffey et al., 1992; Johnson-Greene, Adams, Gilman, Kluin et al., 1997). One implication of alcohol-related cerebellar degeneration is that impaired coordination associated with cerebellar pathology may complicate recovery of ambulation after disabling illness and may contribute to increased risk of falls.

Overall, problem drinking has been associated with specific neuropathological changes in the brain and correlated cognitive impairments, primarily in the domain of executive functioning. However, the permanence of cognitive and metabolic changes in chronic alcoholics has been the subject of much debate. Johnson-Greene, Adams, Gilman, Kluin et al. (1997) found in a small sample of patients with severe chronic alcoholism that abstinence was associated with improved performance on neuropsychological tests of general and executive functioning, as well as recovery of local cerebral metabolic rates for glucose measured using positron emission tomography. The implication of these findings is that problem drinking may worsen cognitive changes associated with aging and contribute to brain trauma and illness, though there are indications of at least partial recovery with abstinence.

Psychological manifestations of alcohol abuse

Alcohol use appears to have a strong relationship to psychological states, such as depression, which is experienced by many elderly. It has been recognized for some time that psychological illness can adversely affect performance on neuropsychological measures. In particular, there is a growing body of literature focusing on the detrimental impact of depression on neuropsychological performance (Basso & Bornstein, 1999; Rohling, Green, Allen, & Iverson, 2003). Deficits have been noted on more challenging tasks, including those involving executive functioning, problem solving, memory, and attention. There is also empirical support to suggest that depression and age have a synergistic relationship and that depression can produce differentially worse impairments in elderly patients (Boone et al., 1995; King, Caine, & Cox, 1993; King, Cox, Lyness, & Caine, 1995).

Research has revealed that patients with histories of alcohol abuse have a higher prevalence of comorbid psychological disorders than the general population (Helzer & Pryzbeck, 1988; Hesselbrock, Hesselbrock, Tennen, Meyer, & Workman, 1983; Ross, Glaser, & Germanson, 1988; Weisman, Meyers, & Harding, 1980). Specifically, anxiety and depression are frequently associated with chronic alcoholism (Grant, Adams, & Reed, 1986; Løberg, 1981; Merikangas & Gelernter, 1990). In many patients who abuse alcohol, initially high levels of depressive symptoms have been found to decrease after several weeks of abstinence (Brown et al., 1995; Brown & Schuckit, 1988; Dackis, Gold, Pottash, & Sweeney, 1986; Schuckit & Hesselbrock, 1994). However, despite improvement following abstinence, many patients with a history of alcohol abuse continue to experience elevated levels of emotional distress and may meet diagnostic criteria for a mood or other psychiatric disorder (Schuckit et al., 1985; Schuckit, Irwin, & Brown, 1990; Schukit, Irwin, & Smith, 1994).

Patients with comorbid alcohol and psychiatric disorders have heightened severity of alcohol problems (Helzer & Pryzbeck, 1988), increased utilization of treatment services (Ross et al., 1988), and increased relapse rates after treatment (Booth, Yates, Petty, & Brown, 1991; Brown, Irwin, & Schuckit, 1991; Overall, Reilly, Kelley, & Hollister, 1985). Psychological conditions have also been implicated in the initiation and maintenance of alcohol abuse, as alcohol has been implicated as a form of self-medication (Kuschner, Sher, & Beitman, 1990; Weiss & Rosenberg, 1985). These findings are particularly important considering the strong link between depression and recovery from disabilities (Parikh, Lipsey, Robinson, & Price, 1990; Turner & Noh, 1988; Turner & Wood, 1985; Westbrook & Viney, 1982) and the high prevalence of depression in elderly medical patients (Blazer, 1989; Kessler, Foster, Webster, & House, 1992; Koenig et al., 1991; Langer, 1994; Mulsant & Ganguli, 1999), particularly those with stroke (Sinyor, Amato, & Kaloupek, 1986).

There has been more modest research examining the relationship between emotional states and neuropsychological test performance in patients with alcohol abuse. Goldstein, Shelly, Mascia, and Tarter (1985) demonstrated a significant correlation only for a subset of patients with alcoholism who had "psychotic" profiles on the MMPI and measures of neuropsychological functioning. Though this was the first study to show an association between neuropsychological functioning and emotional functioning in persons who abuse alcohol, the use of the MMPI to classify broad profile types was a shortcoming of this investigation. In another study, Johnson-Greene, Adams, Gilman, and Junck (2002) conducted a factor analytic study of the MMPI that showed a relationship between emotional distress and executive dysfunction measured with the Halstead Category Test. This study suggests that there is an association between measures of affective and cognitive functioning in persons with chronic alcohol abuse.

Treatment considerations

Once alcohol problems have been identified in the elderly there are several treatment options that have been shown to be effective. At risk drinkers may benefit from simple, brief interventions that focus on education, assessment, and feedback on the potential for future alcohol-related consequences. Problem drinkers, on the other hand, may benefit from use of contracting, goal setting, and other behavior modification techniques to help curtail drinking. In fact, brief interventions have been successful in reducing consumption in 10–30% of nondependent problem drinkers (Flemming,

Barry, Manwell, Johnson, & London, 1997). Motivational interviewing techniques have also been shown to be effective with problem drinkers (Miller & Rollnick, 1991). The underlying premise for all intervention strategies is to avoid approaches that blame or punish the drinker and focus more on education and mutual exploration of behavior change options. There remains an ongoing debate over the goal of alcohol interventions, with some clinicians promoting abstinence and others focusing on harm reduction as a means of reducing alcohol-related consequences.

Drug abuse

Illicit substance abuse

Epidemiological data suggest that as individuals age, the incidence of illicit drug abuse decreases. Rates of illicit substance abuse are highest in individuals aged 18–25 and tend to decrease steadily across age groups. According to the National Household Survey on Drug Abuse (NHSDA) completed in 2000, an estimated 568,000 individuals aged 55 or older reported past-month illicit drug use (SAMHSA, 2001). This represents approximately 1% of older adults in the United States. Thus, although the rate of illicit substance abuse is significantly lower in this cohort than in younger age groups, it is evident that the problem of substance abuse affects a considerable number of older Americans. The most commonly abused substances by older Americans were marijuana and psychotherapeutic agents used nonmedically, according to the NHSDA report. Use of illicit street drugs is relatively rare in the elderly population and is generally considered a problem of special populations such as elderly prisoners and individuals with a long-term history of opiate addiction (Rosenberg, 1995).

Several reasons have been cited for age-related declines in illicit drug abuse. One theory is the "maturing out" hypothesis, where factors related to the aging process and to duration of substance abuse lead to decreased drug utilization. Such factors include progression to different developmental stages in life, physical limitations, decreased income, risk of criminal prosecution, and mortality related to substance abuse (Allen & Landis, 1997; Gomberg, 1999; Rosenberg, 1995). Similar to the problem noted in elderly problem drinking, underdetection of substance abuse in elderly individuals has also been cited as a reason for the observed decrease in illicit substance abuse over time (Allen & Landis, 1997). Although rates of illicit substance abuse in the elderly are comparatively low, the problem of illicit substance abuse in the elderly is projected to grow as the baby boom generation ages, as there will be a larger number of elderly persons who were exposed to illicit substance abuse in early adulthood (Patterson & Jeste, 1999).

Cognitive effects of illicit substance use

To date, there are no studies addressing the neurocognitive sequelae of illicit substance abuse in the elderly. Studies that have been conducted to determine the lasting neuropsychological effects of substance abuse have been carried out with younger participants and have often been mired with methodological problems such as failure to control for premorbid developmental issues, demographics (age, education), duration of substance abuse, polysubstance use, exposure to adulterants, route of administration, and comorbid medical and psychiatric conditions. Thus, findings of these studies have often been inconclusive or at least equivocal. A review of the literature addressing chronic neuropsychological impairments associated with various classes of illicit substances was completed by Carlin and O'Malley (1996). There is no evidence to suggest that chronic cognitive consequences of drug abuse would be significantly different in the elderly. However, research has neither confirmed nor refuted this postulation. Perhaps as the prevalence of substance abuse in the elderly population increases there will be more research focused on this problem, leading to improved understanding of the neuropsychological and functional consequences of drug abuse specific to elderly patients. Future research in this area will need to control for the cognitive and physiological effects of normal aging in addition to the methodological hurdles noted above.

Prescription and over-the-counter medications

Compared to use of illicit substances, utilization of prescription and over-the-counter (OTC) medications increases dramatically as individuals age. A number of factors combine to increase the risk for misuse or abuse of medication as well as the risk for experiencing adverse medication-related events in elderly patients, such as adverse drug interactions. First, the number of medications taken on a daily basis by elderly individuals is very high. Second, the types of medications prescribed to these patients can often be habit forming (e.g., sedative-hypnotics, opioid analgesics) and are associated with greater impairment of alertness and cognition. Third, age-related pharmacokinetic and pharmacodynamic changes are known to occur, and are often implicated when elderly individuals experience adverse medication-related events. Finally, cognitive changes that can accompany aging can contribute to accidental misuse or abuse of medication.

Epidemiology of medication abuse in older adults

Approximately 35% of all drug prescriptions written in the United States are for older adults (Baum, Kennedy, & Forbes, 1985; Pollock, 1998). The most commonly prescribed drugs are cardiovascular medications, diuretics, antibiotics, analgesics, and psychoactive drugs (Gomberg, 1999). Older Americans are also the largest consumer group of nonprescription medication, with estimates suggesting that approximately two-thirds of individuals over the age of 60 take at least one OTC medication per day (Abrams & Alexopoulos, 1988). Overall, the average number of medications taken by elderly individuals on a daily basis ranges from four to eight (Allen & Landis, 1997). Because the number of medications typically used by older Americans is high, the potential for adverse drug reactions, drug interactions, and accidental as well as overt misuse of medication is elevated, with subsequent cognitive and functional decline possibly resulting.

Classes of medication

In addition to increased use of medications by the elderly, the classes of medications prescribed to these patients is also an important factor contributing to the risk for accidental or overt misuse of medication. Use of centrally acting psychoactive drugs is especially high in the elderly population, with an estimated 25% of all individuals over the age of 55 using this class of medication (Beardsley, Gardocki, Larson, & Hidalgo, 1988). This statistic is particularly important as individuals over the age of 55 report abusing psychotherapeutic agents more frequently than any other drugs (SAMHSA, 2001).

Of the psychoactive medications, sedative-hypnotics are the most commonly prescribed. In fact, benzodiazepines comprise 17–23% of all prescriptions in the elderly (D'Archangelo, 1993). This is not surprising given the affective and behavioral disturbances commonly reported by elderly individuals. Epidemiological studies suggest that the prevalence of anxiety disorders in older Americans is approximately 5.5% (Regier et al., 1998). This figure, however, is considered by many to be low as Generalized Anxiety Disorder was not included in overall anxiety disorder prevalence estimates (Hybels & Blazer, 2003). The prevalence of anxiety symptoms is considered to be even higher in hospitalized or homebound elderly patients than in their less medically compromised counterparts (Bruce & McNamara, 1992; Kvaal, Macijauskiene, Engedal, & Laake, 2001). The prevalence of anxiety symptoms in elderly patients becomes especially important in light of epidemiological research that shows approximately one-fourth of individuals with anxiety disorders also suffer from a substance abuse disorder (Regier et al., 1990).

With respect to behavioral disturbances, sleep changes are among the most common problems in the elderly. Sleep difficulties are known to increase with advancing age and are often associated with the presence of somatic or psychiatric diseases that are disruptive to sleep (Schneider, 2002). Approximately 57% of individuals over the age of 60 report sleep complaints (Foley et al., 1995). Prescription and OTC sedative-hypnotics continue to be commonly utilized to address the sleep problems characteristic of this population. Because they can be habit forming, the potential for misuse or abuse of sedative-hypnotics is high in the elderly population.

Pain is another issue commonly reported by the elderly during visits to medical care providers (Freedman, 2002). There are few epidemiological studies exploring the prevalence of chronic pain in elderly patients, though there is considerable anecdotal evidence to support the claim that chronic pain is highly prevalent in this population. In one epidemiological study in an Australian sample, it was reported that 70% of community-dwelling elderly expected to experience pain with advancing age, and 47% reported actual pain (Helme, Andrews, & Allen, 1992). Given the frequency of pain complaints in elderly patients, opioid analgesics are often prescribed to help ameliorate these symptoms. Potential adverse effects of sedative-hypnotic and opioid analgesic use or misuse by elderly patients will be further addressed in the following sections.

Sedative-hypnotics

Although well warranted in many cases, use of sedative-hypnotics can be especially problematic in the elderly population, as these drugs can be habit-forming and are therefore at high risk for misuse. Benzodiazepine use has been associated with a host of adverse events in older patients. For example, there is an increased risk for falls (Leipzig, Cumming, & Tinetti, 1999; Ray, Thapa, & Gideon, 2000), hip fracture (Cumming & Le Couteur, 2003; Wang, Bohn, Glynn, Mogun, & Avorn, 2001), incontinence (Landi et al., 2002), and involvement in motor vehicle accidents (Hemmelgarn, Suissa, Huang, Boivin, & Pinard, 1997; McGwin, Sims, Pulley, & Roseman, 2000) in elderly individuals using benzodiazepines. The risk of delirium is also elevated in hospitalized elderly patients using benzodiazepines (Francis, Martin, & Kapoor, 1990; Gray, Lai, & Larson, 1999).

Cognitive changes associated with acute and long-term benzodiazepine use have been well documented. In a study by Foy et al. (1995), a temporal and dose-dependent association between benzodiazepine use and decline in the Mini Mental State Exam (MMSE) score was established. Specifically, greater declines in MMSE were found in hospitalized patients whose use of benzodiazepines had been recent. Furthermore, in those patients with positive urinalyses who had reported taking higher doses of benzodiazepine medication (5 mg or more), the odds ratio for cognitive impairment was greater. In addition to decline on general measures of cognition such as the MMSE, researchers have consistently reported impairments in psychomotor speed and delayed memory associated with acute use of benzodiazepines (Greenblatt et al., 1991).

Studies examining the cognitive effects of chronic benzodiazepine use have consistently reported that long-term benzodiazepine use is associated with cognitive decline. Specific cognitive deficits reported in association with long-term benzodiazepine use include impairments in immediate and delayed memory, attention, processing speed, working memory, and visual-spatial skills (Golombok, Moodley, & Lader, 1988; Gorenstein, Paulo, Bernik, Pompeia, & Marcourakis, 1995). Research has also established a generalized cognitive effect of long-term benzodiazepine use. For example, in a meta-analytic study, Barker, Greenwood, Jackson, and Crowe (2004) found significantly greater impairment in each of 12 cognitive domains assessed in long-term benzodiazepine users compared with controls. Given the potential for adverse physical consequences, the potential for short- and long-term cognitive impairment associated with benzodiazepine use, and the potential for abuse of these habit-forming medications, close monitoring is required when using this class of medication with elderly patients. It is suggested that benzodiazepine use in the elderly not exceed four consecutive months (SAMHSA, 1998).

Studies have also investigated the cognitive effects of OTC sedative-hypnotic medications in the elderly. One medication in common use for its sedative-hypnotic qualities in the elderly is diphenhydramine (common brand names are Benadryl, Genahist, Sominex, and Uni-Hist). After controlling for age and gender, diphenhydramine use is associated with an increased risk for cognitive decline as measured by the MMSE in nondemented elderly individuals, and the relationship between severity of cognitive decline and diphenhydramine use appears to be dose dependent (Agostini, Leo-Summers, & Inouye, 2001; Basu, Dodge, Stoehr, & Ganguli, 2003). Again, these findings support the need for close monitoring of medications used for their sedative-hypnotic qualities in elderly patients.

Opioid analgesics

Opioid analgesic medications have a high risk for abuse compared to other medications, and although beneficial in many instances, their use can be associated with adverse events in the elderly. For example, use of opioid analgesic medication by elderly patients increases their risk for respiratory depression (Cepeda et al., 2003), constipation (Staats, Markowitz, & Schein, 2004), and delirium (Davis & Srivastava, 2003). The potential for developing acute neurocognitive effects other than delirium also exists. Specific cognitive findings associated with acute opioid analgesic use include slowed reaction time and psychomotor speed as well as impairments in working and visual memory (Banning, Sjogren, & Kaiser, 1992; Bruera, Macmillan, Hanson, & Macdonald, 1989). Oxycodone, a medication frequently used for treatment of chronic pain, has been shown to produce deficits similar to those related to other opioid analgesics. These deficits include impairment in psychomotor speed, logical reasoning, and hand-eye coordination (Zacny & Gutierrez, 2003).

This section has offered a brief overview of select prescription and OTC medications. For a more comprehensive review, see Stein and Strickland (1998) and Chapter 15 in this volume.

Physiological changes and risk for cognitive decline

A third consideration with respect to medication-associated cognitive decline in elderly patients is the physiological changes that accompany aging. Elderly patients are especially vulnerable to the development of acute confusional states given the physiological changes that affect the body's utilization of medication. Age-related pharmacokinetic and pharmacodynamic changes increase the risk of adverse drug reaction/neurotoxicity with many classes of drugs.

Pharmacokinetics is a term used to describe the plasma concentration of a drug in the body at a given time. Absorption, distribution, metabolism, and clearance of a drug are all aspects of pharmacokinetics, and each can be affected in a unique way by the aging process. Specifically, absorption can be reduced as age advances due to the possible development of dysphagia, age-associated declines in gastric emptying and intestinal motility, increased gastric pH, reductions in absorptive surface area, ingestion of drugs that inhibit absorption (e.g. anticholinergics, antacids), and development of liver, pancreas, or intestinal disease (Zubenko & Sunderland, 2000). Distribution is affected by age-related changes in body composition. As individuals age, the percentage of body fat increases and total water content decreases. Therefore, if a drug is lipophilic (as are most psychotropics), the body will store the drug for a longer period of time, increasing the half-life of the drug and resulting in drug accumulation. In contrast, if a drug is hydrophilic (e.g., lithium), the volume of distribution of that drug will diminish, the half-life of that drug will be shorter, and the window for maintaining appropriate levels will be much smaller.

Metabolism of drugs in the body occurs either through oxidation, reduction, or conjugation. This biotransformation takes place largely in the liver, which is central to the metabolism of virtually all drugs, but especially to the metabolism of psychotropic medications (Lee, 1995; Zubenko & Sunderland, 2000). In elderly patients, metabolism of drugs is a key consideration, as the aging process is associated with a 25–35% decrease in liver size and a 40% decrease in blood flow to the liver (Turnheim, 2003; Zeeh & Platt, 2002). Decreased drug metabolism is associated mainly with the decreased blood flow, as less blood that contains the drug reaches the liver to be cleared (Turnheim, 2003). Thus, aging is associated with a reduction in the rate of metabolism. Finally, clearance of drugs is also affected by the aging process, particularly those drugs eliminated by the kidneys. As with the liver, aging produces a decrease in renal blood flow and glomerular filtration which can lead to decreased drug clearance and subsequent increases in drug serum levels (Turnheim, 2003).

The pharmacodynamic properties of many medications can also be affected by the aging process. *Pharmacodynamics* is a broad term that refers to the biochemical and physiologic effects of drugs and their mechanisms of action. Age-related pharmacodynamic changes may take place at the receptor level, the signal-transduction level, or may occur as the homeostatic mechanisms of the body become less efficient (Turnheim, 2003). As the body ages, the number of dopaminergic, GABAergic, and cholinergic neurons and receptors in the CNS decreases (Turnheim, 2003; Wong, Young, Wilson, Metzler, & Gjedde, 1997). Thus, serum concentrations of drugs acting on these receptors may remain elevated in elderly patients, making the elderly more vulnerable to development of extrapyramidal symptoms and cognitive decline related to drug ingestion.

Anticholinergic effects of medications are of great relevance with respect to elderly patients, as they are cited as one of the most common causes of delirium in the elderly (Cole, 2004). A recent study has established a direct link between serum anticholinergic activity and cognitive impairment in elderly patients (Mulsant et al., 2003). It has been suggested that cognitive impairment results from anticholinergic toxicity with such frequency because many medications have anticholinergic side effects, and increased use of multiple medications can produce an additive effect resulting in cognitive impairment (Tune, 2001). Homeostatic mechanisms such as postural control, orthostatic circulatory control, and thermoregulation are also progressively reduced in the elderly (Pollock, 1998). Due to this reduction in homeostatic mechanisms, a greater length of time may be required to regain the original steady-state of functioning that may have been disrupted by introduction of a pharmacologic agent. Thus, medication side effects may be more pronounced in the elderly, and they are likely to be at increased risk for adverse events related to medication (Turnheim, 2003).

Increased incidence of cognitive impairment

In addition to increased use of medication and physiological changes that may predispose elderly patients to adverse drug reactions, the increased incidence of cognitive impairment in elderly patients heightens their risk for medication misuse. In those who experience cognitive decline, attention and memory impairment may lead to confusion about which medications to take, when to take them, and how often to take them. Thus, the potential for missing doses or taking extra doses of medication exists. Mismanagement of medication can lead to neurotoxicity, adverse drug reactions, and drug–drug interactions which can precipitate or worsen cognitive decline or delirium.

Assessment and treatment implications

Substance abuse assessment in elderly patients should begin with a thorough clinical interview. With elderly patients, special emphasis should be given to specific medications being taken, medication compliance, number of medical providers prescribing medication, and past history of substance abuse. The clinical interview may yield any of a number of red flags, including polypharmacy, lack of an organized system to track medication administration, use of medications with potential for addiction, use of multiple medical providers, or positive history of past substance abuse. If necessary, current substance abuse status might be clarified through assessment with standardized instruments, though, with the exception of instruments assessing potential alcohol abuse, no instruments specific to substance abuse in an elderly population have been developed.

Treatment of substance abuse in the elderly can vary widely depending upon patient characteristics and circumstances. Recommendations might include consultation with medical providers to minimize polypharmacy, reduction in number of providers prescribing medications or appointment of one physician as a coordinator to enhance medication monitoring, and use of a pillbox or other aide in medication administration to strengthen compliance and ensure proper dosing of medications. It is important to note that most elderly individuals who have substance abuse issues do not intend to abuse medications from the outset. Blaming should be avoided in favor of open discussion and education. Treatment modalities are similar to those utilized in the treatment of alcohol abuse. Though not widely available, an increasing number of substance abuse treatment programs aimed at elderly individuals are emerging. Research has demonstrated that elderly patients are likely to be compliant with and respond well to formalized age-specific treatment programs (Allen & Landis, 1997; Stewart & Oslin, 2001).

Conclusions

Many older adults intentionally or unintentionally misuse or abuse alcohol, illicit drugs, or prescription or OTC medications. Misuse or abuse of such substances may both result from and contribute to neurocognitive deficits. Neuropsychologists must assess prior and current substance use as part of any neuropsychological evaluation. In addition, neuropsychologists should be knowledgeable of and be prepared to discuss treatment options with their patients and those involved in their patients' lives.

Acknowledgements

This chapter was supported in part by a grant provided to the first author from the National Institute of Alcohol Abuse and Alcoholism (NIAAA), No. K23AA013898.

References

Abrams, R. C., & Alexopoulos, G. S. (1988). Substance abuse in the elderly: Over-the-counter and illegal drugs. *Hospital and Community Psychiatry, 39*, 822–829.

Adams, K. M., Gilman, S., Koeppe, R. A., Kluin, K. J., Brunberg, J. A., Dede, D., et al. (1993). Neuropsychological deficits are correlated with frontal hypometabolism in positron emission tomography studies of older alcoholic patients. *Alcoholism: Clinical and Experimental Research, 17*, 205–210.

Adams, K. M., Gilman, S., Koeppe, R. A., Kluin, K., Johnson-Greene, D., Berent, S., & Lohman, M. (1995). Frontal lobe hypometabolism measured using [18F] FDG PET among older alcoholic patients. *Neuropsychology, 9*, 275–280.

Adams, W. L., Barry, K. L., & Fleming, M. F. (1996). Screening for problem drinking in older primary care patients. *Journal of the American Medical Association, 276*, 1964–1967.

Adams, W. L., & Cox, N. S. (1995). Epidemiology of problem drinking among elderly people. *International Journal of Addictions, 30*, 1469–1492.

Agostini, J. V., Leo-Summers, L., & Inouye, S. K. (2001). Cognitive and other adverse effects of diphenhydramine use in hospitalized older patients. *Archives of Internal Medicine, 161,* 2091–2097.

Allen, D. N., & Landis, R. K. B. (1997). Substance abuse in elderly individuals. In P. D. Nussbaum (Ed.), *Handbook of neuropsychology and aging* (pp. 111–137). New York: Plenum Press.

American Psychiatric Association. (1994). *Diagnostic and statistical manual of mental disorders* (4th ed.). Washington, DC: Author.

Babor, T. F., de la Fuenta, J. R., Saunders, J., & Grant, M. (1992). *AUDIT: The Alcohol Use Disorders Identification Test: Guidelines for its use in primary health care.* Geneva, Switzerland: World Health Organization.

Banning, A., Sjogren, P., & Kaiser, F. (1992). Reaction time in cancer patients receiving peripherally acting analgesics alone or in combination with opioids. *Acta Anaesthesiologica Scandinavica, 36,* 480–482.

Barker, M. J., Greenwood, K. M., Jackson, M., & Crowe, S. F. (2004). Persistence of cognitive effects after withdrawal from long-term benzodiazepine use: A meta-analysis. *Archives of Clinical Neuropsychology, 19*(3), 437–454.

Bassett, S. S., Chase, G. A., Folstein, M. F., & Reiger, D. A. (1998). Disability and psychiatric disorders in an urban community: Measurement, prevalence, and outcomes. *Psychological Medicine, 28,* 509–517.

Basso, M. R., & Bornstein, R. A. (1999). Neuropsychological deficits in psychotic versus non-psychotic unipolar depression. *Neuropsychology, 13,* 69–75.

Basu, R., Dodge, H., Stoehr, G. P., & Ganguli, M. (2003). Sedative-hypnotic use of diphenhydramine in a rural, older adult, community-based cohort: Effects on cognition. *American Journal of Geriatric Psychiatry, 11,* 205–213.

Baum, C., Kennedy, D. L., & Forbes, M. B. (1985). Drug utilization in the geriatric age group. In S. R. Moore & T. W. Teal (Eds.), *Geriatric drug use: Clinical and social perspectives* (pp. 63–69). New York: Pergamon.

Beardsley, R. S., Gardocki, G. L., Larson, D. B., & Hidalgo, J. (1988). Prescribing of psychotropic medication by primary care physicians and psychiatrists. *Archives of General Psychiatry, 45,* 1117–1119.

Bernstein, R. (1995, May). *Sixty-five plus in the United States* (Statistical brief). Washington, DC: US Census Bureau.

Blazer, D. (1989). The epidemiology of depression in late life. *Geriatric Psychiatry, 22,* 35–52.

Blow, F. C., Brower, K. J., Schulenberg, J. E., Demo-Dananberg, L. M., Young, J. P., & Beresford, T. P. (1992). The Michigan Alcohol Screening Test—Geriatric version (MAST-G): A newly elderly-specific screening instrument. *Alcoholism: Clinical and Experimental Research, 16,* 372.

Bombardier, C., & Rimmele, C. (1998). Alcohol use and readiness to change after spinal cord injury. *Archives of Physical Medicine and Rehabilitation, 79,* 1110–1115.

Boone, K. B., Lesser, I. M., Miller, B. L., Wohl, M., Berman, N., Lee, A., et al. (1995). Cognitive functioning in older depressed outpatients: Relationship of presence and severity of depression to neuropsychological test scores. *Neuropsychology, 9,* 390–398.

Booth, B. M., Yates, W. R., Petty, F., & Brown K. (1991). Patient factors predicting early alcohol-related readmissions for alcoholics: Role of alcoholism severity and psychiatric co-morbidity. *Journal of Studies on Alcohol, 52,* 37–43.

Brennan, P. L., Kagay, C. R., Geppert, J. J., & Moos, R. H. (2000). Elderly Medicare inpatients with substance use disorders: Characteristics and predictors of hospital readmissions over a four-year interval. *Journal of Studies on Alcohol, 61*(6), 891–895.

Brown, S. A., Inaba, R. K., Gillin, J. C., Schuckit, M. A., Stewart, M. A., & Irwin, M. R. (1995). Alcoholism and affective disorder: Clinical course of depressive symptoms. *American Journal of Psychiatry, 152*, 45–52.

Brown, S. A., Irwin, M., & Schuckit, M. A. (1991). Changes in anxiety among abstinent male alcoholics. *Journal of Studies on Alcohol, 52*, 55–61.

Brown, S. A., & Schuckit, M. A. (1988). Changes in depression among abstinent alcoholics. *Journal of Studies on Alcohol, 49*, 412–417.

Bruce, M. L., & McNamara, R. (1992). Psychiatric status among the homebound elderly: An epidemiologic perspective. *Journal of the American Geriatrics Society, 40*, 561–566.

Bruera, E., Macmillan, K., Hanson, J., & Macdonald, R. N. (1989). The cognitive effects of the administration of narcotic analgesics in patients with cancer pain. *Pain, 39*, 13–16.

Bucholz, K. K., Sheline, Y. I., & Helzer, J. E. (1995). The epidemiology of alcohol use, problems, and dependence in elders: A review. In T. Beresford & E. Gomberg (Eds.), *Alcohol and aging* (pp. 19–41). New York: Oxford University Press.

Carlin, A. S., & O'Malley, S. (1996). Neuropsychological consequences of drug abuse. In I. Grant & K. M. Adams (Eds.), *Neuropsychological assessment of neuropsychiatric disorders* (2nd ed., pp. 486–503). New York: Oxford University Press.

Cepeda, M. S., Farrar, J. T., Baumgarten, M., Boston, R., Carr, D. B., & Strom, B. L. (2003). Side effects of opioids during short-term administration: Effect of age, gender, and race. *Clinical Pharmacology and Therapeutics, 74*(2), 102–112.

Charlifue, S., & Gerhart, K. (1991). Behavioral and demographic predictors of suicide after spinal cord injury. *Archives of Physical Medicine and Rehabilitation, 72*, 488–492.

Christian, J. C., Reed, T., Carmelli, D., Page, W. F., Norton, J. A., & Breitner, J. C. S. (1995). Self-reported alcohol intake and cognition in aging twins. *Journal of Studies on Alcohol, 56*, 414–416.

Clay, S. W. (1997). Comparison of AUDIT and CAGE questionnaires in screening for alcohol use disorders in elderly primary care outpatients. *Journal of the American Osteopathic Association, 10*, 588–592.

Coffey, C. E., Wildinson, W. E., Parashos, L. A., Soady, S. A. R., Sullivan, R. J., Patterson, L. J., et al. (1992). Quantitative cerebral anatomy of the aging human brain: A cross-sectional study using magnetic resonance imaging. *Neurology, 42*, 527–536.

Cole, M. G. (2004). Delirium in elderly patients. *American Journal of Geriatric Psychiatry, 12*, 7–21.

Corrigan, J. D. (1995). Substance abuse as a mediating factor in outcome from traumatic brain injury. *Archives of Physical Medicine and Rehabilitation, 76*, 302–309.

Corrigan, J. D., Rust, E., & Lamb-Hart, G. (1995). The nature and extent of substance abuse problems in persons with traumatic brain injury. *Journal of Head Trauma Rehabilitation, 10*, 29–46.

Courville, C. B. (1955). *Effects of alcohol in the central nervous system of man.* Los Angeles: San Lucas Press.

Cumming, R. G., & LeCouteur, D. G. (2003). Benzodiazepines and risk of hip fracture in older people: A review of the evidence. *CNS Drugs, 17*, 825–837.

Dackis, C. A., Gold, M. S., Pottash, A. L., & Sweeney, D. R. (1986). Evaluating depression in alcoholics. *Psychiatry Research, 17*, 105–109.

D'Archangelo, E. (1993). Substance abuse in later life. *Canadian Family Physician*, *39*, 1986–1993.

Davis, M. P., & Srivastava, M. (2003). Demographics, assessment and management of pain in the elderly. *Drugs and Aging*, *20*, 23–57.

Dikmen, S., Donovan, D., Loberg, T., Machmer, J., & Temkin, N. (1993). Alcohol use and its effects on neuropsychological outcome in head injury. *Neuropsychology*, *7*, 296–305.

Elie, M., Cole, M. G., & Primeau, F. J. (1998). Delirium risk factors in elderly hospitalized patients. *Journal of General Internal Medicine*, *13*, 204–212.

Ewing, J. A. (1984). Detecting alcoholism: The CAGE Questionnaire. *Journal of the American Medical Association*, *252*, 1905–1907.

Fauerbach, J. A., Engrav, L., & Kowalske, K. (2001). Barriers to employment among working-aged patients with major burn injury. *Journal of Burn Care Rehabilitation*, *22*, 26–34.

Fink, A., Hays, R. D., Moore, A. A., & Beck, J. C. (1996). Alcohol-related problems on older persons: Determinants, consequences, and screening. *Archives of Internal Medicine*, *156*, 1150–1156.

Fleming, M. F., Barry, K. L., Manwell, L. B., Johnson, K., & London, R. (1997). Brief physician advice for problem alcohol drinkers: A randomized controlled trial in community-based primary care practices. *Journal of the American Medical Association*, *277*, 1039–1045.

Foley, D. J., Monjan, A. A., Brown, S. L., Sinonsick, E. M., Wallace, R. B., & Blazer, D. G. (1995). Sleep complaints among elderly persons: An epidemiologic study of three communities. *Sleep*, *18*, 425–432.

Foy, A., O'Connell, D., Henry, D., Kelly, J., Cocking, S., & Halliday, J. (1995). Benzodiazepine use as a cause of cognitive impairment in elderly hospital inpatients. *Journal of Gerontology: Medical Sciences*, *50A*, M99–M106.

Francis, J., Martin, D., & Kapoor, W. N. (1990). A prospective study of delirium in hospitalized elderly. *Journal of the American Medical Association*, *263*, 1097–1101.

Freedman, G. M. (2002). Chronic pain: Clinical management of common causes of geriatric pain. *Geriatrics*, *57*(5), 36–41.

Freund, G. (1982). The interaction of chronic alcohol consumption and aging on brain structure and function. *Alcoholism Clinical and Experimental Research*, *6*, 13–21.

Goldstein, G., Shelly, C., Mascia, G. V., & Tarter, R. E. (1985). Relationships between neuropsychological and psychopathological dimensions in male alcoholics. *Addictive Behavior*, *10*, 365–372.

Golombok, S., Moodley, P., & Lader, M. (1988). Cognitive impairment in long-term benzodiazepine users. *Psychological Medicine*, *18*, 365–374.

Gomberg, E. S. L. (1995). Older women and alcohol use and abuse. In M. Galanter (Ed.), *Recent developments in alcoholism: Vol. 12. Alcoholism and women* (pp. 61–79). New York: Plenum Press.

Gomberg, E. S. L. (1999). Substance abuse in the elderly. In P. J. Ott & R. E. Tarter (Eds.), *Sourcebook on substance abuse: Etiology, epidemiology, assessment, and treatment* (pp. 113–125). Needham Heights, MA: Allyn & Bacon.

Gorenstein, C., Paulo, B., Bernik, M. A., Pompeia, S., & Marcourakis, T. (1995). Impairment of performance associated with long-term use of benzodiazepines. *Journal of Psychopharmacology*, *9*, 313–318.

Grant, I., Adams, K. A., & Reed, R. (1986). Intermediate-duration (subacute) organic mental disorder of alcoholism. In I. Grant (Ed.), *Neuropsychiatric correlates of alcoholism* (pp. 37–60). Washington, DC: American Psychiatric Press.

Gray, S. L., Lai, K. V., & Larson, E. B. (1999). Drug-induced cognition disorders in the elderly: Incidence, prevention, and management. *Drug Safety, 21*, 101–122.

Greenblatt, D. J., Harmatz, J. S., Shapiro, L., Engelhardt, N., Gouthro, T. A., & Shader, R. I. (1991). Sensitivity to triazolam in the elderly. *New England Journal of Medicine, 324*, 1691–1698.

Grobmyer, S. R., Maniscalco, S. P., Purdue, G. F., & Hunt, J. L. (1996). Alcohol, drug intoxication, or both at the time of burn injury as a predictor of complications and mortality in hospitalized patients with burns. *Journal of Burn Care Rehabilitation, 17*, 532–539.

Harper, C., Sheedy, D., Halliday, G., Double, K., Dodd, P., Lewohl, J., & Kril, J. (1998). Neuropathological studies: The relationship between alcohol and aging. In E. Gomberg, A. Hegedus, & R. Zucker (Eds.), *Alcohol problems and aging research* (Monograph 33) (pp. 117–134). Bethesda, MD: US Department of Health and Human Services.

Harper, C. G., & Kril, J. (1989). Patterns of neuronal loss in the cerebral cortex in chronic alcoholic patients. *Journal of Neurological Science, 92*, 81–89.

Harper, C. G., & Kril, J. (1991). If you drink your brain will shrink: Neuropathological considerations. *Alcohol and Alcoholism, 1*(Suppl.), 375–380.

Heinemann, A., Goranson, N., Ginsburg, K., & Schnoll, S. (1989). Alcohol use and activity patterns following spinal cord injury. *Rehabilitation Psychology, 34*, 191–206.

Heinemann, A., Keen, M., Donohue, R., & Schnoll, S. (1988). Alcohol use in persons with recent spinal cord injuries. *Archives of Physical Medicine and Rehabilitation, 69*, 619–624.

Helme, R. D., Andrews, P. V., & Allen, F. (1992). Medication use by elderly people resident in public housing in Melbourne. *Proceedings of the Australian Association of Gerontologists, 27*, 30–33.

Helzer, J. E., & Pryzbeck, T. R. (1988). The co-occurrence of alcoholism with other psychiatric disorders in the general population and its impact on treatment. *Journal of Studies on Alcohol, 49*, 219–224.

Hemmelgarn, B., Suissa, S., Huang, A., Boivin, J. F., & Pinard, G. (1997). Benzodiazepine use and the risk of motor vehicle crash in the elderly. *Journal of the American Medical Association, 278*, 27–31.

Hesselbrock, M. N., Hesselbrock, V. M., Tennen, H., Meyer, R. E., & Workman, K. L. (1983). Methodological considerations in the assessment of depression in alcoholics. *Journal of Consulting and Clinical Psychology, 51*, 399–405.

Higgins, J. P., Wright, S. W., & Wrenn, K. D. (1996). Alcohol, the elderly, and motor vehicle crashes. *American Journal of Emergency Medicine, 14*, 265–267.

Hobbs, F. B. (1995). *The elderly population* (Statistical brief). Washington, DC: US Census Bureau.

Holroyd, S., & Currie, L. (1997). A descriptive study of elderly community-dwelling alcoholic patients in the rural south. *American Journal of Geriatric Psychiatry, 5*, 221–228.

Holroyd, S., & Duryee, J. J. (1997). Substance use disorders in a geriatric psychiatry outpatient clinic: Prevalence and epidemiologic characteristics. *American Journal of Geriatric Psychiatry, 5*, 221–228.

Hybels, C. F., & Blazer, D. G. (2003). Epidemiology of late-life mental disorders. *Clinical Geriatric Medicine*, *19*(4), 663–696.

Jernigan, T. L., Butters, N., DiTriaglia, G., Schafer, K., Smith, T., Irwin, M., et al. (1991). Reduced cerebral grey matter observed in alcoholics using magnetic resonance imaging. *Alcoholism Clinical and Experimental Research*, *15*, 418–427.

Jernigan, T. L., Schafer, K., Butters, N., & Cermak, L. S. (1991). Magnetic resonance imaging of alcoholic Korsakoff's patients. *Neuropsychopharmacology*, *4*, 175–186.

Johnson-Greene, D., Adams, K. M., Gilman, S., & Junck, L. (2002). Relationship between neuropsychological and emotional functioning in severe chronic alcoholism. *The Clinical Neuropsychologist*, *16*, 300–309.

Johnson-Greene, D., Adams, K. M., Gilman, S., Kluin, K., Junck, L., Martorello, S., & Heumann, M. (1997). Impaired upper limb coordination in alcoholic cerebellar degeneration. *Archives of Neurology*, *54*, 436–439.

Johnson-Greene, D., Adams, K. M., Gilman, S., Koeppe, R. A., Kluin, K., Junck, L., & Lohman, M. (1997). Effects of abstinence and relapse upon neuropsychological function and cerebral glucose metabolism in severe chronic alcoholism. *Journal of Clinical and Experimental Neuropsychology*, *22*, 378–385.

Jurkovich, G. J., Rivera, F. P., Gurney, J. G., Seguin, D., Fligner, C. L., & Copass, M. (1992). Effects of alcohol intoxication on the initial assessment of trauma patients. *Annals of Emergency Medicine*, *21*, 704–708.

Kaplan, C., & Corrigan, J. (1992). Effect of blood alcohol level on recovery from severe closed head injury. *Brain Injury*, *6*, 337–349.

Kelley, D., & Lynch, J. (1992). Burns in alcohol and drug users result in longer treatment times with more complications. *Journal of Burn Care Rehabilitation*, *13*, 218–220.

Kemp, B., Brumel-Smith, K., & Ramsdell, J. (1990). *Geriatric rehabilitation*. Boston: Little Brown Co.

Kessler, R. C., Foster, C., Webster, P. S., & House, J. S. (1992). The relationship between age and depressive symptoms in two national surveys. *Psychological Aging*, *7*, 119–126.

King, D. A., Caine, E. D., & Cox, C. (1993). Influence of depression and age on selected cognitive functions. *The Clinical Neuropsychologist*, *7*, 443–453.

King, D. A., Cox, C., Lyness, J. M., & Caine, E. D. (1995). Neuropsychological effects of depression and age in an elderly sample: A confirmatory study. *Neuropsychology*, *9*, 399–408.

Kiwerski, J., & Krasuski, M. (1992). Influence of alcohol intake on the course and consequences of spinal cord injury. *International Journal of Rehabilitation Research*, *15*, 240–245.

Koenig, H. G., Meador, K. G., Shelp, F., Goli, V., Cohen, H. J., & Blazer, D. G. (1991). Major depressive disorder in hospitalized medically ill patients: An examination of young and elderly male veterans. *Journal of the American Geriatrics Society*, *39*, 881.

Kril, J., & Harper, C. G. (1989). Neuronal counts from four cortical regions of alcoholic brains. *Acta Neuropathologia*, *79*, 200–204.

Kuschner, M. G., Sher, K. J., & Beitman, B. D. (1990). The relation between alcohol problems and the anxiety disorders. *American Journal of Psychology*, *147*, 685–695.

Kvaal, K., Macijauskiene, J., Engedal, K., & Laake, K. (2001). High prevalence of anxiety symptoms in hospitalized geriatric patients. *International Journal of Geriatric Psychiatry*, *16*(7), 690–693.

Landi, F., Cesari, M., Russo, A., Onder, G., Sgadari, A., & Bernabei, R., on behalf of the Silvernet-HC Study Group. (2002). Benzodiazepines and risk of urinary incontinence in frail older persons living in the community. *Clinical Pharmacology and Therapeutics, 72,* 729–734.

Langer, K. G. (1994). Depression in disabling illness: Severity and patterns of self-reported symptoms in three groups. *Journal of Geriatric Psychiatry and Neurology, 7,* 121.

Lee, W. M. (1995). Drug-induced hepatotoxicity. *New England Journal of Medicine, 333,* 1118–1127.

Leipzig, R. M., Cumming, R. G., & Tinetti, M. E. (1999). Drugs and falls in older people: A systematic review and meta-analysis: I. Psychotropic drugs. *Journal of the American Geriatrics Society, 47,* 30–39.

Leuchter, A. F., Dunkin, J. J., Lufkin, R. B., Anzai, Y., Cook, I. A., & Newton, T. F. (1994). Effect of white matter disease on functional connections in the aging brain. *Journal of Neurology, Neurosurgery, and Psychiatry, 57,* 1347–1354.

Løberg, T. (1981). MMPI-based personality subtypes of alcoholics. *Journal of Studies on Alcohol, 42,* 766–782.

McGwin, G., Jr., Sims, R. V., Pulley, L., & Roseman, J. M. (2000). Relations among chronic medical conditions, medications, and automobile crashes in the elderly: A population-based case-control study. *American Journal of Epidemiology, 152,* 424–431.

Merikangas, K. R., & Gelernter, C. S. (1990). Comorbidity for alcoholism and depression. *Psychiatric Clinics of North America, 13,* 613–632.

Miller, W. R., & Brown, S. (1997). Why psychologists should treat alcohol and drug problems. *American Psychologist, 52,* 1269–1279.

Miller, W. R., & Rollnick, S. (1991). *Motivational interviewing.* New York: Guilford Press.

Mulsant, B. H., & Ganguli, M. (1999). Epidemiology and diagnosis of depression in late life. *Journal of Clinical Psychiatry, 60*(Suppl. 20), 9–15.

Mulsant, B. H., Pollock, B. G., Kirshner, M., Shen, C., Dodge, H., & Ganguli, M. (2003). Serum anticholinergic activity in a community-based sample of older adults. *Archives of General Psychiatry, 60,* 198–203.

Oslin, D. W., Streim, J. E., Parmelee, P., Boyce, A. A., & Katz, I. R. (1997). Alcohol abuse: A source of reversible functional disability among residents of a VA nursing home. *International Journal of Geriatric Psychiatry, 12,* 825–832.

Overall, J. E., Reilly, E. L., Kelley, J. T., & Hollister, L. E. (1985). Persistence of depression in detoxified alcoholics. *Alcoholism Clinical and Experimental Research, 9,* 331–333.

Parikh, R. M., Lipsey, J. R., Robinson, R. G., & Price, T. R. (1990). Post-stroke depression: Impact on daily living over two years. *Archives of Neurology, 47,* 785–790.

Patterson, T. L., & Jeste, D. V. (1999). The potential impact of the baby-boom generation on substance abuse among elderly persons. *Psychiatric Services, 50,* 1184–1188.

Pfefferbaum, A., Lim, K. O., Zipursky, R. B., Mathalon, D. H., Rosenbloom, M. J., Lane, B., et al. (1992). Brain grey and white matter volume loss accelerates with aging in chronic alcoholics: A quantitative MRI study. *Alcoholism Clinical and Experimental Research, 16,* 1078–1089.

Pollock, B. G. (1998). Psychotropic drugs and the aging patient. *Geriatrics, 53*(Suppl. 1), S20–S24.

Ray, W. A., Thapa, P. B., & Gideon, P. (2000). Benzodiazepines and the risk of falls in nursing home residents. *Journal of the American Geriatrics Society, 48*, 682–685.

Regier, D. A., Farmer, M. E., Rae, D. S., Locke, B. Z., Keith, S. J., Judd, L. L., & Goodwin, F. K. (1990). Comorbidity of mental disorders with alcohol and other drug abuse. *Journal of the American Medical Association, 264*, 2511–2518.

Regier, D. A., Kaelber, C. T., Rae, D. S., Farmer, M. E., Knauper, B., Kessler, R. C., et al. (1998). Limitations of diagnostic criteria and assessment instruments for mental disorders: Implications for research and policy. *Archives of General Psychiatry, 55*, 109–115.

Reid, M. C., & Anderson, P. A. (1997). Geriatric substance abuse disorders. *Medical Clinics of North America, 81*, 999–1016.

Rivara, F., Jurkovich, G., Gurney, J., Seguin, D., Flinger, C., Ries, R., et al. (1993). The magnitude of acute and chronic alcohol abuse in trauma patients. *Archives of Surgery, 128*, 907–913.

Rohling, M. L., Green, P., Allen, L. M., & Iverson, G. L. (2003). Depressive symptoms and neurocognitive test scores in patients passing symptom validity tests. *Archives of Clinical Neuropsychology, 17*, 205–222.

Rosenberg, H. (1995). The elderly and the use of illicit drugs: Sociological and epidemiological considerations. *International Journal of the Addictions, 30*, 1925–1951.

Ross, H. E., Glaser, F. B., & Germanson, T. (1988). The prevalence of psychiatric disorders in patients with alcohol and other drug problems. *Archives of General Psychiatry, 45*, 1023–1031.

Schneider, D. L. (2002). Insomnia: Safe and effective therapy for sleep problems in the older patient. *Geriatrics, 57*, 24–35.

Schuckit, M. A., & Hesselbrock, V. (1994). Alcohol dependence and anxiety disorders: What is the relationship? *American Journal of Psychiatry, 15*, 1723–1734.

Schuckit, M. A., Hesselbrock, V. M., Tipp, J., Nurnberger, J. I., Anthenelli, R. M., & Crowe, R. R. (1985). The prevalence of major anxiety disorders in relatives of alcohol dependent men and woman. *Journal of Studies on Alcohol, 56*, 309–317.

Schuckit, M. A., Irwin, M., & Brown, S. A. (1990). The history of anxiety symptoms among 171 primary alcoholics. *Journal of Studies on Alcohol, 51*, 34–41.

Schuckit, M. A., Irwin, M., & Smith, T. (1994). One-year incidence rate of major depression and other psychiatric disorders in 239 alcoholic men. *Addiction, 89*, 441–445.

Sinyor, D., Amato, P., & Kaloupek, D. (1986). Post-stroke depression: Relationship to functional impairment, coping strategies, and rehabilitation outcome. *Stroke, 17*, 1102–1107.

Smith, J. W. (1995). Medical manifestations of alcoholism in the elderly. *International Journal of Addictions, 30*, 1749–1798.

Soderstrom, C., Smith, G., Dischinger, P., McDuff, D., Hebel, J., Golick, D., et al. (1997). Psychoactive substance abuse disorders among seriously injured trauma center patients. *Journal of the American Medical Association, 277*, 1769–1774.

Staats, P. S., Markowitz, J., & Schein, J. (2004). Incidence of constipation associated with long-acting opioid therapy: A comparative study. *Southern Medical Journal, 97*, 129–134.

Stein, R. A., & Strickland, T. L. (1998). A review of the neuropsychological effects of commonly used prescription medications. *Archives of Clinical Neuropsychology, 13*, 259–284.

Stewart, D., & Oslin, D. W. (2001). Recognition and treatment of late-life addictions in medical settings. *Journal of Clinical Geropsychology, 7*(2), 145–158.

Substance Abuse and Mental Health Services Administration. (1998). *Substance abuse among older adults: Treatment Improvement Protocol (TIP) Series 26* (DHHS Publication No. SMA 98-3179). Rockville, MD: Author.

Substance Abuse and Mental Health Services Administration. (2001). *Summary of findings from the 2000 National Household Survey on Drug Abuse* (NHSDA Series: H-13, DHHS Publication No. SMA 01-3549). Rockville, MD: Author.

Tune, L. E. (2001). Anticholinergic effects of medication in elderly patients. *Journal of Clinical Psychiatry, 62*(Suppl. 21), 11–14.

Turner, R. J., & Noh, S. (1988). Physical disability and depression: Longitudinal analysis. *Journal of Health and Social Behavior, 29*, 23–37.

Turner, R. J., & Wood, D. W. (1985). Depression and disability: The stress process in a chronically strained population. In J. R. Greenley (Ed.), *Research in community and mental health* (Vol. V, pp. 77–109). Greenwich, CT: JAI Press.

Turnheim, K. (2003). When drug therapy gets old: Pharmacokinetics and pharmaco-dynamics in the elderly. *Experimental Gerontology, 38*, 843–853.

US Senate Special Committee on Aging. (1987–1988). *Aging America, 1988: Trends and projections.* Washington, DC: US Department of Health and Human Services.

Wang, P. S., Bohn, R. L., Glynn, R. J., Mogun, H., & Avorn, J. (2001). Hazardous benzodiazepine regimens in the elderly: Effects of half-life, dosage, and duration on risk of hip fracture. *American Journal of Psychiatry, 158*, 892–898.

Weisman, M. M., Meyers, J. K., & Harding, P. S. (1980). Prevalence and psychiatric heterogeneity of alcoholism in United States urban community. *Journal of Studies on Alcoholism, 41*, 672–681.

Weiss, K. J., & Rosenberg, D. J. (1985). Prevalence of anxiety disorder among alcoholics. *Journal of Clinical Psychiatry, 46*, 3–5.

Westbrook, M. T., & Viney, L. L. (1982). Psychological reactions to the onset of chronic illness. *Social Science and Medicine, 16*, 899–905.

Wiggins, R. C., Gorman, A., Rolsten, C., Samorajski, T., Ballinger, W. E. J., & Freund, G. (1988). Effects of aging and alcohol on the biochemical composition of histologically normal human brain. *Metabolism and Brain Disease, 3*, 67–80.

Wong, D. F., Young, D., Wilson, P. D., Metzler, C. C., & Gjedde, A. (1997). Quantification of neuroreceptors in the living human brain: III. D_2-like dopamine receptors: Theory, validation, and changes during normal aging. *Journal of Cerebral Blood Flow and Metabolism, 17*, 316–330.

Zacny, J. P., & Gutierrez, S. (2003). Characterizing the subjective, psychomotor, and physiological effects of oral oxycodone in non-drug-abusing volunteers. *Psychopharmacology, 170*, 242–254.

Zeeh, J., & Platt, D. (2001). The aging liver: Structural and functional changes and their consequences for drug treatment. *Gerontology, 48*, 121–127.

Zubenko, G. S., & Sunderland, T. (2000). Geriatric psychopharmacology: Why does age matter? Harvard Review of Psychiatry, 7, 311–333.

17 Neuropsychologists as family service providers after the onset of neurological disorders in older adults

Laura A. Taylor, Lee A. Livingston, Jeffrey S. Kreutzer, and Deborah D. West

With advances in health care, the population of elderly persons is growing world-wide. As the population ages, rates of geriatric neuropsychological disorders also increase, including Alzheimer's disease, Parkinson's disease, traumatic brain injury (TBI), cerebrovascular accidents (CVA), and brain tumors. Concomitant problems often include depression, anxiety, neurobehavioral problems, substance misuse, pain, sleep problems, safety issues, and impairments in judgment.

Increasingly, family members are taking on caregiving roles for their elderly relatives. Research reveals that the vast majority of elderly individuals 65 years or older continue to live in the community, with the assistance of family and friends (American Association of Retired Persons, 1997; National Alliance for Caregiving, 1997; Stevens, Walsh, & Baldwin, 1993; Wallhagen, 1992; Wilson & Trost, 1987). A recent report by the National Alliance for Caregiving and the American Association of Retired Persons (2004) estimates approximately 44.4 million American adults (21% of the adult population) are providing care to another adult on an unpaid basis. The 2004 report was based upon a national survey in which 1237 caregivers were interviewed. Results revealed that 79% of the individuals receiving care are 50 years and older, with a mean age of 75. Within this sample, the primary problems necessitating care among adults ages 50 and older included the following: Alzheimer's disease, dementia, or other condition resulting in mental confusion (25%); aging (15%); diabetes; cancer; and heart disease.

Many families have difficulty coping with the increasing burdens and stress associated with caring for and supporting elderly relatives with neuropsychological disorders. Neuropsychologists are in a unique position to evaluate, support, and treat geriatric patients and their family members. This chapter will review the literature on the family members' responses to neuropsychological disorders, family members' needs, the neuropsychologist's role in helping families, family assessment issues, and methods of intervention. Much of the information presented in this chapter will be focused on the primary caregiver.

Family issues, reactions, and needs

Family life cycle issues

The impact of neurological illness and injury on a family depends greatly upon the stage in which the individual family members are within their life cycle (Barth, 1996). For example, middle-aged children of elderly patients are in the prime of caring for their immediate family, often including young children or adolescents. Focused on the needs of their offspring, middle-aged adults may feel unprepared to provide additional care and attention to an elderly parent with neuropsychological problems. Similarly, an older person is often looking forward to or enjoying retirement after focusing on his or her career for decades. Being diagnosed with a neurological condition can have devastating effects on the patient, his or her siblings, or a spouse. Expectations of having years of satisfying retirement may be dashed when an elderly relative requires full-time care and daily living assistance. Hopes and plans for the future are prematurely lost when disability precedes the natural life cycle for such a circumstance.

Defining extended families and their roles

Shifts in typical roles and responsibilities of family members are often necessitated by the caregiving needs of an elderly relative with neurological problems. To facilitate change in family roles, clinicians may encourage the inclusion of extended family members in long-term care provision. Clinicians help to redefine and reassign family responsibilities in therapy or family meetings. Fortifying an extended network of family members provides the primary caregiver or caregivers with access to respite and additional means of emotional support (Kreutzer, Zasler, Camplair, & Leininger, 1990).

Family reactions

Delineating the sociocultural aspects of the American caregiver offers context for appreciating the needs and reactions of family members providing informal care to geriatric patients with neurological illness or injury. Of the millions of unpaid family caregivers in America, the typical caregiver profile is a 46-year-old woman spending an average of 20 hours or more per week providing in-home care to an elderly person (National Alliance for Caregiving & AARP, 2004). The majority of these women balance numerous responsibilities at work and at home, including housekeeping, managing finances, transporting the patient to appointments, providing home-health care, and encouraging recreational and social opportunities.

Among the first to describe the relationship between the sequelae of neurological illness or injury and family adjustment, Lezak (1978, 1986, 1988) proposed that treatment providers be alert for common family reactions, the role of family expectations, and the prevalence of depression. Another early finding reported in the scientific literature is that family members are often more disturbed by disruptions to the patient's personality than to physical changes (Brooks & Aughton, 1979; Lezak, 1978; Thomsen, 1984). Specifically, neurobehavioral (Ergh, Rapport, Coleman, & Hanks, 2002) and affective difficulties (Miller, Berrios, & Politynska, 1996) demonstrated by persons with neurological illness or damage appear related to psychological distress for primary caregivers and families. Remarkably, studies examining caregiver distress and recency of brain injury (Kreutzer, Gervasio, & Camplair, 1994) or severity of neurological trauma (Knight, Devereux, & Godfrey, 1998; McKinlay, Brooks, Bond, Martinage, & Marshall, 1981; Rosenbaum & Nanjenson, 1976) have generally failed to find a strong association between these factors.

Family caregivers are apt to incur increased problems with their physical functioning and health (Draper, Poulos, Poulos, & Ehrlich, 1996; Pinquart & Sorensen, 2003; Stone, Cafferata, & Singh, 1987). In addition to an increased risk for physical disease, elderly caregivers have a higher mortality rate compared to their noncaregiving peers (Schulz & Beach, 1999; Schulz, O'Brien, Bookwala, & Fleissner, 1995). Loss of sleep, exhaustion, and fatigue are commonly reported by primary caregivers due to the overwhelming burden of providing constant care to elderly relatives (Schur & Whitlatch, 2003).

Psychological and emotional functioning is another important area in caregiver research. For example, Morgan and Laing (1991) investigated factors related to perceived emotional burden in spouses providing informal care to patients with Alzheimer's disease. These researchers found shock, disbelief, and denial were associated with an increased sense of caregiver burden. History of a loving marital relationship was correlated with a lower sense of burden and stress for spouses in the study. Hirschfeld (2003) also investigated the reactions of family members caring for elderly relatives with neurological illness such as Alzheimer's disease, multi-infarct dementia, or other chronic brain syndromes. Feelings of resentment, helplessness, hopelessness, and guilt were major areas of family tension in this sample of caregivers. Maintaining a sense of mutuality (i.e., reciprocity and gratification from the relationship with the impaired person) and finding meaning in the caregiving role were factors mediating negative reactions of family members. In a meta-analysis of 84 caregiving research articles, Pinquart and Sorensen (2003) discovered the largest differences between caregivers and noncaregivers in regard to perceived levels of depression, general subjective well-being, stress, and self-efficacy.

Family needs

The 2004 report on caregiving conducted by the National Alliance for Caregiving and the American Association of Retired Persons highlighted the unmet needs of caregivers. Among the most commonly reported unmet needs were setting aside time for oneself (35%), balancing responsibilities at work and home (29%), and dealing with emotional distress and physical stress

(29%). Other needs included: help ensuring safety of the person for whom they are providing care (30%); finding activities to engage in with the person for whom they are caring (27%); talking with health care professionals (22%); and making decisions about end-of-life issues (20%).

Several studies have been conducted examining the needs of family members providing care to elderly individuals with Alzheimer's disease (Beisecker, Chrisman, & Wright, 1997; Bowd & Loos, 1996; Fortinsky & Hathaway, 1990; Francis & Munjas, 1992; Smith, Lauret, Peery, & Mueller, 2001; Wackerbath & Johnson, 2002). Information was cited among the most important needs. In Fortinsky and Hathaway's (1990) survey of 120 caregivers, primary needs were reported to be caregiving assistance services; assistance from health care professionals; support groups; and information about respite, support, and care. During interviews with 39 family caregivers, Francis and Munjas (1992) learned that urban families were in need of assistance with legal protection, planning, and supervision. Bowd and Loos (1996) indicated that the 68 rural caregivers they surveyed reported needing education and support more than assistance with tasks. Information needs were cited as most important among the 114 family caregivers interviewed by Beisecker et al. (1997). Information was requested in the following areas: disease course, available treatments and services, legal and financial issues, research, and the caregiver's personal needs.

Smith et al. (2001) conducted semistructured interviews with 45 caregivers and found that caregivers reported a variety of needs, including the following: financial, housing, and legal assistance; medical assistance for themselves and/or the patient; emotional support; spiritual guidance; and information. In a survey of 128 family members providing care to individuals with Alzheimer's disease, Wackerbath and Johnson (2002) found that information and support needs were described by caregiving family members. Among the information needs, education about health care coverage and ways to find the best care were cited as most important. Diagnosis, treatment, and financial/legal information were also highlighted, followed by general information about the disease. Support needs primarily centered on the care receiver (e.g., providing emotional support to the care receiver and understanding their emotional reactions). Female caregivers were more likely than male caregivers to describe needs for support from others and time for self as important.

Research on the needs of families following TBI have been examined extensively (Campbell, 1988; Engli & Kirsivali-Farmer, 1993; Grant & Bean, 1992; Junque, Bruna, & Mataro, 1997; Kolakowsky-Hayner, Miner, & Kreutzer, 2001; Kosciulek & Pichette, 1996; Kreutzer, Serio, & Berquist, 1994; Mathis, 1984; Mauss-Clum & Ryan, 1981; Moules & Chandler, 1999; Serio, Kreutzer, & Gervasio, 1995; Sinnakaruppan & Williams, 2001; Stebbins & Leung, 1998). However, the studies have not focused solely on geriatric patients with TBI. Findings from these studies reveal that families of individuals with TBI commonly report the need for reassurance and maintenance of hope, communication with professionals, emotional support, respite, information about resources, and honest and complete health information (Campbell, 1988; Grant & Bean, 1992; Kosciulek & Pichette, 1996; Kreutzer et al., 1994; Mathis, 1984; Witol, Sander, & Kreutzer, 1996). Family needs have been shown to fluctuate over time (Kolakowsky-Hayner et al., 2001; Witol et al., 1996) and are often related to the patient's neurobehavioral status (Serio et al., 1995). In addition, researchers have found that family members describing higher levels of unmet needs are significantly more likely to report higher rates of psychiatric symptoms and lower perceived quality of life (Moules & Chandler, 1999).

The role of neuropsychologists in helping families

Clinical neuropsychologists are skilled at meeting the needs of families who are dealing with neuropsychological illness or injury in a geriatric family member. Because clinical neuropsychologists have extensive knowledge about the sequelae and course of neuropsychological conditions, they are able to educate family members about long-term sequelae and prognosis and to provide strategies to deal with the sequelae. In addition, neuropsychologists assess the cognitive and emotional impact of caregiving and life changes on family members. Results from comprehensive evaluations may then be used to develop treatment plans and recommendations to improve family members' functioning and enhance their ability to care for their elderly loved one. The neuropsychologist is also an expert in providing individual, marital, group, and family therapy or making appropriate referrals for such services.

Clinical neuropsychologists are often called upon to provide services to geriatric patients with neuropsychological conditions and their families. Family evaluation and intervention is often requested when concerns arise about the family members' reactions to the condition and their ability to care for the patient. Consider the following situations:

- A 75-year-old gentleman, with a long history of vascular problems, was evaluated and diagnosed with dementia. Two years later their physician referred the gentleman's wife for evaluation of memory decline, concentration problems, and emotional distress associated with her role as primary caregiver for her husband. The couple had limited support, and no respite care was available. Comprehensive neuropsychological evaluation of the gentleman's wife was conducted. She was diagnosed with Cognitive Disorder NOS secondary to cognitive and functional impairments and Adjustment Disorder with Mixed Anxiety and Depressed Mood. Psychotherapy and respite services were recommended.
- A 73-year-old man, 18 months status post CVA, was recently discharged from an assistive living facility because staff felt he could safely live in the community. Although he could manage basic self-care activities,

continued problems with more complex self-care activities, such as financial management and driving, were evident. Neuropsychological evaluation was conducted at the request of his 45-year-old daughter. She expressed concerns about her father's ability to live independently in a rural community with limited supports. History of forgetting to turn off appliances raised concerns about fire safety. The patient's driving abilities and competency to manage his finances were also questioned. Neuropsychological evaluation corroborated his daughter's concerns. Feedback was provided to the patient and his daughter, and long-term care options and safety issues were discussed. The patient's daughter requested individual therapy to enhance her ability to cope with her role as caregiver.

- A family was referred by their attorney for comprehensive psychological testing secondary to concerns about their emotional response to the mother's severe TBI following a motor vehicle accident. The family included the husband, one adult daughter, and three adult sons. The children were unable to provide necessary care in the home and expressed guilt about the possibility of putting their mother in a nursing home. Psychological testing was conducted to evaluate the nature and extent of emotional impact of the injury on individual family members. All family members endorsed symptoms of depression and anxiety, which were impacting vocational and interpersonal functioning. Individual psychotherapy, family therapy, and support group attendance were recommended.

- A 65-year-old woman was referred for neuropsychological assessment by her neurosurgeon following diagnosis with a stage IV glioblastoma multiforme. Her husband of 25 years and primary caregiver requested that the neuropsychologist help get his wife "back to normal." Evaluation was conducted to ascertain cognitive and functional status. The patient was found to have profound dementia and to be unable to manage basic self-care activities (e.g., toileting). A feedback session was held with the patient and her husband. During the meeting, recommendations for addressing cognitive and functional limitations were discussed. In addition, the neuropsychologist focused on the husband's need to know that he was doing everything he could to help his wife. The husband was encouraged to take care of himself so he would be able to care for his wife. Social support, respite, and strategies to cope with loss and change were highlighted.

Each of these scenarios provides examples of situations in which comprehensive, holistic neuropsychological evaluation would likely yield valuable information about emotional, cognitive, and adaptive functioning. The results would assist in treatment planning and prognostication regarding future service needs.

Neuropsychological assessment

Depending on the setting and situation, family assessment may be quantitative and qualitative, relying on a combination of record reviews, interviews, observations, and standardized assessment tools (Kreutzer, Kolakowsky-Hayner, Demm, & Meade, 2002). Self-assessment is also encouraged by asking family members to review and respond to questionnaires, either in writing or during the course of discussions. Comprehensive assessment enables the clinician to gain an understanding of: (a) the patient's illness or neurological injury and course of recovery; (b) the patient's psychological, neuropsychological, and neurobehavioral functioning; (c) family members' emotional well-being; (d) family members' and patient's coping and problem-solving strategies and their effectiveness; and (e) family history and cultural dynamics.

Neuropsychologists are often called upon to conduct comprehensive neuropsychological evaluations to assess the sequelae of geriatric neuropsychological disorders and the impact on patient functioning. Findings provide the basis for determining recommendations, providing appropriate referrals, and developing treatment plans. In addition, results elucidate steps family members may take to optimize the geriatric patient's functioning and ensure the appropriate level of care and supervision.

Evaluation of the impact of the neuropsychological injury or illness on the family, particularly those in caregiving roles, is also critical. Neuropsychological and psychological assessment may be necessary to evaluate the functioning of family members. Comprehensive neuropsychological evaluation involves several steps: (a) clarification of the referral question; (b) records review; (c) clinical interview; (d) behavioral observation; and (e) standardized testing to assess cognitive, neurobehavioral, and emotional functioning and judgment and safety issues. The following sections will describe techniques to evaluate the functioning of both the geriatric patient and family members.

Clarification of the referral question

Identifying issues of concern and clarifying referral questions are among the first tasks faced by the neuropsychologist. In doing so, the neuropsychologist is able to ensure that the evaluation directly answers the questions posed by the referral source. The examiner must determine if the referring party is primarily interested in patient functioning, family functioning, or both. Referral sources should be educated about the impact of geriatric neuropsychological disorders on the family. In some situations, the neuropsychologist may determine that evaluation of the family is warranted and suggest referral of family members for evaluation or treatment in the neuropsychological report.

Table 17.1 Common referral questions relating to evaluation and treatment of family members of geriatric patients

---

- How have family members reacted to the patient's condition? Describe the emotional status of immediate family members including siblings and children. Are family members using adaptive or maladaptive coping mechanisms?
- Describe the needs of individual family members. What types of supports or services would be appropriate? What services best address the personal needs of individuals in the family?
- What kinds of support and education programs would benefit family members?
- Which family members should or should not be involved in treatment?
- What can be done to stabilize the patient's marital relationship?
- What was the family member's level of psychological and cognitive functioning before the onset of the geriatric patient's neuropsychological condition? Address issues relating to previous emotional disturbance and interpersonal relationships.
- Is the family a good support system for the patient and for each other? How are family members helping the patient or contributing to present difficulties?
- Are the family members willing and capable of providing care and supervision? What obstacles may hinder optimal care provision (e.g., family members' health, cognitive, or emotional status; transportation, housing, financial, or insurance issues)?
- Does the individual have adequate support from family, friends, and community resources? If not, what community support services could be recommended? Are respite services needed?
- What are the family's expectations regarding recovery, prognosis, and the patient's ability to return to previous activities (e.g., work, driving)?
- Do the family members understand the nature of the patient's condition and need for care, especially with regard to safety issues?
- Is the family eligible for special services, programs, or benefits?
- How have family members' academic and vocational potential been affected by the geriatric patient's neuropsychological illness or injury? Would additional educational or occupational support be of benefit?

Referral for neuropsychological evaluation or treatment may come from a diversity of sources, including professionals and family members. Table 17.1 depicts common referral questions received from professionals seeking neuropsychological services for families of geriatric patients. The sample referral questions elucidate the complex issues and questions which neuropsychologists typically address in evaluating and treating families of geriatric patients.

Oftentimes, referrals may come directly from the families of geriatric patients. In every evaluation, identification of the family's primary concerns and questions is necessary to ensure the evaluation directly addresses their needs. Table 17.2 depicts questions commonly posed by family members. The questions highlight family members' needs for education about prognosis and long-term care.

Table 17.2 Common questions posed by family members of geriatric patients

- What is the patient's prognosis?
- What areas of functioning are impaired and to what extent?
- How has the patient's status changed over time? Is their condition getting worse, improving, or staying the same?
- Will the patient be able to return to work, drive, manage finances, and/or live independently?
- What level of supervision will be required currently and long term?
- What services are available to help our family address the needs of the geriatric patient (e.g., respite, support groups, financial assistance)?
- What treatments are recommended to help the patient adapt to their neuropsychological condition (e.g., therapy, medication consultation)?
- Could interaction effects of medications be negatively impacting their functioning?
- Is the patient eligible for special services, programs, or benefits?

Records review

The evaluation process is based upon information gathered in part through review of records. Review of records provides guidance for the interview, test selection, diagnostic formulation, and treatment planning. Review of medical records provides information about health status before and after condition onset. In addition, review of mental health records provides information about emotional issues and substance use pre- and postcondition onset. Identification of health and emotional concerns fosters accurate diagnosis and referral. Medical and mental health records also indicate treatments and medications which have been effective in the past. Review of academic and vocational records will elucidate the patient's and/or family member's level of premorbid functioning. Establishing premorbid functioning level provides the basis for judging current impairment levels.

Behavioral observation

During the course of the evaluation, the examiner observes behaviors that are not readily tapped by quantitative assessment methods, including the following: appearance, eye contact, gait/ambulation, motor abilities, initiation, processing speed, mental status, orientation, alertness, affect, mood, receptive and expressive language abilities, judgment, insight, self-awareness, work habits, level of motivation and effort, stamina, and persistence. Family communication and interaction patterns may also be observed.

Clinical interview

The clinical interview is typically conducted with the geriatric patient and one or more family members or caregivers. Through the interview, the examiner gathers information about the primary concerns of the patient and family members or other caregivers. Identification of their concerns allows for appropriate test selection. The interview also provides information about the patient's level of self-awareness.

Quantitative assessment of cognitive functioning

Neuropsychological assessment is a holistic process that involves assessment of a broad range of cognitive functioning areas, including the following: attention and concentration, sensory and motor abilities, learning and memory, visuoperception and visuoconstructional abilities, language, and reasoning. Identification of cognitive deficits often provides the basis for developing compensatory strategies which may be employed by the patient and family members to optimize functioning.

Occasionally, concerns will be raised about family members' ability to provide care for the geriatric patient. Cognitive functioning may need to be assessed to ascertain if the family member of the geriatric patient has memory deficits or other cognitive impairments, which impact his or her ability to provide appropriate care. In these situations, neuropsychological assessment of the family member may be requested. The reader is referred to Lezak's (1995) seminal text on neuropsychological assessment for a comprehensive review of methods used to assess cognitive and neuropsychological functioning, and to Chapters 2 and 3 of this volume for assessment methods specific to geriatric neuropsychology.

Special issues in the comprehensive assessment of the geriatric patient

Judgment and safety issues are often the primary concerns of referral sources and family members. In particular, questions often arise surrounding the geriatric patient's ability to live independently, drive, and/or manage finances and medications. In assessing judgment and safety issues, the examiner is encouraged to ask patients and their family members about functioning. Doing so allows for comparison of responses in circumstances where the patient's judgment or self-awareness is questionable. The Judgment and Safety Screening Inventory (JASSI) (Kreutzer, West, & Marwitz, 2001) was designed to assess concerns about the following areas of functioning: travel; financial management; interpersonal functioning; food and kitchen; use of appliances, tools, and utensils; household issues; medications and alcohol; fire safety; and firearm safety. Patient and informant versions permit comparisons of informant responses to ascertain the patient's self-awareness. Figure 17.1 depicts the section of the JASSI that assesses financial functioning.

Quantitative assessment devices are often used to assess patient's ability to carry out activities of daily living. For example, the Independent Living Scales (Loeb, 1996) assesses abilities in the following areas: memory/orientation, financial management, managing home and transportation, health and

FINANCIAL

(*If the patient does not manage their own money, tell us what your concerns would be if they* **did** *manage their own money.*)	CONCERN LEVEL			
	None	Little	Much	Very
1. Misplacing wallet	⓪	①	②	③
2. Misplacing checkbook	⓪	①	②	③
3. Misplacing credit cards	⓪	①	②	③
4. Losing money	⓪	①	②	③
5. Failing to record checks in checkbook	⓪	①	②	③
6. Forgetting to pay bills	⓪	①	②	③
7. Easily talked into giving away money	⓪	①	②	③
8. Giving others personal financial information	⓪	①	②	③
USE THE SPACE BELOW FOR COMMENTS OR OTHER CONCERNS IN THIS AREA:	8 ITEM TOTAL:			

Figure 17.1 Excerpt from the informant version of the Judgment and Safety Screening Inventory. Reproduced with permission of the authors (Kreutzer et al., 2001).

safety, and social adjustment. Patients are evaluated based upon their knowledge about instrumental activities of daily living and their ability to carry out activities such as filling out a check or counting change. Use of quantitative devices may be particularly helpful when patients or family members are resistant to believing that the patient's ability to carry out activities of daily living is impaired. They may question others' reports about their abilities, but may have difficulty refuting objective test findings.

Assessment of geriatric patients' neurobehavioral and emotional functioning is also critical. With neuropsychological disorders, neurobehavioral and personality changes are common. In addition, geriatric patients often have difficulty adjusting to functional and cognitive changes and have increased risk of emotional difficulties. Common instruments used to evaluate emotional functioning include the Beck Depression Inventory (Beck, Rush, Shaw, & Emery, 1979), the Brief Symptom Inventory (Derogatis, 1975), the Hamilton Depression Rating Scale (Hamilton, 1967), and the Minnesota Multiphasic Personality Inventory (Hathaway & McKinley, 1989). However, these measures rely on self-report, which may be compromised secondary to cognitive and self-awareness deficits. As such, corroboration from family members and records is important. Comparison of patient and family reports on assessment instruments is helpful. The Neurobehavioral Functioning Inventory (NFI; Kreutzer, Seel, & Marwitz, 1999) is an 83-item measure designed to examine the frequency of neurobehavioral difficulties following TBI. Information is gathered about functioning in six domains: depression, somatic symptoms, memory/attention, communication, aggression, and motor functioning. Patient and family versions are available to permit comparisons of responses.

Special issues in the comprehensive assessment of family members

Given the critical role family members play in caring for their elderly relatives, assessment of their functioning is vital. Evaluation should address the following areas: changes in family roles and responsibilities; impact on family members' relationships; existing supports and additional support needs; family members' needs; emotional impact of the geriatric patient's condition on the family; stress; health status; and sleep. Understanding these areas will allow the neuropsychologist to ensure family members have the support needed to continue performing their critical caregiving role. Written recommendations may be offered to optimize family functioning and increase family supports. In offering recommendations, special care should be taken to help family members understand that they will be unable to provide optimal support if they do not take care of themselves and seek support in managing increasing responsibilities.

During the evaluation, care should be taken to understand the impact of the geriatric patient's condition on each relative. Each family member should be asked about changes in their roles and responsibilities (e.g., work, child care, household responsibilities). The family should be asked about changes in family members' relationships with each other, the geriatric patient, extended family, friends, and other supports. Information about relationships will elucidate current support networks. In addition, asking about access to community resources and support services will guide referral and development of recommendations. Table 17.3 depicts questions that help identify the changing roles of family members and their reactions to the geriatric patient's condition.

Assessment of family members' needs is another important step toward ensuring that recommendations are appropriate and helpful. The interview should incorporate questions focusing on the family's needs for education,

Table 17.3 Questions used to assess family change and family reactions

- How did you feel when you first learned that your family member was ill/injured?
- How did you feel when you realized that your family member's condition might have long-term effects?
- How have other family members reacted to your family member's condition?
- How have you helped to support other family members?
- What impact has your family member's condition had on your daily responsibilities (e.g., work responsibilities and hours, time with friends, activities, financial situation, household responsibilities)?
- What impact has your family member's condition had on your relationship with him/her?
- What impact has your family member's condition had on your relationships with other family members and friends?
- Which changes have been the most difficult for you?
- How has your family member's condition affected your plans for the future?

support, health care services, assistance with responsibilities, respite, and referral. The Family Needs Questionnaire (Kreutzer, 1988) is a 40-item self-report instrument which was originally developed for use with families of patients with brain injury to assess their perceived needs. The measure was designed to assess the importance of specific needs and the extent to which needs have been met. A factor analytic investigation conducted with families of TBI survivors (Serio, Kreutzer, & Witol, 1997) revealed six independent factors comprising six scales: Health Information, Emotional Support, Instrumental Support, Professional Support, Community Support Network, and Involvement with Care. The measure has also proved helpful in illuminating the needs of spinal cord injury survivors (Meade, Taylor, Kreutzer, Marwitz, & Thomas, 2004).

Family members' emotional functioning is often an area of concern following diagnosis of an elderly relative with a neurological condition. Research reveals that depression and feelings of anger are commonly reported among family caregivers of geriatric patients (Anthony-Bergstone, Zarit, & Gatz, 1988; Drinka, Smith, & Drinka, 1987; Gallagher, Rose, Rivera, Lovett, & Thompson, 1989; Haley, Levine, Lane-Brown, Berry, & Hughes, 1987). Depression and anger have been found to have a negative effect on caregivers' level functioning, and depression has been found to be associated with limited support networks, decreased perception of adequacy, and conflictual interpersonal relationships (Cohen & Willis, 1985; Fiore, Becker, & Coppel, 1983; Rivera, Rose, Futterman, Lovett, & Gallagher-Thompson, 1991). Given the negative effects of emotional distress on caregiving abilities, emotional status should be closely monitored. Common devices used to assess family members' emotional functioning include the Beck Depression Inventory (Beck et al., 1979), the Brief Symptom Inventory (Derogatis, 1975), the Hamilton Depression Rating Scale (Hamilton, 1967), and the Minnesota Multiphasic Personality Inventory (Hathaway & McKinley, 1989).

Caregiving is often accompanied by an increase in the level of stress secondary to increasing responsibilities. Stress levels should be monitored on a regular basis. Family members may be asked to rate their level of stress on a 1 (no stress) to 10 (extreme stress) scale. In addition, measures such as the "13-Item Stress Test" may also be administered to ascertain the level of stress family members are experiencing (Kreutzer & Kolakowsky-Hayner, 1999).

Caregivers who experience health and sleep problems are more likely to decide to institutionalize their family members (Bergman-Evans, 1994). For this reason, assessment of caregivers' sleep patterns and levels of fatigue are critical. In addition, regular monitoring of their medical status is also needed and should be strongly recommended.

Recommendations and treatment planning

The primary aim of comprehensive assessment of geriatric patients and their family members is the development of practical, feasible recommendations and treatment plans. Recommendations should focus of identifying strategies and interventions to enhance patients' and families' emotional well-being and optimize functioning. Referral for medical care, psychological or psychiatric intervention, support, and community services are commonly included. Table 17.4 depicts recommendations to optimize the functioning of geriatric patients. These sample recommendations may provide guidance to family members and referral sources about strategies they may employ to enhance the well-being of the geriatric patient. Table 17.5 illustrates sample recommendations that may be offered to family members providing care to elderly relatives. The recommendations are intended to optimize family members' functioning so they may provide optimal care for their elderly family members.

Treatment options

Psychological treatment of patients with neurological disorders and their family members often involves a series of steps (Kreutzer et al., 2002). Treatment often begins with assessment, a continuing process that necessarily serves as the basis of effective family interventions. Consideration of alternative treatment approaches and modalities that adequately address the family's difficulties is paramount. Practical issues such as financial concerns, personal schedules, and other potential barriers are attended to at the beginning of treatment. Next, treatment providers facilitate discussions with family members to help identify goals and priorities. The wishes and personal preferences of patients and their families should guide this process. During the course of treatment, clinicians often revisit goals to revise them as the family's situation and priorities change.

   The willingness of family members to participate, the severity of patients' neurobehavioral problems, individual distress levels, and the nature of identified problems affect therapy modality choice. Practical issues such as the availability of transportation and the need to coordinate multiple schedules are also influential. Family members can choose to participate in one or more therapy modality depending on their needs and desires. Following are descriptions of the most commonly used treatment modalities.

Treatment modalities

Family therapy

This typically involves the elderly person and several family members. The approach provides a forum for constructive discussion of frustrations, where individuals are encouraged to take an active problem-solving approach (Kreutzer et al., 1990). Family therapy may emphasize grief reduction, improving affect, communication and social skills, behavior management, and ongoing education. The therapist commonly works with families to reassign roles and responsibilities, aid in stress reduction, and restructure the

Table 17.4 Sample recommendations for optimizing functioning of the geriatric patient

Attention, orientation	• Minimize distractions in the environment (e.g., turn off the radio or television).
	• Monitor stress levels and emotional well-being; seek intervention should stress levels increase, since emotional difficulties can decrease cognitive abilities.
	• Praise the patient for paying attention.
	• Work on tasks in short sessions and take frequent breaks.
	• Vary activities to maintain interest.
	• Call the patient's name and make eye contact with him/her prior to giving instructions.
	• Use short, uncomplicated sentences when speaking to the patient.
Behavioral issues	• Establish clear rules and set firm behavioral limits.
	• Avoid focusing on negative behavior as attention may be rewarding.
	• Allow decision-making input, especially in decisions related to him/her.
	• Consult him/her and offer choices concerning care and treatment whenever feasible.
	• Complex or numerous choices will likely be confusing. Use a directive, but supportive, approach, and provide simple choices.
	• Encourage self-help to the extent he/she is capable: avoid doing too much of what he/she can do independently.
	• Explain unusual procedures or activities in advance.
	• When the patient is agitated, provide reassurance in a pleasantly modulated tone of voice; avoid shouting or speaking harshly.
	• Avoid assigning the patient tasks beyond his/her capability.
	• Provide continued reassurance that effort is most important and ultimately brings success.
	• Provide regular feedback regarding apparent improvements, large or small.
Communication	• Keep instructions short and simple.
	• Pause frequently and obtain feedback on comprehension (e.g., whether he/she is looking at you or appears confused; asking him/her to repeat back what you said).
	• Repeat key information and/or write down key points.
	• Talk to him/her in a natural manner that is typical for speaking to other adults.
	• Include him/her in conversations whenever possible and ask for his/her opinions.
	• With aphasia, encourage any type of communication (e.g., speech, gesturing, pointing, drawing).
	• Allow the patient plenty of time to finish talking.
Daily living	• Incorporate structured routines into daily activities, setting specific times for eating and sleeping, chores, exercise, and relaxation.

(continued)

Table 17.4   (contd.)

	• Arrange for participation in a structured day treatment program. • Assist the patient in developing interests and hobbies to give him/her a sense of accomplishment and diminish boredom. • Increase patient's participation in physical exercise, with doctor's approval. • Remember increasing efforts will not necessarily result in improved performance. Beyond a certain point, encouraging the patient to act may hinder performance. • Important activities (e.g., financial management) should be scheduled at times when the patient is most energetic and alert. • Repeat pertinent information about surroundings (e.g., date; location if different from home). • Introduce and explain nonroutine activities to avoid confusion (e.g., why he/she must go to the doctor).
Financial	• Consult with a certified financial planner to address long-term strategies for ensuring the security of funds. • Take steps to formally appoint a legal guardian to assist with financial management and decisions regarding expenditures. • Monitor expenditures and receipts regularly.
Health	• Seek continued medical follow-up to address physical symptoms. • Ask health providers to write down instructions and simplify treatment regimens, if possible. • Maintain a journal of medical visits including: current symptoms for which consultation is being sought, appointment date, doctor's name, and medications or treatments prescribed. • Request coordination of services by a single physician (e.g., phychiatrist) with a holistic perspective. • Maintain communication with the patient's physician regarding optimal exercise, self-care, activity, and diet. • Monitor food intake to ensure nutritional needs are being met. • Medication administration must be closely supervised. Use of individual "dose-packs," blister packs, or medication organizer may prove helpful.
Initiation and persistence	• Give directions to start the task (e.g., "It's time to take your bath. Let's get into to the bathtub now."). • Choose things he/she enjoys doing (e.g., a bubble bath instead of a shower). • Break tasks down into small, simple steps. • Avoid asking open-ended questions (e.g., "What do you want to do now?"). Instead provide two or three clear choices (e.g., "Would you rather take a bath or a shower?") • Offer a reward for starting a task. • Praise completion of each step during a task rather than waiting until he/she has completed it. • Encourage the patient to persist especially with challenging tasks. • Allow adequate time for the patient to complete a given task on his/her own, being careful to avoid overresponding to illegitimate complaints of fatigue or helplessness.

Table 17.4 (contd.)

	• Talk the patient through a structured problem solving approach (i.e., clearly state the problem, identify and evaluate options, and choose a course of action).
Memory	• Orient the patient to day, date, time, and location on a regular basis.
	• A watch with day/date function can facilitate time orientation.
	• View news or other educational programs, read magazine/newspaper articles, listen to radio programs, and discuss content with the patient.
	• Write a chronological biography or personal history time line to enhance his/her fund of personal information.
	• Review pictures and mementos and discuss events relevant to the family's history.
	• Purchase and help the patient use a daily planner or organizer, such as those found in office supply or variety stores.
	• Set up a home information center, or a prominent place where new information is clearly posted (e.g., a bulletin board for phone messages, reminder lists, family calendar).
	• Set aside planning time. Routinely take time during the day or week to go over tasks that need to be completed and new information.
	• Use watch alarms or kitchen timers as a reminder to complete important tasks, such as taking medication.
	• Use step-by-step checklists. Post written checklists for doing certain activities, such as the steps for using the washing machine.
Safety	• Driving or operating machinery must be prohibited: he/she poses a significant risk to himself/herself and to others by getting behind the wheel of a car.
	• Do not leave him/her unsupervised for more than a few minutes.
	• Establish and review procedures for responding to fire, police, or medical emergency: consider motor problems in the event of fire or other emergency requiring rapid escape from the house.
	• Post emergency telephone numbers where they can be easily seen.
	• Monitor him/her carefully when he/she is climbing stairs.
	• Place nonskid bath mats on the floors and adhesive strips in the tub. Use gritty, waterproof paint on outdoor steps.
	• Install handrails by the toilet, bath, and stairs.
	• Clear walking paths of telephone and electric cords and all clutter.
	• Place phones, preferably cordless, in as many rooms as possible and use an answering machine to avoid rushing to answer the phone.
	• Secure wall-to-wall carpeting and remove small area rugs layered on top of carpeting.
	• Keep often-used items in cabinets that can be easily reached without using a step stool.
	• Install a railing on both sides of the staircase.

(continued)

Table 17.4 (contd.)

- Mark first and last stair steps with brightly colored tape.
- Make sure there is a light switch at the top and bottom of the staircase.
- Regularly check batteries in smoke detectors.
- Install gas detectors, if using natural gas for heating.
- Check expiration dates on all perishable foods and discard food once it has passed the expiration date.
- Take care in using toxic chemicals, reading labels carefully and ensuring they are used and stored only in well-ventilated areas.

Table 17.5 Sample recommendations for optimizing family members' functioning

Emotional distress/stress	Caregiver stress secondary to the demands of the care giving role warrants intervention:
	• Individual counseling would likely prove helpful in decreasing emotional distress, enhancing coping skills, and providing training in stress management and relaxation.
	• Psychiatric medication management appears warranted to address symptoms of depression and anxiety.
	• Build and utilize support systems (e.g., discussing frustrations with family and close friends).
	• Explore and take advantage of respite opportunities.
	• Support group involvement is recommended to increase support and understanding about the patient's condition.
	• Education regarding the nature and extent of cognitive impairments would increase family members' understanding of the patient's condition.
	• Contact local and/or national groups and associations for support, information, and resources (e.g., National Family Caregivers Association, National Quality Caregiving Coalition, Brain Injury Association of America).
	• Taking time to get physical exercise and eating a healthy diet are important for staying healthy and fulfilling caregiving responsibilities.
	• Develop interests or hobbies and increase involvement in social and recreational activities.
	• Family counseling will likely offer an avenue for promoting effective communication among family members and increasing support.
	• Family members would likely benefit from instruction in behavioral management strategies to decrease behavioral acting out by the patient.
Fatigue	The family member is describing significant problems with fatigue, insomnia, and frequent and early morning awakening. Sleep problems hinder the family member's ability to care for the patient adequately. The following strategies are recommended to enhance sleep and improve functioning:
	• Be alert to signs and symptoms of becoming overtired.
	• Learn to pace oneself to prevent fatigue.

Table 17.5   (contd.)

	• Practice healthy sleeping habits to restore energy and improve stamina (e.g., go to bed at the same time each night, avoid consuming caffeine, smoking, or exercising right before bed). • Take frequent breaks to prevent overtiring. • Talk with your physician about sleep medications that may prove helpful.
Memory problems/ cognitive decline	Concern is expressed about the caregiver's cognitive functioning. He/she reports memory problems and often forgets to take his/her own medications. The caregiver may have difficulty providing care given his/her own difficulties. Alternative placement should be considered to ensure safety of both the caregiver and his/her family member.

---

family into an effective team. Neuropsychologists are also adept at facilitating family discussions about moving an elderly relative with neurological problems into a skilled nursing center or other assisted living environment. This topic is discussed in greater detail later in this chapter.

Marital therapy

This method includes the older person with the neurological condition and his or her spouse or significant other. Many techniques applicable to the treatment of family problems are relevant and useful in marital therapy (Kreutzer et al., 1990). Therapy objectives frequently include improving communication, empathy, mutual support, reciprocity, and satisfaction. Couples are taught skills in marital therapy to enhance the quality of their relationship, based on deficits identified during the assessment process. Marital therapy is ideal for addressing relationship issues that couples are uncomfortable discussing with extended family members, such as sexuality or other intimacy concerns.

Individual therapy

This form of therapy may be the most conducive to the discussion of highly sensitive, personal issues with the patient. Concerns about dependency, anxiety about the future, and daily coping difficulties are appropriate for individual therapeutic work. Patients are also free to explore intense feelings of guilt, anger, fear, and grief in individual counseling sessions. Family members, caregivers, or friends may be involved in the patient's individual therapy as appropriate.

Individual psychotherapy may also be appropriate for family members independent of the geriatric patient's treatment. Individual therapy provides a forum for discussing common reactions, such as ambivalence or frustration the family member does not wish to disclose in front of the patient in family treatment sessions.

Group therapy

Group therapy often involves family members from different families, and it facilitates learning from interactions, feedback, and recollections of others' experiences. Meetings can be organized specifically to provide education, referral, support, or skill-building opportunities. The participation of persons with neurological dysfunction may or may not be encouraged. Gallagher-Thompson (1994) described a psychoeducational approach to group treatment for caregivers of patients with Alzheimer's disease. This program, emphasizing enhancement of coping skills to deal with negative affect, resulted in reports of reduced depression and severity of anger.

Bibliotherapy

This often serves as a complement to other modalities and is perhaps the most commonly provided family therapy modality. Written information, covering topics of import to patients and families, is provided or recommended over the course of treatment. Professionals, elderly persons with neurological disease or damage, and family members often contribute recommendations from self-help and consumer-focused literature. Bibliotherapy is relatively inexpensive, and literature is available to address a wide variety of topics (Kreutzer et al., 2002).

Support groups

For elderly patients with neurological conditions are a valuable community resource. Support groups for family members, caregivers, and friends of geriatric persons with neuropsychological difficulties are also available in most communities. Information about medical and psychological issues faced by groups of people with similar difficulties is provided in the support group format. Participants often discuss local resources such as medical and rehabilitation treatment providers, financial services, and opportunities for respite. Support groups are also an important source of emotional support. People commonly report that participating in support groups is vital to their well-being and positive adjustment. People without the resources or ability to attend support groups may benefit from online, web-, and telephone-based sources of education and support (Glueckauf & Loomis, 2003).

Psychoeducation

Providing education to families is an important part of neuropsychological treatment. Rehabilitation providers should be aware of the current treatments for the illnesses their patients develop and be forthcoming with information during family sessions (Barth, 1996). In sessions or during family meetings, therapists model the appropriate way to discuss issues related to a relative's neurological condition with one another, with treatment professionals, and with concerned friends or acquaintances (Barth, 1996).

Neuropsychologists and other rehabilitation specialists commonly deal with questions of prognosis. From both a practical and an emotional standpoint, families want and need to know the anticipated course of their relative's illness or injury (Weiner & Svetlik, 1996). The course and outcome invariably depend on a number of factors, including the etiological basis for the neurological condition, preexisting physical status of the patient, and timeliness or quality of medical intervention. For example, dementia associated with Alzheimer's or Parkinson's disease typically demonstrates a progressive course of gradual deterioration (Thommessen et al., 2002). In contrast, strokes often produce an acute insult to the integrity of cerebral functioning (Read, 1996). Dementia related to cardiovascular disease (i.e., neurological deficits caused by multiple cerebral infarcts, subcortical ischemic lesions, or diffuse small vessel disease) usually presents with a stepwise deterioration of functioning. Prognostication and psychoeducation help families adjust to their loved one's neurological condition and prepare for the patient's future care needs.

In addition to preparing caregivers for the more unusual neurobehavioral difficulties that a geriatric patient with neurological problems may exhibit, Weiner and Svetlik (1996) recommended educating family members about common defense mechanisms. Psychoeducation about the spectrum of psychological phenomena and normal coping mechanisms (e.g., denial and projection) may help to enhance caregivers' empathy for their elderly relatives. For example, an elderly person with a neurological illness or injury, unaware of cognitive deficits, may blame caregivers for his or her difficulties performing routine daily living tasks. Patients may exhibit paranoia and accuse the caregiver of "hiding" personal property that the patient misplaced or lost. Health care providers may wish to recommend that commonly used objects be placed conspicuously to prevent arguments between caregiver and patient about "disappearing" items.

Primary treatment methods

Therapists working with families in a psychotherapeutic context enlist a number of methods and strategies to facilitate successful intervention. Levesque and Gendron (2003) described several such treatment techniques utilized in family intervention. The techniques consisted of listening, normalizing, problem solving, reframing, and effective communication.

Listening

The first tool for creating a therapeutic relationship with families involves nonjudgmental listening. From initial assessment throughout the therapeutic process, clinicians facilitate the exploration of family stress, reactions, and coping mechanisms. Listening communicates the clinician's desire to understand the viewpoints and feelings of individual family members. Family members are allowed to express their thoughts and feelings without the therapist providing a preemptive solution to problems. Therapists can better judge the effectiveness of currently employed problem-solving strategies and offer constructive advice on approaches they have yet to utilize.

Normalizing

Normalizing refers to facilitating patients' and family members' recognition of the universality of upsetting situations. For example, families facing problems associated with neurological decline of an elderly parent, spouse, sibling, or grandparent are often reassured by understanding they are not alone in their distress. Treatment providers often make use of normalizing in psychotherapy. Support groups and group therapy are also useful in providing normalizing experiences for patients, family members, and caregivers. Individuals learn how to cope with distressing life experienced from the wisdom shared by others in these formats.

Problem solving

Problem-solving skills are often directed at the changeable aspects of situations faced by the family. The six-step process involves the following: (1) identify the problem, (2) generate alternative solutions, (3) select a solution and evaluate associated pros and cons, (4) plan and rehearse implementation of the solution, (5) try out the solution, and (6) evaluate the outcome. Problem-solving strategies can be helpful to reduce the frequency of behaviors that family members consider particularly difficult or challenging. For example, a clinician may address an elderly patient's aggression towards his or her spouse by identifying triggers related to aggressive outbursts and problem solving with the family to identify prevention techniques.

Reframing

Reframing refers to "finding a different way to think about the situation, or creating an alternative meaning for it, so that the emotion generated by the unchangeable aspects of a stressful event may be more easily managed" (Levesque & Gendron, 2003, p. 305). In circumstances that are not amenable to problem-solving approaches, reframing the meaning of difficulties may benefit the family.

To guide the reframing process, neuropsychological treatment providers teach family members to consider emotionally difficult situations in terms of helpful versus unhelpful behavior. Therapists may help caretakers cope with interpersonal and behavior problems by instructing them in specific reframing techniques. Therapy goals include enhancing awareness of automatic thoughts, identifying unhelpful aspects of thought processes, and replacing unhelpful thoughts with realistic expectations (Beck et al., 1979).

Clinicians can also address caregivers' reluctance to ask for help by using reframing techniques. For example, with caregivers who are afraid of being perceived as selfish, clinicians can advocate for taking care of oneself in order to care better for others. Reminding a family member that asking for support exudes confidence in another person's ability to provide help may also diminish resistance. Focusing on potential benefits of having someone else provide caregiving on a temporary basis is likely to reduce a family member's maladaptive beliefs.

Effective communication

Neuropsychologists who work with family members providing direct caregiving to neurologically compromised elders strive to improve communication skills by a number of means. The quality of communication between the caregiver and elderly person may have deteriorated along with the patient's neurological condition. Maladaptive styles of communication often contribute to erosion of family functioning and dissatisfaction with the relationship. A family member may also fail to recognize when the time has come to ask for additional support from others within or outside the immediate family network. A number of factors, such as discomfort asking others for help or difficulties identifying resources for support, may interfere with help-seeking.

According to Levesque and Gendron (2003), caregivers tend to rely on a rational style of communication with persons suffering compromised neurological functioning. They often use logical reasoning or arguing to obtain cooperation from their loved one. As the patient has an organically based cognitive impairment, rational styles of communication are unlikely to be effective. Instead, caregivers are encouraged to use distraction, humor, and similar strategies to deescalate arguments with elderly persons with neurological disorders. Clinicians may also instruct caregivers to use short, simple sentences or to provide choices when communicating with the patient to decrease arguments and confusion.

Caregivers or family members may voice a number of concerns or reservations about asking others for support in caring for a loved one with neurological injury or illness. When therapists are alert to signs of resistance to seeking additional support, they may intervene by offering encouragement to caregivers. Clinicians are encouraged to listen for statements such as the following:

- "My friends used to come by and offer to help. They don't anymore. They must be sick of me asking for help."
- "Nobody cares about anyone else. It's every man, woman, and child for themselves."
- "Asking for help makes you look like you can't handle things on your own. It's a sign of weakness."
- "I'm tired of asking for help. I'm sick of being a burden."
- "My friends and family have more important things to do than worry about me."

Knowing how, when, and where to ask for help

Therapists can promote positive attitudes about asking for help by exploring the associated benefits with caregivers. Family members are encouraged to consider a number of constructive aspects of asking for help. For example, such behavior lets others know their support and involvement is valued. Asking for help with specific problems also increases the likelihood of receiving constructive assistance. Communicating needs with others provides an opportunity to build relationships with people who care. Caregivers should be assured that asking for help shows recognition of limitations and lets people who care about them know how they are doing. Being a member of a team may give relatives of elderly patients the chance to help others later. Reminding caregivers that asking for support will not only decrease their frustration level but also improve their ability to handle multiple responsibilities is another potential benefit.

Promoting effective communication skills is essential to helping family members be receptive to receiving support from others. Clinicians can help caregivers recognize when to ask for help and learn how they may best communicate their needs. In terms of timing, caregivers are encouraged to ask for help before problems become overwhelming. Identifying persons the caregiver trusts to ask for support is also important. Clinicians may facilitate identification of specific difficulties faced by family members in caretaking roles. By understanding problems in concrete ways, practical solutions become more clear and conquerable. Families are then able to ask people with the appropriate skills or resources to deal with identified difficulties. Family members are advised to make others comfortable with declining or accepting requests for help. Thanking the other person for listening to problems, even if they are unable or willing to help, is an important way to maintain good relationships.

Greatest challenges for geriatric patients and their families

After an elderly person receives a neurological diagnosis, family members confront a number of common difficulties. To circumvent potential problems, clinicians may teach patients and family members helpful strategies. Setting reasonable goals, remaining patient and learning to deal with neurological complications, and managing crises and stress are examples of such strategies. The most typical challenges faced by families and elderly patients are described in the following section.

Setting reasonable goals

To set reasonable goals for living with neurological compromise, one must appreciate the neurobehavioral difficulties likely to be encountered over time. Patients may have a diversity of symptoms, depending on their neurological condition. For example, persons with Alzheimer's disease tend to have cognitive (short-term memory loss, disorientation, distractibility, inability to perform complex activities of daily living), physical (slow gait), and emotional (social withdrawal, denial, and anxiety) problems in the disease's early stages (Reisberg, 1996). In later stages, difficulties with recent and remote memory, agitation, paranoia, aphasia, and performance of routine tasks of daily living emerge. Symptoms of early cognitive decline also become more pronounced.

To set reasonable goals, family members and patients are encouraged to implement the following strategies: (1) set goals considering the elderly person's recent progress and individual strengths; (2) recognize the patient's challenges and assets when developing goals; (3) ask trusted professionals, friends, or family members for input about whether or not goals are reasonable; (4) break down long-range plans into incremental steps that gradually progress towards an ultimate goal; (5) give themselves and the patient credit for accomplishing small steps along the way to achieving large goals; (6) remember that most people set their goals too high and need help carrying out complicated plans; (7) keep in mind daily challenges, available resources, and limitations and imperfections; (8) to avoid being overwhelmed, focus on the most important things necessary to accomplish today and tomorrow; and (9) make a "to do" list, number goals in order of priority, and work on the highest priorities first.

Maintaining patience with the recovery process

With acquired neurological injury, many patients are encouraged by a period of rapid recovery experienced within the first 6–18 months. However, improvement following acquired neurological injury may span years, even decades. For elderly patients, however, neurological recovery may be slower and less complete than the recovery experienced by younger patients. In general, geriatric patients have higher rates of mortality and poorer long-term functional outcome following traumatic injury due to a combination of pre-existing medical conditions and less physiologic reserve (Jacobs, 2003).

Neuropsychological treatment providers offer education to elderly patients and family members about prognosis and the course of recovery from brain injury and neurological illness. Patients are encouraged to realize that recovery may be a long process and that solving big problems often takes time. Viewing recovery on a daily basis and avoiding comparison of functioning to a time before neurological compromise is another beneficial coping strategy for patients and families to acquire. Because taking on too much too soon can easily lead to failure, patients and their families are reminded to take things slowly after neurological insult or the onset of a disease process. Pushing the patient too hard or being overly critical can be detrimental to recovery efforts. Along this line of reasoning, a focus on accomplishments and progress instead of failures is also beneficial. Clinicians offer support in times of setbacks and reinforce the fact that people are not perfect and everyone makes mistakes. Encouraging patients and families to learn from mistakes can help them overcome barriers that impede optimal functioning.

Managing crises and stress

One of the most stressful situations many older adults and families face is providing daily care to a relative with disability (Longino & Mittlemark, 1996). A multitude of problems and stressors must be managed by patients and their families after neurobehavioral difficulties appear. A primary role of treatment providers is to facilitate stress management for families. Providing a framework and teaching skills for successful coping is crucial. Stress management techniques commonly consist of strategies such as deep breathing, taking a break from the stressor, and engaging in relaxing activities.

In treatment, establishing that everyone has limits and many people require support in times of crisis builds the requisite foundation for stress management. Identifying indicators of stress overload is helpful during the initial stages of treatment. Patients and families are instructed to check their "pressure gauge" to monitor stress on a routine basis (Kreutzer, Gourley, & West, 1999). Patients and families may be taught effective problem-solving skills, such as brainstorming and trying out alternative solutions to problems. Clinicians may also assist patients and families with developing back up plans to cope with particular stressors.

Managing intense emotions

Geriatric patients with neurological conditions and their families may have intense emotions of grief, anger, fear about the future, and guilt. Strong feelings are not only common, but also anticipated reactions to the psychological trauma associated with neurological impairment. As a first step in treatment, patients and families are encouraged to recognize and monitor intense feelings. Clinicians help their patients recognize the power they have over strong emotional reactions. By learning to focus on solving problems, patients and families can gain control over their negative emotions and work toward making things better. The following strategies are associated with successful management of intense emotions: (1) talk with trusted others about feelings and positive ways to cope; (2) recognize the difference between thoughts and feelings; (3) avoid making decisions when strong emotions are present; (4) remember that intense emotions can undermine even the best problem solving efforts; (5) stop the cycle of escalating emotions before feelings get too intense; (6) try to understand the point of view of others; think about how they may respond to intense reactions, rash behaviors, or harsh words; (7) avoid saying the first thing that comes to mind; take a break, count to ten, or breathe deeply and think about what to say before responding; (8)

remember that nobody can solve all their problems by themselves; and (9) recognize the difficulties and challenges faced by caregivers and the hard work involved in making things better.

Specific problems arising from reactions such as guilt or blame may be circumvented with appropriate intervention. These emotional reactions can interfere with caregivers getting the help they need from others. Clinicians often work with caregivers to facilitate attitudes conducive for soliciting support. Family members and patients are encouraged to recognize when they are feeling guilty or blaming others. People are likely to respond better to the positive attitude of a caregiver or patient seeking support than to persons with a defeatist attitude. Therefore, reminding caregivers and patients that optimism is crucial for success can be beneficial. Clinicians also help reconstruct family members' beliefs when they become preoccupied with other people's faults and problems. Encouraging patients and families to consider what can be done to improve their situation will diminish their inclination to criticize others.

Living with a family member who is very different

Neurological problems can have devastating effects on the personality and behavioral characteristics of elderly patients. In the case of progressive illnesses such as Alzheimer's disease, a person's personality may slowly change over a matter of months and years. Acute damage related to stroke or traumatic injury can result in rapid and dramatic changes to the patient. Whether the personality of a patient changes gradually or quickly, family members often have difficulties relating to this "new person."

Neuropsychologists may focus their interventions on helping others understand the neurobehavioral aspects of the patient's particular condition. As different processes of disease or damage manifest themselves in unique ways, clinicians may provide education about what changes to expect. Realizing that personality and behavior changes have a neurological basis and that these difficulties should not to be taken personally can be a relief to perplexed caregivers, family members, or friends.

Normalizing reactions such as denial, anger, sadness, and a mixture of painful feelings can be helpful. Communicating that these types of emotional reactions are common diminishes the shame people may be experiencing. Allowing caregivers to express ways in which they miss the "old" person, the way things once were, or their hopes for the future can help them move past grief and focus on improving their relationships. In most circumstances, positive qualities of the patient still exist. Therapists can help caregivers and others recognize aspects of the person they continue to admire. Realizing that a patient's irritability or anger may be an expression of his or her frustration and confusion can help the caregiver develop empathy and depersonalize problematic behaviors. Talking with other family members may also help diffuse frustration and negative feelings about the patient.

Consulting with medical providers

As caregivers, families report that a primary need is having adequate medical information about the patient's condition and support from medical providers (Bowd & Loos, 1996; Wackerbath & Johnson, 2002). Caregivers may be reluctant to consult with the patient's physician for a number of reasons. Some may fear appearing stupid by asking questions. Others may feel the doctor is "too busy" to adequately address their concerns. Wishing to avoid having the patient's doctor think they have little trust in his or her care, many people avoid asserting their need for relevant information about progress or prognosis (Kreutzer & Kolakowsky-Hayner, 1999).

Neuropsychologists can help families obtain information and support vital to the care of their loved one. Encouraging family members to ask questions of the patient's treatment providers is an important role of clinicians. Caregivers, family members, and friends should be advised to adopt strategies similar to the following to make the most of consultations with doctors and to enhance their understanding of medical and rehabilitation services: (1) write down important questions as soon as they are thought of; keep a running list that new questions are added to; (2) keep questions organized and in a safe place; a "treatment notebook" may help patients and families keep track of ongoing treatments, medications, side effects, or symptoms; (3) bring the questions to every doctor's appointment; (4) write down the answers to questions, so they may be reviewed later; (5) ask for copies of medical records to keep in a notebook or binder; and (6) attend appointments with the patient if memory problems are a concern.

Coping with losses and changing demands and roles

Facilitating successful transitions in family members' roles from spouse, sibling, or child to caregiver is an important goal of psychotherapeutic interventions. Family members express their distress about losses and changing demands and roles they experience as caregivers in a number of ways. Therapists may hear statements from family members similar to the following: (1) "I miss the way things used to be"; (2) "He's more like my child than my husband"; (3) "I have to take care of everything on my own now—work, the kids, the house, and our finances. It's just too much"; and (4) "We had plans for the future; now, it looks like they'll never happen."

Abrupt behavioral changes often alert clinicians of coping difficulties experienced by family caregivers. Problems with irritability, restlessness, ability to sit still, or changes in weight may be obvious to clinicians. Caregivers may also report more subtle difficulties such as insomnia, low energy, fatigue, and social withdrawal, common problems for people overwhelmed by stress.

To help family members deal with the strain of caregiving, clinicians provide advice and offer strategies likely to enhance well-being. Neuropsychologists working with families that are in a caretaking capacity may encourage them to develop new plans for the future based on changing expectations and needs. Helping family members recognize that worry is a natural human tendency that can be redirected with focused attention facilitates this process. Caregivers learn to pay attention to positive aspects of situations such as their accomplishments, strengths, and resources. Normalizing family members' reactions to rapid life changes and increased demands of caregiving is often beneficial.

Balancing needs of the caregiver and patient

Most persons providing informal caregiving services work outside the home in addition to their caretaking responsibilities (National Alliance for Caregiving & American Association of Retired Persons, 2004). Under these circumstances, "caregiver burn-out" is likely to be a significant problem. Helping the family caregiver recognize signs of severe stress is an important first step. Clinicians working with families may have heard statements from caregivers similar to these: (1) "How much longer can I keep going like this?" (2) "I can't take much more of this! I can't go on living this way"; (3) "Everything is going wrong"; (4) "Nobody else seems to care; it's all up to me to do everything"; and (5) "No one understands what I'm going through."

Neuropsychologists working with families of geriatric patients are cognizant of the impact neurological conditions have on the entire family system. In a time of medical crisis for elderly relatives, families tend to shift their focus to caring for the relative and overlooking personal needs and responsibilities. Clinicians often emphasize the importance of self-care in order to enhance caregiving of others in therapy. Reminding caregivers to pace themselves, take breaks, and ask for help is also helpful to prevent stress overload. Helping caregivers develop a schedule that balances work, providing care to their loved one, and participating in activities outside the home may be crucial for maintaining emotional well-being and coping with stress. Therapists encourage family members to be careful not to take on additional responsibilities at work if giving up occupational pursuits is not an option. Family members may benefit from referral to respite services in their community.

Recognizing limitations as a caregiver

Family members' financial, emotional, and physical resources may be depleted by the constant responsibilities of caregiving. The tendency to overlook a caregiver's limitations (e.g., physical frailty, cognitive decline, or emotional maladjustment) is often associated with a family's desire to provide home-based care. Financially, providing informal care to elderly relatives can be extremely draining on family income or savings (Weinberger et al., 1993). Emotionally, caregivers of geriatric patients with neurological illnesses experience an increased level of stress, strain, anxiety, and depression compared to noncaregiving persons (Quayhagen et al., 2000; Schulz et al., 2003; Weiner & Svetlik, 1996). Emotional problems such as depression and anxiety may also be ignored in the course of the constant demands of caregiving. Physical limitations due to chronic pain, complex medical conditions, inability to lift or transfer a patient safely, or difficulty providing for basic hygiene needs (dressing, bathing, toileting, etc.) may interfere with the provision of adequate care. Primary caregivers experiencing age-related cognitive decline may be unaware of their own deficits in thinking. Attuned to the tendency of caregivers to ignore their own limitations and needs, clinicians commonly seek to provide early intervention before personal and family resources are overwhelmed.

When safety concerns take precedence over desire to optimize the patient's independence

Family members often seek recommendations for addressing an elderly patient's capacity and competency to perform routine and complex activities of daily living. Evaluating mental status (i.e., alertness, orientation, and sensorium) and higher cognitive functioning skills of judgment, mental flexibility, and planning are vital to forming appropriate treatment recommendations. In addition, a person's ability to perform routine activities of living such as self-care/hygiene, cooking, and light housework is important, and his or her ability to safely continue performing such activities should be maximized. Complex tasks of daily living like driving, shopping, and managing finances may also be a focus of neuropsychological treatment. Getting input from an objective third party can be helpful in determining a patient's true level of capacity when self-awareness is a question.

Post-assessment feedback sessions are valuable to communicate with the patient and family about capacity issues. Neuropsychologists working with family members help communicate assessment findings in a way that is acceptable to the geriatric patient. Problem-solving strategies to maintain optimal independence may also be the focus of family meetings. Developing plans for enhancing recreation and opportunities for socialization may compensate for the removal of privileges such as driving. Family members are advised to seek a driving evaluation from their local Department of Motor Vehicles if questions about safety and driving remain. Neuropsychologists working with older patients should stress the importance of maintaining personal safety and public welfare above all other things, including a desire for independence.

Transitioning to nursing home care

Placing an older relative in a nursing home is an emotionally challenging and difficult decision, often seen as a last resort. According to Stone et al. (1987), family members reserve consideration of nursing home placement for when the patient's needs exceed the limits of the caregiver. Gold, Reis, Markiewicz, and Andres (1995) described factors related to caregivers' decisions to terminate home-based care of their older family member with dementia in favor of nursing home placement. Reasons cited for ending home caregiving included change in the patient's condition (81%), caregiver exhaustion (30.4%), wandering (24.6%), incontinence (18.8%), inability to be left alone (17.4%), aggression (14.5%), illness of another family member or conflicting family needs (11.6%), and caregiver illness (10.1%).

Ryan and Scullion (2000) also investigated the experience of caregivers when faced with placing an elderly family member in a nursing home. They found that family members procrastinated as long as possible before making this decision. A period of prolonged home-based care and a crisis usually precipitated a nursing home placement. Caregivers participating in the Ryan and Scullion study reported common difficulties, including having ambivalent feelings (i.e., a mixture of guilt and relief), receiving inadequate support from health care professionals, and feeling they had no choice in the decision-making process.

Neuropsychological treatment providers are adept at facilitating family discussions about moving an elderly patient into a skilled nursing center or other assisted living environment. Assessing the resources and limitations of family members, taking into consideration the individual needs and preferences of all parties involved, and developing a plan to facilitate the transition are common strategies utilized during family sessions. Clinicians are also skilled in helping families cope with the emotional turmoil surrounding this decision. Sadness, guilt, fear, and anger are examples of intense emotions family members are apt to experience as they approach making a final decision. The decision to place an elderly patient into a nursing facility may be destigmatized by health care providers exerting their expertise into the process. Families are often relieved from the burden of guilt when a professional recommends nursing home placement for their older relative with neurological difficulties.

End-of-life issues

As people age, there is a natural transition from focus on time spent living to time remaining until death. The "crisis of finitude" typically occurs for persons during the fifth decade of life and later (Cohler & Nakamaura, 1996). Neurological illness or injury may cause significant disruption to the expectations and plans of individuals and families in their elder years. Instead of enjoying retirement (e.g., traveling, visiting grandchildren, and pursuing hobbies), individuals, couples, or families may be faced with issues of mortality prematurely. Yet, little attention has been paid in the research literature to the impact on caregivers of providing end-of-life care to family members with progressive neurological illnesses (Schulz et al., 2003).

Schulz et al. (2003) investigated the impact of end-of-life on 217 caregivers involved in the Resources for Enhancing Alzheimer's Caregiving Health (REACH) study. They found that caregivers exhibited high levels of depressive symptoms during the year before the patient's death. Within 3 months of the death, however, caregivers had clinically significant declines in the level of depressive symptomatology. Additionally, 72% of caregivers reported that the death was a personal relief, and over 90% reported the death was a relief to the patient. Zisook and Shuchter (1996) described the adaptive capacities of bereaved elderly persons as a testament to their resiliency in that most people are able to grieve loss, reengage, and function adequately in their daily lives.

For the minority of bereaved elderly caregivers demonstrating a period of significant maladjustment following the death of a relative, additional psychological treatment may be warranted. Neuropsychologists experienced in working with elderly caregivers commonly differentiate between normal and pathological grieving and provide appropriate intervention. Although grief is a highly individualized process, clinicians address a number of dimensions in therapy, including emotional and cognitive experiences, coping skills, adaptive functioning, and enhancing relationships of the bereaved (Zisook & Shuchter, 1996). Provision of early and relevant psychological and psychiatric interventions often averts preventable complications of prolonged bereavement faced by caregivers.

A final comment

Evaluating the cognitive and psychomotor abilities of patients with neurological disorders has been the traditional role of neuropsychologists. With more neuropsychologists working in rehabilitation settings, the role of neuropsychology has expanded. Many neuropsychologists are evaluating patients' psychological and neurobehavioral status. Many are developing and implementing treatment plans and serving as consultants to rehabilitation teams.

Research has revealed and substantiated the importance of family involvement in rehabilitation. Investigators have consistently reported that the lives of individual family members are often tragically affected by the patient's injury or illness. Clearly, caring for an elderly person with a neuropsychological condition precipitates drastic changes in the caregiver's role, responsibilities, and life plans. Consequent to drastic life changes are symptoms of emotional distress, including despair, frustration, anxiety, and social isolation.

Clinicians are encouraged to develop their skills in evaluating the needs and reactions of family members. By doing so, they have a greater opportunity to benefit caring family members as well as the patient.

References

American Association of Retired Persons. (1997). *A profile of older Americans: 1997.* Washington, DC: Author.

Anthony-Bergstone, C., Zarit, S., & Gatz, M. (1988). Symptoms of psychological distress among caregivers of dementia patients. *Psychology and Aging, 3*, 245–248.

Barth, J. C. (1996). Chronic illness and the family. In F. Kaslow (Ed.), *Handbook of relational diagnosis and dysfunctional family patterns* (pp. 496–508). Toronto, Canada: John Wiley & Sons.

Beck, A. T., Rush, A. J., Shaw, B. F., & Emery, G. (1979). *Cognitive therapy of depression*. New York: Guilford.

Beisecker, A. E., Chrisman, S. K., & Wright, L. J. (1997). Perceptions of family caregivers of persons with Alzheimer's disease: Communication with physicians. *American Journal of Alzheimer's Disease, 12*, 73–83.

Bergman-Evans, B. (1994). A health profile of spousal Alzheimer's caregivers: Depression and physical health characteristics. *Journal of Psychosocial Nursing, 32*(9), 25–30.

Bowd, A., & Loos, C. (1996). Needs, morale, and coping strategies of caregivers for persons with Alzheimer's disease in isolated communities in Canada. *American Journal of Alzheimer's Disease, 11*, 32–39.

Brooks, D., & Aughton, M. (1979). Psychological consequences of blunt head injury. *International Rehabilitation Medicine, 1*, 160–165.

Campbell, C. H. (1988). Needs of relatives and helpfulness of support groups in severe head injury. *Rehabilitation Nursing, 13*(6), 320–325.

Cohen, S., & Willis, T. A. (1985). Stress, social support, and buffering hypothesis. *Psychological Bulletin, 98*, 310–357.

Cohler, B., & Nakamura, J. (1996). Self and experience across the second half of life. In J. Sadavoy, L. Lazarus, L. Jarvik, & G. Grossberg (Eds.), *Comprehensive review of geriatric psychiatry* (2nd ed., pp. 153–194). Washington, DC: American Psychiatric Press.

Derogatis, L. R. (1975). *Brief Symptom Inventory*. Baltimore: Clinical Psychometric Research.

Draper, B., Poulos, R., Poulos, C., & Ehrlich, F. (1996). Risk factors for stress in elderly caregivers. *International Journal of Geriatric Psychiatry, 11*(3), 227–231.

Drinka, T. J., Smith, J., & Drinka, P. J. (1987). Correlates of depression and burden for informal caregivers of patients in a geriatrics referral clinic. *Journal of the American Geriatrics Society, 35*, 522–525.

Engli, M., & Kirsivali-Farmer, K. (1993). Needs of family members of critically ill patients with and without acute brain injury. *Journal of Neuroscience Nursing, 25*(2), 78–85.

Ergh, T., Rapport, L., Coleman, R., & Hanks, R. (2002). Predictors of caregiver and family functioning following traumatic brain injury: Social support moderates caregiver distress. *Journal of Head Trauma Rehabilitation, 17*(2), 155–174.

Fiore, J., Becker, J., & Coppel, D. (1983). Social network interactions: A buffer or a stress? *American Journal of Community Psychology, 11*, 423–439.

Fortinsky, R., & Hathaway, T. (1990). Information and service needs among active and former family caregivers of persons with Alzheimer's disease. *The Gerontologist, 30*, 604–609.

Francis, G. M., & Munjas, B. A. (1992). Needs of family caregivers and persons with Alzheimer's disease. *American Journal of Alzheimer's Care Research, 7*, 23–31.

Gallagher, D., Rose, J., Rivera, P., Lovett, S., & Thompson, L. W. (1989). Prevalence of depression in family caregivers. *The Gerontologist, 29*, 449–456.

Gallagher-Thompson, D. (1994). Clinical intervention strategies for distressed caregivers: Rationale and development of psychoeducational approaches. In E. Light, G. Niederehe, & B. Lebowitz (Eds.), *Stress effects on family caregivers of Alzheimer's patients* (pp. 260–277). New York: Springer.

Glueckauf, R. L., & Loomis, J. S. (2003). Alzheimer's caregiver support online: Lessons learned, initial findings and future directions. *Neurorehabilitation, 18*, 135–146.

Gold, D. P., Reis, M., Markiewicz, D., & Andres, D. (1995). When home caregiving ends: A longitudinal study of outcomes for caregivers of relatives with dementia. *Journal of the American Geriatrics Society, 43,* 10–16.

Grant, J., & Bean, C. (1992). Self-identified needs of informal caregivers of head-injured adults. *Family and Community Health, 15*(2), 49–58.

Haley, W. E., Levine, E. G., Lane-Brown, S., Berry, J., & Hughes, G. (1987). Psychological, social and health consequences of caring for a relative with senile dementia. *Journal of the American Geriatrics Society, 35,* 405–411.

Hamilton, M. (1967). Development of a rating scale for primary depressive illness. *British Journal of Social and Clinical Psychology, 6,* 278–296.

Hathaway, S. R., & McKinley, J. C. (1989). *Minnesota Multiphasic Personality Inventory–2 (MMPI-2): Manual for administration and scoring.* Minneapolis, MN: University of Minnesota Press.

Hirschfeld, M. (2003). Home care versus institutionalization: Family caregiving and senile brain disease. *International Journal of Nursing Studies, 40*(5), 463–469.

Jacobs, D. (2003). Special considerations in geriatric injury. *Current Opinions in Critical Care, 9*(6), 535–539.

Junque, C., Bruna, O., & Mataro, M. (1997). Information needs of the traumatic brain injury patient's family members regarding the consequences of injury and associated perception of physical, cognitive, emotional and quality of life changes. *Brain Injury, 11*(4), 251–258.

Knight, R., Devereux, R., & Godfrey, H. (1998). Caring for a family member with a traumatic brain injury. *Brain Injury, 8,* 197–210.

Kolakowsky-Hayner, S. A., Miner, K. D., & Kreutzer, J. S. (2001). Long-term life quality and family needs after traumatic brain injury. *Journal of Head Trauma Rehabilitation, 16*(4), 374–385.

Kosciulek, J., & Pichette, E. (1996). Adaptation concerns of families of people with head injuries. *Journal of Applied Rehabilitation Counseling, 27*(2), 8–13.

Kreutzer, J. S. (1988). *Family Needs Questionnaire.* Richmond, VA: Rehabilitation Research and Training Center on Severe Traumatic Brain Injury, Medical College of Virginia.

Kreutzer, J. S., Gervasio, A., & Camplair, P. (1994). Patient correlates of caregiver's distress and family functioning after traumatic brain injury. *Brain Injury, 8,* 211–230.

Kreutzer, J. S., Gourley, G., & West, D. (1999). *Getting better (and better) after brain injury: A guide for survivors.* Richmond, VA: National Resource Center for Traumatic Brain Injury.

Kreutzer, J. S., & Kolakowsky-Hayner, S. (1999). *Getting better (and better) after brain injury: A guide for family, friends, and caregivers.* Richmond, VA: National Resource Center for Traumatic Brain Injury.

Kreutzer, J. S., Kolakowsky-Hayner, S., Demm, S., & Meade, M. (2002). A structured approach to family intervention after brain injury. *Journal of Head Trauma Rehabilitation, 17,* 349–367.

Kreutzer J. S., Seel, R. T., & Marwitz, J. H. (1999). *The Neurobehavioral Functioning Inventory.* San Antonio, TX: Psychological Corporation.

Kreutzer, J. S., Serio, C. D., & Berquist, S. (1994). Family needs after brain injury: A quantitative analysis. *Journal of Head Trauma Rehabilitation, 9*(3), 104–115.

Kreutzer, J. S., West, D. D., & Marwitz, J. H. (2001). *Judgment and Safety Screening Inventory: Administration manual.* Richmond, VA: National Resource Center for Traumatic Brain Injury.

Kreutzer, J. S., Zasler, N., Camplair, P., & Leininger, B. (1990). A practical guide to family intervention following adult traumatic brain injury. In J. Kreutzer & P. Wehman (Eds.), *Community integration following traumatic brain injury* (pp. 249–286). Baltimore: Paul Brookes.

Levesque, L., & Gendron, M. (2003). Taking care of the caregivers. In R. Mulligan, M. van der Linden, & A. Juillerat (Eds.), *The clinical management of early Alzheimer's disease: A handbook*. Mahwah, NJ: Lawrence Erlbaum Associates, Inc.

Lezak, M. (1978). Living with the characterologically altered brain injured patient. *Journal of Clinical Psychiatry, 39,* 592–598.

Lezak, M. (1986). Psychological implications of traumatic brain damage for the patient's family. *Rehabilitation Psychology, 31*(4), 241–250.

Lezak, M. (1988). Brain damage is a family affair. *Journal of Clinical and Experimental Neuropsychology, 10*(1), 111–123.

Lezak, M. D. (1995). *Neuropsychological assessment* (3rd ed.). New York: Oxford University Press.

Loeb, P. A. (1996). *Independent Living Scales: Manual*. San Antonio, TX: Psychological Corporation.

Longino, C., Jr., & Mittlemark, M. (1996). Sociodemographic Aspects. In J. Sadavoy, L. Lazarus, L. Jarvik, & G. Grossberg (Eds.), *Comprehensive review of geriatric psychiatry* (2nd ed., pp. 135–158). Washington, DC: American Psychiatric Press.

Mathis, M. (1984). Personal needs of families of critically ill patients with and without brain injury. *Journal of Neurosurgical Nursing, 16,* 36–44.

Mauss-Clum, N., & Ryan, M. (1981). Brain injury and the family. *Journal of Neurosurgical Nursing, 13,* 165–169.

McKinlay, W., Brooks, D., Bond, M., Martinage, D., & Marshall, M. (1981). The short-term outcome of severe blunt head injury as reported by relatives of injured persons. *Journal of Neurology, Neurosurgery, and Psychiatry, 44,* 527–533.

Meade, M. A., Taylor, L. A., Kreutzer, J. S., Marwitz, J. H., & Thomas, V. (2004). A preliminary study of acute family needs after spinal cord injury: Analysis and implications. *Rehabilitation Psychology, 49*(2), 150–155.

Miller, E., Berrios, G., & Politynska, B. (1996). Caring for someone with Parkinson's disease: Factors that contribute to distress. *International Journal of Geriatric Psychiatry, 11,* 263–268.

Morgan, D. G., & Laing, G. P. (1991). The diagnosis of Alzheimer's disease: Spousal perspectives. *Qualitative Health Research, 1*(3), 370–387.

Moules, S., & Chandler, B. J. (1999). A study of the health and social needs of carers of traumatically brain injured individuals served by one community rehabilitation team. *Brain Injury, 13*(12), 983–993.

National Alliance for Caregiving. (1997). *Family caregiving in the US: Findings from a national survey.* Washington, DC: National Alliance for Caregiving and American Association of Retired Persons.

National Alliance for Caregiving & American Association of Retired Persons. (2004). *Caregiving in the U.S.* Retrieved April 5, 2004, from http://assets.aarp.org/rgcenter/il/ us_caregiving.pdf

Pinquart, M., & Sorensen, S. (2003). Differences between caregivers and noncaregivers in psychological health and physical health: A meta-analysis. *Psychology and Aging, 18*(2), 250–267.

Quayhagen, M., Quayhagen, M. P., Corbeil, R., Hendrix, R., Jackson, J. E., Synder, L., & Bower, D. (2000). Coping with dementia: Evaluation of four non-pharmacologic interventions. *International Psychogeriatrics, 12*(2), 249–265.

Read, S. (1996). Vascular dementias. In J. Sadavoy, L. Lazarus, L. Jarvik, & G. Grossberg (Eds.), *Comprehensive review of geriatric psychiatry* (2nd ed., pp. 459–477). Washington, DC: American Psychiatric Press.

Reisberg, B. (1996). Alzheimer's disease. In J. Sadavoy, L. Lazarus, L. Jarvik, & G. Grossberg (Eds.), *Comprehensive review of geriatric psychiatry* (2nd ed., pp. 401–458). Washington, DC: American Psychiatric Press.

Rivera, P. A., Rose, J. M., Futterman, A., Lovett, S., & Gallagher-Thompson, D. (1991). Dimensions of perceived social support in clinically depressed and non-depressed female caregivers. *Psychology and Aging, 6*, 232–237.

Rosenbaum, M., & Nanjenson, T. (1976). Changes in the life patterns and symptoms of low mood as reported by wives of severely brain injured soldiers. *Journal of Consulting and Clinical Psychology, 44*, 881–888.

Ryan, A., & Scullion, H. (2000). Nursing home placement: An exploration of the experiences of family carers. *Journal of Advanced Nursing, 32*(5), 1187–1195.

Schulz, R., & Beach, S. (1999). Caregiving as a risk factor for mortality: The caregiver health effects study. *Journal of the American Medical Association, 282*, 2215–2219.

Schulz, R., Mendelsohn, A., Haley, W., Mahoney, D., Allen, R., Zhang, S., et al. (2003). End-of-life care and the effects of bereavement on family caregivers of persons with dementia. *New England Journal of Medicine, 349*(20), 1936–1942.

Schulz, R., O'Brien, A., Bookwala, J., & Fleissner, K. (1995). Psychiatric and physical morbidity effects of dementia caregiving: Prevalence, correlates, and causes. *The Gerontologist, 35*, 771–791.

Schur, D., & Whitlatch, C. (2003). Circumstances leading to placement: A difficult caregiving decision. *Lippincott's Case Management, 8*(5), 187–195.

Serio, C. D., Kreutzer, J. S., & Gervasio, A. H. (1995). Predicting family needs after brain injury: Implications for intervention. *Journal of Head Trauma Rehabilitation, 10*(2), 32–45.

Serio, C. D., Kreutzer, J. S., & Witol, A. D. (1997). Family needs after traumatic brain injury: A factor analytic study of the Family Needs Questionnaire. *Brain Injury, 11*(1), 1–9.

Sinnakaruppan, I., & Williams, D. M. (2001). Family carers and the adult head-injured: A critical review of carers' needs. *Brain Injury, 15*(8), 653–672.

Smith, A. L., Lauret, R., Peery, A., & Mueller, T. (2001). Caregiving needs: A qualitative exploration. *The Clinical Gerontologist, 24*(1/2), 3–26.

Stebbins, P., & Leung, P. (1998). Changing family needs after brain injury. *Journal of Rehabilitation, 64*(4), 15–22.

Stevens, G. L., Walsh, R. A., & Baldwin, B. A. (1993). Family caregivers of institutionalized and noninstitutionalized elderly individuals. *Nursing Clinics of North America, 28*(2), 349–362.

Stone, R., Cafferata, G. L., & Singh, J. (1987). Caregivers of the frail elderly: A national profile. *The Gerontologist, 27*, 616–626.

Thommessen, B., Aarsland, D., Braekhus, A., Oksengaard, A., Engedal, K., & Laake, K. (2002). The psychosocial burden on spouses of the elderly with stroke, dementia and Parkinson's disease. *International Journal of Geriatric Psychiatry, 17*, 78–84.

Thomsen, I. V. (1984). The patient with severe blunt head trauma: A 10–15 year second follow-up. *Journal of Neurology, Neurosurgery, and Psychiatry, 47*, 260–268.

Wackerbath, S. B., & Johnson, M. M. S. (2002). Essential information and support needs of family caregivers. *Patient Education and Counseling, 47*(2), 95–100.

Wallhagen, M. (1992). Caregiving demands: Their difficulty and effects on the well-being of elderly caregivers. *Scholarly Inquiry for Nursing Practice: An International Journal, 6*(2), 111–133.

Weinberger, M., Gold, D. T., Divine, G. W., Cowper, P. A., Hodgson, L. G., Schreiner, P. J., & George, L. K. (1993). Expenditures in caring for patients with dementia who live at home. *American Journal of Public Health, 83*(3), 338–341.

Weiner, M. F., & Svetlik, D. (1996). Dealing with family caregivers. In M. Weiner (Ed.), *The dementias: Diagnosis, management, and research* (2nd ed., pp. 233–250). Washington, DC: American Psychiatric Press.

Wilson, N. L., & Trost, R. (1987). A family perspective on aging and health. *Health Values, 11*(2), 52–57.

Witol, A. D., Sander, A. M., & Kreutzer, J. S. (1996). A longitudinal analysis of family needs following traumatic brain injury. *Neurorehabilitation, 7*, 175–187.

Zisook, S., & Shuchter, S. (1996). Grief and bereavement. In J. Sadavoy, L. Lazarus, L. Jarvik, & G. Grossberg (Eds.), *Comprehensive review of geriatric psychiatry* (2nd ed., pp. 529–592). Washington, DC: American Psychiatric Press.

18 Decision-making capacity in the impaired older adult

Paul J. Moberg and Maureen Gibney

The right of capable persons to make decisions about their own care and safety is an integral presumption of legal and ethical practice in the United States. Rooted in respect for autonomy, the ceding of decisions to capable persons is articulated in the construct of informed consent. Landmark federal legislation (the Patient Self-Determination Act; Beauchamp & Childress, 1994) and many practitioner ethics codes, including the American Psychological Association's *Ethical Principles of Psychologists and Code of Conduct* (2002; "Ethics Code" in the following discussion) mandate that clinicians honor the individual's right to autonomy. This "personal rule of the self … is free from both controlling interferences of others and from personal limitations that prevent meaningful choice, such as inadequate understanding" (Beauchamp & Childress, 1994, p. 121). How does the ethical practitioner proceed, however, when there is a question of inadequate understanding—when capacity itself is in question? Evaluating the integrity or impairment of a patient's decision-making capacity will frequently be the task of the geriatric neuropsychologist.

Decision-making capacity is, not surprisingly, a complex construct. The 1982 report of the President's Commission for the Study of Ethical Problems in Medicine and Biomedical and Behavioral Research identified three requirements "to greater or lesser degree" for capacity: "(1) possession of a set of values and goals …; (2) the ability to communicate and to understand information; and (3) the ability to reason and to deliberate about one's choices" (Jonsen, Veatch, & Walters, 1998, pp. 473–475). The Commission articulated the decision-specific nature of capacity, noted its dimensional characteristics, and noted the need for variable stringency depending on the importance of the potential outcomes. This increased rigor in decisional capacity demonstration, however, must not serve to preclude patients from exercising their judgment, if the patient demonstrates the requisite appreciation and rationality, and the Commission affirmed the right of capable persons to make decisions that might appear "wrong" to evaluators (Jonsen et al., 1998, p. 474).

Although decision-making capacity is decision specific, it has been argued that there are shared decisional abilities that are underlying, regardless of the particulars of a decision. Grisso and Appelbaum (1998, pp. 31–32) offered four "functional abilities," derived from studying writings in law, medical ethics, clinical practice, and empirical investigation, and policy statements from key commissions, on which capacity assessments should focus. The four functional abilities are: (a) expressing a choice, (b) understanding information required for the decision, (c) appreciating how the information given pertains to the person's own life, and (d) logical reasoning using the information.

As noted, the President's Commission articulated the need to observe a variable stringency in determining capacity depending on the importance of potential outcomes. Drane (1984; see also Buchanan & Brock, 1990, pp. 48–57) described a hierarchical approach to determining capacity to consent to treatment that takes into account the discernible risks and benefits in a given treatment decision, assigning three standards of stringency. The most liberal standard is applied when the benefit outweighs the risk for the patient's choice compared to other possible choices and when the decisions are "objectively in the patient's best interests" (p. 926). If the benefit to risk ratio is equivalent for all choices, then a higher standard is employed. When the patient's choices are riskier than would be the case for alternative choices, when they "fly in the face of both professional and public rationality," (p. 927) then the most stringent standard is imposed.

Although the President's Commission included in its report the observation that capacity is decision specific, in practice that characteristic may sometimes be difficult to recognize. A recent report (Ganzini, Volicer, Nelson, & Derse, 2003) of the most common misunderstandings about decisional capacity encountered by consultation-liaison psychiatrists, geriatricians, and geriatric psychologists who receive requests to evaluate patients for capacity is illuminating. Ganzini et al.'s respondents reported that the most frequent error made by clinicians seeking consultation was viewing incapacity as global rather than decision-specific.

For neuropsychologists, discerning which decision and which decisional capacity are at issue will guide the investigation. An inquiry into the capacity of a person to refuse surgery will differ from that facing the evaluator asked if one frail elder can manage money or another can assert a capable acceptance of fall risk rather than move to a care setting (Macciocchi & Stringer, 2001, caution that in considering potential risk and harm, the evaluator must be aware of actuarial constraints on forming predictions from symptoms as a matter of ethical practice).

In general, the strategy for evaluation will be similar regardless of the decision in question: (a) clarify the referral question and determine if the person receiving the consultation request is competent to address the question; (b) plan the assessment and address cultural considerations and ethical issues such as informed consent and confidentiality; (c) conduct the assessment; (d) communicate the results; and (e) recommend any additional evaluations or interventions that might enhance capacity or address temporal limitations on the evaluation findings (Baker, Lichtenberg, & Moye, 1998; Department of

Veterans Affairs, 1997). Addressing the ethical imperative of informed consent, the 2002 revision of the Ethics Code included new language (Standard 9.03a) exempting psychologists from obtaining informed consent when "one purpose of the testing is to evaluate decisional capacity," in recognition of "the fact that the term 'consent' refers to a person's legal status to make autonomous decisions based on age, mental capacity, or the legal decision under consideration" (Fisher, 2003, p. 191).

The evaluation in most settings will address, in addition to the specific decisional capacity at issue, the person's cognition, mood, environmental supports, and functional limitations that may not be centrally mediated. A person's inability to complete a task may reflect executional rather than decisional incapacity, for instance, and the evaluator's responsibility may include identifying or recommending further exploration of needed adaptations and environmental supports so execution of the capable person's decisions is possible. Awareness of the special sensory-motor, medical, normative, and cultural concerns in the assessment of older persons is essential, regardless of the particular referral question triggering the assessment.

Measurement concerns

Central to the question of evaluation is measurement. Perhaps the most thoroughgoing measurement issue facing psychologists consulted for decision-making capacity evaluation is whether or not to use a specific decision-making capacity instrument and, if so, which one to select. Strongly arguing against the employment of a "capacimeter" are Kapp and Mossman (1996), who articulated potential sources of error in the application of a standard instrument and instead recommended the adoption of clinical practice parameters. Edelstein (2000) countered that while practice guidelines are useful they "do not preclude the biases and vicissitudes of clinical judgment often associated with nonstandardized and informal assessment methods" (p. 8). An extensive critique of the research literature on assessment of capacity to consent to treatment and research participation by Kim, Karlawish, and Caine (2002) noted, among other findings, the analytic difficulties presented by research in which the definition of capacity, comparison of normative versus clinical judgment and of formal instruments, and the degree of leniency or stringency adopted by the examiners differ study by study.

Despite methodological challenges, the empirical investigation of decision-making capacity has yielded substantial information about the occurrence of impairment in clinical populations and in older persons with and without dementing illness. Marson, Ingram, Cody, and Harrell (1995) assessed persons with mild to moderate Alzheimer's disease (AD) and a group of healthy older persons with a vignettes-based instrument (the Capacity to Consent to Treatment Instrument, CCTI). Five legal standards for capacity to consent to medical treatment were investigated: (a) knowing that a decision is to be made, (b) making a reasonable decision, (c) understanding the personal and future impact of the choice selected, (d) demonstrating logical reasoning in the decision making, and (e) comprehension of the treatment context and choices. The authors reported that healthy persons and those with mild and moderate dementia performed similarly under the first two, least difficult, standards. The performance of persons with AD was significantly lower than that of the group of healthy persons on the last three of the five standards, with most healthy controls performing well for all five standards. The authors cautioned that "the process of understanding and responding to a hypothetical medical problem will always differ from that associated with a personal medical problem," but they noted that standardized assessment with vignettes can assess those abilities essential to capacity (p. 6).

Dymek, Atchison, Harrell, and Marson (2001) assessed persons with Parkinson's disease with overall mild cognitive impairment and healthy controls using the CCTI and neuropsychological instruments. The healthy control group was competent for all legal standards using a statistical determination, while the Parkinson's disease group demonstrated increasing impairment as the complexity of the standard rose (30% statistically determined to be marginally incapable or incapable for the first standard, 80% for the fifth). "Declines in simple executive function, and to a lesser extent memory" appeared to be particularly vulnerable (p. 22).

Moye, Karel, Azar, and Gurrera (2004) evaluated healthy controls and older persons with dementia due to differing etiologies. Participants were given the MacArthur Competence Tool for Treatment (MacCAT-T; Grisso & Appelbaum, 1998), the Hopemont Capacity Assessment Instrument (HCAI; Edelstein, 2000), and the CCTI, with specific reference to the standards of understanding, appreciation, reasoning, and expression of a treatment choice, the assessment of which differs across instruments. The dementia group performed worse than the control group for understanding as assessed by all three capacity instruments, although most of those with mild dementia did not demonstrate impairment. All participants scored within the normal range on the MacCAT-T measurement of appreciation, a substantial percentage of the control adults fell within the impaired range on the HCAI appreciation assessment, and the group with dementia demonstrated impairment for appreciation on the CCTI. The dementia group demonstrated impairment for reasoning on the CCTI; subscores for MacCAT-T reasoning varied; and on average, there was no significant difference between the dementia and control group for reasoning on the HCAI. Finally, expression of treatment choice was intact for all conditions, although some control participants had difficulty with the HCAI requirement of expressing a choice for the person described in the vignette because "they could not make a choice on behalf of another" (Moye et al., 2004, p. 7).

In summary, the empirical literature yields guidance about the vulnerability of particular clinical populations (in the studies cited above, persons with Alzheimer's disease or Parkinson's disease) to impaired decisional capacity. In clinical practice, however, any individual patient referred with a "high-risk" diagnosis may have preserved capacity to weigh and communicate decisions. The neuropsychologist who acknowledges the desirability of including standardized measures or structured interviews within the capacity evaluation will nonetheless confront the issue that there currently is no consensus protocol for the evaluation of cognition, mental health status, or specific capacity questions when decisional capacity is at issue for a particular patient. There are many measures assessing capacity domains for specific clinical and legal questions and for specific populations, but no uniform standard for the selection of instruments appropriate for both the context and population characteristics of specific capacity questions. The theoretical and practice concerns that this lack of uniformity raises are outside the scope of this chapter, but the reader is referred to the analysis and compilation offered in the second edition of *Evaluating Competencies: Forensic Assessments and Instruments* (Grisso, 2003) for a rich discussion of measurement characteristics.

Decision-making capacity evaluation in clinical contexts

Specific concerns to be addressed in clinical capacity evaluations include characterizing the person's neuropsychological status, assessing the four decisional abilities articulated by Grisso and Appelbaum (1998), and evaluating the patient's ability to use clearly presented medical information to weigh a decision. If there are remediable deficits in the person's cognitive presentation, providing compensation for them may be important for determining capacity. For instance, if there is a significant memory disorder but the patient is able to self-monitor and use reminders, information about the choices can be written out for ready reference. If there is expressive language disorder in the context of relatively preserved comprehension, consultation with a speech and language pathologist for the strategic use of aids can allow for the determination of the person's decisional abilities and decisional capacity within the situational demands the patient is facing.

Although occasionally a physician will request an evaluation when the patient is in agreement but the person's family is opposed to the recommendation, typically referrals for evaluation of a patient's decision-making capacity will be triggered by the patient's disagreement with a clinical recommendation, such as a course of treatment or increased supervision for safety. Sometimes the patient will have agreed with a recommendation but then is inconsistent in that agreement.

One question that may arise in the referral or assessment is how transient the attenuated capacity may be. Particularly in cases of delirium or significant psychiatric disorder, there may be constraints on the person's understanding, judgment, or communication that are potentially resolvable with improvements in the person's health status. In these instances, if treatment for the capacity-impairing condition itself is at issue, the consultant may find decision-making capacity to be currently compromised, and it may be necessary for a surrogate decision maker to be consulted in the treatment planning. In other cases, however, there may not be a need for immediate intervention and the treatment team may be able to continue the treatment the patient has already accepted (such as intervention for new suspiciousness or severe depression), offering support while continuing in a noncoercive way to present their concerns to the patient. If the patient's substantially disrupted capacity continues, a process for proxy decision making can still be invoked whether the patient concurs with or continues to object to the recommended treatment. If in the interim the patient has recovered adequate capacity, the institution of surrogate decision making can be averted. Often, in geriatric neuropsychology, the presenting issue is not the question of transient challenges to decisional capacity but rather a dementing illness, usually in the mild through moderate stages, in which there is no clear uniform incapacity for substantial decisions, such as participation in treatment with potential risk or transfer to a long-term care facility, and the patient is in disagreement with the recommendation.

Decision-making capacity and guardianship

While there often is overlap between clinical concerns and referral to potential guardianship, as for instance a hospital's seeking court intervention for a patient with impaired decisional capacity who has no proxy decision-maker, the mechanisms for determination of clinical and civil incapacity are distinct. A judge is the determiner of a legal status of incapacity, and many specific capacities are recognized in law, each of which "must be approached and analyzed discretely" (Marson, 2001, p. 269). Legal descriptions of impairment have included "incompetence," "incapacity," and "disability," but three essential components of capacity, however it is termed, are common to state laws: "(1) disorders/disabilities; (2) decision-making/communicating impairment; and (3) functional impairment" (Anderer, 1990a, pp. 3–4). In order to deprive someone of self-rule, it must be demonstrated that "the respondent's functional impairment endangers his or her physical health or safety or may lead to the waste or dissipation of his or her property" (Anderer, 1990b, p. 108).

Although guardianship may be sought in order to provide medical treatment, a question about the person's ability to safely live at home or manage money may frequently be the reason a neuropsychologist is asked to do a decision-making capacity evaluation. Buchanan and Brock (1990) argued that there should be an even greater respect paid to autonomy when living arrangements or how the person manages money is at issue, because of their importance and because "many decisions about the use of an individual's financial resources or about where and how to live are more clearly questions of personal preference, about which there is no objectively correct answer, than are decisions about medical care" (p. 78). They noted that viewing financial decision-making capacity as decision specific is particularly challenging because financial matters often involve other persons, who need to know that the person with whom they are negotiating and interacting contractually is able to reliably participate in financial decisions.

Clinical rating scales of capacity

Almost every practitioner making judgments concerning decisional capacity utilizes some form of interview, but remarkably little is known about the threshold used by clinicians for such judgments. Although there are a number of measures that have been used to assess functional status in patients, there are fewer that directly address the issue of capacity or competency. Below is a list of standardized clinical rating scales that are commonly used to assess capacity or competency. While not exhaustive, we sought to include those measures that are widely used, are well validated, and specifically address the issue of capacity.

MacArthur Competence Assessment Tool

The MacArthur Competence Assessment Tool (MacCAT-T) was developed to meet the need for a practical tool that would help obtain and organize information about patients' decision-making abilities (Grisso & Appelbaum, 1998). It is perhaps one of the most widely used of the structured interview scales in the competency literature. The MacCAT-T is a structured interview that takes approximately 15–20 minutes to complete. This scale is based on the four areas of decisional capacity related to generally applied legal standards for competence and consent to treatment and research. These four areas include: (a) understanding relevant information, (b) appreciation of the implication of the information for one's own situation, (c) reasoning with the information in a decisional process, and (d) evidencing a choice. The MacCAT-T interview covers the following specific domains: (a) understanding of disorder, (b) appreciation of disorder, (c) understanding of treatment risks/discomforts, (d) appreciation of treatment, (e) alternative treatments, (f) reasoning, and (g) expressing a choice. The MacCAT-T does not yield a total score, but rather four general subscales (i.e., Understanding, Appreciation, Reasoning, Expressing a Choice). Field studies revealed intraclass correlations (ICC) to be quite good for Understanding (ICC = .99), Appreciation (ICC = .87), and Reasoning (ICC = .91) subscales for three independent raters. The MacCAT-T has been used in a number of competence studies in AD and shown to have good predictive validity (Karlawish, Casarett, & James, 2002; Kim & Caine, 2002; Kim, Caine, Currier, Leibovici, & Ryan, 2001).

Capacity to Consent to Treatment Instrument

The Capacity to Consent to Treatment Instrument (CCTI; Marson, Cody, Ingram, & Harrell, 1995; Marson, Ingram et al., 1995) is an instrument used to assess consent capacity in older healthy controls and patients with mild and moderate AD. The CCTI utilizes two clinical vignettes that each present a hypothetical medical problem (i.e., neoplasm, atherosclerotic heart disease) and symptoms, and two treatment options with associated risks and benefits.

The administration of the CCTI approximates an informed consent dialogue and requires the patient to process both oral and written information concerning the medical problem at hand as well as the treatment options and associated risks and benefits. After presentation of these vignettes, the patient is asked to answer questions designed to test consent capacity under four established legal standards drawn from case law: (a) LS1—Simply evidencing/communicating a treatment choice; (b) LS3—Appreciating the practical and anticipated consequences of a treatment choice; (c) LS4—Providing rational reasons (pro and con) for a treatment choice; and (d) LS5—Understanding the treatment situation, and treatment choices, and respective risks/benefits. In addition, questions concerning consent-related ability are also asked (LS2—What constitutes a reasonable choice?). The CCTI assigns each patient one of three outcomes (i.e., capable, marginally capable, incapable) for each standard. Reliability coefficients for the CCTI vignettes were reported to be around .93. A review of validation studies of the CCTI is presented in Marson and Harrell (1999).

Hopemont Capacity Assessment Interview

The Hopemont Capacity Assessment Interview (HCAI; Edelstein, 2000) is a semistructured interview designed to aid in the assessment of medical and financial decision making among nursing home residents. The HCAI is broadly based on the aforementioned Grisso and Appelbaum (1998) criteria. This measure uses a number of orally presented vignettes to assess competency, some describing medical situations requiring decisions (i.e., nonlife-threatening eye infection, life-threatening respiratory or cardiac arrest), while others deal with day-to-day financial decisions (i.e., purchase of a soft drink, loan of a substantial amount of money to a relative for a questionable cause). Prior to the presentation of these vignettes, brief definitions of the concepts of risk, benefit, and choice are presented to the patient and a series of questions concerning their meaning are asked. The scoring of the HCAI utilizes a criterion-referenced approach, with a 3-point scoring system being used (i.e., 0 = inadequate, 1 = questionable, 2 = adequate). The HCAI has been shown to be comparable to the MacCAT-T and CCTI in older patients with dementia (Moye et al., 2004).

The aforementioned measures constitute some of the more commonly used competence assessment tools. A number of other more recent measures also deserve attention, such as the Hopkins Competency Assessment Test (HCAT; Janofsky, McCarthy, & Folstein, 1991) and the Aid to Capacity Evaluation (ACE; Etchells et al., 1999).

In addition to more global competency measures, neuropsychologists are often brought into the evaluation process when there is a question about the patient's ability to conduct her or his financial affairs. In general, the literature has suggested that such assessments include formal tests of knowledge of income, assets, expenses, ability to write checks and balance account statements, etc., as well as an appreciation of how bills are paid, and consideration of financial problems and financial needs (Anderer, 1990b). The following measures are a sampling of tasks used to assess these functions in elderly patients.

Financial Capacity Instrument

The Financial Capacity Instrument (FCI; Griffith et al., 2003; Marson et al., 2000) is a companion instrument to the CCTI that directly assesses the decisional skills associated with financial dealings. In their development of this instrument, the authors identified the main domains of everyday financial activity. The inclusion criteria for these domains were: (a) theoretical relevance to independent functioning of community-dwelling older adults, (b) clinical relevance to health care professionals who treat older adults and evaluate financial capacity, and (c) general relevance to extant and prior state statutory criteria for financial competency. Using these criteria, the authors identified six initial domains of financial activity: (a) basic monetary skills, (b) financial conceptual knowledge, (c) cash transactions, (d) checkbook management, (e) bank statement management, and (f) financial judgment. From these initial criteria, the FCI was derived, consisting of 18 financial ability tests (tasks), 9 domains (activities), and 2 total scores. The FCI takes approximately 40–45 minutes to administer to patients with dementia.

Measure of Awareness of Financial Skills

Another clinical measure specifically targeting financial capacity is the Measure of Awareness of Financial Skills (MAFS; Cramer, Tuokko, Mateer, & Hultsch, 2004). The MAFS is a three-part scale consisting of a participant questionnaire, an informant questionnaire, and a performance-based measure. Based on an review of the financial capacity and awareness literature, the authors constructed 19 objectives judged to be important for assessing financial skills in a given patient. One main objective of the MAFS was to include both participant–informant and participant–performance comparison methods in the assessment process. As such, the MAFS includes: (a) a 34-item participant questionnaire consisting of questions pertaining to financial management (questions address the patient's self-rating of ability to balance a checkbook, count money, write checks, financial capability, and knowledge and awareness of various financial consequences), (b) a parallel informant questionnaire in which the same questions concerning the patient are posed to the informant, and (c) a performance measure consisting of six financial tasks that were selected to parallel the aforementioned questions (e.g., counting money, balancing a checkbook). Internal consistency estimates for patient and informant questionnaires were described as high (.92 and .97, respectively), and convergent validity analysis showed that higher levels of unawareness as detailed on the MAFS were associated with poorer cognitive skills as measured on an abbreviated neuropsychological battery. Discriminant validity analysis revealed that performance on the MAFS was not related to social desirability or neuroticism. A follow-up validation study of the MAFS (van Wielingen, Tuokko, Cramer, Mateer, & Hultsch, 2004) examined this scale's use in a sample of 42 community-dwelling individuals with dementia. Results revealed that severity of global cognitive impairment and executive dysfunction were significantly related to poorer awareness on the MAFS. In addition, significantly less awareness of financial ability was seen with more complex as compared to simple tasks. The MAFS differs from the FCI in that the MAFS also measures the patient's ability to understand the situation, including its financial risks, benefits, and alternatives (i.e., awareness).

While there are other financial capacity instruments available in the literature (e.g., Goel, Grafman, Tajik, Gana, & Danto, 1997; Lowenstein et al., 1989), the previously discussed tasks offer a balance between specific performance-based approaches and clinician/caregiver/patient ratings. As noted earlier, a comprehensive review and compilation of clinical rating scales and measures is offered in the second edition of *Evaluating Competencies: Forensic Assessments and Instruments* (Grisso, 2003).

Neuropsychological assessment of capacity

From a neuropsychological perspective, the assessment of decisional capacity involves a complex set of neurocognitive functions as well as noncognitive factors. The patient must comprehend and encode what is said, process and manipulate this information, weigh the risk–benefit ratios of the possible choices, and communicate a decision in a cohesive and clear manner. While neuropsychological assessment is often at the core of most comprehensive competency assessments, there has been little agreement on what measures best discriminate between competent or incompetent patients or how these measures relate to real-life assessment or clinical ratings of capacity. The following is a general overview of some of the research detailing neuropsychological performance in relation to competence or capacity.

In one of the earliest studies examining the neuropsychological correlates of competency, Marson, Cody et al. (1995) and Marson, Ingram et al. (1995) examined 29 patients with probable AD and 15 healthy elderly controls. Using a brief neuropsychological battery and the CCTI, the authors showed that only semantic (Animal Naming) and phonemic (Controlled Oral Word Association [COWA]; Benton & Hamsher, 1978) word-list generation tasks significantly predicted status on LS4 of the CCTI. Notably, measures of verbal reasoning and memory were not related to CCTI measures.

In a follow-up study, Marson, Chatterjee, Ingram, and Harrell (1996) examined 29 patients with probable AD and 15 healthy controls. They found that in the AD group, simple auditory comprehension (Auditory Comprehension Screen [SAC]; Eisenson, 1954) was associated with the capacity to evidence a treatment of choice (LS1, the minimal standard). Phonemic word-list generation (COWA) predicted the capacity to appreciate the "consequences of a treatment choice" (LS3), while measures of conceptualization (Conceptualization subscale from the Mattis Dementia Rating Scale [MDRS]; Mattis, 1976) and confrontation naming (Boston Naming Test [BNT]; Kaplan, Goodglass, & Weintraub, 1983) together predicted the patient's ability to "understand the treatment situation and choices" (LS5, the most stringent standard). Notably, using discriminant function analysis, the authors found that the best predictor of LS1 for all subjects was confrontation naming, while visuomotor tracking (Trails A) best predicted LS3 and LS5 performance.

Bassett (1999) examined the neuropsychological predictors of competence in 20 persons with AD and 20 healthy controls utilizing a financial capacity questionnaire, a competency test for medical decision making, and a battery of neuropsychological measures selected to reflect the cognitive processes theoretically related to competency. Results indicated that AD patients performed worse than controls on both competency measures. Only performance on the Trail Making Test, Part A (Reitan, 1958) and Word-List Recall from the Consortium to Establish a Registry for Alzheimer's Disease (CERAD; Morris et al., 1989) were significantly correlated with competency measures. Notably, Trails A predicted over 85% of the variance in competency scores and discriminated competent from not competent AD patients with 77–82% accuracy.

Dymek, Marson, and Harrell (1999) assessed 82 patients with probable or possible AD on the CCTI. In the exploratory phase of the experiment, a principal components analysis revealed that the CCTI is composed of two orthogonal factors: (a) Verbal Conceptualization/Reasoning and (b) Verbal Memory. In the validation phase, principal components analysis of individual factor scores and neuropsychological test performance supported and further elaborated the described two-factor structure. Specifically, measures of conceptualization, executive function, language, semantic memory and attention loaded significantly on the CCTI reasoning/conceptualization factor whereas immediate and delayed verbal recall indices loaded on the verbal memory factor of the CCTI. These findings suggest that consent capacity in an AD population is a multidimensional construct represented by neurocognitive factors of verbal reasoning and verbal memory. The authors further hypothesized that measures of verbal conceptualization/reasoning and verbal memory are likely to be sensitive to declining treatment consent capacity in older adults with AD.

In a follow-up study examining 20 patients with Parkinson's disease (PD) and 20 healthy controls, Dymek et al. (2001) used the CCTI and a battery of neuropsychological measures to define those cognitive functions related to competency in patients suffering from subcortical pathology. Results showed that relative to controls, PD patients showed more compromise (marginally capable or incapable) on the CCTI, with simple measures of executive function (i.e., Executive Interview [EXIT]; Royall, Mahurin, & Gray, 1992) and, to a lesser extent, memory and orientation (i.e., Memory Subscale from the Mattis Dementia Rating Scale [MDRS]; Mattis, 1976) predicting competency performance on the CCTI. Notably, the CCTI competency predictor profiles of the PD and AD groups seemed to differ insofar as executive dysfunction was the preeminent predictor of competency for the PD group, whereas a variety of cognitive functions predicted CCTI competency in patients with AD. Overall, these studies of neuropsychological functions with regard to capacity, while not specifying a specific test or tests to determine these judgments, highlight the importance of memory and executive functions in core aspects of this concept.

Summary and conclusions

Elderly patients with cognitive impairment are at increased risk for having impaired decisional abilities and pose a significant challenge to the evaluating neuropsychologist. Patients in this population often have significant medical and neuropsychiatric comorbidity and inevitably are faced with difficult treatment decisions. For neuropsychologists, discerning which decision and which decisional capacity are at issue will guide the investigation and the tools used. For emphasis, the terms used to define the targets of decisional capacity assessments (Marson, Dymek, & Karlawish, 2001) are summarized in Table 18.1.

Table 18.1 Terms used to define the targets of decisional capacity assessments

---

1. *Decisional capacity.* This term is related to the patient's ability to understand and comprehend treatment information, to reason, and to appreciate the consequences of choices made. In general, this term is related to the person's decision-making processes. In this case, a neuropsychologist may utilize neuropsychological and psychological tests to discern a given patient's decisional abilities.

2. *Competency.* This concept relates to whether the neuropsychologist decides a patient is capable of carrying out a specific act (e.g., consent to a risky surgical procedure) or set of activities (e.g., handling her or his financial affairs). The clinician will use the assessment of the patient's decision-making abilities in forming this judgment. In this framework, both decisional capacity and competency are *clinical judgments* made by the neuropsychologist.

3. *Legal competency.* In contrast to the aforementioned, this term relates to the decision made by a judge or other legal professional about whether or not a given patient has the ability under the law to carry out a specific act or series of activities. The neuropsychologist's typical role in this process is to define the patient's decisional skills and abilities and to form a judgment concerning how these skills or abilities affect the patient's functioning in a given area or areas. The judge then utilizes this information along with other legal factors to arrive at a finding concerning competency.

Source: From Marson et al. (2001).

In general, it is helpful to think of the capacity evaluation as consisting of both clinical (i.e., interview) and neuropsychological (testing) components. That is, a thoughtful and comprehensive capacity evaluation should include both structured clinical interview scales designed to test capacity as well as objective neuropsychological measures that have been shown to be sensitive to decisional abilities in populations at risk for impaired decisional capacity.

As seen in the above text, assessment of capacity is complex and multifaceted. That is, there is no one measure of capacity from either a clinical rating scale or neuropsychological standpoint. Cognitive, emotional, and subjective factors contribute significantly to this process, highlighting the rich process that occurs when assessing a given patient's capacity. These factors are not yet clearly delineated, but it is evident that the neuropsychologist must balance the quantitative aspects of this process (i.e., objective neuropsychological and clinical assessment) with the less easily defined needs and hopes of the patient. The subjective components of the process are to be further studied and may provide insights into the decision-making processes of patients suffering from neurological and psychiatric illness. The careful assessment of such subjective aspects, the "noncognitive" contributions to capacity and consent, may in the future receive guidance from neuropsychological researchers, whose work has already provided valuable information about many of the theoretical and practice concerns in capacity evaluation.

Acknowledgement

This work was supported in part by National Institutes of Health Grants MH63381 (PJM) and P30-AG010124-12 (Alzheimer's Disease Center) and Parkinson's Disease Research, Education, and Clinical Center (PADRECC) at the Philadelphia VA Medical Center.

References

American Psychological Association. (2002). Ethical principles of psychologists and code of conduct. *American Psychologist, 57*, 1060–1073.

Anderer, S. J. (1990a). *Determining competency in guardianship proceedings.* Washington, DC: Division for Public Services, American Bar Association.

Anderer, S. J. (1990b). A model for determining competency in guardianship proceedings. *Mental and Physical Disability Law Report, 14*, 107–114.

Baker, R. R., Lichtenberg, P. A., & Moye, J. (1998). A practice guideline for assessment of competency and capacity of the older adult. *Professional Psychology: Research and Practice, 29*, 149–154.

Bassett, S. S. (1999). Attention: Neuropsychological predictor of competency in Alzheimer's disease. *Journal of Geriatric Psychiatry and Neurology, 12*, 200–205.

Beauchamp, T. L., & Childress, J. F. (1994). *Principles of biomedical ethics* (4th ed.). New York: Oxford University Press.

Benton, A., & Hamsher, K. (1978). *Multilingual Aphasia Examination.* Iowa City, IA: University of Iowa.

Buchanan, A. E., & Brock, D. W. (1990). *Deciding for others: The ethics of surrogate decision making*. Cambridge, UK: Cambridge University Press.

Cramer, K., Tuokko, H. A., Mateer, C. A., & Hultsch, D. F. (2004). Measuring awareness of financial skills: Reliability and validity of a new measure. *Aging and Mental Health, 8*(2), 161–171.

Department of Veterans Affairs. (1997). *Assessment of competency and capacity of the older adult: A practice guideline for psychologists*. Milwaukee, WI: National Center for Cost Containment.

Drane, J. F. (1984). Competency to give informed consent: A model for making clinical assessments. *Journal of the American Medical Association, 252*, 925–928.

Dymek, M. P., Atchison, P., Harrell, L., & Marson, D. C. (2001). Competency to consent to medical treatment in cognitively impaired patients with Parkinson's disease. *Neurology, 56*, 17–24.

Dymek, M. P., Marson, D. C., & Harrell, L. (1999). Factor structure of capacity to consent to medical treatment in patients with Alzheimer's disease: An exploratory study. *Journal of Forensic Neuropsychology, 1*(1), 27–48.

Edelstein, B. (2000). Challenges in the assessment of decision-making capacity. *Journal of Aging Studies, 14*, 423–437.

Eisenson, J. (1954). *Examining for aphasia*. New York: Psychological Corporation.

Etchells, E., Darzins, P., Silberfeld, M., Singer, P. A., McKenny, J., Naglie, G., et al. (1999). Assessment of patient capacity to consent to treatment. *Journal of General Internal Medicine, 14*, 27–34.

Fisher, C. B. (2003). *Decoding the Ethics Code: A practical guide for psychologists*. Thousand Oaks, CA: Sage.

Ganzini, L., Volicer, L., Nelson, W., & Derse, A. (2003). Pitfalls in assessment of decision-making capacity. *Psychosomatics, 44*, 237–243.

Goel, V., Grafman, J., Tajik, J., Gana, S., & Danto, D. (1997). A study of the performance of patients with frontal lobe lesions in a financial planning task. *Brain, 120*, 1805–1822.

Griffith, H. R., Belue, K., Sicola, A., Krzywanski, S., Zamrini, E., Harrell, L., & Marson, D. C. (2003). Impaired financial abilities in mild cognitive impairment: A direct assessment approach. *Neurology, 60*(3), 449–457.

Grisso, T. (2003). *Evaluating competencies: Forensic assessments and instruments*. New York: Plenum Press.

Grisso, T., & Appelbaum, P. S. (1998). *Assessing competence to consent to treatment: A guide for physicians and other health care professionals*. New York: Oxford University Press.

Janofsky, J. S., McCarthy, R. J., & Folstein, M. F. (1991). The Hopkins Competency Assessment Test: A brief method for evaluating patients' capacity to give informed consent. *Hospital and Community Psychiatry, 43*, 132–136.

Jonsen, A. R., Veatch, R. M., & Walters, L. (Eds.). (1998). *Source book in bioethics: A documentary history*. Washington, DC: Georgetown University Press.

Kaplan, E., Goodglass, H., & Weintraub, S. (1983). *Boston Naming Test*. Philadelphia: Lea & Febiger.

Kapp, M. B., & Mossman, D. (1996). Measuring decisional capacity: Cautions on the construction of a "capacimeter". *Psychology, Public Policy, and Law, 2*, 73–95.

Karlwish, J. H., Casarett, D. J., & James, B. D. (2002). Alzheimer's disease patients' and caregivers' capacity, competency, and reason to enroll in an early-phase

Alzheimer's disease clinical trial. *Journal of the American Geriatrics Society, 50,* 2019–2024.

Kim, S. Y. II., & Caine, E. D. (2002). Utility and limits of the Mini Mental State Examination in evaluating consent capacity in Alzheimer's disease. *Psychiatric Services, 53*(10), 1322–1324.

Kim, S. Y. H., Caine, E. D., Currier, G. W., Leibovici, A., & Ryan, J. M. (2001). Assessing the competence of persons with Alzheimer's disease in providing informed consent for participation in research. *American Journal of Psychiatry, 158,* 710–717.

Kim, S. Y. H., Karlawish, J. H. T., & Caine, E. D. (2002). Current state of research on decision-making competence of cognitively impaired elderly persons [Electronic version]. *American Journal of Geriatric Psychiatry, 10,* 151–165.

Loewenstein, D. A., Amigo, E., Duara, R., Guterman, A., Hurwitz, D., Berkowitz, N., et al. (1989). A new scale for the assessment of functional status in Alzheimer's disease and related disorders. *Journal of Gerontology, 44,* 114–121.

Macciocchi, S. N., & Stringer, A. Y. (2001). Assessing risk and harm: The convergence of ethical and empirical considerations. *Archives of Physical Medicine and Rehabilitation, 82*(Suppl. 2), 1–7. Retrieved July 4, 2004, from Archives of Physical Medicine and Rehabilitation Online.

Marson, D. C. (2001). Loss of competency in Alzheimer's disease: Conceptual and psychometric approaches [Electronic version]. *International Journal of Law and Psychiatry, 24,* 267–283.

Marson, D. C., Chatterjee, A., Ingram, K. K., & Harrell, L. E. (1996). Toward a neurologic model of competency: Cognitive predictors of capacity to consent in Alzheimer's disease using three different legal standards. *Neurology, 46*(3), 666–672.

Marson, D. C., Cody, H. A., Ingram, K. K., & Harrell, L. E. (1995). Neuropsychological predictors of competency in Alzheimer's disease using a rational reasons legal standard. *Neurology, 52*(10), 955–959.

Marson, D. C., Dymek, M., & Karlawish, J. (2001). Competency to consent to medical treatment in cognitively impaired patients with Parkinson's disease [Letter, reply]. *Neurology, 56,* 1782–1783.

Marson, D. C., & Harrell, L. E. (1999). Executive dysfunction and loss of capacity to consent to medical treatment in patients with Alzheimer's disease. *Seminars in Clinical Neuropsychiatry, 4*(1), 41–49.

Marson, D. C., Ingram, K. K., Cody, H. A., & Harrell, L. E. (1995). Assessing the competency of patients with Alzheimer's disease under different legal standards: A prototype instrument. *Archives of Neurology, 52,* 949–954.

Marson, D. C., Sawrie, S. M., Snyder, S., McInturff, B., Stalvey, T., Boothe, A., et al. (2000). Assessing financial capacity in patients with Alzheimer disease: A conceptual model and prototype instrument. *Archives of Neurology, 57,* 877–884.

Mattis, S. (1976). Dementia rating scale. In R. Bellack & B. Karasu (Eds.), *Geriatric psychiatry* (pp. 77–121). New York: Grune & Stratton.

Morris, J. C., Heyman, A., Mohs, R. C., Hughes, J. P., van Belle, G., Fillenbaum, G., et al. (1989). The Consortium to Establish a Registry for Alzheimer's Disease (CERAD). *Neurology, 39,* 1159–1165.

Moye, J., Karel, M. J., Azar, A. R., & Gurrera, R. J. (2004). Capacity to consent to treatment: Empirical comparison of three instruments in older adults with and without dementia. *The Gerontologist, 44,* 166–175.

Reitan, R. (1958). Validity of the Trail Making Test as an indication of organic brain damage. *Perceptual and Motor Skills, 8*, 271–276.

Royall, D., Mahurin, R., & Gray, K. (1992). Bedside assessment of executive cognitive impairment: The Executive Interview. *Journal of the American Geriatrics Society, 40*, 1221–1226.

Van Wielingen, L. E., Tuokko, H. A., Cramer, K., Mateer, C. A., & Hultsch, D. F. (2004). Awareness of financial skills in dementia. *Aging and Mental Health, 8*(4), 374–380.

19 Ethical issues in geriatric neuropsychology

Shane S. Bush and Thomas A. Martin

The transition into late adulthood, like other developmental transitions, is associated with physical, psychological, and social changes. Like other life transitions, late adulthood offers opportunity for growth and changes that enrich life. The shift in medicine and social sciences in recent years from an illness-oriented, disease model of aging toward a more functional model of health and wellness reflects the positive aspects of aging (Beckingham & Watts, 1995; Bowling, 1993; Kaplan & Strawbridge, 1994; Myers, 1992). However, aging, like other developmental stages, is not without potential factors that mitigate against successful adjustment (Coleman, 1992).

In contrast to earlier developmental stages, a primary challenge in late adulthood is coping with loss (Myers, 1999; Waters & Goodman, 1990). For example, losses in the areas of sensory abilities, motor skills, cognition, or long-term relationships are more common in older adults. Such losses may be accompanied by negative emotional changes (Erikson, 1963; Erikson, Erikson, & Kivnick, 1986; Lebowitz et al., 1997). In addition, medical problems, physical pain, and medication usage occur with greater frequency in older adults. These physical and psychosocial changes may result in increased dependence on others for assistance with daily tasks and decisions that were previously completed independently. From a clinical perspective, the developmental changes of late life pose unique professional and ethical challenges for neuropsychologists who work with geriatric populations (Hays, 1999).

Advanced consideration of the ethical issues that may arise during the practice of geriatric neuropsychology and the ways to approach ethical challenges better prepares neuropsychologists to proceed in a manner that advances the welfare of the recipients of their services. Although the ethical choices one makes are indelibly linked to the theoretical principles relevant in the decision-making context, this chapter strives to provide a practical approach for evaluating and addressing the ethical challenges that may be encountered in a geriatric neuropsychology practice. As the salient ethical issues are discussed, several case examples are provided to illustrate the application of a decision-making model within specific contexts.

Ethical decision making

Determining how to approach an ethical dilemma may be facilitated by drawing upon an ethical decision-making model. A variety of ethical decision-making models have been proposed, including general models (e.g., Canadian Psychological Association, 2000; Haas & Malouf, 2002; Kitchener, 2000; Koocher & Keith-Spiegel, 1998) and those applied to health care settings (Hanson, Kerkhoff, & Bush, 2005) and forensic practice (Bush, Connell, & Denney, in press). Knapp and Vandecreek (2003) reviewed the general ethical decision-making models and determined that they shared five common steps: (a) identification of the problem, (b) development of alternatives, (c) evaluation of alternatives, (d) implementation of the best option, and (e) evaluation of the results. Knapp and Vandecreek also noted that, despite their value, these models did not adequately consider emotional and situational factors or the need for an immediate response in some situations.

Due to the limitations found in previous models, Bush et al. (in press) proposed an eight stage model that expanded upon previously developed models to provide a more comprehensive approach to ethical decision making. The eight stages consist of the following: (a) identify the problem, (b) consider the significance of the context and setting, (c) identify and utilize resources, (d) consider personal beliefs and values, (e) develop possible solutions to the problem, (f) consider the potential consequences of various solutions, (g) choose and implement a course of action, and (h) assess the outcome and implement changes as needed.

Application of this model occurs within the framework of positive ethics, which requires a shift from an emphasis on misconduct and disciplinary action to an emphasis on the pursuit of one's highest ethical potential (Handelsman, Knapp, & Gottlieb, 2002). That is, selecting the optimal ethical option often requires more than simply avoiding ethical misconduct (risk management); it requires a commitment to pursuing the highest ethical principles available to health care providers. Additionally, positive ethics requires practicing in a manner that is preferable or aspirational, not simply according to what is required or permissible.

Salient ethical issues: An overview

The ethical concerns of neuropsychologists have been found to vary somewhat from the concerns of psychologists in general. Pope and Vetter (1992) surveyed 1319 members of the American Psychological Association (APA) and requested examples of ethical dilemmas that the psychologists encountered in their work. Fifty-one per cent (679) of the surveyed members replied, from which 703 ethical dilemmas were obtained. The dilemmas were grouped into 23 general categories representing the ethical and practice areas of concern. The top three categories of concern for psychologists in general were confidentiality, dual relationships, and financial issues. Forensic issues ranked fifth, issues related to assessment ranked ninth, and professional competence ranked eleventh.

In contrast to the general membership of APA, neuropsychologists prioritize ethical challenges somewhat differently. In a review of ethically challenging vignettes elicited from members of the American Board of Clinical Neuropsychology, the greatest percentage (56%) of ethical problems involved aspects of assessment practices (Brittain, Francis, & Barth, 1995). Brittain, Francis, McSweeny, Fisher, and Barth (1997) surveyed the membership of the National Academy of Neuropsychology, obtaining 456 responses. The respondents expressed greatest concern about examiner competence, assessment issues (inappropriate use of tests), and conflict between law and ethics. Dual relationship issues ranked tenth, confidentiality ranked eleventh (see Martelli, Zasler, & Grayson, 1999, for the complete list). Fifty per cent of the respondents indicated that the APA Ethics Code (1992 version) was insufficient to address ethical problems in neuropsychology.

In 1995, Binder and Thompson published a seminal article on neuropsychology ethics. They examined the 1992 APA Ethics Code and its applicability to neuropsychology. Their article focused on the following ethical issues: competence; multiple relationships; validity of test results and test interpretation; documentation of assessment results; records and confidentiality; forensic activities; avoiding harm in general, including informed consent issues, minimizing psychological discomfort, response validity, and examiner bias; supervision of subordinates; and fees. These issues were examined, and recommendations were provided.

Morgan (2002, 2005) and McSweeny (2005) have written about ethical issues in geriatric neuropsychology specifically, emphasizing the need for professional competence, the unique assessment considerations, and the importance of respect for people's rights and dignity, all aimed at the promotion of the client's welfare. Additional authors have explored ethical issues in neuropsychology in practice settings in which geriatric patients are frequently encountered, such as acute medical settings (Pinkston, 2005; Wilde, 2005; Wilde, Bush, & Zeifert, 2002) and rehabilitation settings (DeLuca, 2005; Johnson-Greene, 2005; Swiercinsky, 2002).

Application of general ethical principles to geriatric neuropsychology

Ethical principles represent the morality underlying the appropriate practice of a profession (Beauchamp & Childress, 2001). The ethical principles function as an analytic framework for guiding the ethical behavior of the members of the profession. The biomedical ethical principles espoused by Beauchamp and Childress have been widely referenced in ethical decision making in a variety of health care contexts and have been integrated into the most recent version of the APA Ethics Code (2002b). They proposed four core biomedical ethical principles: respect for autonomy, nonmaleficence, beneficence, and justice. Briefly, respect for autonomy refers to valuing the right to self-determination based on sufficient understanding of the circumstances of one's life. Nonmaleficence refers to causing no harm through one's professional choices or actions. Beneficence refers to contributing to the welfare of others through the performance of positive acts, rather than merely by refraining from harmful acts. Justice in this context refers to distributive justice; that is, fair opportunity to obtain at least a decent minimum of available health care resources.

With regard to the General Principles of the current APA Ethics Code (2002b), the principle of autonomy is found in General Principle E, Respect for People's Rights and Dignity. The principles of Beneficence and Nonmaleficence were combined to comprise General Principle A. Distributive justice is represented by General Principle D, Justice. The General Principles of the APA Ethics Code also include Fidelity and Responsibility (Principle B) and Integrity (Principle C). These latter principles (Fidelity and Responsibility, and Integrity) are more consistent with virtue ethics, representative of the character of the practitioner, than they are of ethics grounded in principles. Thus, the APA Ethics Code has incorporated both the ethics of principles and of virtues. Although the General Principles of the APA Ethics Code are considered aspirational, it would seem difficult to justify choosing not to practice in a manner consistent with the highest ideals of the profession.

Determination of a preferred choice or course of action can often be facilitated by considering the general ethical principles underlying the situation. However, ethical principles may conflict with each other, creating dilemmas. In such situations, an attempt should be made to determine the overriding moral obligation. Unfortunately, as Beauchamp and Childress (2001) stated, "Often no straightforward movement from theory or principles to particular judgments is available in these contexts. Theory and principles are only starting points and general guides for the development of norms of appropriate conduct. They are supplemented by paradigm cases of right action, empirical data, organizational experience, and the like" (p. 2). In addition to ethical principles, geriatric neuropsychologists must consider other sources of ethical authority, such as published articles and chapters, guidelines, and position papers. Choice of action will also be determined by jurisdictional laws.

In addition to moral principles that conflict with each other, "conflicts between moral requirements and self-interest sometimes produce a practical dilemma rather than a moral dilemma" (Beauchamp & Childress, 2001, p. 11). Conflicts between moral requirements and self-interests may be as challenging to negotiate as conflicts between two or more moral principles. To the extent possible, neuropsychologists working with older adults should, through continuing education and consultation with colleagues, attempt to anticipate potential dilemmas that may arise and determine in advance how such dilemmas may be managed. Despite one's best efforts to anticipate such situations, unique variations or ethical challenges will inevitably arise. When confronting such situations, identifying and weighing the fundamental ethical principles that are involved tends to be a good place to start.

Select topics of ethical concern in geriatric neuropsychology

Geriatric neuropsychologists have many sources of moral, professional, ethical, and legal authority from which to draw when faced with ethical challenges. In addition to the general ethical principles described above, the APA Ethical Standards provide guidelines for professional behavior in a number of general areas. The Standards are enforceable for members of APA and for psychologists whose state psychology boards have adopted the APA Ethics Code for their professional guidelines. Because the Code was designed to apply in a general manner to psychologists across professional contexts, specific application of the Code is dependent upon supplementary resources, such as guidelines of professional organizations, published articles and chapters, and jurisdictional laws. In this chapter an attempt has been made to present and examine the Ethical Standards that may be most relevant and challenging to neuropsychologists working with older adults.

Professional competence

Professional competence is based on the general bioethical principle of nonmaleficence (General Principle A, Beneficence and Nonmaleficence; Ethical Standard 3.04, Avoiding Harm). In order to minimize the potential for harming patients, neuropsychologists must possess the requisite specialized knowledge and skills to perform the requested services (APA Ethical Standard 2.01, Boundaries of Competence, subsections a and b; Association of State and Provincial Psychology Boards [ASPPB], 2005, Section III A1, Limits on Practice). Competence in geriatric neuropsychology consists of four components, as follows.

First, the geriatric neuropsychologist must have adequate education, training, and experience in neuropsychology. Competence in neuropsychology is readily identified through board certification "by way of an accepted, rigorous peer review process sponsored by a nonprofit professional organization that has standing within a given professional field" (Sweet, Grote, & van Gorp, 2002, p. 114). Although board certification does not imply competence in all areas of neuropsychology and, in fact, is not required for practice, the specialized education, training, and experience required for board certification provide an appropriate standard for neuropsychological competence. Although competence in neuropsychology is a beginning, additional education and training are needed. As the APA Presidential Task Force on the Assessment of Age-Consistent Memory Decline and Dementia (1998) stated, "competence in conducting clinical interviews and administering, scoring, and interpreting psychological and neuropsychological tests is necessary, but may not be sufficient" (section II. 3A).

Second, the geriatric neuropsychologist must have appropriate education, training, and experience in gerontology. Late adulthood represents a distinct developmental stage with unique issues and concerns. Neuropsychologists working with older adults must be familiar with the unique issues of the neuropsychologically asymptomatic members of this population. Familiarity with the more common medical disorders experienced by older adults and the potential neuropsychological side effects of the medications used to treat them is essential.

Third, geriatric neuropsychologists must possess in-depth understanding of the neuropathology and psychopathology of older adults. Such understanding includes knowledge of how the neuropathology and psychopathology evidenced by older adults translate into performance on measures of cognitive and psychological functioning. In addition, competence in this area includes knowledge of potential treatment options for the various disorders, including psychological, pharmacologic, and rehabilitative options. It may be necessary to offer information or treatment recommendations for family members and other caregivers, as well as the patient. Geriatric neuropsychologists should be able to discuss these issues with appropriate parties and to make referrals as needed.

Fourth, geriatric neuropsychologists must be able to demonstrate the integration of their competence in neuropsychology, gerontology, and the neuropathology and psychopathology of older adults. Competent neuropsychological assessment and treatment of geriatric patients must be based on appropriate education, supervised training, and experience with the population to whom, and in the setting in which, services are offered. For example, data collection methods, tests, and normative data will differ depending on the specific geriatric populations assessed and the contexts in which evaluations are performed.

Competence is not a static trait. Attainment of board certification does not guarantee that the psychologist will maintain competence in the years following awarding of the diploma (Binder & Thompson, 1995). Rapid advances are being made in geriatric medicine, neuroimaging, and other areas of relevant inquiry, and geriatric neuropsychologists have a responsibility to remain current with emerging information (APA Ethical Standard 2.03, Maintaining Competence; ASPPB Section A2, Maintaining Competence). The following scenario (Scenario A) highlights several relevant ethical issues related to professional competence in the practice of geriatric neuropsychology.

After relocating to a new city, a neuropsychologist enters into a group psychology practice that caters to young and middle age adults. After several weeks of practice, he is informed by the owner of practice that they have received a referral to assess the neuropsychological ability of a 78-year-old woman to continue living independently. Her medical history is remarkable for advanced arthritis, congestive heart failure, and cognitive decline. She has an eighth grade education. Despite very limited experience with older adults, the neuropsychologist, wanting to accommodate the owner of the practice, accepts the referral. On the day of the evaluation the patient arrives in the company of her grandson. After taking a thorough history from the patient and her grandson, the neuropsychologist introduces them to the clinic's psychometrist and requests that the clinic's standard full-day test battery be administered. Three hours later, the psychometrist meets with the neuropsychologist and reports that the patient appears anxious and is having difficulty completing many test items. He invited the grandson into the room for the past hour to serve as a calming presence for the patient, with some benefit. Moreover, the psychometrist admits that he has no experience testing geriatric patients and is frustrated by the patient's frequent requests for breaks. He also expresses doubts that she will be able to complete the full-day evaluation as scheduled given her current pace. The neuropsychologist has other patients scheduled for the rest of the afternoon and is unsure how to proceed.

Application of the decision-making model can help identify the relevant ethical issues and possible courses of action:

(a) Identify the problem. The neuropsychologist realizes that he is now in the middle of a situation that exceeds his level of professional competence. He must decide whether or not to continue with the evaluation, given his limited experience with geriatric patients and the actions and reaction of a psychometrist with no geriatric testing experience.

(b) *Consider the significance of the context and setting.* In the clinical psychology group practice, the neuropsychologist is without immediate access to a colleague who can offer advice and potentially assume responsibility for the evaluation. However, in contrast to many medical settings, there is less urgency to complete the evaluation in one day.

(c) *Identify and utilize resources.* The neuropsychologist is familiar with the ethical and legal guidelines surrounding his dilemma, having reviewed the APA Ethics Code, the ASPPB Code of Conduct, the Standards for Educational and Psychological Testing (SEPT; American Educational Research Association, American Psychological Association, National Council on Measurement in Education, 1999), and state laws in a recent continuing education course on ethics. Recalling that the various resources were generally consistent with regard to the issues of concern in this case, he reflects on the relevant sections of the APA Ethics Code for guidance. The neuropsychologist realizes that he lacks adequate education, training, and experience to perform geriatric evaluations and that he should not have accepted this referral (Standard 2.01, Boundaries of Competence). In addition, he realizes that his psychometrist is not qualified to work with older adults (Standard 2.05, Delegation of Work to Others). Nevertheless, having missed the initial opportunity to decline the referral, the neuropsychologist understands that he is obligated to resolve the matter in the best interests of the patient. In deciding whether or not to proceed with the evaluation, the psychologist confronts ethical dilemmas and questions related to beneficence and nonmaleficence (Principle A). More specifically, if he discontinues the evaluation, will the welfare of the patient be compromised by his inability to identify her possible need for supervision (Standard 3.04, Avoiding Harm)? Conversely, if he renders an opinion regarding her ability to live independently given the data that has been collected, can he harm the patient (Standards 9.01, Bases for Assessments; 9.02, Use of Assessments; 9.06, Interpreting Assessment Results)? Although the neuropsychologist considers conferring with his practice partners, their lack of expertise in geriatric neuropsychology limits their ability to be of assistance. Consultation with an experienced geriatric neuropsychologist will likely help the neuropsychologist select an appropriate course of action.

(d) *Consider personal beliefs and values.* Through consideration of his own personal beliefs and values, the neuropsychologist begins to appreciate how his desire to please his new colleagues influenced his decision to accept a referral that he was not competent to perform. Additionally, he realizes that his preference to err on the side of caution regarding the patient's possible need for supervision, if inadequately supported, will result in a loss of independence that can adversely impact her quality of life (Principle E, Respect for People's Rights and Dignity).

(e) *Develop possible solutions to the problem.* The neuropsychologist understands that the evaluation can not be continued at that time and that a report cannot be generated based on the data collected to that point. He considers the following courses of action: (1) rescheduling the remainder of the evaluation for another day, while obtaining supervision from a qualified colleague in the interim; and (2) referring the patient to a qualified neuropsychologist.

(f) *Consider the potential consequences of various solutions.* The neuropsychologist, very competent with younger adults, considers that he may be able to salvage the evaluation by obtaining consultation with a qualified colleague. By doing so, he will eliminate the need for the patient to begin another evaluation, enhance his professional skills, and please his new employer. However, postponing the evaluation until he is able to obtain adequate consultation could potentially harm the patient by delaying the identification of any safety concerns. In contrast, by referring the patient to a qualified neuropsychologist, he will ensure that an appropriate evaluation is performed and that appropriate decisions are made regarding the patient's welfare. He can provide the geriatric neuropsychologist with the information obtained during the clinical interview in order to reduce redundancy, and he can provide the geriatric neuropsychologist with the list of tests administered (and data if requested) so that potential practice effect issues can be anticipated. However, the patient and her grandson will need to present for another evaluation session, and the patient's reaction to such a requirement cannot be anticipated. In addition, the esteem of the neuropsychologist's colleagues may be adversely affected.

(g) *Choose and implement a course of action.* The neuropsychologist decides that it will be in the best interest of the patient if he refers her to another neuropsychologist. He then meets with the patient and her grandson and informs them of the need for the referral. He promises to help them find a qualified examiner. The neuropsychologist subsequently works with the referring physician's office to locate a qualified geriatric neuropsychologist who is willing to evaluate the patient. Additionally, he (with patient authorization; Standard 4.05, Disclosures) contacts the geriatric neuropsychologist to discuss the particulars of the case.

(h) *Assess the outcome and implement changes as needed.* The evaluation by the geriatric neuropsychologist goes smoothly, and the referral question is appropriately addressed.

Human relations

Despite the unique issues often experienced by many geriatric patients, it is advisable for neuropsychologists to avoid making assumptions based solely on the patient's age (Standard 3.01, Unfair Discrimination). For example, when meeting for the first time with an 86-year-old patient who is accompanied by her 60-year-old son, it may be tempting to initially address the son and to request background information from him. However, failure to appropriately consider the patient's ability to accurately answer questions would reflect a lack of appreciation of her right to be involved in discussions that may have substantial implications for her independence, treatment, and care (General Principle E, Respect for People's Rights and Dignity). In addition, failure to consider the patient's ability to understand that she is being discussed in her presence may damage rapport and diminish the value of subsequent neuropsychological services.

Informed consent

The right to be fully informed regarding the proposed neuropsychological services and to consent to, or decline, participation as a result of that information is based on the principle of autonomy. With some exceptions as described below, neuropsychologists inform patients or examinees of the nature and purpose of the services, fees, involvement of third parties, potential risks, and limits of confidentiality, and provide an opportunity for questions and answers (Standards 3.10, Informed Consent; 9.03, Informed Consent in Assessments; and 10.01, Informed Consent to Therapy; APA Presidential Task Force on the Assessment of Age-Consistent Memory Decline and Dementia, 1998).

For individuals with questionable capacity to provide consent or for those mandated for services, information about the nature and purpose of the proposed services should still be provided, and it is generally appropriate to seek the individual's assent. Presenting the limitations on confidentiality and the implications of failing to participate may be of particularly value to the examinee. With individuals who have been deemed incompetent to make medical decisions, including consenting to neuropsychological services, and for whom a surrogate decision-maker has been appointed, the surrogate decision-maker should be fully informed and determine whether or not the services proceed. At all times, the neuropsychologists should keep the rights and welfare of the examinee or patient at the forefront of professional decision making. The consent/assent process, whether written or oral, should be documented.

The extent to which potential implications of neuropsychological evaluations are conveyed must be carefully considered. As Binder and Thompson (1995) stated, some patients "would choose not to undergo a neuropsychological examination if they fully understood that an abnormal result could jeopardize their normal prerogatives to make important decisions" (p. 39). For example, in the case of a neuropsychological evaluation that is requested to determine a 72-year-old man's cognitive capacity to manage medications, pay bills, or engage in other instrumental activities of daily living, informing him that the results may be used to remove him from his home or otherwise reduce his independence may limit the extent to which he agrees to participate with the evaluation.

In addition to possible refusal to participate, achievement of informed consent may interfere with the validity of the neuropsychological findings. Some patients may be less disclosing about psychosocial variables, premorbid history, and perceived deficits when made aware of the potential ramifications of their participation (Fisher, Johnson-Greene, & Barth, 2002). Providing less specific information about the purpose of the evaluation may increase both the chances of participation and the likelihood of valid results, which may ultimately promote the health and safety of the patient, consistent with the principle of beneficence. Geriatric neuropsychologists should prepare to face and work through difficult ethical challenges that pit beneficence against autonomy (APA, 2004). To the extent possible, it is important to balance protection of older adults' safety and well-being with their right to make their own decisions regarding the direction of their lives.

Although the neuropsychologist's personal values cannot (and perhaps should not) be removed entirely from ethically challenging situations, the ability to identify one's own values and to separate them from the values of the patient may be necessary in order to promote the patient's autonomy. In some cases, preserving a patient's independence may be worth accepting some level of substandard living or some risk of patient self-injury (Norris, Molinari, & Ogland-Hand, 2002). The issues may become more complex when (a) cognitive capacity is variable or uncertain; (b) selection or appointment of the substitute decision-maker is unresolved or the surrogate appears to be pursuing an agenda that is inconsistent with the best interests of the patient; (c) pressures from multiple involved parties, such as family members, legal representatives or authorities, and institutions, conflict; and/or (d) the issues involve death and dying. In such situations, it may be natural, and perhaps necessary, for the neuropsychologist to assume a paternalistic stance, consistent with medical tradition. Paternalism reflects a protective, beneficent position that overrides the preferences of another (Beauchamp & Childress, 2001). As such, paternalism represents a conflict between beneficence and autonomy. Great care should be taken any time that a neuropsychologist considers interfering with a patient's right to hold views, make choices, and take actions based upon his or her own values or beliefs. As noted by Macciocchi and Stringer (2002), constraints on autonomy due to beneficence must be supported by strong clinical evidence rather than conjecture. That is, a paternalistic stance should be considered only when neuropsychological evidence of incapacity is clear and convincing.

It is important for neuropsychologists to access colleagues and other available resources to help clarify the relevant issues, provide an uninvolved perspective, and offer assistance with choosing a course of action. To the extent that these concerns arise in the context of health care teams, families, or other systems, neuropsychologists may be particularly well suited to apply their knowledge and skills in a manner that serves to educate and facilitate communication among all parties.

To the extent that family members or others are closely involved in the life, care, or decision making of the geriatric patient, all parties may need to be clear about the role of the neuropsychologist, who the patient is, the probable uses of information obtained, and the nature of confidentiality (Standards 3.07, Third-Party Requests for Services, and 4.02, Discussing the Limits of Confidentiality). Agreement regarding who will be informed of the results of a neuropsychological evaluation is particularly important. It is not uncommon for family members who provide transportation to the evaluation and pay for neuropsychological services to expect to be informed of the examination findings. However, the examinee with capacity to make such decisions may ask that unfavorable results be withheld from family members. Careful discussion and clarification regarding the parameters of the evaluation with all involved parties at the outset of neuropsychological services may serve to avoid such conflicts.

HIPAA and informed consent

The Privacy Rule, which is one of the four components of the Health Insurance Portability and Accountability Act (HIPAA) of 1996, took effect April 14, 2003. This federal legislation was intended to simplify and protect the confidentiality of electronic billing and transmission of health information and to provide increased patient access to their medical records, including the right of patients to amend their medical records to clarify errors. Although those goals may seem straightforward and consistent with ethical practice, the legislation evolved into a complex series of administrative rules, with exceptions for certain settings. Of particular relevance to geriatric neuropsychologists performing evaluations in the context of competency determinations, personal injury litigation, or other forensic questions is the caveat that because such services are designed to serve a legal purpose, they do not constitute health services (Connell & Koocher, 2003). And, information compiled in anticipation of use in *civil*, *criminal*, and *administrative* proceedings is not subject to the same right of review and amendment as is health care information in general (§164.524[a][1][ii]; US Department of Health and Human Services, 2003). Thus, HIPAA and the privacy rules included therein do not seem to apply to geriatric neuropsychological evaluations performed in legal contexts.

It seems likely that most practicing neuropsychologists have now adopted or modified consent forms to reflect the general provisions of HIPAA. However, general forms that specify rights for patients in clinical contexts may be misleading to individuals undergoing neuropsychological evaluations for legal purposes. In order for consent to be informed, both verbal review of consent issues and the forms reflecting consent-related information, including that related to HIPAA, must be tailored to the context in which neuropsychological services are provided. Due to the need to consider and prioritize state laws, federal laws, and ethical guidelines, neuropsychologists are advised to consult legal counsel when adopting procedures and forms for topics such as informed consent.

Cooperation with other professionals

Neuropsychologists who perform evaluations to address questions of dementia often do so in a multidisciplinary context. The potential influence of medical, neurological, and/or psychiatric influences on cognitive functioning frequently requires contributions from a variety of medical professionals. Neuropsychologists have a responsibility to facilitate necessary evaluations (APA Presidential Task Force on the Assessment of Age-Consistent Memory Decline and Dementia, 1998) or to cooperate with such professionals if the multidisciplinary evaluation process is already underway (Standard 3.09, Cooperation with Other Professionals). However, such consultation should be performed with sensitivity to confidentiality issues. Neuropsychologists do not share with others personal information obtained in the course of an evaluation that is not pertinent to the referral question (Standard 4.04, Minimizing Intrusions on Privacy).

Institutional practice

Geriatric neuropsychologists often perform services as consultants to, or employees of, institutions. Such institutions include the following: (a) community-based settings, such as senior centers or home-based services; (b) outpatient settings, such as mental health or primary care clinics; (c) day treatment or partial hospital programs; (d) inpatient medical, psychiatric, or rehabilitation hospitals; and (e) long-term care settings, such as skilled nursing facilities and assisted living centers (APA Presidential Task Force on the Assessment of Age-Consistent Memory Decline and Dementia, 1998). Geriatric neuropsychologists should be aware that the level of impairment and functional ability of examinees is likely to vary between settings, and different practices may be required in each setting. In addition, variations on the ethical obligations owed may be found across settings.

Consistent with the principle of autonomy and the right of individuals to accept or decline services, neuropsychologists have a responsibility before services are provided and as needed after services have commenced to establish the parameters of proposed neuropsychological services with all relevant parties (Standard 3.11, Psychological Services Delivered to or Through Organizations). Neuropsychologists must clarify with all parties who the client will be and what the neuropsychologist's role will be with the client and other involved parties, provide information about the purpose and nature of the proposed services, describe the probable uses of the information obtained and who will have access to the information, and clarify limits of confidentiality. If jurisdictional laws or organizational rules prohibit the provision of such information, involved individuals are informed accordingly. Knowledge of the financing and reimbursement systems that govern the operations of the facilities in which one works is an aspect of professional competence due to the potential for such factors to affect service delivery or patient financial responsibility.

Conflicts may arise between the best interests of the older adult and the needs or interests of the staff or management of the institution in which the services are provided. Although ethical challenges are best resolved by serving the best interests of the patient, it may be difficult to establish what the best interests of the patient are when professionals disagree. Determination of *best interests* requires a comparative assessment made by one person for another who is unable to make that determination independently (Beauchamp & Childress, 2001). To promote the best interests of a patient, the neuropsychologist must make a quality of life determination, selecting the option that offers the greatest benefit from among the available options. The neuropsychologist, in an attempt to protect the patient's well-being, must assess the risks and benefits of various options, taking into consideration the patient's comfort level and potential restoration or loss of function. Making such determinations for another is a great responsibility and should, to the extent possible, be based on an understanding of the patient's values and preferences. Family members and prior documentation from the patient may be of considerable value in this process. Conflicts between ethics and organizational demands should be clarified, with a commitment to the Ethics Code emphasized and an attempt made to resolve the conflict in a manner that is consistent with the Ethics Code (Standard 1.03).

Privacy and confidentiality

Privacy refers to the right of individuals to choose how much of their personal information may be shared with others. Privacy is a fundamental human right; it is essential to ensure one's dignity and freedom of self-determination (Koocher & Keith-Spiegel, 1998) and is based on the principle of respect for autonomy (Beauchamp & Childress, 2001). *Confidentiality* is based on the right to privacy and poses limits on the release of patient information to others. Geriatric neuropsychologists, like all psychologists, have a primary ethical obligation, with some exceptions, to protect information obtained from or related to patients (Standard 4.01, Maintaining Confidentiality). Recipients of neuropsychological services must understand at the outset of the relationship the nature and limits of confidentiality (Standards 4.02, Discussing the Limits of Confidentiality, and 4.05, Disclosures). In addition to being an ethical requirement, confidentiality is based on statutes or case law in some jurisdictions, with legal implications for the practitioner if confidentiality is inappropriately violated. *Privilege* is a related legal concept that allows certain relationships protection from disclosure in legal proceedings. Privilege belongs to the patient; that is, the patient controls when information may be revealed. In some jurisdictions, privilege applies to the psychologist–patient relationship (Behnke, Perlin, & Bernstein, 2003).

Neuropsychologists working with older adults are aware that family members, caregivers or companions, and others are often involved in the lives of patients. In addition, evaluation and treatment services are often interdisciplinary in nature, involving a number of health care professionals. The potential involvement of others creates rich opportunities for gathering and exchanging information about the patient in order to better understand and serve the patient, but such involvement also increases the potential for violations of the patient's privacy. Family members and other health care professionals may pressure the neuropsychologist to discuss evaluation results or treatment progress; however, legally competent geriatric patients have a right to expect adherence to confidentiality until they provide consent for the information to be shared (APA, 2004). Designation of who will receive neuropsychological information about the patient is typically specific to certain family members or professionals. Neuropsychologists may need to educate those who are involved in the patient's life but have not been authorized to receive patient information about confidentiality requirements. In addition, it may be important to discuss confidentiality issues with the patient in private. The following scenario (Scenario B) illustrates confidentiality challenges that may occur in geriatric neuropsychology.

Mr. Jones, 79 years old, widowed, and living alone, is referred for a neuropsychological evaluation by his neurologist as part of a comprehensive multidisciplinary dementia evaluation; however, the various medical professionals are not part of the same group, working instead within separate practices in the region. Mr. Jones is brought for an initial interview by his daughter. He is legally competent to provide consent. He authorizes the neuropsychologist to interview and eventually release evaluation results to his daughter and to the referring neurologist. Clinical interview reveals that Mr. Jones has a rocky relationship with his son and fears that his son is trying to take his home and money. Nevertheless, Mr. Jones is forced to rely on his son for maintenance around the house and for transportation. Mr. Jones arrives for a subsequent testing session with his daughter, but he is brought to the feedback session by his son. The neuropsychologist invites Mr. Jones into the office, at which point the son says, "You want me in there too, right Dad?" Mr. Jones, looking rather uncomfortable, says, "Uh, ya, I guess," and the son comes in. After the feedback session, the neuropsychologist discusses the results with the neurologist and sends a report. Three days later, Mr. Jones' internist calls, saying he had been faxed a copy of the report by the neurologist and wanted to discuss one of the recommendations. In addition, Mr. Jones' grandson calls and wants to meet to find out why no recommendation was made for Mr. Jones to have a live-in companion.

As Scenario B illustrates, there exist a variety of potential threats to the privacy of patient information, particularly for some older patients who rely on family members or others for assistance. As stated in the ASPPB Code of Conduct, "In a situation in which more than one party has an appropriate interest in the professional service rendered by the psychologist to a client or clients, the psychologist shall, to the extent possible, clarify to all parties prior to rendering the services the dimensions of confidentiality and professional responsibility that shall pertain in the rendering of services" (Section E3, Services Involving More Than One Interested Party). Clinicians are well-served by anticipating the more common types of threats to confidentiality in their practice settings and by taking steps in advance to avoid problems.

In Scenario B, the neuropsychologist, having not anticipated the problems, may apply the ethical decision-making model as follows:

(a) *Identify the problem.* Mr. Jones' physician and grandson both want to discuss the results of the neuropsychological evaluation, but the neuropsychologist has not received authorization to discuss the information with either person.

(b) *Consider the significance of the context and setting.* In the context of a multidisciplinary evaluation, discussion among professionals is essential for Mr. Jones' welfare. However, since the evaluation was performed on an outpatient basis with professionals who practice independently of each other, a universally applied consent form was not used. Instead, each clinician was responsible for addressing foreseeable issues related to the exchange of information. Providing education to Mr. Jones' grandson may benefit Mr. Jones and his family.

(c) *Identify and utilize resources.* The neuropsychologist refers to the APA Ethics Code and to state laws. A call is also placed to a trusted colleague. The neuropsychologist determines that sharing information to promote Mr. Jones' welfare is consistent with the principle of beneficence. However, sharing information without considering Mr. Jones' wishes constitutes a failure to respect autonomy. Standards 4.01

(Maintaining Confidentiality) and 4.05 (Disclosures) and state law require the neuropsychologist to obtain Mr. Jones' consent before discussing the results of the evaluation with others.

(d) *Consider personal beliefs and values.* The neuropsychologist believes in open communication among parties with an interest in Mr. Jones' neuropsychological state and welfare. He believes that such communication will advance the understanding of Mr. Jones' welfare by those involved in his life. In the neuropsychologist's mind, all of the requirements and paperwork are excessive and only serve to delay the "right" course of action.

(e) *Develop possible solutions to the problem.* The neuropsychologist considers the following: (1) returning the calls to discuss the case; (2) returning the calls but stating that he was not permitted to discuss the case due to confidentiality requirements; (3) returning the calls and referring the callers to the neurologist; (4) returning the doctor's call but not the grandson's call; (5) calling Mr. Jones to ask his permission to discuss the results with the physician and/or the grandson, and to have such permission in writing if granted; and, (6) returning no calls regarding this case.

(f) *Consider the potential consequences of various solutions.* The neuropsychologist suspects, and has confirmed while consulting the resources, that any discussion of Mr. Jones' results with others must be authorized by Mr. Jones. He dismisses the option of avoiding the problem by not calling.

(g) *Choose and implement a course of action.* The neuropsychologist contacts Mr. Jones and discusses the requests to share the results of the evaluation. Mr. Jones has questions about who wants the information and for what purposes. Mr. Jones agrees to come in to the neuropsychologist's office to discuss release of information in more detail. He then signs releases to have the neuropsychological results shared with all pertinent health care professionals and family members.

(h) *Assess the outcome and implement changes as needed.* The neuropsychologist returns the calls and provides reports to the other clinicians involved in the interdisciplinary evaluation.

This dilemma was resolved quickly and easily; however, had the neuropsychologist not been able to reach Mr. Jones, the pressure from others to discuss the results would likely have increased. Thus, the importance of anticipating potential problems with confidentiality and addressing them in advance during the informed consent process is emphasized.

Assessment

Thorough assessment of cognitive, psychiatric, or behavioral symptoms in older adults is preferably interdisciplinary in nature (APA, 2004). As part of such a process, neuropsychologists may employ those methods that are

deemed necessary to answer referral questions. The use of neuropsychological tests may represent the most important and unique contribution that
neuropsychologists can make to the assessment of dementia and age-
related cognitive decline (APA Presidential Task Force on the Assessment
of Age-Consistent Memory Decline and Dementia, 1998). In the selection
of assessment methods, neuropsychologists must strive to be familiar with
the theory, research, and application of potential methods with older
adults, and to select instruments that are psychometrically appropriate for
this population (APA, 2004; Ethical Standard 9.02, Use of Assessments;
SEPT Standard 12.3).

In recent years, an increasing number of neuropsychological tests have
been developed with higher age ranges in mind. In addition, geriatric norms
have been developed for measures previously applicable only to younger
adults. However, situations still arise in which assessment of geriatric patients
requires modification of standardized measures or procedures or in which
representative norms are unavailable (see Chapter 5 in this volume). Geriatric
neuropsychologists must strive to develop skill in tailoring evaluations to
accommodate both the specific characteristics of the patient and the context
in which the evaluation is performed (APA, 2004). Neuropsychologists working with older adults must also be familiar with the problems inherent in
using assessment instruments created for younger persons.

Many newly developed tests require or offer as an option computer administration. Some older examinees may be less familiar and comfortable with
computers than are younger examinees. Before administering tests via computer, neuropsychologists should assess the examinee's level of comfort with
such procedures, substitute paper-and-pencil versions of tests when indicated, and describe any limits to interpretation based on the use of information technology (Browndyke, 2005; Schatz, 2005). Neuropsychologically
vulnerable patients are particularly entitled to increased protection from the
potential negative effects of technology use (Bush, Naugle, & Johnson-
Greene, 2002).

Response validity determinations

In the interpretation of assessment results, which may include computer-
generated analyses, neuropsychologists are responsible for considering the
purpose of the evaluation, situational factors, and personal characteristics of
the examinee that may impact the accuracy of the interpretation (Standard
9.06, Interpreting Assessment Results). For most evaluations, an initial step
in the interpretation process is making a determination regarding the validity
of the information and data obtained from the examinee.

There are many reasons why the information or data may not be a valid
representation of the examinee's actual neuropsychological status. Such reasons include "sensory deficits, fatigue, medication side effects, physical illness
and frailness, discomfort or disability, poor motivation, financial disincentives,

depression, anxiety, not understanding the test instructions, and lack of inter-est" (APA Presidential Task Force on the Assessment of Age-Consistent Memory Decline and Dementia, 1998). Additional reasons include distrust of medical professionals and opposition to the purpose of the evaluation.

Within the contexts in which many geriatric evaluations are performed, malingering may occur relatively infrequently. However, as noted above, other factors may also affect response validity and subsequently contribute to the development of inaccurate conclusions regarding the patient's actual level of neuropsychological functioning. Thus, the assumption that symptom validity assessment outside of forensic contexts is unnecessary reflects a limited appre-ciation of the various factors that may compromise the validity of a patient's responses and performance. Neuropsychologists in any setting must "attempt to assess these sources of error and to limit and control them to the extent that they are able" (APA Presidential Task Force on the Assessment of Age-Consistent Memory Decline and Dementia, 1998). Neuropsychologists have traditionally offered a statement similar to the following, "The patient appeared to put forth good effort on the tests; therefore, the results are con-sidered valid for interpretation." Such statements reflect an attempt, however limited, to address the issue of response validity.

The manner in which response validity is assessed will vary depending on the context of the evaluation. Assessment of response validity may include specific tests, indices, observations, comparisons, and/or other procedures. Determination of how to assess response validity is determined by the clini-cian given the unique context of the evaluation and the characteristics of the examinee. When symptom validity tests are used, selection of the tests, as with other measures, must be made based on the fit between the characteris-tics of the standardization sample and the individual being evaluated.

Discussing limitations of interpretations

When the measures or procedures employed in a neuropsychological evalua-tion of older adults differ from the group on which they were developed or established, it is necessary to indicate any significant limitations of the inter-pretation (Standard 9.06, Interpreting Assessment Results; SEPT Standard 12.19). It seems likely that most competent neuropsychologists would agree that under such circumstances, results should be interpreted cautiously or conservatively. However, there has been little discussion in the literature or relevant professional guidelines about what "interpreted with caution" means or how it should be conveyed in a report.

Geriatric neuropsychologists may struggle with the question of what to conclude about the results of evaluations for which appropriate measures or norms do not exist. It may be argued that such measures should never have been selected. However, consider the case of a 92-year-old college educated woman with hemiparesis of her dominant hand and difficulty hearing. A neuropsychological evaluation of this patient would likely require use of measures that were not developed on similar people. In addition, administration procedures would likely require modification. The following series of questions is posed to stimulate thought and discussion about this issue.

How should the neuropsychologist in this case describe the limitations of the results? Does the neuropsychologist offer a diagnostic impression but indicate that "the results were interpreted with caution?" What would such a statement mean? Would it mean the neuropsychologist adjusted the interpretive ranges (e.g., mild impairment) down/up by a certain amount (e.g., 1 standard deviation)? If so, how can that be justified? Does it mean that the neuropsychologist has little confidence in the diagnosis or conclusions? If not, then how were the results interpreted cautiously? Such a statement may have little value for other neuropsychologists; however, would it be sufficient for most readers of the report? If so, would that satisfy the ethical obligation to indicate limitations of the interpretation?

According to the ASPPB Code of Conduct, "The psychologist shall include in his/her report of the results of a formal assessment procedure for which norms are available, any deficiencies of the assessment norms for the individual assessed and any relevant reservations or qualifications which affect the validity, reliability, or other interpretation of results" (Section H3, Reservations Concerning Results). In addition, according to the Standards for Educational and Psychological Testing (American Educational Research Association, American Psychological Association, National Council on Measurement in Education, 1999), "if no normative or validity studies are available for the population at issue, test interpretations should be qualified and presented as hypotheses rather than conclusions" (p. 131). It is not sufficient to merely state that "caution" was used in the test interpretation; the examiner must state explicitly the manner in which deviations from standardized testing conditions or normative samples may have impacted the test results or interpretation (Iverson & Slick, 2003). Rather than writing "interpreted with caution," it may be more informative to offer a statement to the effect that the patient's current test results likely underrepresent his or her neuropsychological potential.

In addition to determining how to convey in the report the limits of the interpretation, to what extent should the potential for such limitations be included in the informed consent process? Are geriatric neuropsychologists obligated to inform potential examinees that although neuropsychological tests can be administered, the results might not offer an accurate representation of their neuropsychological functioning? Would it be a fair allocation of resources, beneficial for the patient, and respectful of patient autonomy if the neuropsychologist failed to provide this information and proceeded with the evaluation anyway? In the section that addresses the use of innovative services and techniques, the ASPPB Code of Conduct states, "The psychologist shall inform clients of the innovative nature and the known risks associated with the services, so that the client can exercise freedom of choice concerning such services" (Section A3, Adding New Services and Techniques).

In this section, a number of questions have been raised but few clear answers have been provided. Geriatric neuropsychologists represent a variety of practice settings, patient populations, and professional and lay audiences. As such, specific recommendations will not apply to all readers. Neuropsychologists working with older adults must consider the questions above in the context of their specific professional activities and establish practices that provide potential recipients of their services with as much specific information as is needed to meet both the goals of the evaluation and the requirements of professional ethics.

The following scenario (Scenario C) highlights several ethical issues related to the neuropsychological assessment of older persons in an inpatient medical stetting.

A neuropsychologist employed at a rehabilitation hospital is asked to assess the cognitive status of a 73-year-old man who is now ventilator dependent secondary to advanced chronic obstructive pulmonary disease. Following a review of medical records, the neuropsychologist learns that the patient's wife passed away several years ago and that he lives alone. The patient has a 47-year-old daughter who provided the patient with considerable assistance prior to his hospitalization. The results of the neuropsychological evaluation will have direct implications for discharge planning. During a clinical interview, the patient presents as depressed and moderately confused, with his participation in the interview compromised by fatigue and difficulty speaking due to his tracheostomy tube. Attempts to have the patient communicate through writing are minimally successful as the patient frequently becomes frustrated and appears to lose his train of thought. Despite attempts to inform the patient about the nature and purpose of the evaluation, the neuropsychologist is uncertain if the patient fully understands the particulars of the evaluation. Nonetheless, after the patient's psychiatrist enters the room and reassures the patient that he needs to participate in the evaluation, the patient appears to agree to undergo the testing.

Application of the decision-making model can help identify the relevant ethical issues and possible courses of action:

(a) *Identify the problem.* Despite the patient's apparent agreement to participate, the neuropsychologist remains unsure about whether or not it is appropriate to proceed. The neuropsychologist is concerned both about the patient's level of understanding of the evaluation process and the ability to administer tests to this patient in the manner in which they were standardized. The neuropsychologist is faced with questions related to informed consent and the appropriate use of assessment instruments. Specifically, does the patient possess an appropriate understanding of the particulars of the evaluation to make an informed decision regarding his desire to participate? Has the patient been afforded sufficient opportunity to ask questions? Should the neuropsychologist contact the patient's daughter for permission to proceed with testing? Will the patient's need for special accommodations lead to the inappropriate use of the assessment measures the neuropsychologist is planning to employ?

(b) *Consider the significance of the context and setting.* Working in an inpatient medical setting, the neuropsychologist is used to completing evaluations as soon as possible. However, in reviewing this case the neuropsychologist recognizes that there are no extenuating circumstances that required immediate completion of the evaluation. In contrast, extenuating circumstances may necessitate delaying the evaluation. The neuropsychologist understands that the multidisciplinary treatment approach employed by the hospital means that there are several colleagues available who can offer preliminary insight into the patient's cognitive status and communication ability.

(c) *Identify and utilize resources.* The neuropsychologist reviews the relevant sections of the APA Ethics Code, the Standards for Educational and Psychological Testing, and state laws, and he consults with a colleague who has experience working with geriatric patients in a medical setting. Through these avenues, the neuropsychologist is able to clarify the relevant ethical and legal issues and determine possible courses of action. He realizes that his primary responsibility is to insure that his actions do not result in inappropriate decisions or treatment recommendations for the patient; instead, the evaluation should ultimately facilitate treatment and promote the patient's welfare (General Principle A, Beneficence and Nonmaleficence). The neuropsychologist also understands that, to the extent possible, the patient should be involved in making the decisions that govern his medical procedures and care and his discharge (General Principle E, Respect for People's Rights and Dignity; Standards 3.10, Informed Consent, and 9.03, Informed Consent in Assessments; SEPT Standard 8.4). However, the extent of the patient's understanding of the information provided by the neuropsychologist and other treatment team members is unknown. The patient does not have a designated surrogate decision-maker. The neuropsychologist is also aware that standard administration of the test battery typically utilized on the unit will not be possible with this patient, yet any adaptations made will not be supported by research (Standard 9.02, Use of Assessments; SEPT Standards 10.2, 10.10, and 10.11). Nevertheless, the neuropsychologist believes that clinically valuable information can be gained by selecting and adapting tests to accommodate this patient.

(d) *Consider personal beliefs and values.* The neuropsychologist reflects on the personal value placed on autonomy. In addition, considerable appreciation is maintained for the dictum, "First, do no harm." The neuropsychologist would much rather conduct no evaluation and provide no treatment recommendations to the team than perform an inappropriate evaluation and draw inaccurate conclusions or make recommendations that are inconsistent with the best interests of the patient. Determining how to optimize autonomy, do no harm, and assist the patient remains the challenge.

(e) *Develop possible solutions to the problem.* Concerned that the patient has not made an informed decision regarding his desire to participate in the evaluation and that the patient's expressive language difficulties may invalidate his assessment findings, the neuropsychologist considers the following courses of action: (1) continue with the evaluation as scheduled; (2) meet with relevant treatment team members and the patient's daughter to gain insight into the patient's functioning and obtain assistance with determining the patient's desire to participate in the evaluation; and (3) refuse to conduct the evaluation at his time.

(f) *Consider the potential consequences of various solutions.* The neuropsychologist considers the following potential consequences: (1) continuing with the evaluation may result in the neuropsychologist's ability to answer important referral questions, or it may result in the collection of invalid data and the generation of inappropriate conclusions; (2) obtaining additional information from the treatment team and the patient's daughter may facilitate neuropsychological decision making, or it may result in the collection of multiple subjective opinions that are of little value after a period of unnecessary delay; (3) refusing to conduct the evaluation may result in the neuropsychologist not taking action that is potentially harmful, but the absence of the neuropsychological evaluation may result in other team members making decisions about the patient's care that are not fully informed and thus may run counter to the patient's wishes or interests.

(g) *Choose and implement a course of action.* Having reviewed the relevant written resources and spoken with a colleague, the neuropsychologist chooses to delay the evaluation in order to consult with team members and call the patient's daughter. The attending physician agrees with the plan. The patient's speech and respiratory therapists report that the patient appears depressed, with variable cognition and willingness to participate in treatment. However, they indicate that the patient is less fatigued and better able to tolerate his speaking valve in the mornings. The neuropsychologist is unable to reach the patient's daughter. The following morning the neuropsychologist meets with the patient, explains the purpose and nature of the evaluation, and seeks the patient's assent to undergo the evaluation. The patient appears more alert and more relaxed and appears to agree to undergo the evaluation, although the extent of the patient's understanding of the potential implications of the evaluation remains undetermined. The neuropsychologist is of the opinion that failure to modify test administration to meet this patient's needs, despite a lack of research to support such modifications, will be less harmful than administering the tests in the manner in which they were standardized and interpreting the results according to norms that were based on very different populations. As a result, test administration is modified. Test results suggest that the patient is experiencing memory and receptive language difficulties and moderate depression. Following completion of the evaluation, the neuropsychologist is careful to report the manner in which test administration was modified and the limitations of the test results, interpretation, and recommendations.

(h) *Assess the outcome and implement changes as needed.* The neuropsychologist completes the assessment and contributes useful information to the treatment team. Plans are made for serial assessments, to include integration of the findings of other team members and information from the patient's daughter.

Neuropsychological treatment

Psychotherapy

Older adults respond to psychotherapy to a degree similar to younger patients, and they benefit from a variety of forms of psychological treatment (APA, 2004). No single modality of therapy has emerged as preferable. Clinicians may adapt traditional treatments or provide therapies that have been developed specifically for use with older adults, such as reminiscence therapy. What seems clear is the importance of possessing specialized skills in treating older adults (Pinquart & Soerensen, 2001). As is required by the Ethics Code, "Where scientific or professional knowledge in the discipline of psychology establishes that an understanding of factors associated with age … is essential for effective implementation of their services or research, psychologists have or obtain the training, experience, consultation, or supervision necessary to ensure the competence of their services, or they make appropriate referrals" (Standard 2.01, Boundaries of Competence, subsection b).

The cohort comprised of today's older adults may have less familiarity with psychological services or may harbor more negative beliefs or feelings about mental health issues compared to subsequent cohorts (APA, 2004). Neuropsychologists working with older adults must be sensitive to the potential for such attitudes to impact the working relationship or receptivity to neuropsychological services in general and take extra care to educate the patient about the services proposed and their implications (General Principle E, Respect for People's Rights and Dignity). Interestingly, when older adults are educated about potential treatments for depression, including psychopharmacologic and psychotherapeutic approaches, they tend to prefer psychologically-based treatments (APA, 2002a).

Depending on the patient and the context, a primary goal of psychotherapy at this stage of the lifecycle may be continued psychological growth. However, because many of the disorders of late adulthood are recurrent or chronic, the clinical objectives may consist of symptom management and rehabilitative maximization of function (Knight & Satre, 1999). Neuropsychologists have an ethical obligation to facilitate patient understanding of the goals of treatment and to manage expectations appropriately (Standard 10.01a, Informed Consent to Therapy). Balancing the potential benefits of maintaining hope for progress in an individual patient or family facing an unfavorable prognosis can be a particularly challenging moral and professional endeavor for clinicians.

Depression and end-of-life issues

Depression is one of the most common psychiatric disorders experienced by older adults, and it is associated with suicide (APA, 2002a). Older adults, and men in particular, have the highest rates of suicide of any age group. Although comprehensive coverage of end-of-life choices is beyond the scope of this chapter, neuropsychologists working with older patients who are considering suicide, including assisted suicide, should be aware of the complex moral, ethical, professional, and legal issues involved and the resources that are available to guide clinicians in what may be the most professionally and emotionally trying experiences for neuropsychologists (see, for example, APA's *Depression and Suicide in Older Adults Resource Guide*, 2002a; and APA Working Group on Assisted Suicide and End-of-Life Decisions, 2000). The APA Working Group on Assisted Suicide and End-of-Life Decisions reported the following (section 1):

> Sweeping advances in public health, biomedical sciences, and clinical medicine … may significantly extend life but may also confront dying individuals, their families, and health care providers with a prolonged period of dying that involves complex choices about end-of life care. These changes have resulted in the need to address end-of-life decision-making from many perspectives including medical, legal, ethical, moral, spiritual, economic, and psychosocial dimensions. There is likely to be an increasingly sophisticated demand for psychosocial services in dealing with end-of-life decisions. Furthermore, the specific issue of assisted suicide promises to become one of the most contentious and difficult social issues of our time … In a diverse society with a variety of social and cultural values as well as a history of unequal access to medical care, issues surrounding dying and death become more complicated than in more homogeneous societies. Those working with dying persons and their families must be aware of the enormous inequities in access to and quality of health care and of the influence of profound differences in beliefs, values, and self concepts of disenfranchised people on end-of-life decision-making.

Cognitive rehabilitation and training

Until recent years, treatments such as cognitive rehabilitation or memory training have been considered limited in their usefulness for individuals with age-related cognitive decline and dementia (APA, 2004). Instead, treatments such as environmental restructuring and the use of compensatory memory aids and other strategies have been preferred. However, recent research has provided support for the value of cognitive activity and exercise in late life (Ball et al., 2002; Hofmann, Hock, Kuhler, & Muller-Spahn, 1996; Moore, Sandman, McGrady, & Kesslak, 2001; Wilson et al., 2002). When one considers recommending or providing treatments that are less well established, it is particularly important to weigh the potential benefits against the potential risks and costs and to involve the patient or the surrogate decision-maker in the decision-making process (Bush & Martin, 2004). The use of innovative treatments is consistent with ethical practice in those instances in which the potential costs and risks are minimal (nonmaleficence), the potential for benefit exists (beneficence), and expectations can be carefully managed.

Serving special populations

The 1992 APA Ethics Code included a standard (2.04c, Use of Assessment in General and With Special Populations) that addressed assessment issues as they pertain to special populations based on factors such as gender, age, race, ethnicity, national origin, religion, sexual orientation, disability, language, or socioeconomic status. Although this standard was not included in the current Ethics Code (2002b), the essential points of the standard can be found elsewhere in the Ethics Code. Neuropsychologists must still be familiar with the proper applications of the measures they employ, recognize limits to the certainty with which diagnostic or other statements can be made with special populations, and make adjustments in administration or interpretation as needed (Standards 9.02, Use of Assessments, and 9.06, Interpreting Assessment Results). Age is specified in the Ethics Code (General Principle E, Respect for People's Rights and Dignity; Standard 3.01, Unfair Discrimination) among those factors that are essential to consider in professional activities.

Ethical practice requires particular attention to the welfare of vulnerable patients. Physical frailty, cognitive impairment, cultural and linguistic diversity, disability, and other characteristics of the patient may increase vulnerability to inappropriate and potentially harmful conclusions and/or care by neuropsychologists insensitive to the relevance and importance of such factors. In addition, a combination of these factors in a given patient increases the demand on the neuropsychologist to exercise care in each step of the evaluation and treatment process (see Chapter 6 in this volume).

Personal and societal biases exist toward some groups with which neuropsychologists have professional contact, and neuropsychologists are not immune from such biases. Neuropsychologists must be aware of how biases regarding age, gender, ethnicity, and other patient characteristics may interfere with objective evaluation and recommendations (APA Presidential Task Force on the Assessment of Age-Consistent Memory Decline and Dementia, 1998; APA General Principles D, Justice, and E, Respect for

People's Rights and Dignity, and Standard 3.01, Unfair Discrimination). Geriatric neuropsychologists must strive to overcome any such biases or refer the patient to another clinician.

Health promotion

Neuropsychologists may contribute to the health and well-being of older adults and other special populations through the development of psycho-educational programs, involvement in community-based prevention programs, and advocacy within health care and political systems (APA, 2004). Consistent with the principle of beneficence, neuropsychologists can combine their clinical and consultation skills with familiarity with relevant research to promote the health and well-being of groups of individuals that extend well beyond the numbers that most neuropsychologists can reach in a clinical practice.

Conclusions

Neuropsychologists providing professional services to older adults may find their responsibilities to be nearly as ethically challenging as they are personally and professionally rewarding. When working with older adults, ethical challenges may tax the morality of both the professional and the profession. As stated by Beauchamp and Childress (2001), "No moral theorist or professional code of ethics has successfully presented a system of moral rules free of conflicts and exceptions, but this fact is not cause for either skepticism or alarm" (p. 15). In fact, neuropsychologists, armed with their education, training, experience, and ethical resources, may be particularly well equipped to face such conflicts and exceptions. Ethical decision-making models, such as the one described in this chapter, help provide a context from which dilemmas can be addressed. Yet, despite the value of models, codes, and guidelines, "often what counts most in the moral life is not consistent adherence to principles and rules, but reliable character, good moral sense, and emotional responsiveness" (Beauchamp & Childress, 2001, p. 26).

Hays (1999) requested that "practitioners working with geriatric clients advocate for an ethic for elderly that respects their dignity but also afford them the protection they deserve" (p. 662). We would add that in the attempt to strike the balance between dignity and protection, geriatric neuropsychologists consider the fit between their own beliefs and values and the settings in which they work, striving to anticipate potential ethical challenges and to address them as early and as directly as possible.

References

American Educational Research Association, American Psychological Association, National Council on Measurement in Education. (1999). *Standards for educational and psychological testing*. Washington, DC: American Educational Research Association.

American Psychological Association. (1992). Ethical principles of psychologists and code of conduct. *American Psychologist, 47*, 1597–1611.

American Psychological Association. (2002a). *Depression and suicide in older adults resource guide*. Retrieved May 28, 2004, from http://www.apa.org/pi/aging/depression.html

American Psychological Association. (2002b). Ethical principles of psychologists and code of conduct. *American Psychologist, 57*(12), 1060–1073.

American Psychological Association. (2004). Guidelines for psychological practice with older adults. *American Psychologist, 59*(4), 236–260.

American Psychological Association, Presidential Task Force on the Assessment of Age-Consistent Memory Decline and Dementia. (1998). *Guidelines for the evaluation of dementia and age-related cognitive decline*. Washington, DC: American Psychological Association.

American Psychological Association Working Group on Assisted Suicide and End-of-Life Decisions. (2000). *Report of the Board of Directors of APA from the Working Group on Assisted Suicide and End-of-Life Decisions*. Retrieved May 28, 2004, from http://www.apa.org/pi/aseol/section1.html

Association of State and Provincial Psychology Boards. (1990). *ASPPB code of conduct, revised*. Retrieved June 10, 2005, from www.asppb.org/publications/model/conduct.aspx

Ball, K., Berch, D. B., Helmers, K. F., Jobe, J. B., Leveck, M. D., Marsiske, M., et al. (2002). Effects of cognitive training interventions with older adults. *Journal of the American Medical Association, 288*(18), 2271–2281.

Beauchamp, T. L., & Childress, J. F. (2001). *Principles of biomedical ethics* (5th ed.). New York: Oxford University Press.

Beckingham, A. C., & Watts, S. (1995). Daring to grow old: Lessons in healthy aging and empowerment: Learning to live at all ages. *Educational Gerontology, 21*, 479–495.

Behnke, S. H., Perlin, M. L., & Bernstein, M. (2003). *The essentials of New York Mental Health Law*. New York: W. W. Norton & Company.

Binder, L., & Thompson, L. (1995). The ethics code and neuropsychological assessment practices. *Archives of Clinical Neuropsychology, 10*, 27–46.

Bowling, C. L. (1993). The concepts of successful and positive aging. *Family Practice, 10*, 449–453.

Brittain, J. L., Francis, J. P., & Barth, J. T. (1995). Ethical issues and dilemmas in neuropsychological practice reported by ABCN diplomates. *Advances in Medical Psychotherapy, 8*, 1–22.

Brittain, J. L., Francis, J. P., McSweeny, A. J., Fisher, J. M., & Barth, J. T. (1997) *Ethics in Neuropsychology: Where are we now*. Workshop presented at the annual meeting of the National Academy of Neuropsychology, Las Vegas, NV.

Browndyke, J. N. (2005). Ethical challenges with the use of information technology and telecommunications in neuropsychology, part I. In S. S. Bush (Ed.), *A casebook of ethical challenges in neuropsychology* (pp. 179–189). New York: Psychology Press.

Bush, S., Naugle, R., & Johnson-Greene, D. (2002). The interface of information technology and neuropsychology: Ethical issues and recommendations. *The Clinical Neuropsychologist, 16*(4), 536–547.

Bush, S. S., Connell, M. A., & Denney, R. L. (in press). *Ethical issues in forensic psychology*. Washington, DC: American Psychological Association.

Bush, S. S., & Martin, T. A. (2004, July). *Balancing bioethical principles in computer-based memory treatment*. Poster presentation at the ninth international conference on Alzheimer's Disease and Related Disorders, Philadelphia, PA.

Canadian Psychological Association. (2000). *Canadian code of ethics for psychologists* (3rd ed.). Ottawa, Ontario: Author.

Coleman, P. G. (1992). Personal adjustment in later life: Successful aging. *Reviews in Clinical Gerontology*, *2*, 67–78.

Connell, M., & Koocher, G. (2003). HIPAA and forensic practice. *American Psychology Law Society News*, *23*(2), 16–19.

DeLuca, J. (2005). Ethical challenges in neuropsychology in rehabilitation settings, part I. In S. S. Bush (Ed.), *A casebook of ethical challenges in neuropsychology* (pp. 97–103). New York: Psychology Press.

Erikson, E. H. (1963). *Childhood and society*. New York: Norton.

Erikson, E. H., Erikson, J. M., & Kivnick, H. Q. (1986). *Vital involvement in old age*. New York: Norton.

Fisher, J. M., Johnson-Greene, D., & Barth, J. T. (2002). Examination, diagnosis, and interventions in clinical neuropsychology in general and with special populations: An overview. In S. Bush & M. Drexler (Eds.), *Ethical issues in clinical neuropsychology* (pp. 3–22). Lisse, The Netherlands: Swets & Zeitlinger.

Haas, L., & Malouf, J. (2002). *Keeping up the good work: A practitioner's guide to mental health ethics* (3rd ed.). Sarasota, FL: Professional Resource Press.

Handelsman, M., Knapp, S., & Gottlieb, M. (2002). Positive ethics. In R. Snyder & S. Lopez (Eds.), *Handbook of positive psychology* (pp. 731–744). New York: Oxford University Press.

Hanson, S. L., Kerkhoff, T. R., & Bush, S. S. (2005). *Health care ethics for psychologists: A casebook*. Washington, DC: American Psychological Association.

Hays, J. R. (1999). Ethics of treatment in geropsychology: Status and challenges. In M. Duffy (Ed.), *Handbook of counseling and psychotherapy with older adults* (pp. 662–676). New York: John Wiley & Sons.

Hofmann, M., Hock, C., Kuhler, A., & Muller-Spahn, F. (1996). Interactive computer-based cognitive training in patients with Alzheimer's disease. *Journal of Psychiatric Research*, *30*, 493–501.

Iverson, G. L., & Slick, D. J. (2003). Ethical issues associated with psychological and neuropsychological assessment of persons from different cultural and linguistic backgrounds. In I. Z. Schultz & D. O. Brady (Eds.), *Psychological injuries at trial* (pp. 2066–2087). Chicago: American Bar Association.

Johnson-Greene, D. (2005). Ethical challenges in neuropsychology in rehabilitation settings, part II. In S. S. Bush (Ed.), *A casebook of ethical challenges in neuropsychology* (pp. 104–110). New York: Psychology Press.

Kaplan, G. A., & Strawbridge, W. J. (1994). Behavioral and social factors in healthy aging. In R. P. Abeles, H. C. Gift, & M. G. Ory (Eds.), *Aging and quality of life* (pp. 57–78). New York: Springer.

Kitchener, K. S. (2000). *Foundations of ethical practice, research, and teaching*. Mahwah, NJ: Lawrence Erlbaum Associates, Inc.

Knapp, S., & Vandecreek, L. (2003). *A guide to the 2002 revision of the American Psychological Association's Ethics Code*. Sarasota, FL: Professional Resource Press.

Knight, B. G., & Satre, D. D. (1999). Cognitive behavioral psychotherapy with older adults. *Clinical Psychology: Science and Practice*, *6*, 188–203.

Koocher, G. P., & Keith-Spiegel, P. (1998). *Ethics in psychology: Professional standards and cases* (2nd ed.). New York: Oxford University Press.

Lebowitz, B. D., Pearson, J. L., Schneider, L. S., Reynolds, C. F., III, Alexopoulos, G. S., Bruce, M. L., et al. (1997). Diagnosis and treatment of depression in late life:

Consensus statement update. *Journal of the American Medical Association, 278*(14), 1186–1190.

Macciocchi, S. N., & Stringer, A. Y. (2002). Assessing risk and harm: The convergence of ethical and empirical considerations. *Archives of Physical Medicine and Rehabilitation, 82*(Suppl. 2), S15–S19.

Martelli, M. F., Zasler, N. D., & Grayson, R. (1999). Ethical considerations in impairment and disability evaluations following acquired brain injury. In V. R. May & M. F. Martelli (Eds.), *Guide to functional capacity evaluation with impairment rating applications. Midlothian, VA*: NADEP Publications.

McSweeny, A. J. (2005). Ethical challenges in geriatric neuropsychology, part I. In S. S. Bush (Ed.), *A casebook of ethical challenges in neuropsychology* (pp. 147–152). New York: Psychology Press.

Moore, S., Sandman, C. A., McGrady, K., & Kesslak, J. P. (2001). Memory training improves cognitive ability in patients with dementia. *Neuropsychological Rehabilitation, 11*(3/4), 245–261.

Morgan, J. (2002). Ethical issues in the practice of geriatric neuropsychology. In S. S. Bush & M. L. Drexler (Eds.), Ethical issues in clinical neuropsychology (pp. 87–101). Lisse, The Netherlands: Swets & Zeitlinger.

Morgan, J. (2005). Ethical challenges in geriatric neuropsychology, part II. In S. S. Bush (Ed.), A casebook of ethical challenges in neuropsychology (pp. 153–158). New York: Psychology Press.

Myers, J. E. (1992). Wellness, prevention, development: The cornerstone of the profession. *Journal of Counseling and Development, 71*, 136–139.

Myers, J. E. (1999). Adjusting to role loss and leisure in later life. In M. Duffy (Ed.), *Handbook of counseling and psychotherapy with older adults* (pp. 41–56). New York: John Wiley & Sons.

Norris, M. P., Molinari, V., & Ogland-Hand, S. (Eds.). (2002). *Emerging trends in psychological practice in long-term care*. Binghampton, NY: Haworth Press.

Pinkston, J. B. (2005). Ethical challenges in neuropsychology in medical settings, part I. In S. S. Bush (Ed.), *A casebook of ethical challenges in neuropsychology* (pp. 65–70). New York: Psychology Press.

Pinquart, M., & Socrensen, S. (2001). How effective are psychotherapeutic and other psychosocial interventions with older adults? A meta analysis. *Journal of Mental Health and Aging, 7*, 207–243.

Pope, K. S., & Vetter, V. A. (1992). Ethical dilemmas encountered by members of the APA: A national survey. *American Psychologist, 47*, 397–411.

Schatz, P. (2005). Ethical challenges with the use of information technology and telecommunications in neuropsychology, part II. In S. S. Bush (Ed.), *A casebook of ethical challenges in neuropsychology* (pp. 190–197). New York: Psychology Press.

Sweet, J. J., Grote, C., & van Gorp, W. G. (2002). Ethical issues in forensic neuropsychology. In S. S. Bush & M. L. Drexler (Eds.), *Ethical issues in clinical neuropsychology* (pp. 103–133). Lisse, The Netherlands: Swets & Zeitlinger.

Swiercinsky, D. P. (2002). Ethical issues in neuropsychological rehabilitation. In S. S. Bush & M. L. Drexler (Eds.), *Ethical issues in clinical neuropsychology* (pp. 135–163). Lisse, The Netherlands: Swets & Zeitlinger.

US Department of Health and Human Services. (2003). *Public Law 104-191: Health Insurance Portability and Accountability Act of 1996*. Retrieved November 24, 2003, from http://www.hhs.gov/ocr/hipaa/

Waters, E. B., & Goodman, J. (1990). *Empowering older adults: Practical strategies for counselors*. San Francisco: Jossey-Bass.

Wilde, E. A. (2005). Ethical issues in neuropsychology in medical settings, part II. In S. S. Bush (Ed.), A casebook of ethical challenges in neuropsychology (pp. 71–80). New York: Psychology Press.

Wilde, E. A., Bush, S. S., & Zeifert, P. (2002). Ethical issues in neuropsychology in medical settings. In S. S. Bush & M. L. Drexler (Eds.), *Ethical issues in clinical neuropsychology* (pp. 195–221). Lisse, The Netherlands: Swets & Zeitlinger.

Wilson, R. S., Mendes de Leon, C. F., Barnes, L. L., Schneider, J. A., Bienias, J. L., Evans, D. A., & Bennett, D. A. (2002). Participation in cognitively stimulating activities and risk of incident Alzheimer disease. *Journal of the American Medical Association, 287*, 742–748.

Appendix: Resources for the practice of geriatric neuropsychology

General information and support services

Administration on Aging
330 Independence Avenue, SW
Washington, DC 20201
Tel: (202) 619-0724
Website: http://www.aoa.gov/index.asp

Aging Network Services
4400 East-West Hwy.
Bethesda, MD 20814
Tel: (301) 657-4329
Website: http://www.agingnets.com

Alliance for Aging Research
2021 K Street, NW, Suite 305
Washington, DC 20006
Tel: (202) 293-2856
Website: http://www.agingresearch.org

American Association of Homes & Services for the Aging
901 E Street, NW, Suite 500
Washington, DC 20004-2011
Tel: (202) 783-2242
Website: http://www.aahsa.org

American Association of Retired Persons (AARP)
601 E Street, NW
Washington, DC 20049
Tel: (800) 424-3410
Website: http://aarp.org

American Dietetic Association
120 S. Riverside Plaza, Suite 2000
Chicago, IL 60606-6995
Tel: (800) 366-1655
Website: http://www.eatright.org

American Federation for Aging Research
70 West 40th Street, 11th Floor
New York, NY 10018
Tel: (212) 703-9977
Website: http://www.afar.org

American Geriatrics Society Foundation for Health in Aging
The Empire State Building
350 Fifth Avenue, Suite 801
New York City, NY 10118
Tel: (800) 563-4916
Website: http://www.healthinaging.org

American Senior Fitness Association
PO Box 2575
New Smyrna Beach, FL 32170
Tel: (904) 423-6634
Website: http://www.seniorfitness.net

American Society for Geriatric Dentistry
211 East Chicago Avenue, 5th Floor
Chicago, IL 60611
Tel: (312) 440-2660

American Society of Consultant Pharmacists
1321 Duke Street
Alexandria, VA 22314-3516
Tel: (800) 355-2727
Website: http://www.ascp.com

American Society on Aging
833 Market Street, Suite 511
San Francisco, CA 94103-1824
Tel: (415) 974-9600
Website: http://www.asaging.org

Americans with Disabilities Act
US Department of Justice
950 Pennsylvania Avenue, NW
Civil Rights Division
Disability Rights Section—NYAV
Washington, DC 20530
Tel: (800) 514-0301
Website: http://www.ada.gov

Assisted Living Federation of America
10300 Eaton Place, Suite 400
Fairfax, VA 22030
Tel: (703) 691-8100
Website: http://www.alfa.org

Center for Medicare and Medicaid Services
7500 Security Building
Baltimore, MD 21244-1850
Tel: (877) 267-2323
Website: http://www.medicare.gov/

Eldercare Locator
Tel: (800) 677-1116
Website: http://www.eldercare.gov

FirstGov for Seniors
Website:
http://www.firstgov.gov/Topics/Seniors.shtml

Gerontological Society of America
1030 15th St. NW, Suite 250
Washington, DC 20005
Tel: (202) 842-1275
Website: http://www.geron.org/

Goodwill Industries International
9200 Rockville Pike
Bethesda, MD 20814
Tel: (800) 741-0186
Website: http://www.goodwill.org

Meals on Wheels Association of America
203 S. Union Street
Alexandria, VA 22314
Tel: (703) 548-5558
Website: http://www.mowaa.org

National Association for Continence
PO Box 8310
Spartanburg, SC 29305-8310
Tel: (800) 252-3337
Website: http://www.nafc.org

National Committee for Prevention of Elder Abuse
UMASS Memorial Health Care
119 Belmont Street
Worcester, MA 01605
Tel: (508) 334-6166
Website: http://www.preventelderabuse.org

National Council on Aging
409 Third St., SW, Suite 200
Washington, DC 20024
Tel: (202) 479-1200
Website: http://www.ncoa.org

National Easter Seals Society
230 W. Monroe St.
Chicago, IL. 60606
Tel: (800) 221-6827
Website: http://www.easterseals.com

National Institute on Aging
Building 31, Room 5C27, 31 Center Dr.
Bethesda, MD 20892-2292
Tel: (800) 222-2225
Website: http://www.nih.gov/nia

Sexuality Information and Education Council of the United States
130 West 42nd Street, Suite 350
New York, NY 10036
Tel: (212) 819-9770
Website: http://www.siecus.org

Alzheimer's disease

Alzheimer's Association
919 N. Michigan Ave., Suite 1100
Chicago, IL 60611
Tel: (800) 272-3900
Website: http://www.alz.org

Alzheimer's Disease Education and Referral Center
National Institute on Aging
PO Box 8250
Silver Spring, MD 20907-8250
Tel: (800) 438-4380
Website: http://www.alzheimers.org

Aphasia

American Speech Language Hearing Association (ASHA)
10801 Rockville Pike
Rockville, MD 20852-3279
Tel: (800) 638-8255
Website: http://www.asha.org

Aphasia Hope Foundation
2436 West 137th Street
Leawood, KS 66224
Tel: (866) 449-5804
Website: http://aphasiahope.org

National Aphasia Association
29 John St., Suite 1103
New York, NY 10038
Tel: (800) 922-4622
Website: http://www.aphasia.org

Arthritis

Arthritis Foundation
PO Box 7669
Atlanta, GA 30357-0669
Tel: (800) 283-7800
Website: http://www.arthritis.org

Arthritis Society
393 University Avenue, Suite 1700
Toronto, Ontario M5G 1E6
Tel: (416) 979-7228
Website: http://www.arthritis.ca

National Arthritis, Musculoskeletal, & Skin Disease Information Clearing House
National Institutes of Health
1AMS Circle
Bethesda, MD 20892-3675
Tel: (877) 226-4267
Website: http://www.nih.gov/niams

National Osteoporosis Foundation
1232 22nd Street NW
Washington, DC 20037-1292
Tel: (800) 223-9994
Website: http://www.nof.org

Assisted living

American Association of Homes and Services for the Aging
2519 Connecticut Avenue, NW
Washington, DC 20008-1520
Tel: (202) 783-2242
Website: http://www.aahsa.org

Assisted Living Federation of America
11200 Waples Mill Road, Suite 150
Fairfax, VA 22030
Tel: (703) 691-8100
Website: http://www.alfa.org

National Center for Assisted Living
1201 L Street, NW
Washington, DC 20005
Tel: (202) 824-4444
Website: http://www.ncal.org

Ataxia

National Ataxia Foundation
2600 Fernbrook Lane, #119
Minneapolis, MN 55447
Tel: (612) 553-0020
Website: http://www.ataxia.org

Brain injury

Brain Injury Association of America
105 N. Alfred St.
Alexandria, VA 22314
Tel: (800) 444-6443
Website: http://www.biausa.org

Brain Injury Services
10340 Democracy Lane, Suite 305
Fairfax, VA 22030
Tel: (800) 425-4641
Website: http://www.braininjurysvcs.org

Caregiving

Children of Aging Parents
1609 Woodbourne Road, Suite 302A
Levittown, PA 19057-1511
Tel: (800) 227-7294
Website: http://www.caps4caregivers.org

Family Caregiver Alliance
180 Montgomery Street, Suite 1100
San Francisco, CA 94108
Tel: (800) 445-8106
Website: http://www.caregiver.org

National Alliance for Caregiving
4720 Montgomery Lane, 5th Floor
Bethesda, MD 20814
Website: http://www.caregiving.org/

National Family Caregivers Association
10400 Connecticut Avenue, Suite 500
Kensington, MD 20895-3944
Toll free: 1-800-896-3650
Tel: 301-942-6430
Fax: 301-942-2302
E-mail: info@thefamilycaregiver.org
Website: http://www.nfcacares.org/

National Quality Caregiving Coalition (NQCC)
Rosalynn Carter Institute for Caregiving
750 First Street, NE
Washington, DC 20002-4242
Tel: 202-336-5606
Fax: 202-336-5919
Website: http://www.nqcc.us/

Well Spouse Foundation
63 W. Main Street, Suite H
Freehold, NJ 07728
Tel: (800) 838-0879
Website: http://www.wellspouse.org

Diabetes

American Diabetes Association
1701 North Beauregard Street
Alexandria, VA 22311
Tel: (800) 342-2383
Website: http://www.diabetes.org/home.jsp

National Diabetes Education Program
One Diabetes Way
Bethesda, MD 20814-9692
Tel: (301) 496-3583
Website: http://www.ndep.nih.gov

Hearing/vision impairment

Alexander Graham Bell Association for the Deaf
3417 Volta Place, NW
Washington, DC 20007
Tel: (202) 337-5220
Website: http://www.agbell.org

American Association of the Deaf-Blind (AADB)
814 Thayer Avenue
Silver Spring, MD 20910
Tel: (800) 735-2258
Website: http://www.aadb.org

American Council of the Blind (ACB)
1155 15th Street NW, Suite 720
Washington, DC 20005
Tel: (800) 424-8666
Website: http://www.acb.org

American Foundation for the Blind (AFB)
11 Penn Plaza, Suite 300
New York, NY 10001
Tel: (800) 232-5463
Website: http://www.afb.org

American Tinnitus Association
PO Box 5
Portland, OR 97207
Tel: (800) 634-8978
Website: http://www.ata.org

Association of Late-Deafened Adults, Inc. (ALDA)
1145 Westgate Street, Suite 206
Oak Park, IL 60301
Tel/fax: (877) 348-7537
Website: http://www.alda.org

Foundation for Glaucoma Research
200 Pine Street, Suite 200
San Francisco, CA 94104
Tel: (415) 986-3162
Website: http://www.glaucoma.org

National Institute on Deafness and Other Communication Disorders
1 Communication Ave.
Bethesda, MD 20892-3456
Tel: (800) 241-1044
Website: http://www.nidcd.nih.gov/

Legal assistance

American Bar Association Commission on Law and Aging
740 15th Street, NW, 8th Floor
Washington, DC 20005
Tel: (202) 662-8690
Website: http://www.abanet.org/aging

Legal Services for the Elderly
130 West 42nd Street, 17th Floor
New York, NY 10036
Tel: (212) 391-0120
Website: http://www.lsny.org

National Academy of Elder Law Attorneys
1604 North Country Club Road
Tucson, AZ 85716
Tel: (520) 881-4005
Website: http://www.naela.org/

National Senior Citizens Law Center
1101 14th Street, NW, Suite 400
Washington, DC 20005
Tel: (202) 289-6976
Website: http://www.nsclc.org

Mental health

American Association of Geriatric Psychiatry
7910 Woodmont Ave., Suite 1050
Bethesda, MD 20814-3004
Tel: (301) 654-7850
Website: http://www.aagpgpa.org

American Psychological Association
750 First St., NE
Washington, DC 20002-4242
Tel: (202) 336-5500
Website: http://www.apa.org

Anxiety Disorder Education Program
National Institute of Mental Health
5600 Fishers Lane, Rm. 7C-02
Rockville, MD 20857
Tel: (800) 647-2642
Website: http://www.nimh.nih.gov/
healthinformation/anxietymenu.cfm

Anxiety Disorders Association of America
11900 Parklawn Dr., Suite 100
Rockville, MD 20852-2624
Tel: (301) 231-9350
Website: http://www.adaa.org

Depression and Related Affective Disorders Association (DRADA)
Meyer 3-181, 600 N. Wolfe St.
Baltimore, MD 21287-7381
Tel: (410) 955-4647
Website: http://www.drada.org/

Depression Awareness Recognition and Treatment Education Program
National Institute of Mental Health
5600 Fishers Lane
Rockville, MD 20857
Tel: (800) 421-4211
Website: http://www.nimh.nih.gov/
healthinformation/depressionmenu.cfm

National Alliance for the Mentally Ill (NAMI)
200 N. Glebe Rd., Suite 1015
Arlington, VA 22203-3754
Tel: (800) 950-6264
Website: http://www.nami.org

National Anxiety Foundation
3135 Custer Dr.
Lexington, KY 40517
Website: http://www.lexington-on-line.
com/naf.html

National Institute of Mental Health/Public Inquiries
6001 Executive Blvd., Room 8184, MSC 9663
Bethesda, MD 20892-9663
Tel: (301) 443-4513
Website:
http://www.nimh.nih.gov/about/index.cfm

National Mental Health Association
1021 Prince St.
Alexandria, VA 22314
Tel: (800) 969-6642
Website: http://www.nmha.org

Pain

American Chronic Pain Association
PO Box 850
Rocklin, CA 95677
Tel: (916) 632-0922
Website: http://www.theacpa.org

American Pain Society
4700 West Lake Avenue
Glenville, IL 60025-1489
Tel: (847) 375-4715
Website: http://www.ampainsoc.org/

International Association for the Study of Pain
IASP Secretariat
909 NE 43rd St., Suite 306
Seattle, WA 98105-6020
Tel: (206) 547-6409
Website: http://www.iasp-pain.org

National Chronic Pain Outreach Association
PO Box 274
Millboro, VA 24460-9606
Tel: (540) 862-9437
Website: http://www.chronicpain.org

Parkinson's disease

American Parkinson Disease Association
1250 Hylan Blvd.
Staten Island, NY 10305-1946
Tel: (800) 223-2732
Website: http://www.apdaparkinson.com

Muhammad Ali Parkinson Research Center
Barrow Neurological Institute
Phoenix, AZ 85013
Tel: (800) 273-8182
Website: http://www.maprc.com

National Parkinson Foundation
1501 NW Ninth Ave.
Miami, FL 33136
Tel: (800) 327-4545
Website: http://www.parkinson.org

Parkinson's Action Network
818 College Ave., Suite C
Santa Rosa, CA 95404
Tel: (800) 850-4726
Website: http://www.parkinsonsaction.org/

Parkinson's Disease Foundation
710 W. 168th St., 3rd Floor
New York, NY 10032
Tel: (800) 457-6676
Website: http://www.pdf.org/

Parkinson's Institute
1170 Morse Ave.
Sunnyvale, CA 94089
Tel: (800) 786-2958
Website: http://www.parkinsonsinstitute.org

United Parkinson Foundation
833 W. Washington Blvd.
Chicago, IL 60607
Tel: (312) 733-1893
E-mail: UPF_ITF@msn.com

Sleep disorders

American Sleep Disorders Association
6301 Bandel Rd., #101
Rochester, MN 55901
Tel: (507) 287-6006

National Sleep Foundation
729 15th Street, NW, 4th Floor
Washington, DC 20005
Tel: (888) 637-7533
Website: http://www.sleepfoundation.org

Stroke

American Heart Association's Stroke Connection
7272 Greenville Ave.
Dallas, TX 75231
Tel: (800) 553-6321
Website: http://www.strokeassociation.org

National Institute of Neurological Disorders and Stroke
Office of Scientific and Health Reports
PO Box 5801
Bethesda, MD 20824
Tel: (800) 352-9424
Website: http://www.ninds.nih.gov

National Stroke Association
9707 E. Easter Lane
Englewood, CO 80112
Tel: (800) 787-6537
Website: http://www.stroke.org

Index